Current Research in Systemic Lupus Erythematosus

Current Research in Systemic Lupus Erythematosus

Editor: Carrie Kane

FOSTER ACADEMICS

www.fosteracademics.com

www.fosteracademics.com

FOSTER ACADEMICS

Cataloging-in-Publication Data

Current research in systemic lupus erythematosus / edited by Carrie Kane.
p. cm.
Includes bibliographical references and index.
ISBN 978-1-63242-916-2
1. Systemic lupus erythematosus. 2. Systemic lupus erythematosus--Research. 3. Autoimmune diseases. I. Kane, Carrie.
RC924.5.L85 C87 2020
616.772-dc23

Foster Academics,
118-35 Queens Blvd., Suite 400,
Forest Hills, NY 11375, USA

ISBN 978-1-63242-916-2 (Hardback)

Contents

Preface

The main aim of this book is to educate learners and enhance their research focus by presenting diverse topics covering this vast field. This is an advanced book which compiles significant studies by distinguished experts in the area of analysis. This book addresses successive solutions to the challenges arising in the area of application, along with it; the book provides scope for future developments.

Systemic lupus erythematosus is an autoimmune disease characterized by fever, painful and swollen joints, chest pain, swollen lymph nodes, red rash, etc. This condition is caused because the immune system of the body attacks many healthy tissues of the body. It is believed to arise due to a combination of genetic and environmental factors. Some of the risk factors associated with the incidence of this disease are vitamin D deficiency, female sex hormones, smoking, certain infections and sunlight. It can be diagnosed through serologic testing. Clinically indirect immunofluorescence is the most widely used method. Testing for complement system levels, liver enzymes, electrolytes and kidney function, and complete blood count also aid in the diagnosis. The treatment of systemic lupus erythematosus involves the use of corticosteroids and anti-malarial drugs. Some forms of lupus nephritis may require intermittent cytotoxic drugs. This book brings forth some of the most innovative concepts and elucidates the unexplored aspects of systemic lupus erythematosus. It presents researches and studies performed by experts across the globe. Through this book, we attempt to enlighten the readers about the new concepts in the diagnosis and treatment of systemic lupus erythematosus.

It was a great honour to edit this book, though there were challenges, as it involved a lot of communication and networking between me and the editorial team. However, the end result was this all-inclusive book covering diverse themes in the field.

Finally, it is important to acknowledge the efforts of the contributors for their excellent chapters, through which a wide variety of issues have been addressed. I would also like to thank my colleagues for their valuable feedback during the making of this book.

Editor

1

Patterns of Ambulatory Medical Care Utilization and Rheumatologist Consultation Predating the Diagnosis of Systemic Lupus Erythematosus

Ning-Sheng Lai[1,2☯], Tzung-Yi Tsai[3,4,5☯], Malcolm Koo[3,6], Kuang-Yung Huang[1,2], Chien-Hsueh Tung[1], Ming-Chi Lu[1,2]*

1 Division of Allergy, Immunology and Rheumatology, Dalin Tzu Chi Hospital, Buddhist Tzu Chi Medical Foundation, Chiayi, Taiwan, **2** School of Medicine, Tzu Chi University, Hualien, Taiwan, **3** Department of Medical Research, Dalin Tzu Chi Hospital, Buddhist Tzu Chi Medical Foundation, Chiayi, Taiwan, **4** Department of Nursing, Tzu Chi College of Technology, Hualien, Taiwan, **5** Department of Environmental and Occupational Health, College of Medicine, National Cheng Kung University, Tainan, Taiwan, **6** Dalla Lana School of Public Health, University of Toronto, Toronto, Ontario, Canada

Abstract

Objective: To investigate the records of ambulatory medical care from patients predating the diagnosis of systemic lupus erythematosus (SLE) using nationwide, population-based claims data.

Methods: The frequencies and costs of ambulatory medical care utilization in 337 newly-diagnosed SLE cases between 2004 and 2010, identified from Taiwan's National Health Insurance Research Database, were compared with 1,348 controls who were frequency matched for sex, age, and the catastrophic illness certificate application year of the cases.

Results: Patients with SLE had a median frequency of ambulatory medical care utilization compared with controls one year prior to the index date (22 vs. 2, $P<0.001$). The differences were significant throughout all eight annual periods. Similarly, the inflation-adjusted costs of ambulatory medical care utilization in patients with SLE increased annually over the study period, from a median of US$18 eight years prior to the index date to US$680 one year prior to the index date. Diseases of the respiratory system (International Classification of Diseases, Ninth Revision, Clinical Modification [ICD-9-CM] codes 460–519), digestive system (ICD-9-CM codes 520–579), musculoskeletal system and connective tissue (ICD-9-CM codes 710–739, excluding 710.0), and skin and subcutaneous tissue (ICD-9-CM codes 680–709) were the top four common causes of visits in the 0.5 to 2 year period preceding the index date and percentages of SLE patients suffered from these disorders increased progressively over the study period. Only 56.4% of the patients with SLE had consulted a rheumatologist and most of the serology tests were done within one year predating the index date.

Conclusions: Increased frequencies and costs of ambulatory care utilization among Taiwanese patients with SLE occurred several years predating their definitive SLE diagnosis. When multisystemic disorders are presented in young female patients, the possibility of SLE should be considered and screened with tools such as the antinuclear antibody test.

Editor: Arvind Chopra, Center for Rheumatic Diseases, India

Funding: This work was supported by a grant from the Dalin Tzu Chi Hospital, Buddhist Tzu Chi Medical Foundation (DTCRD101-E-08), Taiwan. The funder had no role in study design, data collection and analysis, decision to publish, or preparation of the manuscript.

Competing Interests: The authors have declared that no competing interests exist.

* Email: e360187@yahoo.com.tw

☯ These authors contributed equally to this work.

Introduction

Systemic lupus erythematosus (SLE) is a complex systemic autoimmune disease with a wide range of clinical features that involve almost every organ systems in the body. The peak age of onset is around late teens and early 40 s with a women-to-men ratio of 9:1. In addition, people of African or Asian descent are at particular risk for developing SLE and exhibit more severe clinical manifestations compared with those of European descent [1]. Genetic, epigenetic, environmental, hormonal, and immunoregulatory factors all contribute to the development of SLE [2].

SLE is notoriously challenging to diagnose because of its heterogeneous clinical presentation and the lack of good biomarkers [3]. Although SLE is characterized by the presence of several autoantibodies [4,5], there exists a long preclinical phase from the development of autoimmunity to its clinical onset [6]. The gradual sequential development of autoantibodies takes many years preceding the clinical onset of SLE [6–9]. Moreover, clinical criteria of SLE, including arthritis and serositis, skin, hematological system and renal disorder, are also noted several years predating the diagnosis of SLE [4,7,10]. In addition, the severity of the SLE clinical manifestations during the pre-SLE period can fluctuate and many laboratory tests and imaging studies are often needed before a definitive diagnosis of SLE can be made. For these reasons, general practitioners may not suspect the early phase of SLE in their patients and delay a referral to a rheumatologist. Therefore, it is critical to assess the preclinical phase of SLE. However, due to the low incidence of SLE and its highly variable initial manifestations, it is highly inefficient and difficult to assess the preclinical phase of SLE using a cohort study design. Although a case control design is more efficient and feasible to conduct, the results are highly susceptible to recall bias in patients with SLE. Hence, we used an alternative approach based on the claim data of ambulatory medical care to investigate the general health conditions among patients predating the diagnosis of SLE.

Our previous study showed that the frequencies and costs of ambulatory visits in patients gradually increased as the time approaching the diagnosis of rheumatoid arthritis [11]. Yet, to our knowledge, no studies have reported the clinical disorders in a systematic manner among patients with SLE predating the diagnosis of SLE using population-based data. Therefore, the aim of this study was to investigate the pattern of ambulatory medical care utilization over an eight-year period in patients predating the diagnosis of SLE using a nationwide, population-based claim database.

Patients and Methods

Study design

This was a retrospective comparison study using nationwide, population-based cohort data.

Data sources

This study is based on the Longitudinal Health Insurance Database 2000 (LHID2000) of the Taiwan's National Health Insurance Research Database (NHIRD), provided by the Taiwan National Health Research Institute. LHID2000 contains comprehensive utilization and enrollment information from 1996 to 2010 for a randomly selected sample of one million beneficiaries registered in 2000, representing approximately 5% of Taiwan's population. The NHIRD consists of de-identified secondary data of inpatient and ambulatory medical care services of all enrollees of the National Health Insurance (NHI) scheme. The NHI is a single-payer compulsory health insurance program instituted in 1995 and covers over 99% of the Taiwan's population [12].

Under the NHI scheme, insured individuals afflicted with any of the 30 categories of catastrophic illness, specified by the Bureau of NHI, can apply for catastrophic illness certificates. If approved, these patients are exempted from co-payments when seeking medical care related to their catastrophic illness. The issuance of certificates is validated through careful review of medical records, laboratory studies, and imaging studies by at least two specialists.

The study protocol was reviewed and approved by the institutional review board of the Dalin Tzu Chi Hospital, Buddhist Tzu Chi Medical Foundation (No. B10104020). Since the NHIRD files contain only de-identified secondary data, the need for informed consent from individual subjects was waived.

Study subjects

Cases of SLE were identified from the catastrophic illness patients file of the NHIRD with corresponding International Classification of Diseases, Ninth Revision, Clinical Modification (ICD-9-CM) code 710.0. Review of application of catastrophic illness certificates by the Bureau of NHI is based on the 1997 American College of Rheumatology (ACR) revised criteria for the classification of SLE [13]. We excluded patients under the age of 18 years and those with a catastrophic illness certificates issued for autoimmune diseases other than SLE. The date of application of catastrophic illness certificates in approved patients was considered as the index date in the analysis. For each SLE case, four controls were randomly selected from the LHID2000 with frequency-matching for 10-year age interval, sex, and the year of the index date (index year). The index date for each of the control was assigned by using the date of a randomly selected ambulatory visit for a given index year. A total of 337 SLE patients and 1,348 controls were included in the data analysis.

Study variables

In this study, the costs of ambulatory medical care including physician consultation fees (Western medicine, dentistry, and traditional Chinese medicine), visits to emergency departments, medical procedures, pharmacy expenditure, laboratory diagnosis tests, imaging examination, and rehabilitation therapy, were charged according to the payment schedule of the NHI. All cost figures were converted to US dollars based on annual exchange rates and were further adjusted to 2010 dollars using Taiwan's consumer price index to take into the account of inflation.

The study subjects were retrospectively traced back up to eight years preceding the index date when examining the frequencies and costs of ambulatory medical care utilization. The frequencies and costs of the ambulatory medical care utilization on the index date itself were excluded from the analysis. The main causes of the ambulatory medical care utilization were defined by the use of principal diagnosis of the ICD-9-CM coding system [14]. In addition, we obtained frequencies of hospitalization of the study subjects from the LHID2000 with discharged day prior to the index date. Information on whether medical tests including antinuclear antibodies (ANA) via indirect immunoflorescence assay, complete blood count (CBC), alanine aminotransferase (ALT), creatinine (Cre), and chest X-ray had been performed on the study subjects were also obtained from the LHID2000. The geographic location in which the subjects resided were categorized into north, central, south, and east regions. The Deyo adaptation of the Charlson Comorbidity Index (CCI) [15] was used to quantify the subject's comorbidity patterns based on their medical records six months prior to the beginning of the eight-year study period.

Statistical analysis

Data were expressed as mean and standard deviation (SD) or median with interquartile range, as appropriate. Chi-square test and Wilcoxon rank-sum test were used to compare the characteristics between patients with SLE and controls. The frequencies and costs of ambulatory medical care utilization between the two groups were compared using Wilcoxon rank-sum test.

Trends in the frequencies of ambulatory medical care utilization across the eight annual periods were evaluated using generalized estimating equations (GEE) with Poisson log-linear link function. GEE was used to take into the account the statistical dependency of multiple observations for each subject over time. Incident rate ratios were estimated with GEE using the frequency at eight year preceding the index date as the reference category. Trends in the costs of ambulatory medical care utilization were evaluated using GEE with log link function with gamma distribution. Cost ratios were estimated using the cost data at eight year preceding the index date as the reference category. Analyses of frequencies and costs of medical care utilization using GEE were adjusted for age, sex, and CCI. All statistical analyses were conducted using SAS statistical software, version 9.2 for Windows (SAS Institute Inc., Cary, USA). A $P<0.05$ was considered statistically significant.

Results

Demographic data of patients with SLE and controls

Since age and sex were frequency matched between cases and controls, no significant differences were observed in these two variables between the cases and controls. In addition, no significant differences were observed in geographical regions and CCI between cases and controls (Table 1).

Frequency and cost of ambulatory medical visits

We found that SLE patients, prior to diagnosis of SLE, used ambulatory medical services more frequently compared with controls (Table 2). Even after tracing back as far as eight years before the index date, there was still a significant higher median frequency of ambulatory visits in patients with SLE compared with controls (1 vs. 0, $P<0.001$). The differences in median frequency of ambulatory visits gradually increased as the period approached the index date. The differences in the median frequency of ambulatory visits between the patient with SLE and controls became largest (22 vs. 2, $P<0.001$) one year prior to the index date.

Similarly, the inflation-adjusted costs of ambulatory health care utilization were significantly higher in patients with SLE compared with controls predating index date. Compared with the controls, the median cost of annual ambulatory visits was significantly higher in patients with SLE (US$18 vs. US$0, $P<0.001$) eight years prior to the index date. The differences between the two groups gradually increased as the time approaching the diagnosis of SLE and became largest in the year just before the index date (US$680 vs. US$27, $P<0.001$) (Table 2).

We observed significant trends of higher frequencies of visits over the eight-year study period in both patients with SLE and controls. However, the changes over time were more prominent in patients with SLE compared with controls as shown by the larger magnitude of the slope ($\beta=0.10$ vs. $\beta=0.04$) (Table 3). Regarding the costs of ambulatory medical utilization, significant trends of higher costs were also observed in both patients with SLE and controls. The changes over time was greater in patient with SLE compared with controls ($\beta=0.20$ vs. $\beta=0.06$) (Table 4). Over the eight-year period, the annual costs of ambulatory care visits showed nearly a quadruple increase in patients with SLE but only elevated 49% in controls.

Principal causes of ambulatory medical care utilization during the 0.5 to 2 years preceding the index date

To investigate the early and subtle clinical disorders before the apparently onset of SLE, we compared the principle causes of ambulatory medical visits in patients with SLE and controls in the 0.5 to two years period before the index date. We found that ambulatory visits were significantly higher in almost all categories of clinical disorders involving various organ systems in patients with SLE compared with controls. The top four common diseases categories leading to ambulatory medical visits were diseases of the respiratory system (ICD-9-CM codes 460–519), digestive system (ICD-9-CM codes 520–579), musculoskeletal system and connective tissue (ICD-9-CM codes 710–739, excluding 710.0), and skin and subcutaneous tissue (ICD-9-CM codes 680–709) (Table 5).

Among the disorders of the respiratory systems, the frequencies for ambulatory visits for acute respiratory infections (ICD-9-CM codes 460–466), other diseases of the upper respiratory tract (ICD-9-CM codes 470–478), pneumonia and influenza (ICD-9-CM codes 480–488), chronic obstructive pulmonary disease and allied conditions (ICD-9-CM codes 490–496), and pleurisy (ICD-9-CM codes 511) were significantly higher in patients with SLE. Among the disorders of the digestive systems, ambulatory visits for disease of oral cavity, salivary glands, and jaws (ICD-9-CM codes 520–529), diseases of the esophagus, stomach, and duodenum (ICD-9-CM codes 520–529), noninfectious enteritis and colitis (ICD-9-CM codes 555–558), other diseases of intestines and peritoneum(ICD-9-CM codes 560–569), liver diseases (ICD-9-CM codes 570–573), and diseases of gall bladder/biliary tract/pancreas (ICD-9-CM codes 574–577) were significantly more frequent in patients with SLE. Among the diseases of the musculoskeletal system and connective tissue (710–739, but excluding SLE), the frequencies for ambulatory visits for arthropathies (ICD-9-CM codes 711–719), spine disorders (ICD-9-CM codes 720–724), disorder of tendon, brusa, muscle and fascia (ICD-9-CM codes 725–729), and osteopathies and chondropathies (ICD-9-CM codes 730–733) were significantly higher in patients with SLE. Among the diseases of the skin and subcutaneous tissue, ambulatory visits for infection of skin and subcutaneous tissue (ICD-9-CM codes 680–686), inflammatory conditions of skin and subcutaneous tissue (ICD-9-CM codes 690–698), and other diseases of skin and

Table 1. Characteristics of the patients with systemic lupus erythematosus and controls.

		Group, mean ±SD or number (%)		*p*
		SLE	Controls	
		n = 337	n = 1,348	
Age at enrollment (years)		37.4±18.2	37.4±18.1	0.997
Sex (% female)		293 (86.9)	1159 (86.0)	0.646
Geographical region				0.123
	North	152 (45.1)	413 (50.4)	
	Central	88 (26.1)	207 (25.3)	
	South	90 (26.7)	175 (21.4)	
	East	7 (2.1)	24 (2.9)	
Charlson Comorbidity Index		0.09±0.39	0.05±0.38	0.947

SD, standard deviation; SLE, systemic lupus erythematosus.

Table 2. Frequencies and costs of ambulatory medical care utilization in patients with systemic lupus erythematosus and controls over an eight-year period preceding the index date.

Years preceding index date	Annual frequencies of ambulatory medical care utilization		*P*	Annual costs of ambulatory medical care utilization		*P*
	Patients with SLE	Controls		Patients with SLE	Controls	
	n = 337	n = 1,348		n = 337	n = 1,348	
8	8.31±13.23	4.04±9.63	<0.001	232±697	98±454	<0.001
	(1, 0–13)	(0, 0–3)		(18, 0–251)	(0, 0–47)	
7	9.74±12.80	4.95±10.76	<0.001	289±1450	107±288	<0.001
	(5, 0–15)	(0, 0–6)		(82, 0–293)	(0, 0–94)	
6	12.15±13.64	6.05±11.79	<0.001	398±1488	135±407	<0.001
	(8, 1–18)	(0, 0–9)		(142, 13–407)	(0, 0–145)	
5	14.41±13.18	7.30±12.74	<0.001	520±2000	186±848	<0.001
	(11, 5–20)	(1, 0–10)		(218, 73–453)	(12, 0–204)	
4	16.03±13.61	7.86±12.45	<0.001	632±2404	208±903	<0.001
	(13, 6–23)	(2, 0–12)		(243, 93–542)	(16, 0–225)	
3	16.81±13.27	8.10±12.83	<0.001	750±2420	216±893	<0.001
	(14, 6–23)	(2, 0–12)		(265, 110–632)	(20, 0–220)	
2	17.47±15.18	7.84±12.72	<0.001	760±2460	218±949	<0.001
	(13, 6–25)	(1, 0–12)		(291, 109–751)	(27, 0–230)	
1	25.23±15.24	8.07±13.05	<0.001	1134±2503	216±897	<0.001
	(22, 15–32)	(2, 0–12)		(680, 419–1186)	(27, 0–230)	

Values are mean ± standard deviation and (median, 25th–75th percentile).
Costs were converted to US dollars based on annual exchange rates and adjusted to 2010 figures based on Taiwan's consumer price index.
SLE, systemic lupus erythematosus.

subcutaneous tissue (ICD-9-CM codes 700–709) were significantly more frequent in patients with SLE. In addition, most of the patients with SLE had already suffered from three or more organ systems disorders compared with controls (96.1% vs. 44.1%, $P<0.001$) during the 0.5 to 2 years preceding the index date.

Percentages of ambulatory medical care utilization in patients with SLE and controls for four common systemic disorders over the eight-year study period

We investigated the annual percentages of the four most common disorders leading to ambulatory medical care utilization in patients with SLE during the pre-SLE period. We found that the percentages of patients with SLE suffering from these four diseases were all significantly higher than controls over the study period. Moreover, the differences increased the closer the year was to the index date (Fig. 1). One year before the diagnosis of SLE, 77.2% of the patients with SLE suffered from diseases of the respiratory system, 67.1% from diseases of the digestive system, 53.4% from diseases of the musculoskeletal system and connective tissue (excluding SLE), and 57.6% from diseases of the skin and subcutaneous tissue.

Percentages of patients who had received medical tests that might be associated with clinical manifestations of SLE

Annual percentages of medical tests performed including ANA, CBC, Cre, ALT and chest X-ray over the eight-year period preceding the index date were calculated. Although patients with SLE had received these tests more frequently compared with controls during the entire eight-year study period, most of the patients with SLE only received these tests within the one year period before the index date (Fig. 2).

Percentages of hospitalization in patients with SLE and controls over the eight-year study period

Even after tracing back as far as eight years before the index date, there were still a small but significantly higher percentages of hospitalization in patients with SLE compared with controls (7.4% vs. 3.3%, $P<0.001$) (Table 6). The differences were similar over the entire study period except one year prior to the index date where the largest difference was observed between patient with SLE and controls (49.6% vs. 4.1%, $P<0.001$).

Percentages of rheumatologist consultation before the index date

Although there were small but significantly higher percentages of consultations to rheumatologist in patients with SLE eight years predating the index date compared with controls, only 56.4% of the patients with SLE had ever consulted a rheumatologist within one year preceding the diagnosis of SLE (Table 7). In contrast, just one year after the definitive diagnosis of SLE, the percentage of consultations to a rheumatologist increased drastically to 85.8% (Table 7).

Discussion

Using a nationwide, population-based health claim database, we reported a systematic analysis of clinical course of SLE disorders predating the diagnosis of SLE. To our knowledge, this is the first overall analysis of the clinical course of SLE conducted in an Asia

Table 3. Trends in annual frequencies of ambulatory medical care utilization over an eight-year period preceding the index date.

Years preceding index date	Patients with SLE				Controls			
	β	IRR	95% CI	P	β	IRR	95% CI	P
8	Reference year				Reference year			
7	0.02	1.02	0.89–1.16	0.746	0.04	1.04	0.95–1.13	0.346
6	0.09	1.09	0.96–1.24	0.187	0.11	1.11	1.02–1.22	0.028
5	0.13	1.14	0.99–1.30	0.052	0.20	1.22	1.12–1.33	0.013
4	0.20	1.22	1.07–1.41	0.004	0.25	1.28	1.17–1.42	0.001
3	0.25	1.28	1.12–1.47	<0.001	0.26	1.29	1.18–1.42	<0.001
2	0.28	1.32	1.15–1.52	<0.001	0.27	1.31	1.19–1.44	<0.001
1	0.63	1.96	1.64–2.15	<0.001	0.29	1.34	1.22–1.48	<.001
	$\beta=0.10$; trend test $P<0.001$				$\beta=0.04$; trend test $P=0.001$			

Estimates were adjusted for age, sex and Charlson Comorbidity Index using generalized estimating equation with a Poisson log-linear function.
SLE, systemic lupus erythematosus; IRR, incident rate ratio; 95% CI, 95% confidence interval.

Table 4. Trends in annual costs of ambulatory medical care utilization over an eight-year period preceding the index date.

Years preceding index date	Patients with SLE				Controls			
	β	Cost ratio	95% CI	P	β	Cost ratio	95% CI	P
8	Reference year				Reference year			
7	0.20	1.21	0.86–1.77	0.286	0.05	1.00	0.93–1.19	0.940
6	0.44	1.55	1.09–2.26	0.014	0.08	1.08	0.90–1.29	0.415
5	0.59	1.81	1.10–3.01	0.013	0.26	1.29	1.06–1.58	0.009
4	0.79	2.21	1.43–3.39	<0.001	0.32	1.38	1.14–1.67	0.001
3	0.93	2.53	1.66–3.69	<0.001	0.37	1.44	1.20–1.74	<0.001
2	0.96	2.58	1.76–3.89	<0.001	0.39	1.49	1.22–1.84	<0.001
1	1.39	3.92	2.90–5.30	<0.001	0.40	1.49	1.23–1.80	<0.001
	$\beta=0.20$; trend test $P<0.001$				$\beta=0.06$; trend test $P=0.013$			

Estimates were adjusted for age, sex and Charlson Comorbidity Index using generalized estimating equation with log link function and gamma distribution. Costs were converted to US dollars based on annual exchange rates and adjusted to 2010 figures based on Taiwan's consumer price index.
SLE, systemic lupus erythematosus; 95% CI, 95% confidence interval.

Table 5. Causes of ambulatory medical care utilization in patients with systemic lupus erythematosus and controls during the period 0.5 to 2 years preceding the index date.

Diagnosis (ICD-9-CM code)		Group, mean ±SD		p
		Patients with SLE	Controls	
		n = 337	n = 1,348	
Diseases of the respiratory system (460–519)		7.24±9.70	3.66±7.20	<0.001
	Acute respiratory infections (460–466)	5.78±7.06	3.09±6.35	<0.001
	Other diseases of the upper respiratory tract (470–478)	0.67±2.09	0.31±1.52	<0.001
	Pneumonia and influenza (480–488)	0.36±2.34	0.14±0.78	<0.001
	Chronic obstructive pulmonary disease and allied conditions (490–496)	0.37±1.09	0.09±0.84	<0.001
	Pleurisy (511)	0.02±0.20	0.00±0.02	0.010
	Pneumonitis (515–517)	0	0	NA
Diseases of the digestive system (520–579)		5.78±6.99	2.66±5.03	<0.001
	Disease of oral cavity, salivary glands and jaws (520–529)	3.26±3.49	1.60±3.35	<0.001
	Disease of esophagus, stomach, and duodenum (530–537)	1.20±3.22	0.54±2.50	<0.001
	Noninfectious enteritis and colitis (555–558)	0.52±1.42	0.22±0.85	<0.001
	Other diseases of intestines and peritoneum (560–569)	0.33±1.17	0.22±1.94	<0.001
	Liver diseases (570–573)	0.36±1.67	0.06±0.46	<0.001
	Diseases of gall bladder/biliary tract/pancreas (574–577)	0.10±0.08	0.01±0.22	<0.001
Diseases of the musculoskeletal system and connective tissue (710–739)*		4.35±7.48	1.22±4.21	<0.001
	Athropathies (711–719)	1.87±4.45	0.33±1.84	<0.001
	Spine disorders (720–724)	0.73±2.16	0.49±2.10	<0.001
	Disorder of tendon, brusa, muscle and fascia (725–729)	1.08±2.63	0.36±1.57	<0.001
	Osteopathies and chondropathies (730–733)	0.15±1.11	0.02±0.19	<0.001
Diseases of the skin and subcutaneous tissue (680–709)		3.89±5.90	0.91±2.84	<0.001
	Infection of skin and subcutaneous tissue (680–686)	0.51±1.67	0.09±0.66	<0.001
	Inflammatory conditions of skin and subcutaneous tissue (690–698)	2.24±4.21	0.41±1.70	<0.001
	Other diseases of skin and subcutaneous tissue (700–709)	1.15±2.35	0.40±1.73	<0.001
Disorders of the eye and adnexa (360–379)		2.01±3.38	0.68±2.46	<0.001
Diseases of female genital organ (610–629)†		1.93±4.45	1.11±3.39	0.001
Diseases of the circulatory system (390–459)		1.68±5.37	0.63±3.09	<0.001
Diseases of the blood and blood-forming organs (280–289)		1.22±4.61	0.04±0.53	<0.001
Endocrine, nutritional and metabolic diseases, and immunity disorders (240–279)		1.22±3.78	0.45±2.51	<0.001
Infectious and parasitic diseases (001–139)		0.99±2.56	0.37±1.71	0.001
Diseases of kidney (580–589)		0.82±3.82	0.08±1.47	<0.001
Mental disorders (290–319)		0.80±3.13	0.37±2.67	<0.001
Diseases of urinary system (590–599)		0.59±2.18	0.21±1.06	<0.001
Neoplasms (140–239)		0.55±2.95	0.26±1.79	<0.001
Diseases of the nervous system (320–359)		0.53±2.20	0.13±0.97	<0.001
Diseases of the ear and mastoid process (380–389)		0.22±0.76	0.19±1.11	<0.001

Table 5. Cont.

Diagnosis (ICD-9-CM code)	Group, mean ±SD		P
	Patients with SLE	Controls	
	n = 337	n = 1,348	
Complications of pregnancy, child birth, and the puerperium (630–679)[†]	0.17±1.02	0.11±0.80	0.497
Diseases of male genital organ (600–608)[‡]	0.09±0.45	0.13±0.99	0.497
Number of organ system involved[§]			
1	3 (0.9)	49 (3.6)	0.007
2	9 (2.7)	88 (6.5)	0.010
≥3	324 (96.1)	595 (44.1)	<0.001

*Excluding the ICD-9-CM code 710.0.
[†]Female only (patients with SLE, n = 293; controls, n = 1,172).
[‡]Male only (patients with SLE, n = 44; controls, n = 176).
SD, standard deviation; SLE, systemic lupus erythematosus; NA, not applicable.
[§]Represented as number (%).

population. Previous studies have reported the very early clinical course of SLE but most of them had focused on the appearance of autoantibody [16]. A study on 130 U.S. patients showed that the earliest symptoms associated with the ACR criteria for SLE appeared before the diagnosis were discoid rash and seizures, with a mean onset of 1.7 years before diagnosis. Other symptoms associated with the ACR criteria for SLE including arthritis, skin disorders, hematological disorders, serositis, and renal diseases were also commonly presented prior to the diagnosis of SLE [4]. Moreover, thrombotic events were reported to increase in patients with SLE prior to diagnosis [10]. In addition, a Swedish case-control study of 38 patients with SLE found that ACR defined SLE criteria including arthritis, skin disorder, and serositis appeared prior to diagnosis of SLE [7].

Our study showed that patients with SLE already suffered from diseases of the respiratory, digestive, and musculoskeletal systems and skin tissue (Fig. 2) and multiple system disorders (Table 5) several years preceding the definitive diagnosis of SLE. In addition, most of the patients with SLE only received relevant medical tests just within a one-year period prior to the diagnosis of SLE. ANA is a useful test for the initial differential diagnosis of SLE. We found that only 68% of the patients with SLE had ever received an ANA test from ambulatory medical care services while the remaining patients received the test only during hospitalization. A previous study conducted in Taiwan indicated that the positivity rate of ANA in patients with SLE was over 90% [17]. According to the study by Wichainun et al. [18], the ANA test has a sensitivity of over 90% to detect SLE, which is considerably higher than those from other autoantibodies such as anti-dsDNA and anti-SSA/SSB [19]. Therefore, ANA test is a test of choice for initial screening of SLE among patients with multisystemic disorders. Clinicians should consider the possibility of SLE and arrange screening tests such as ANA test when young female patients are presented with multiple systemic disorders.

We noted that patients with SLE visited ambulatory medical services more frequently as a result of a wide array of different clinical disorders. Diseases of the respiratory systems were the most frequent cause of visit for ambulatory medical care. Chronic interstitial lung diseases, acute lupus pneumonitis, or diffuse alveolar hemorrhage [20], and viral, bacterial, or fungal respiratory tract infection related to impaired immunity [21] are commonly noted in patients with SLE. We found various disorders of the respiratory system increased the ambulatory medical utilization in patient with SLE during pre-SLE period. It should

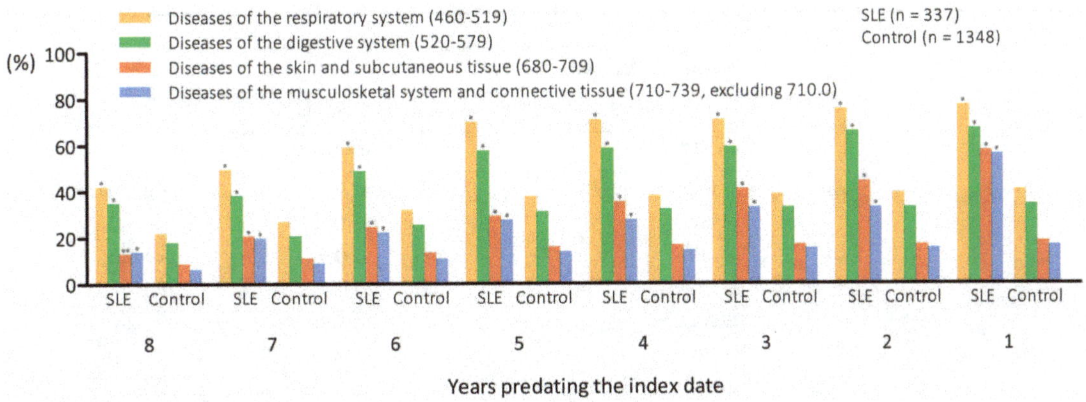

Figure 1. Annual percentages of ambulatory medical care visits for four common systemic disorders in patients with systemic lupus erythematosus and controls over an eight-year period preceding the index date.

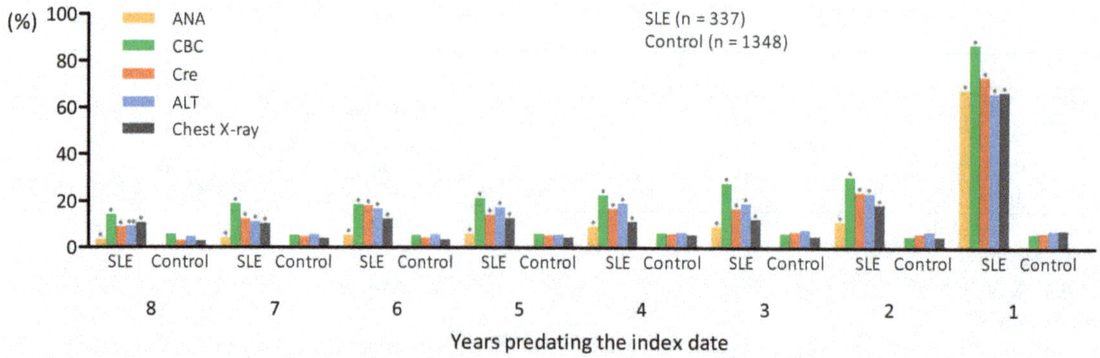

Figure 2. Annual percentages of antinuclear antibodies (ANA) test (via indirect immunofluorescence assay), complete blood count (CBC) test, creatinine (Cre) test, alanine aminotransferase (ALT) test, and chest X-ray from ambulatory medical care services patients with systemic lupus erythematosus and controls over an eight-year period preceding the index date. **P*<0.001, ***P* = 0.002.

be noted that although pleuritis is one of the ACR criteria for SLE, it was rarely reported as a diagnosis during the 0.5 to 2 years preceding the diagnosis of SLE in our study.

For the gastrointestinal disorders, oral ulcer is a common initial presentation of SLE. Other common gastrointestinal disorders associated with SLE itself or the consequence of the medication such as dysphagia, anorexia, nausea, vomiting, hemorrhage, hepatitis, and abdominal pain [22,23] might explain the increased frequency of visit for diseases of the digestive system. Skin and musculoskeletal disorders are both well-known clinical symptoms preceding the diagnosis of SLE [4,7] and common initial presentation of SLE [24,25]. Our findings were consistent with previous reports.

Regarding the diseases of the circulatory system, pericarditis is one of the ACR criteria of SLE but myocarditis, pulmonary hypertension, and valvular heart disease also belong to cardiac involvement of SLE. The ICD-9-CM codes for circulatory diseases (390–459) contain venous thrombosis and vasculitis. The former is well known to develop in patients with SLE prior to the diagnosis [10] and the latter is frequently observed in patients with SLE. Previous studies [4,10] showed that hematological system (such as thrombocytopenia, leucopenia, and lymphopenia) and central nervous system disorders were often noted in patients with SLE predating the diagnosis. Our study revealed similar findings. Furthermore, the results of increased ambulatory medical visits for renal disorder in patients with SLE predating the diagnosis were in line with findings from previous studies [4,7].

Somewhat to our surprise, we found patients with SLE visits ambulatory medical care services more frequently than controls in clinical disorders that are not among the diseases associated with the ACR criteria for classification of SLE. Ocular manifestations in SLE are fairly common, and almost any part of the eye and visual pathway can be affected by SLE. Common ocular manifestations of SLE, including dry eye, scleritis, episcleritis, optic neuritis, retinopathy, and uveitis, may appear as the initial presentation of SLE [24,26]. For the endocrine system, the prevalence of autoimmune thyroid diseases is higher in patients with SLE [27,28] and this could explain our findings. The frequencies of visits for disease of female genital organ, urinary tract, and the ear were also found to be elevated in patients during the pre-SLE period. Although these organ systems could directly be affected by SLE [29,30], the increased visits might also be caused by infections of these organs. A study based on the Taiwan NHI database demonstrated an increased risk of tuberculosis in patients before their diagnosis of SLE [31]. Nevertheless, the risks of other infectious diseases remain to be investigated. Frequencies of visits for neoplasm were also elevated in patients during the pre-SLE period. Patients with SLE had elevated risk for developing

Table 6. Number of patients with systemic lupus erythematosus and controls hospitalized over an eight-year period preceding the index date.

Years preceding index date	Group, number (%)		*P*
	Patients with SLE	Controls	
	n = 337	n = 1,348	
8	25 (7.4)	45 (3.3)	**<0.001**
7	28 (8.3)	53 (3.9)	**<0.001**
6	30 (8.9)	52 (3.9)	**<0.001**
5	32 (9.5)	54 (4.0)	<0.001
4	36 (10.7)	63 (4.7)	<0.001
3	34 (10.1)	56 (4.2)	<0.001
2	30 (8.9)	70 (5.2)	<0.001
1	167 (49.6)	55 (4.1)	<0.001

SLE, systemic lupus erythematosus.

Table 7. Number of patients with systemic lupus erythematosus and controls who had visited a rheumatologist over an eight-year period preceding the index date.

Years preceding index date	Group, number (%)		*P*
	Patients with SLE	Controls	
	n = 337	n = 1,348	
8	25 (7.4)	33 (2.4)	<0.001
7	22 (6.5)	38 (2.8)	<0.001
6	34 (10.1)	45 (3.3)	<0.001
5	39 (11.6)	51 (3.8)	<0.001
4	42(12.5)	62 (4.6)	<0.001
3	47 (13.9)	59 (4.4)	<0.001
2	46 (13.6)	57 (4.2)	<0.001
1	190 (56.4)	61 (4.5)	<0.001
One year after index date	289 (85.8)	114 (8.4)	<0.001

SLE, systemic lupus erythematosus.

cancer late in the diseases course [32] and a concordance development of the SLE and cancer has also been reported [33]. Moreover, the ICD-9-CM codes for neoplasm (140–239) contain not only malignant tumors but also benign tumors. Therefore, additional studies will be needed to clarify this finding.

Findings from this study also showed that many disorders occurred earlier and in a more complex fashion compared with the results from previous studies [4,6]. Such finding might be attributed to the unique medical system in Taiwan and therefore, our results might not be generalizable to other countries. Under the Taiwan's NHI scheme, the out-of-pocket expenses paid by patients for a single ambulatory visit ranges from just US$1.7 in local clinics to US$18.6 in medical centers. The number of annual physician consultations per capita was 13.4 in Taiwan, which was higher than any country in the Organisation for Economic Co-operation and Development (OECD) [34]. In addition, patients in Taiwan can directly consult specialists without the need for a referral from a general practitioner. Therefore, it was not surprised to find that 44.1% of the controls had ambulatory medical visits due to three or more organ system disorders. Chen et al. [14] demonstrated that 79.8% of the general population had consulted more than two specialists within one year. Our study also showed that despite the high frequencies of ambulatory medical visits and the presence of a variety of clinical disorders in patients during their pre-SLE period, relatively few of them had ever consulted a rheumatologist. Even up to just one year preceding the diagnosis of SLE, only about a half of the patients had a rheumatologist consultation. More effort should be put into public health education to increase the public's awareness of SLE and health care providers should consider the possibility of SLE when young female patients are presented with disorders involving multiple organs. Moreover, it is critical to identify pre-SLE patients as early as possible, for example, through the use of questionnaire [35] and screening tools such as the ANA test. Timely treatment for those at elevated risks of developing SLE might help to reduce the high mortality associated with SLE [36].

Several limitations of this study merit attention. First, we were unable to confirm that the application date of the catastrophic illness certificate for SLE was the same date that a patient received his or her definitive diagnosis of SLE. To estimate the lag time between the application date of the catastrophic illness certificate and the definitive diagnosis of SLE, we took the date of the last three consecutive visits with diagnosis of SLE in a given patient as the date of his or her definite diagnosis of SLE. Based on this calculation, we found a mean lag time of only 11.9 days (SD = 29.1 days). Therefore, this relatively short lag time should not materially affect our results. In addition, the diagnosis of SLE in our study was based on the 1997 ACR revised criteria for the classification of SLE [13]. The adoption of the 2012 Systemic Lupus International Collaborating Clinics classification criteria [37] may be able to shorten the period between the onsets of clinical disorders to the final diagnosis of SLE [38]. Furthermore, due to the limitations of our data source, no radiographic reports, serological data (including the complements and autoantibodies), and family history are available.

In conclusion, in this national, population-based study, we found significant increased frequencies and costs of annual ambulatory medical care utilization in SLE patients over a period of at least eight years prior to their definitive diagnosis of SLE. Over the 0.5 to 2 years period preceding the diagnosis of SLE, the frequencies of medical visits related to almost all organ systems were significantly higher in patients with SLE compared with controls. However, only a half of the pre-SLE patients had ever consulted a rheumatologist within one year before their definitive diagnosis of SLE. More effort should be put towards facilitating the recognition of SLE in its early stage.

Acknowledgments

This study is based in part on data from the National Health Insurance Research Database provided by the National Health Insurance Administration, Ministry of Health and Welfare and managed by the National Health Research Institutes. The interpretation and conclusions contained herein do not represent those of the National Health Insurance Administration, Ministry of Health and Welfare or the National Health Research Institutes.

Author Contributions

Conceived and designed the experiments: NSL TYT MK KYH CHT MCL. Performed the experiments: TYT MK. Analyzed the data: NSL TYT MK KYH CHT MCL. Contributed reagents/materials/analysis tools: NSL TYT MCL. Wrote the paper: TYT MK MCL.

References

1. D'Cruz DP, Khamashta MA, Hughes GR (2007) Systemic lupus erythematosus. Lancet 369: 587–596.
2. Tsokos GC (2011) Systemic lupus erythematosus. N Engl J Med 365: 2110–2121.
3. Bertsias GK, Pamfil C, Fanouriakis A, Boumpas DT (2013) Diagnostic criteria for systemic lupus erythematosus: has the time come? Nat Rev Rheumatol 9: 687–694.
4. Heinlen LD, McClain MT, Merrill J, Akbarali YW, Edgerton CC, et al. (2007) Clinical criteria for systemic lupus erythematosus precede diagnosis, and associated autoantibodies are present before clinical symptoms. Arthritis Rheum 56: 2344–2351.
5. Lu R, Robertson JM, Bruner BF, Guthridge JM, Neas BR, et al. (2012) Multiple autoantibodies display association with lymphopenia, proteinuria, and cellular casts in a large, ethnically diverse SLE patient cohort. Autoimmune Dis 2012: 819634.
6. Arbuckle MR, McClain MT, Rubertone MV, Scofield RH, Dennis GJ, et al. (2003) Development of autoantibodies before the clinical onset of systemic lupus erythematosus. N Engl J Med 349: 1526–1533.
7. Eriksson C, Kokkonen H, Johansson M, Hallmans G, Wadell G, et al. (2011) Autoantibodies predate the onset of systemic lupus erythematosus in northern Sweden. Arthritis Res Ther 13: R30.
8. Arbuckle MR, James JA, Kohlhase KF, Rubertone MV, Dennis GJ, et al. (2001) Development of anti-dsDNA autoantibodies prior to clinical diagnosis of systemic lupus erythematosus. Scand J Immunol 54: 211–219.
9. Heinlen LD, McClain MT, Ritterhouse LL, Bruner BF, Edgerton CC, et al. (2010) 60 kD Ro and nRNP A frequently initiate human lupus autoimmunity. PLoS One 5: e9599.
10. McClain MT, Arbuckle MR, Heinlen LD, Dennis GJ, Roebuck J, et al. (2004) The prevalence, onset, and clinical significance of antiphospholipid antibodies prior to diagnosis of systemic lupus erythematosus. Arthritis Rheum 50: 1226–1232.
11. Lai NS, Tsai TY, Li CY, Koo M, Yu CL, et al. (2013) Increased frequency and costs of ambulatory medical care utilization prior to the diagnosis of rheumatoid arthritis: A national population-based study. Arthritis Care Res (Hoboken) 66: 371–378.
12. Cheng SH, Chiang TL (1997) The effect of universal health insurance on health care utilization in Taiwan. Results from a natural experiment. JAMA 278: 89–93.
13. Hochberg MC (1997) Updating the American College of Rheumatology revised criteria for the classification of systemic lupus erythematosus. Arthritis Rheum 40: 1725.
14. Chen TJ, Chou LF, Hwang SJ (2006) Patterns of ambulatory care utilization in Taiwan. BMC Health Serv Res 6: 54.
15. Deyo RA, Cherkin DC, Ciol MA (1992) Adapting a clinical comorbidity index for use with ICD-9-CM administrative databases. J Clin Epidemiol 45: 613–619.
16. Vittecoq O, Goeb V, Le Loët X, Tron F (2005) The preclinical phase of rheumatoid arthritis and lupus. Joint Bone Spine 72: 443–446.
17. Lin YJ, Wan L, Sheu JJ, Huang CM, Lin CW, et al. (2008) G/T polymorphism in the interleukin-2 exon 1 region among Han Chinese systemic lupus erythematosus patients in Taiwan. Clin Immunol 129: 36–39.
18. Wichainun R, Kasitanon N, Wangkaew S, Hongsongkiat S, Sukitawut W, et al. (2011) Sensitivity and specificity of ANA and anti-dsDNA in the diagnosis of systemic lupus erythematosus: a comparison using control sera obtained from healthy individuals and patients with multiple medical problems. Asian Pac J Allergy Immunol 31: 292–298.
19. Bruner BF, Guthridge JM, Lu R, Vidal G, Kelly JA, et al. (2012) Comparison of autoantibody specificities between traditional and bead-based assays in a large, diverse collection of patients with systemic lupus erythematosus and family members. Arthritis Rheum 64: 3677–3686.
20. Torre O, Harari S (2011) Pleural and pulmonary involvement in systemic lupus erythematosus. Presse Med 40: e19–29.
21. Pego-Reigosa JM, Medeiros DA, Isenberg DA (2009) Respiratory manifestations of systemic lupus erythematosus: old and new concepts. Best Pract Res Clin Rheumatol 23: 469–480.
22. Ebert EC, Hagspiel KD (2011) Gastrointestinal and hepatic manifestations of systemic lupus erythematosus. J Clin Gastroenterol 45: 436–441.
23. Sultan SM, Ioannou Y, Isenberg DA (1999) A review of gastrointestinal manifestations of systemic lupus erythematosus. Rheumatology 38: 917–932.
24. Vlachoyiannopoulos PG, Karassa FB, Karakostas KX, Drosos AA, Moutsopoulos HM (1993) Systemic lupus erythematosus in Greece. Clinical features, evolution and outcome: a descriptive analysis of 292 patients. Lupus 2: 303–312.
25. Cerovec M, Anić B, Padjen I, Cikes N (2012) Prevalence of the American College of Rheumatology classification criteria in a group of 162 systemic lupus erythematosus patients from Croatia. Croat Med J 53: 149–154.
26. Sivaraj RR, Durrani OM, Denniston AK, Murray PI, Gordon C (2007) Ocular manifestations of systemic lupus erythematosus. Rheumatology 46: 1757–1762.
27. Pyne D, Isenberg DA (2002) Autoimmune thyroid disease in systemic lupus erythematosus. Ann Rheum Dis 61: 70–72.
28. Kumar K, Kole AK, Karmakar PS, Ghosh A (2012) The spectrum of thyroid disorders in systemic lupus erythematosus. Rheumatol Int 32: 73–78.
29. Jolly M, Patel P (2006) Looking beyond the ordinary: genital lupus. Arthritis Rheum 55: 821–822.
30. Kastanioudakis I, Ziavra N, Voulgari PV, Exarchakos G, Skevas A, et al. (2002) Ear involvement in systemic lupus erythematosus patients: a comparative study. J Laryngol Otol 116: 103–107.
31. Lin YC, Liang SJ, Liu YH, Hsu WH, Shih CM, et al. (2012) Tuberculosis as a risk factor for systemic lupus erythematosus: results of a nationwide study in Taiwan. Rheumatol Int 32: 1669–1673.
32. Bernatsky S, Ramsey-Goldman R, Labrecque J, Joseph L, Boivin JF, et al. (2013) Cancer risk in systemic lupus: an updated international multi-centre cohort study. J Autoimmun 42: 130–135.
33. Lionaki S, Vlachopanos G, Georgalis A, Ziakas P, Gakiopoulou H, et al. (2013) Lupus nephritis and non-Hodgkin lymphoma simultaneously diagnosed in a patient on methimazole. Lupus 22: 95–98.
34. The Organisation for Economic Co-operation and Development (2011) Health at a Glance 2011: OECD Indicators. Available: http://www.oecd.org/health/healthataglance. Accessed 2014 April 4.
35. Spinillo A, Beneventi F, Ramoni V, Caporali R, Locatelli E, et al. (2012) Prevalence and significance of previously undiagnosed rheumatic diseases in pregnancy. Ann Rheum Dis 71: 918–923.
36. Jakes RW, Bae SC, Louthrenoo W, Mok CC, Navarra SV, et al. (2012) Systematic review of the epidemiology of systemic lupus erythematosus in the Asia-Pacific region: prevalence, incidence, clinical features, and mortality. Arthritis Care Res 64: 159–168.
37. Petri M, Orbai AM, Alarcón GS, Gordon C, Merrill JT, et al. (2012) Derivation and validation of the Systemic Lupus International Collaborating Clinics classification criteria for systemic lupus erythematosus. Arthritis Rheum 64: 2677–2686.
38. Pons-Estel GJ, Wojdyla D, McGwin G Jr, Magder LS, Petri MA, et al. (2014) The American College of Rheumatology and the Systemic Lupus International Collaborating Clinics Classification criteria for systemic lupus erythematosus in two multiethnic cohorts: a commentary. Lupus 23: 3–9.

2

The SLE Transcriptome Exhibits Evidence of Chronic Endotoxin Exposure and has Widespread Dysregulation of Non-Coding and Coding RNAs

Lihua Shi[1], Zhe Zhang[2], Angela M. Yu[2], Wei Wang[3], Zhi Wei[3], Ehtisham Akhter[4], Kelly Maurer[1], Patrícia Costa Reis[1], Li Song[1], Michelle Petri[4], Kathleen E. Sullivan[1]*

1 The Division of Allergy Immunology, The Children's Hospital of Philadelphia, Philadelphia, Pennsylvania, United States of America, **2** The Center for Biomedical Informatics, The Children's Hospital of Philadelphia, Philadelphia, Pennsylvania, United States of America, **3** Department of Computer Science, New Jersey Institute of Technology, Newark, New Jersey, United States of America, **4** Division of Rheumatology, Johns Hopkins University School of Medicine, Baltimore, Maryland, United States of America

Abstract

Background: Gene expression studies of peripheral blood mononuclear cells from patients with systemic lupus erythematosus (SLE) have demonstrated a type I interferon signature and increased expression of inflammatory cytokine genes. Studies of patients with Aicardi Goutières syndrome, commonly cited as a single gene model for SLE, have suggested that accumulation of non-coding RNAs may drive some of the pathologic gene expression, however, no RNA sequencing studies of SLE patients have been performed. This study was designed to define altered expression of coding and non-coding RNAs and to detect globally altered RNA processing in SLE.

Methods: Purified monocytes from eight healthy age/gender matched controls and nine SLE patients (with low-moderate disease activity and lack of biologic drug use or immune suppressive treatment) were studied using RNA-seq. Quantitative RT-PCR was used to validate findings. Serum levels of endotoxin were measured by ELISA.

Results: We found that SLE patients had diminished expression of most endogenous retroviruses and small nucleolar RNAs, but exhibited increased expression of pri-miRNAs. Splicing patterns and polyadenylation were significantly altered. In addition, SLE monocytes expressed novel transcripts, an effect that was replicated by LPS treatment of control monocytes. We further identified increased circulating endotoxin in SLE patients.

Conclusions: Monocytes from SLE patients exhibit globally dysregulated gene expression. The transcriptome is not simply altered by the transcriptional activation of a set of genes, but is qualitatively different in SLE. The identification of novel loci, inducible by LPS, suggests that chronic microbial translocation could contribute to the immunologic dysregulation in SLE, a new potential disease mechanism.

Editor: Ludmila Prokunina-Olsson, National Cancer Institute, National Institutes of Health, United States of America

Funding: This work was supported by NIH Grant# 5R01AR058547-05 (www.nih.gov). The funders had no role in study design, data collection and analysis, decision to publish, or preparation of the manuscript.

Competing Interests: The authors have declared that no competing interests exist.

* E-mail: sullivak@mail.med.upenn.edu

Introduction

Systemic lupus erythematosus (SLE) is the quintessential systemic autoimmune disease. The etiopathogenesis is still not fully understood and there are over 20,000 published studies evaluating various aspects of cellular dysfunction in this disease. Over the past 10 years, insights have come from genome-wide association (GWA) studies as well as gene expression studies. In both cases, a type I interferon pathway was implicated [1,2].

One of the hallmarks of lupus is the presence of autoantibodies directed against nucleic acid targets and other nuclear antigens. The process of apoptosis exposes the immune system to nucleic acids and nuclear antigens, particularly when the apoptotic cells are not cleared appropriately and degrade into smaller components [3]. The apoptotic debris are believed to drive much of the type I interferon signature and the type I interferon itself can drive additional apoptosis. Nevertheless, much remains unknown about the pathogenesis of SLE, particularly at the level of nucleic acid accumulation and dysregulated gene expression. Dysregulated gene expression, with the accumulation of aberrant transcripts, could theoretically contribute to apoptosis or increased type I interferon expression and has been shown to mimic lupus [4,5,6,7,8,9].

We utilized next generation sequencing of transcripts (RNA-seq) to characterize the SLE transcriptome in monocytes. Monocytes are a critical cell in SLE. They are implicated in renal damage, which is the major cause of morbidity in SLE, and in atherosclerosis, which is the major cause of mortality in SLE [10,11,12,13]. Monocytes are, therefore, central to the disease process, but are also of interest because they respond to environmental stimuli, alter their function accordingly, and reflect that information back to other immunologically competent cells. They offer the additional advantage of representing a relatively homogeneous population [14]. This is the first RNA-seq study of SLE and we found not only a transcriptome that exhibits quantitative alterations as defined by the level of gene expression, but also qualitative differences with widely altered splicing preferences and non-coding RNA transcription. Some novel transcripts expressed at higher abundance in SLE monocytes were inducible by LPS, known to activate type I interferons [15,16,17]. LPS and microbial products have been demonstrated to accelerate renal disease and induce lupus-like processes in mice [18,19,20,21]. This finding provides an additional perspective from which to understand SLE.

Methods

Patients and cell purification

Investigators at Johns Hopkins University (JHU) School of Medicine obtained written informed consent and HIPAA Authorization of study subjects for all SLE samples. The Institutional Review Board at Johns Hopkins reviewed and approved the study of SLE patients. The use of the anomyzed Red Cross samples was approved by the Red Cross Institutional Review Board. Control samples were obtained from The Center For Aids Research, which supplies blood samples on a fee for service basis. They have obtained consent for the use of the samples and their protocols were approved by the University of Pennsylvania Institutional Review Board.

Primary human monocytes were purified using elutriation and adherence from eight healthy controls and nine SLE patients with no other autoimmunity, as previously described [22,23,24,25]. The purity of monocytes was more than 90% by flow cytometry for CD14 staining. All controls and patients were female and an average of approximately 40 years of age. All SLE patients' disease activity was mild-moderate and no one was on high-level immune suppression (Table S1). All subjects were enrolled in an IRB-approved study and provided informed consent, except the red cross serum samples which were provided as anomyzed discarded samples.

RNA isolation and library preparation

Total RNA was isolated from 2–3 million primary monocytes using the Qiagen RNeasy kit and DNA was removed by on-column DNase digestion (Qiagen, Valencia, CA). This method recovers predominantly RNA species >200 bases. 1 µg of total RNA was used to prepare the library with the SOLiD^{TM} whole transcriptome analysis kit (Applied Biosystems, Foster City, CA), providing strand-specific data. The procedure followed the instructions of the manufacturer. For miRNA validation, we used miRNeasy from Qiagen. Table S2 provides RNA quality and cell count information. The OD 260/280 ratio ranged from 1.8–1.98. RIN scores were not consistently obtained prior to fragmentation but were >7 for those where the RIN was defined. Post fragmentation, the RIN score averaged 2.3. The RNA quality and counts were not different between patients and controls.

RNA abundance validation

qRT-PCR was used to define quantitative differences in RNA abundance. The Clontech Advantage RT for PCR kit (Clontech, Mountain View, CA) was used to generate cDNA. Gene expression was detected by real-time PCR using the TaqMan 9600. Transcript levels were normalized to the 18S or β-actin signal, as has been previously used in SLE studies [26,27,28]. Mature miRNAs were detected with Taqman miRNA assays. Relative quantitation was performed using spiked *Caenorhabditis elegans* miRNA-238 as an exogenous control (Qiagen Syn-cel-miR-238-3p miScript miRNA Mimic). Commercially available primers were purchased from Applied Biosystems for: cel-miR-238 (248 primer for isoform cel-miR-238-3p - MIMAT0000293); hsa-miR-212 (515 primer for isoform hsa-miR-212-3p - MIMAT0000269 and 461768_mat for isoform hsa-miR-212-5p - MIMAT0022695); and *CCR2* (Hs00174150 primer for *CCR2* isoform NM_001123041.2 and Hs00704702_s1* for *CCR2* isoform NM_001123396.1) and from Qiagen for *RND3* (QT00002744),*TSLP* (QT01670809), *RGPD1* (QT01678425), *CD177* (QT02452849), *TUBB1* (QT00049574), and *ITG-B* (QT01003121). Novel loci were detected with custom primers using SYBR green. Primer sequences are listed in the Methods S1. The Mann Whitney U test was used to analyze the differences between SLE and controls.

Endotoxin analyses

MonoMac 6 cells and primary monocytes from healthy donors were stimulated with 100 U/ml α2-interferon (PBL Biomedical Laboratories, Piscataway, NJ), 10 ng/ml γ–interferon (R&D Systems, Inc., Minneapolis, MN), 10 ng/ml tumor necrosis factor (TNF-α) (Sigma, Saint Louis, MO) for 16 hours, or 1 µg/ml of LPS for two hours. SB203580 was used as a p38- MAPK inhibitor by pretreating the cells for 30 minutes at a concentration of 10 µM. SP600125 (Calbiochem, Darmstadt, Germany) was used as a JNK inhibitor at a concentration of 10 µM and U0126 (Cell signaling, Danvers, MA) was used as an ERK inhibitor at a concentration of 10 µM. Cells were harvested after stimulation and RNA was prepared as above. To measure circulating endotoxin, serum samples from 99 SLE patients and 112 Red Cross blood donors were analyzed using the Limulus assay (Thermo Scientific, Rockford, IL). The Wilcoxon method was used to compare the levels across groups.

Bioinformatics

We used the Tophat-Cufflinks pipeline and further refinements [29] to assemble the monocyte transcriptome and detect novel loci and isoforms, followed by mapping short reads to a collection of reference RNA sequences, including isoforms of coding genes, small RNAs, long non-coding RNAs (lncRNAs), and repetitive elements. The number of reads mapped to each transcript was used for evaluating differential expression between control and SLE samples. Data has been submitted to GEO as GSE53419.

The following steps were used in data analysis:

- Use TopHat to align 50 bp sequencing reads to reference genome hg19. TopHat also searched for reads partially mapped to distant locations to identify exon-exon junctions. As a result, TopHat mapped ~22 million reads per sample on average and stored the aligned reads in BAM files. This step did not use any known gene annotation
- Use Cufflinks to assemble transcriptomes of individual samples while using RefSeq gene annotation as reference. On average, Cufflinks reported 65,008 genes and 83,430 transcripts in individual transcriptomes.
- Use Cuffmerge to combine individual transcriptomes, also using RefSeq as reference. The merging improved the reliability of novel loci and isoforms by taking a consensus of individual transcriptomes. Cuffmerge reported 59,887 transcripts of 34,307 genes in a consensus transcriptome.

- Use Cuffcompare to categorize transcripts by comparing the consensus transcriptome to RefSeq annotation. For example, a class "=" transcript had the same exon-exon junctions as a known RefSeq transcripts and a class "u" transcripts had no overlapping to any known genes. As a result, Cuffcompare identified 10,200 novel transcribed loci and 10,313 isoforms including novel exon-exon junctions of known genes.
- Use the gene annotation tracks downloaded from UCSC Genome Browser to evaluate the novelty of the new loci and isoforms reported by Cuffcompare. The tracks were UCSC Genes, Ensembl Genes, GENCODE Genes V12, CCDS, H-Inv 7.0, sno/miRNA and lincRNA Transcripts, including evidence-based gene annotation, computationally generated gene prediction, and collections of non-coding RNAs. The comparison identified 2,280 and 4,000 high novelty loci and isoforms not included in any of the seven annotation tracks.
- Repeat the TopHat-to-Cuffcompare steps without using a reference annotation for assembling and merging transcriptomes. Cuffcompare identified 774 transcripts having the exact same exon-exon junctions as known RefSeq transcripts. These true positives had higher read counts and consistency across samples. Surprisingly, they were also longer and included more exons on average, which presumably made them more difficult to be completely assembled. High read count and high consistency were then used as the criteria to filter the novel loci and isoforms identified by previous steps to obtain 3,725 and 1,327 high-confidence novel loci and isoforms respectively.

Align reads to reference transcriptome using Novoalign. NovoalignCS was used to align reads to a reference transcriptome to obtain the read count per transcript. Each entry of the reference transcriptome was the full sequence of a transcript without introns. The reference transcriptome included all RefSeq transcripts and novel loci/isoforms reported by Cuffmerge, as well as three classes of non-coding RNAs: small RNAs from snoRNABase and miRBase), lincRNAs (UCSC Genome Browser lincRNAs track), and repetitive elements (Repbase).

Reads mapped to the same transcript were counted to define the transcription level. Reads mapped to different RNA classes or transcripts of different genes were excluded. The number of unique reads mapped to different transcripts of the same genes were used as gene-level read count. Only reads mapped to the sense strand were counted, whereas reads mapped to the antisense strand of coding genes were used to quantitate antisense transcription.

Statistical analysis of transcriptional data. We noticed that the fold change of patients and controls was slightly dependent on the baseline expression level ($r = 0.15$, $p < 0.01$), and applied Loess adjustment to remove this bias by assuming an equal amount of total RNA between samples. The global average of patient-control difference was very close to zero (0.4% higher in SLE) after the adjustment.

Statistical analysis of differential expression was performed within R environment using Bioconductor packages. Rsamtools package was used to import aligned reads from BAM files to R environment. Gene-level differential expression between SLE and control samples was analyzed with the Bioconductor EdgeR package. Genes without at least three read counts in at least three samples were excluded.

Gene-gene correlation analysis was performed by the following steps: calculate the correlation coefficients between genes in control and SLE groups separately; convert correlation coefficients to z scores using Fisher's transformation; take the average of z scores, and convert the average z score back to a single combined correlation coefficient r. Enrichment studies utilized DAVID which reports adjusted p values based on the Benjamini Hochberg algorithm [30].

3′ Untranslated analysis. For analysis of the 3′ untranslated regions, RNA-Seq reads were aligned to reference genome (UCSC, hg19) using Tophat 1.3.1 by default parameters for Applied Biosystems' Colorspace format. Uniquely mapped reads were kept for downstream analysis. PolyA_DB together with the 3′ ends of transcripts from UCSC, RefSeq, Aceview annotations were collected as a comprehensive APA database [31]. For each annotated cleavage site, the number of reads in the upstream 200 nt window were computed as the estimation for the expression level of the mRNA isoform terminating at that 3′end. The read count for each isoform was added up in nine case samples and eight control samples, respectively. We required at least 10 reads supporting each isoform resulting in ~6600 APA genes for analysis. The relative ratio of expression at proximal to distal sites, in addition with a p-value, was calculated by Fisher's Exact test using R (http://www.r-project.org/). Relative ratio>2 and p-value<0.01 were used to predict different isoform usage.

Analysis of published gene sets. Five data sets were created from four monocyte GEO data series, GSE15219, GSE19627, GSE5504, and GSE21909 (one from each of the first three and two from GSE21909, which used saline and cortisol for intravenous delivery of LPS). Samples and groups were selected so that each group had matched replicates/donors. (Table 1)

Results

Transcriptome characterization

Monocyte transcriptomes from Nine female SLE patients and eight female healthy controls were studied using RNA-seq. Total RNA was purified from monocytes and used for library preparation. Our first goal in this study was to reconstruct the human monocyte transcriptome using the entire dataset. The Tophat-Cufflinks pipeline reported four major classes of transcripts (Figure S1A), including 10,313 isoforms of known genes and 10,200 transcribed loci not included in the RefSeq annotation. The processed data are given in an excel spreadsheet in Data S1. The novel isoforms had a more complex structure (Figure S1B). On the other hand, the novel loci were shorter on average than known genes and over 97% of them included only one exon.

To further define the monocyte transcriptome, we counted the total number of reads solely aligned to each of the four major RNA classes: coding RNAs, long non coding (lncRNAs), small RNAs, and repetitive elements. Ribosomal RNAs (rRNA) were excluded from this summary. Close to 80% of the non-rRNA reads were mapped to coding RNAs while the other three classes evenly shared the remaining reads (Figure S1C). Small RNAs had the highest molar concentration after read counts were adjusted by the total length of the RNA classes, followed by repetitive elements, coding RNAs, and lncRNAs (Figure S1D). These data were comparable to the distribution seen in other systems [32].

The classifications of transcripts were refined. We identified 4,000 high-novelty isoforms that were not present in seven additional annotated databases and included at least one unknown exon-exon junction, as well as 2,271 high-novelty loci that had no overlap with either exons or introns of any previously reported transcripts. We then defined 1,327 high-confidence isoforms, having at least 10 uniquely mapped reads not mapped to any other genes or isoforms of the same gene in at least six samples, and 3,725 high-confidence novel loci having at least 10 uniquely mapped reads in at least six samples and more than 10× overall sequencing depth. After this refinement, 448 novel isoforms and

Table 1. GEO sources.

	# groups	# replicates
GSE15219	4	2
GSE19627	2	3
GSE5504	4	2
GSE21909_Saline	3	3
GSE21909_Cortisol	3	3

778 novel loci that had both high-novelty and high-confidence were identified. There was no association between high-novelty and high-confidence (Figure S2). We manually examined a subset of the 778 novel loci for protein coding potential and the possibility that they are orthologs of coding genes in other species using BLAST. Most did not exhibit similarity to any annotated genes and the majority had limited protein coding potential (<100 contiguous amino acids). We selected 27 novel loci and validated transcription from all 27 using RT-PCR (Figure S3, Table S3).

Class-specific transcripts in SLE

The major goal of this study was to identify a unique signature of the monocyte transcriptome in SLE as a strategy to improve our understanding of the pathogenic mechanisms. We found that there were a large number of known protein coding genes expressed in normal monocytes, but silenced in SLE (Figure 1A). These genes were highly enriched with ones related to embryo development (p = 6.0E-60), suggesting that SLE monocytes are more differentiated. Antisense transcripts were also more likely to be silenced in SLE (Figure 1B). On the other hand, the numbers of novel loci and novel isoforms transcribed only in patients were 3.95 and 1.49 times higher, respectively, than the numbers of control-specific ones (Figure 1C and 1D).

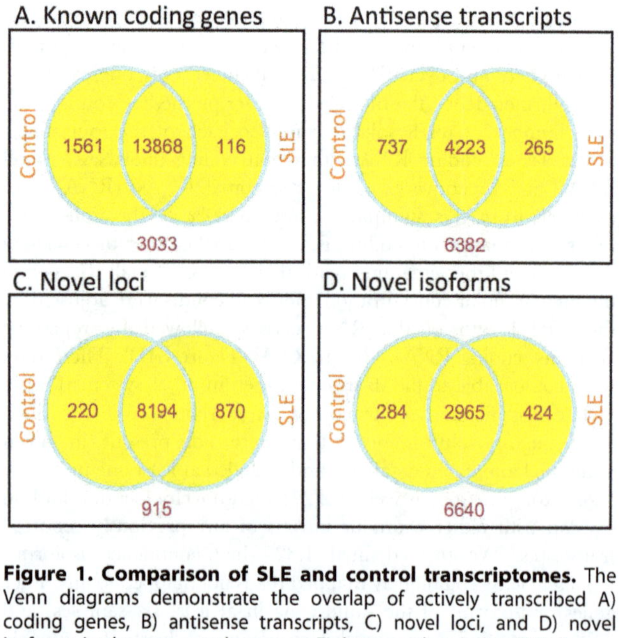

Figure 1. Comparison of SLE and control transcriptomes. The Venn diagrams demonstrate the overlap of actively transcribed A) coding genes, B) antisense transcripts, C) novel loci, and D) novel isoforms in the two sample groups. Eight control and nine SLE libraries were used.

We evaluated the differential expression between the two groups of samples in six classes of genes/transcripts: known RefSeq protein coding genes, novel loci identified by Cufflinks, lncRNAs, small RNAs, repetitive elements, and the antisense transcripts of coding genes. These genes/transcripts were filtered by a statistical analysis, so all the remaining 33,760 (72% of 47,171 total reads) were mapped by at least three sequencing reads in at least three samples. We applied the negative binomial test implemented by the edgeR package of Bioconductor [33] and identified 1,754 differentially expressed genes/transcripts with p values less than 0.01 and a false discovery rate (FDR) of 0.2. Classes of differentially expressed genes (DEGs) are shown in Table S4.

The patient-control difference of total transcription varied dramatically between RNA classes (Figure 2A). Total transcription of both sense and antisense transcripts of known coding genes was reduced by approximately 15% in SLE (p = 5.6E-61 and 7.4E-105 respectively). Total transcription of novel loci was strikingly increased by over 45% in SLE (p<1.0E-300), as SLE patients produced many previously undiscovered transcripts that had low or no transcription in healthy monocytes. Although expression of small RNAs was downregulated by about 5%, expression of 91 pri-miRNAs was dramatically increased by 38% (p = 0.01), whereas the three classes of small nucleolar RNAs were all downregulated in SLE patients (Figure 2B). The overall up-regulation of pri-miRNAs and down-regulation of coding genes jointly suggested a modified miRNA regulatory system in SLE. Subclasses of repetitive elements also had different directions of change in SLE (Figure 2C). All endogenous retroviral (ERV) subclasses were consistently downregulated (p = 4.7E-4 to 3.8E-29). Other retrotransposons such as LTR retrotransposons, SINE, and LINE (L1) elements were variably decreased in SLE patients, while expression of SINE1/7SL elements was increased.

Protein-coding genes

Functional analysis of the protein coding genes identified a large number of pre-defined gene sets whose members were enriched within differentially expressed genes (DEGs), partially listed in Table S5. Most noticeably, DEGs upregulated in SLE were enriched with genes related to immune response and cytokine activity, while the downregulated DEGs were enriched with genes related to cell adhesion and motion. According to Genetic Association Database (GAD), eleven upregulated DEGs were associated with SLE in previous studies (Table S6). In addition, the combined gene set of up- and downregulated DEGs was enriched with potential targets of transcription factors highly relevant to SLE, including AP1 (p = 3.4E-09), E47 (p = 1.1E-8), RFX1 (5.8E-7), IRF1 (p = 1.4E-3), and IRF2 (p = 1.3E-3). We selected six DEGs, five upregulated and one downregulated in SLE, to be validated in new samples using qRT-PCR. Five of the genes were significantly different between controls and patients (p = 0.049 to

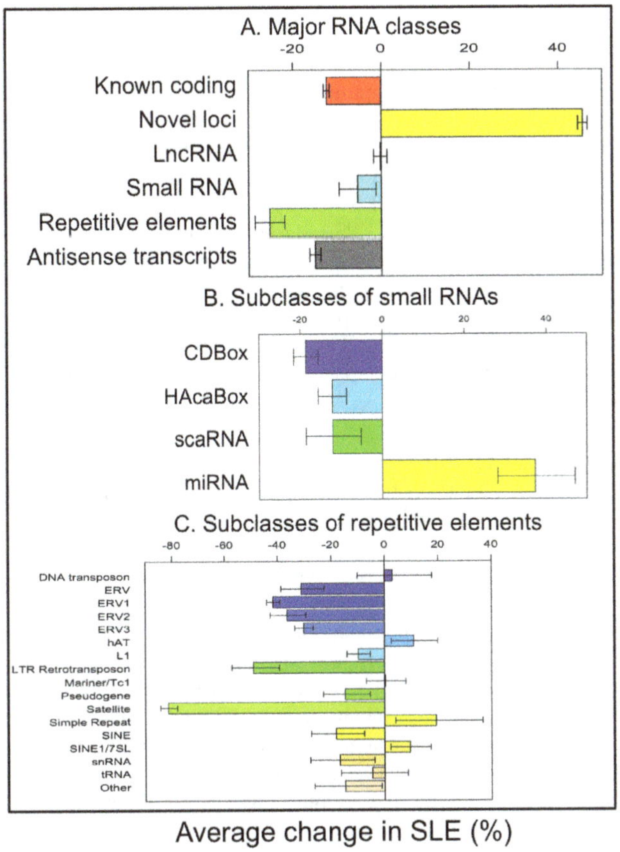

Figure 2. Differential expression of RNA classes. A) The average transcriptional changes of five RNA classes in SLE. B) The average transcriptional change of four sub-classes of small RNAs in SLE. C) The average transcriptional change of 17 subclasses of repetitive elements in SLE. The eight control and nine SLE libraries were used for this analysis. Error bars indicate standard deviation.

0.0001) and all six were changed in the same direction in both patient cohorts (Figure S4).

Polyadenylation

Polyadenylation along with mRNA cleavage and termination are regulated in a gene-specific manner and these steps appear to be particularly important for the regulation of genes involved in inflammation [34,35,36]. Tissue-specific and developmentally-regulated polyadenylation have been described with differentiation favoring longer 3′ UTRs [37,38,39]We examined the structure of the coding genes by defining the 3′ untranslated region for each gene. Sixty-seven genes had longer 3′UTRs in patients compared to controls and 54 genes had shorter 3′UTRs in patients (defined by a ratio of >2.0 and a $p<0.01$). The longer 3′UTR gene set was characterized by pathways centered on NFκB, Akt, UBC and HNF4A. The shorter 3′UTR gene set was characterized by pathways centered on UBC, NFκB, and ERK (Figure S5). As shorter 3′UTRs can escape regulation by miRNAs and the inflammatory pathways implicated by the pathway analysis are concordant with what is known about SLE, these gene sets are notable and may given insight into the SLE process [38,40].

Antisense transcription

We analyzed antisense transcription because of the potential for sense-antisense duplex RNA to drive type I interferon expression and because antisense transcripts can regulate transcription in *cis* [41]. The gene-level read counts of sense and antisense transcripts were positively, but weakly, correlated ($r = 0.19$, $p<0.01$). Overall, examining patients and controls together, the total number of reads mapped to the antisense transcripts was about 1/30 of the total number of reads mapped to the sense transcripts. However, a small set of genes demonstrated much higher antisense transcription than sense transcription (Figure S6), such as *USP5*, a ubiquitin peptidase, and *CMTM5*, a chemokine-like factor gene.

In SLE, some coding genes had significantly changed antisense transcription in the opposite direction of their sense counterparts, most noticeably *IVNS1A BASES* (influenza virus NS1A binding protein), *RACGAP1* (Rac GTPase activating protein 1) and *THBS1* (thrombospondin 1). All three genes had significantly upregulated sense transcripts and significantly downregulated antisense transcripts in SLE. The reversed change of sense and antisense transcripts of these genes suggested that the two transcripts are distinctly regulated.

LncRNA expression

LncRNAs can regulate nearby coding genes as *cis*-regulatory elements. We summarized the correlation of transcription between pairs of lncRNAs and coding genes (Figure S7). When the lncRNAs were located within 100 kb upstream of coding genes, the pairs had a positive correlation on average, regardless of whether the lncRNAs were on the same strand as the coding genes or not. The correlation increased as the distance between lncRNAs and coding genes became closer. On the other hand, when the lncRNAs were located downstream of coding genes, there was no association between the two classes of transcripts if they were on the opposite strands, and a much stronger association if they were on the same strand. The latter might suggest the misclassification of extended 3′ UTR transcription of coding genes as lncRNAs. Although lncRNAs were less likely to change in SLE compared to other RNA classes (Table S4), the locations of some significantly changed lncRNAs suggested their involvement in SLE. For example, both *HIVEP2* itself and a lncRNA about 800 to 1,500 bases upstream of its transcription start site (TSS) were significantly upregulated in SLE, although their RNA abundance was over 50 times different. There were also two significantly upregulated lncRNAs located within 50 kb of each other on chromosome 6 and surrounded by a group of signficantly dysregulated coding genes including *TAGAP*, *FNDC1*, *SOD2*, *WTAP*, and *ACAT2* (Figure S8).

Pri-miRNA expression

Our RNA purification method did not retain miRNAs, however, pri-miRNAs were easily detected and the combination of increased pri-miRNAs and decreased targets suggested an impact of the miRNAs (Figure S9). Two pri-miRNAs, miR 193a and miR-212, were statistically significantly increased in SLE samples with concomitantly diminished target mRNA levels. MiR-193a, regulating k-ras and survival, was increased by 776% ($p = 0.009$) [42]. MiR-212, regulating apoptosis, was increased by 148% ($p = 0.009$) [43]. Thesetwo cellular processes are known to be aberrant in SLE monocytes [44,45].

We validated mature miR-212-3p differential expression in SLE using qRT-PCR on new samples from six controls and 13 SLE patients (Figure S10). An exogenous control was used because we could not identify an miRNA in monocytes that was unaffected by cytokine treatment (data not shown). The expression of miR-212-5p was too low to be detected in this ligation-based detection strategy. The predicted targets of miR-193a-3p, miR-193a-5p and miR-212 were downregulated by 14.0% to 16.7% in SLE, which was more than the average down-regulation of all other genes (Figure S11).

Repetitive element expression

Repetitive elements were globally downregulated in SLE (Figure 2C). A closer look at the downregulated repetitive elements showed that they were predominantly ERV classes and were closely correlated with each other, suggesting that they were co-regulated via an upstream mechanism. Interferon is known to repress retroviral activation and over-expression of interferon in SLE has been documented in several studies [1,2,46,47,48]. Coding genes having the highest positive correlation with the downregulated repetitive elements were potential targets of transcription factors AP1 ($p = 3.0E-8$), E47 ($p = 2.2E-9$), RFX1 ($p = 3.7E-8$), IRF1 ($p = 3.5E-2$), and IRF2 ($p = 4.3E-3$), also supporting an effect of interferons.

Isoform analysis

The proportions of the total reads assigned to each isoform for each gene were compared between the control and SLE samples to evaluate differential isoform transcription. Therefore, this analysis only considered the change of relative isoform abundance while ignoring the gene-level differential expression. This comparison identified 54 genes having one or more isoforms where the relative abundance was significantly changed ($p<0.05$) by at least 5%, such as *CCR2*, *HIVEP1*, *HIVEP2*, *IL1B*, *IL1R2* and *TLR2*. *SNAPC3* encodes a subunit of a protein complex that activates snRNA. It was previously known as having a single isoform, while our Cufflinks assembly identified a novel splicing site within its 3′UTR (Figure S12). The relative abundance of these two alternative transcripts was changed by about 12% with $p = 0.003$.

We observed that isoforms where the relative abundance was increased in SLE had significantly more exons than those with decreased relative abundance (Figure S13). This result indicates higher RNA splicing activity and/or more complex RNA processing in SLE monocytes.

We selected two biologically relevant genes to validate the expression of their novel isoforms in monocytes. Primers were designed to selectively bridge the novel exon-exon junction. *IL1R1* and *IRF8* were both found to include a large intragenic exon by RNA-seq (Figures S14 and S15). These exons have no protein coding potential. For IL1R1, the novel exon is an extra 5′ untranslated region. In both cases, PCR demonstrated incorporation of the novel exon (Figure S16).

Novel loci transcription

92% differentially expressed novel loci had higher transcription in SLE (Table S4). Many of the novel loci formed clusters located close to each other. For example, three of the four novel loci, located within a 5 kb region on chromosome 18, were among the most significantly upregulated transcripts (Figure S17). Another example was a cluster of 26 novel loci located within a 34 kb region on chromosome 8, most of which were significantly upregulated in SLE and none of which were downregulated (Figure S18). We selected 22 novel transcripts upregulated in SLE to be validated in new samples using qRT-PCR. Ten of the transcripts were significantly upregulated ($p = 0.034$ to 0.0006) in SLE (Figure 3A), and only two were not upregulated at all (Figure 3B). The other loci were upregulated without reaching statistical significance (Figure 3B and Figure S19).

The fact that these loci were preferentially or exclusively transcribed in SLE monocytes indicates they are very cell-specific. They were not present in seven annotated gene databases supporting SLE-specificity. To examine potential mechanisms driving expression, we initially treated MonoMac 6 cells with TNF-α, α2-interferon, γ–interferon, or LPS. Time course experiments identified the optimal stimulation time. Only LPS replicated the pattern of expression of novel loci seen in the SLE samples (Figure 4A). These findings were further validated using published datasets and examining concordance. In this analysis, genes over-expressed in SLE were equally likely to be represented in the a2-interferon- and LPS-induced genesets (Figure S20). We then confirmed the effect using monocytes from healthy adult donors (Figure 4B). To understand potential pathways regulating the LPS effect, we utilized p38 (SB203580), ERK (U0126) and JNK (SP600125) inhibitors. The major effect of LPS induction of the novel transcripts was p38 mediated (Figures 4C and 4D, Figures S21 and S22).

Circulating endotoxin

Although endotoxin has been previously implicated in murine lupus models and LPS is known to activate interferon pathways via TLR4, there has been no direct measurement of endotoxin in SLE patients [16,17,18,19,20,21]. We compared, therefore, serum levels from 99 female SLE patients and those from 112 female healthy adult blood donors. This patient set comprised new samples. The SLE patients were 91% female, 46% black, 54% Caucasian, mean age 37.1 years, mean SLEDAI (Systemic Lupus Erythematosus Disease Activity Index) of 2.6 and mean physician global estimate of 0.45. The mean prednisone dose was 9 mg/day. The red cross blood donors were females who were self declared as healthy. SLE patients had significantly higher endotoxin levels compared to controls (Figure 5). When we examined clinical markers for associations with circulating endotoxin levels, we found no association with age, weight, erythrocyte sedimentation rate (ESR), C-reactive protein (CRP), specific organ damage, specific autoantibodies or complete blood count (CBC) parameters. Because LPS/endotoxin can induce type I interferon expression, we examined the concordance of coding genes expressed in SLE, after stimulation with LPS and after stimulation with α-interferon using our prior results and published array results [49,50]. There was substantial overlap, demonstrating that endotoxin can in part mimic the type I interferon signature seen in SLE (Figure S21).

Discussion

With the advent of next-generation sequencing technologies a more comprehensive and accurate transcriptional analysis has become feasible. We report a whole transcriptome analysis of patients with SLE and compare gene expression with that of healthy controls. We detected many instances of SLE-specific alternative splicing, alternative polyadenylation, and novel loci transcription. Splicing and polyadenylation in SLE both favored longer, more complex transcripts.

One of our goals was to identify the transcript abundance of non-coding RNAs, which have been demonstrated in subjects with Aicardi Goutières syndrome, an infantile-onset disorder with features of lupus, and in murine models, to drive a type I interferon signature [51,52,53]. In this study, we found instead decreased expression of many non-coding RNAs. We hypothesize that repression of endogenous retroviral sequences may be mediated by the type I interferon that is known to be overexpressed in SLE patients [54]. One class of non-coding RNA for which expression was clearly induced in SLE patients was that of the pri-miRNAs. These small non-coding RNAs are processed to repress translation and regulate multiple messenger

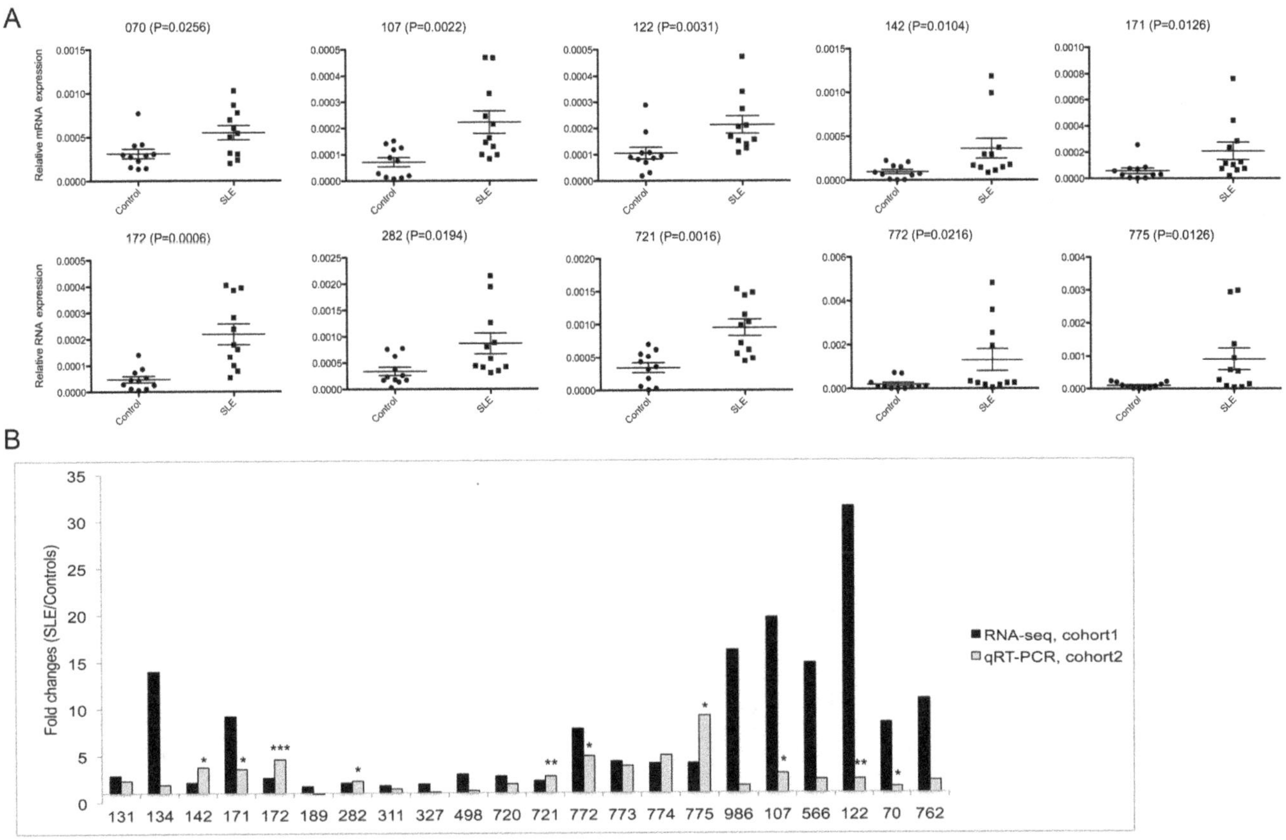

Figure 3. PCR validation in new samples. A) Ten novel loci (70, 107, 122, 142, 171, 172, 282. 721, 772, and 775) were amplified using 11 controls (8 new controls and 3 controls used for the RNA-seq libraries) and 11 new SLE patients. Transcript levels were normalized to β-actin. In each case, the differential expression between SLE and controls was statistically significant with $p<0.05$, according to the Mann-Whitney test. The cross bars indicate mean and standard error. Primers and locations are given in Methods S1. B) There was a good agreement of expression fold changes in SLE between the RNA-seq and qRT-PCR experiments with $p<0.05$ (*), $p<0.01$ (**) or $p<0.001$(***). All but two of 22 tested novel loci were upregulated in both SLE patient cohorts.

RNAs. In our study, two specific pri-miRNAs were significantly upregulated in SLE monocytes compared to healthy controls. In addition, we were able to demonstrate that the targets of these two miRNAs exhibited decreased message levels. These observations suggest that the elevated pri-miRNA levels that we identified in SLE monocytes are functionally relevant.

Among known protein-coding genes, there was evidence of global repression, and many genes downregulated in SLE monocytes were related to cell proliferation and cell adhesion. The genes upregulated in SLE monocytes reflected active inflammation. These observations are concordant with what has been seen using arrays and what is known about monocyte behavior in SLE [1,2,25,55,56,57,58,59]. Monocytes are known to have a shortened life span and to exhibit characteristics related to type I interferon exposure [1,23,45]. The overall repression of gene expression could be consistent with increased differentiation and our previous studies demonstrated altered surface expression of several proteins [14].

The finding of SLE-specific isoforms and polyadenylation was particularly intriguing. The finding of disease-specific isoforms is not unique to this study, but it has not been reported this extensively outside of tumor-specific transcripts. Some studies have found functional effects of autoantibodies directed at nuclear constituents and altered expression of splicing factors and this study raises the question of the mechanism driving altered processing [60,61,62]. Altered expression of splicing factors could also contribute to the pattern observed here [61,62].

This study raises many questions. We examined a cohort of patients with low disease activity to minimize the effect of medications. Whether patients with more severe disease could have a more disturbed transcriptome is not known. This is a relatively small cohort size, and additional studies will be required to replicate these findings. We did not perform extensive validation of the many classes of RNA found to have altered expression, instead capturing a snapshot of the SLE transcriptome in a single cell type and focusing on the breadth of the effect. We validated using new samples from controls and patients for the DEGs and found similar changes in nearly all DEGs, supporting that these effects are consistently seen in the disease. If similar disruptions are found in additional cell types, it would suggest a systematically altered transcriptome. Nevertheless, analyses of isoforms and un-annotated loci is a moving target and additional information is likely to be forthcoming, allowing improved understanding of the regulation of these processes. Monocytes represent a cell type that is uniquely plastic and it may be that effects are magnified in this cell type.

IRF1, IRF2, and RFX1 were previously identified by us as potential regulators of genes with altered histone H4 acetylation [23,24,25]. These transcription factors, now identified as potential regulators of the SLE transcriptome, could integrate inflammatory and interferon signals. The MAP kinase and NFκB pathways were

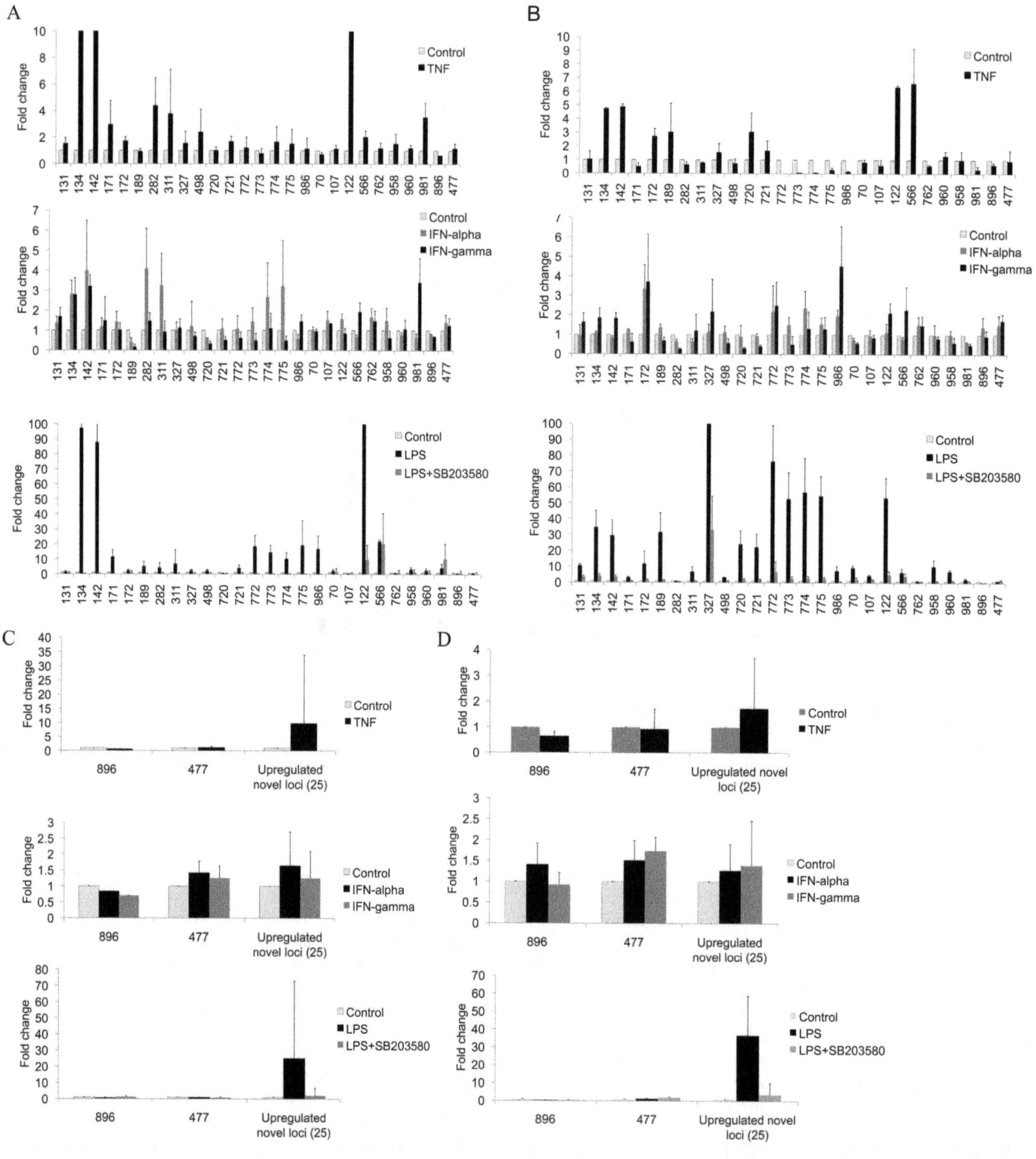

Figure 4. LPS stimulation of monocytes. A) MonoMac 6 cells were stimulated for 16 hours as indicated and qRT-PCR was performed for the novel loci. Only LPS (1 μg/ml) stimulation consistently upregulated these loci. TNF-α (10 ng/ml) led to upregulation of 16/25 (fold change>1.5), αIFN (100 U/ml) led to upregulation of 9/25 (fold change>1.5), γIFN (10 ng/ml) led to upregulation of 5/25 (fold change>1.5), and LPS led to upregulation of 22/25 (fold change>1.5). Three experiments with duplciates or triplicates were averaged. The error bars indicate standard deviation. B) Human primary monocytes were stimulated as above and the abundance of the novel transcripts quantitated by qRT-PCR. TNF-α led to upregulation of 9/25 (fold change>1.5), αIFN led to upregulation of 7/25 (fold change>1.5), γIFN led to upregulation of 9/25 (fold change>1.5), and LPS led to upregulation of 23/25 (fold change>1.5). Pre-treatment of cells with the p38 inhibitor, SB203580 led to markedly diminished induction of expression by LPS. Three experiments with duplciates or triplicates were averaged. The error bars indicate standard deviation. C) The average fold change for the aggregated novel upregulated loci in SLE were calculated for MonoMac 6 cells and D) healthy human primary monocytes stimulated by LPS, TNF-α, αIFN,or γIFN. Locus 896 was down-regulated and locus 477 was not changed in the orignal SLE samples and were included as controls. The error bars indicate standard deviation in C and D.

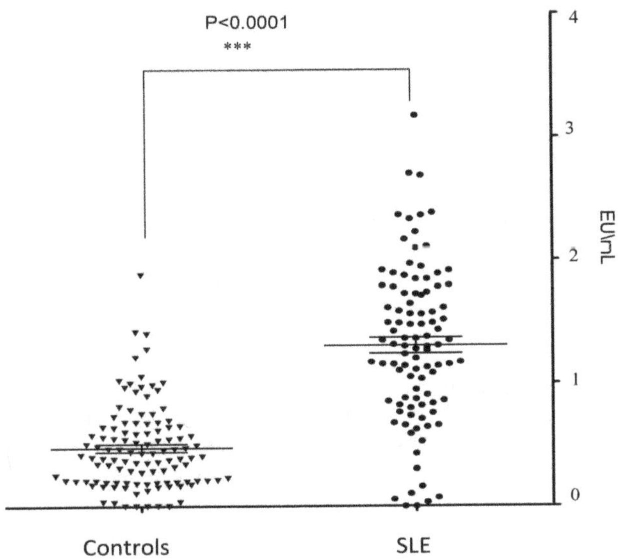

Figure 5. SLE patient circulating endotoxin levels. Circulating endotoxin was quantitated using the Limulus assay. 99 female SLE patients and 112 female Red Cross blood donors were anlayzed. SLE patients had significantly more endotoxin on average than controls ($P < 0.0001$). The cross bars indicate the mean and standard error.

identified as potential regulating pathways in the polyadenylation pattern specific to the SLE samples. These pathways have long been implicated in SLE [63,64,65,66,67,68]. To further implicate the MAP kinase pathway, we found that expression of many novel loci were inducible with LPS and that inducibility could be blocked with the P38 inhibitor, SB203580. The roles of the novel loci are not yet known and we acknowledge that these fall into a bioinformatic limbo. Nevertheless, endotoxin has been implicated in a variety of diseases and induces type I IFN [69,70,71,72,73,74,75,76]. Our findings of significant overlap of the genes induced by LPS/endotoxin, SLE and α-interferon along with increased endotoxin in peripheral blood supports a role for endotoxin in the pathologic gene expression pattern identified here. This is the first RNA-seq study of SLE monocytes and our analysis revealed a surprisingly distorted transcriptome. The strengths of the study include the comprehensive approach to the characterization of the transcriptional landscape, use of a purified cell type, validation of the findings using a new cohort, and a mechanistic insight into the expression of novel loci.

Limitations of this study include a small sample size focused on mild to moderate disease activity. While the low disease activity enabled us to examine patient samples without the perturbation of high-level immune suppression, it may also have limited our findings. The platform used and the sample cell count may also have limited our findings. The libraries were 50 bp single reads and total RNA was used with post-run ribosomal RNA exclusion. Finally, technical aspects such as RNA quality may have limited our ability to identify disease-specific variation in signal. Nevertheless, in spite of these potential limitations, our analyses were robust and identified many changes specific to the SLE transcriptome.

In summary, we found a broadly altered transcriptome. By using a single cell type, we minimized the effects of different cell populations and improved the specificity of our discoveries. The most significant finding of this study was identification of disease-specific novel loci expression, regulated by endotoxin. Circulating endotoxin has been negatively associated with prognosis in a number of diseases and is thought to drive a type of immune exhaustion [77,78]. Whether endotoxin could be responsible for other features of the altered transcriptome or could represent a biomarker for disease severity remains to be determined. While additional studies will be required to determine which features contribute to the pathologic processes in this still enigmatic disease, the importance of this study lies in the identification of multiple features of altered transcription and processing in SLE, a heretofore unappreciated facet of the disease.

Supporting Information

Figure S1 Overall transcriptome characteristics. A) The Tophat-Cufflinks pipeline identified four major classes of transcripts from 17 RNA-seq libraries. RefSeq genes constituted the majority of the transcripts. B) Novel isoforms and loci were different from known transcripts in terms of average length and numbers of exons on average. C) Coding RNA was the most abundant RNA species (except ribosomal RNA) in monocytes based on the count of RNA-seq reads. Non-coding RNA collectively accounted for approximately 20% of total RNA. D) Small RNAs had the highest expression level on average after adjusting read counts for the total length of RNA classes.

Figure S2 High novelty and high confidence novel isoforms and loci. A) Novel isoforms including at least one unknown exon-exon junction or mapped by ≥10 unique reads in at least six libraries were considering as having high-novelty or high-confidence, respectively. B) Novel loci not overlapping any known transcribed region or mapped by ≥10 unique reads in at least six libraries were considering as having high-novelty or high-confidence, respectively. Odds ratios and p values were the result of Fisher's Exact test performed on the overlap.

Figure S3 Validation of novel transcripts. Transcripts were validated for 27 identified novel loci using qRT-PCR (black bars). Primary monocyte RNA was used as the source and control amplifications using non-reverse-transcribed RNA were used as the negative control (No RT bars). Globin, not expected to be expressed in monocytes, was used as an additional negative control. Beta-actin was used for normalization. Most of these novel loci were generally expressed at low levels. The locations of the novel loci are in Methods S1. This represents $n = 1$. Further validation appears in the main text.

Figure S4 Validation of differential gene expression. The differential expression of six coding genes in SLE were validated by qRT-PCR. The samples consisted of 11 controls (including 3 internal validation samples from which the RNA-seq libraries were made) and 11 new SLE patients. Five of the genes were validated as having significant change in SLE. The sixth gene, *CD177*, had the same direction of change in SLE samples but the change did not reach statistical significance. The cross bars indicate mean and standard error according to the Mann-Whitney test.

Figure S5 3′ UTR length networks. A) The genes with longer 3′UTRs in SLE patients were networked using Ingenuity. The two most dominant networks are shown. NFκB, AKT, and UBC are the dominant nodes. B) The genes with shorter 3′UTRs in SLE patients were networked using Ingenuity. The two most dominant networks are shown. MAP kinases and UBC were the dominant nodes. Data output from Ingenuity is shown in the Tables below.

Figure S6 Sense- antisense expression. About 5,000 coding genes had detectable antisense transcription in monocytes. A) The average transcription of antisense transcripts was less than the half of the corresponding sense transcripts; but a small number of antisense transcripts had over ten-fold higher transcription of their sense counterparts. B) The transcription of sense and antisense pairs tended to be positively correlated. The correlation between each pair was first calculated across samples in the control and SLE groups separately, then the two correlation coefficients were combined using Fisher's transformation.

Figure S7 LncRNA association with adjacent transcription. The co-regulation of lncRNAs and their nearby coding genes was dependent on their distance and relative location. The horizontal black line is indicates the average correlation of random pairs of lncRNAs and coding genes. (Oppo: opposite strand.)

Figure S8 Chromosome 6 lncRNA cluster. A cluster of coding genes and lncRNAs located on chr6q25.3 were commonly dysregulated in SLE monocytes. Four coding genes with medium to high transcription levels were all upregulated in SLE while the other coding gene, *FNDC1*, had a very low transcription level and was downregulated in SLE. Both highlighted lncRNAs were significantly upregulated in SLE. Three other lncRNAs within this region had detectable transcription, but no significant changes in SLE. The Table demonstrates the read counts for each locus.

Figure S9 MicroRNA- target correlation. Ten pri-miRNAs and their predicted targets had a negative correlation in monocytes. The correlation was calculated using normalized read counts of pri-miRNAs and target coding genes. The correlation coefficients of each miRNA-target pair were obtained from the control and SLE groups separately and then combined using Fisher's transformation. Each bar represents the average and standard error of correlation coefficients of a target list. Target lists were downloaded from miRBase.

Figure S10 miRNA validation. The increased expression of miR-212-3p in SLE was validated by qRT-PCR with cel-miR-238 as a control. Six new controls and 13 new SLE samples were used.

Figure S11 High expression miRNA target transcript expression. Three miRNAs whose pri-miRNAs had higher expression in SLE were examined for an effect on potential target transcripts. For these three miRNAs, target transcript expression was significantly downregulated on average. While coding genes were generally downregulated in SLE, the target genes tended to be downregulated even more. Target lists were downloaded from miRBase database.

Figure S12 Isoform distribution for *SNAPC3*. A) Cufflinks assembly based on our RNA-seq data identified a novel splicing site within the 3′ UTR of *SNAPC3*. B) The relative abundance of the two isoforms was changed in SLE. C) The difference in relative abundance was statistically significant.

Figure S13 Isoforms with increased expression in SLE are more complex. The isoforms where the relative abundance was increased in SLE had a higher number of exons than those where the relative abundance was decreased ($p = 0.007$). On average, the SLE-favored isoforms had about 0.5 exons more than the control-favored isoforms.

Figure S14 Novel isoforms of IL1R1. Tophat-Cufflinks identified three isoforms of *IL1R1* not included in the RefSeq annotation. Two of them have been included in GENCODE database version 14 (**A&B**), and both had histone patterns at their transcription start sites consistent with expression according to ENCODE histone modification data sets generated from CD14+ monocytes (**C&D**). The other isoform, *TCONS_00030117*, had ~6 kb extra 5′ UTR exon (**E**). According to the ENCODE data, this exon has a strong H3K9me3 footprint (**F**), which is known as a repressive histone modification, suggesting unique transcriptional regulation at this region.

Figure S15 Novel isoform of IRF8. Tophat-Cufflinks identified a novel isoform of *IRF8*, which included a prolonged exon 4. The existence of this isoform was supported by an ENCODE RNA-seq data set generated from 9 cell lines, including lymphoblastoid cell line GM12878. Transcription was detected in GM12878 cross the full gene body of IRF8, but the extended region of exon 4 in the novel isoform had higher transcription level than those of the introns. This isoform is likely an intermediate product of RNA processing and not present in the mature mRNA.

Figure S16 Novel isoform validation. A) Tophat-Cufflinks identified multiple novel isoforms of *IL1R1*, each with a new exon-exon junction in the 5′ UTR. One of the isoforms (in red) was validated by qRT-PCR using a pair of primers across two exons (F4/R4). B) *IRF8* was known to have a single isoform. Tophat-Cufflinks identified a novel isoform, which was validated by qRT-PCR. These gels are representative of three experiments, with comparable results.

Figure S17 Novel transcripts located on Chromosome 18. The detailed annotation of a cluster of novel transcripts located on chromosome 18 using public genomic data. A) Four novel transcripts identified by the Tophat-Cufflinks pipeline in monocytes about 20 kb upstream of coding gene *SERPINB2* are shown. All four transcripts were transcribed at the opposite direction as *SERPINB2*, and three of them were significantly upregulated in SLE by 303% to 671% ($p = 1.3E-6$ to $1.5E-8$). All four transcripts were validated by qPCR. B) These transcripts are not included in commonly used gene annotation databases. Two predicted genes partially overlap with these transcripts, but both are transcribed in the opposite direction. C) Sequences within this region are evolutionarily conserved. D) A very low level of transcription was detected within this region according to an ENCODE RNA-seq data set that measured transcriptomes in nine cell lines, not including monocytes. E) This region has a DNase I hypersensitive site in CD14+ monocytes according to another ENCODE data set. F) Furthermore, an ENCODE data set measuring various histone marks in CD14+ monocytes showed that this region has a nucleosome pattern indicative of active transcription.

Figure S18 Novel transcripts located on Chromosome 8. A cluster of 26 novel transcripts located on chromosome 8 within a

~34 kb region upstream of coding gene *ADAM28*. A) All of the loci are transcribed in the opposite direction of *ADAM28*. B) None of them are included in a common gene annotation databases. Fifteen of these transcripts were significantly upregulated in SLE ($p<0.01$) by 80% to 3435% and none of them were downregulated in SLE. C) Most of the transcripts are located within evolutionarily conserved regions. D) ENCODE data detected very low levels of transcripts within this region in 9 cell lines. E) According to ENCODE data sets generated from monocytes, there is a DNase I hypersensitivity site within this region. F) The same sites showed a histone modification pattern of active nucleosomes.

Figure S19 Differential expression of novel loci. Twelve novel loci were amplified using 11 controls (including three internal validation controls used for the RNA-seq libraries and eight new controls) and 11 new SLE samples using qRT-PCR. All genes were normalized to β-actin. P values according to Mann-Whitney in each case are given in parentheses. Only two failed to demonstrate increased expression in this new SLE cohort. Locations are given in Table S3. The cross bars indicate mean and standard error.

Figure S20 Concordance of LPS, interferon and SLE gene expression. Five LPS data sets were created from four GEO monocyte data series (additional information on methods available in Methods S1). The α-interferon data set is from our previously published work. The coding genes shown to be upregulated in SLE were analyzed for upregulation after LPS stimulation and α-interferon (aIFN) treatment. A) All three LPS data sets demonstrated that LPS treatment also increased expression of the genes shown to be upregulated in SLE. N = the number of unique genes included in the analysis. B) The degree of overlap between SLE-induced genes and aIFN-induced genes was comparable to the degree of overlap between SLE-induced genes and LPS-induced genes.

Figure S21 The effect of different MAP kinase inhibitors on LPS-induced novel loci expression. MonoMac6 cells (above) and primary monocytes (below) were treated with p38 (SB203580), ERK (U0126) and JNK (SP600125) inhibitors for 30 minutes and then stimulated with LPS. The y-axis represents the ratio of the LPS+ inhibitor-treated cells over the LPS alone treated cells, with the horizontal line indicating equivalence. The p38 inhibitor led to most diminished expression of the novel loci. At the right of the graph, loci 477 and 896 were included as controls, which were novel loci that were not altered in SLE. N = 3.

Figure S22 The average of the novel loci expression. The expression levels of the novel loci, demonstrated in Figure S21, were averaged to better highlight the effect of the inhibitors. p38 (SB203580), ERK (U0126) and JNK (SP600125) inhibitors were used to define the role of this pathway on the novel loci expression. A) MonoMac6 cell results from Figure S21 were averaged to demonstrate the overall effect of the MAP kinase inhibitors. B) Similarly, in primary monocytes, the results from Figure S21 were averaged. TNF was used as a positive control for the LPS stimulation in C) MonoMac6 cells and D) primary monocytes.

Table S1 Clinical characteristics of SLE patients.

Table S2 RNA Samples for Libraries.

Table S3 Locations of novel loci.

Table S4 Number of differentially expressed genes/ transcripts in each class.

Table S5 Functional categorization of differentially expressed gene by DAVID.

Table S6 Cross-referencing of genes identified in genetic association studies and significantly upregulated in this study.

Data S1 Processed Data.

Methods S1 Supplemental Methods List.

References S1 Supplemental References List: Tables.

Acknowledgments

The authors would like to acknowledge Stephen Mahoney and Kristen Hunter for SOLiD sample preparation, Juan Perin for alignments and the Red Cross of Philadelphia for the serum samples. The authors gratefully acknowledge advice, guidance and support of Eric Rappaport in the Nucleic Acid Core faciltiy.

Author Contributions

Conceived and designed the experiments: KS. Performed the experiments: L. Shi KM L. Song. Analyzed the data: ZZ AY EA WW ZW PCR. Contributed reagents/materials/analysis tools: MP. Wrote the paper: KS.

References

1. Bennett L, Palucka AK, Arce E, Cantrell V, Borvak J, et al. (2003) Interferon and granulopoiesis signatures in systemic lupus erythematosus blood. Journal of Experimental Medicine 197: 711–723.
2. Kirou KA, Lee C, George S, Louca K, Papagiannis IG, et al. (2004) Coordinate overexpression of interferon-alpha-induced genes in systemic lupus erythematosus. Arthritis Rheum 50: 3958–3967.
3. Casciola-Rosen LA, Anhalt G, Rosen A (1994) Autoantigens targeted in systemic lupus erythematosus are clustered in two populations of surface structures on apoptotic keratinocytes. The Journal of Experimental Medicine 179: 1317–1330.
4. Beck-Engeser GB, Eilat D, Harrer T, Jack HM, Wabl M (2009) Early onset of autoimmune disease by the retroviral integrase inhibitor raltegravir. Proc Natl Acad Sci U S A 106: 20865–20870.
5. Stetson DB, Ko JS, Heidmann T, Medzhitov R (2008) Trex1 prevents cell-intrinsic initiation of autoimmunity. Cell 134: 587–598.
6. Morita M, Stamp G, Robins P, Dulic A, Rosewell I, et al. (2004) Gene-targeted mice lacking the Trex1 (DNase III) 3′→5′ DNA exonuclease develop inflammatory myocarditis. Molecular and Cellular Biology 24: 6719–6727.
7. Gall A, Treuting P, Elkon KB, Loo YM, Gale M Jr, et al. (2012) Autoimmunity initiates in nonhematopoietic cells and progresses via lymphocytes in an interferon-dependent autoimmune disease. Immunity 36: 120–131.
8. Alexander JJ, Saxena AK, Bao L, Jacob A, Haas M, et al. (2002) Prominent renal expression of a murine leukemia retrovirus in experimental systemic lupus erythematosus. Journal of the American Society of Nephrology : JASN 13: 2869–2877.

9. Krieg AM, Steinberg AD (1990) Analysis of thymic endogenous retroviral expression in murine lupus. Genetic and immune studies. The Journal of Clinical Investigation 86: 809–816.
10. Hill GS, Delahousse M, Nochy D, Remy P, Mignon F, et al. (2001) Predictive power of the second renal biopsy in lupus nephritis: significance of macrophages. Kidney Int 59: 304–316.
11. Schiffer L, Bethunaickan R, Ramanujam M, Huang W, Schiffer M, et al. (2008) Activated renal macrophages are markers of disease onset and disease remission in lupus nephritis. J Immunol 180: 1938–1947.
12. Yoshimoto S, Nakatani K, Iwano M, Asai O, Samejima K, et al. (2007) Elevated levels of fractalkine expression and accumulation of CD16+ monocytes in glomeruli of active lupus nephritis. Am J Kidney Dis 50: 47–58.
13. Rho YH, Solus J, Raggi P, Oeser A, Gebretsadik T, et al. (2011) Macrophage activation and coronary atherosclerosis in systemic lupus erythematosus and rheumatoid arthritis. Arthritis care & research 63: 535–541.
14. Rahimi H, Maurer K, Song L, Akhter E, Petri M, et al. (2013) Aberrant regulation of the integrin very late antigen-4 in systemic lupus erythematosus. Lupus in press.
15. Smeekens SP, Ng A, Kumar V, Johnson MD, Plantinga TS, et al. (2013) Functional genomics identifies type I interferon pathway as central for host defense against Candida albicans. Nature communications 4: 1342.
16. Fitzgerald KA, Rowe DC, Barnes BJ, Caffrey DR, Visintin A, et al. (2003) LPS-TLR4 signaling to IRF-3/7 and NF-kappaB involves the toll adapters TRAM and TRIF. The Journal of Experimental Medicine 198: 1043–1055.
17. Richez C, Yasuda K, Watkins AA, Akira S, Lafyatis R, et al. (2009) TLR4 ligands induce IFN-alpha production by mouse conventional dendritic cells and human monocytes after IFN-beta priming. Journal of Immunology 182: 820–828.
18. Shui HA, Ka SM, Wu WM, Lin YF, Hou YC, et al. (2007) LPS-evoked IL-18 expression in mesangial cells plays a role in accelerating lupus nephritis. Rheumatology 46: 1277–1284.
19. Zhai JX, Zhang ZX, Feng YJ, Ding SS, Wang XH, et al. (2012) PDTC attenuate LPS-induced kidney injury in systemic lupus erythematosus-prone MRL/lpr mice. Molecular biology reports 39: 6763–6771.
20. Izui S, Lambert PH, Fournie GJ, Turler H, Miescher PA (1977) Features of systemic lupus erythematosus in mice injected with bacterial lipopolysaccharides: identificantion of circulating DNA and renal localization of DNA-anti-DNA complexes. The Journal of Experimental Medicine 145: 1115–1130.
21. Granholm NA, Cavallo T (1991) Bacterial lipopolysaccharide enhances deposition of immune complexes and exacerbates nephritis in BXSB lupus-prone mice. Clinical and Experimental Immunology 85: 270–277.
22. Garrett S, Dietzmann-Maurer K, Song L, Sullivan KE (2008) Polarization of primary human monocytes by IFN-gamma induces chromatin changes and recruits RNA Pol II to the TNF-alpha promoter. J Immunol 180: 5257–5266.
23. Zhang Z, Maurer K, Perin JC, Song L, Sullivan KE (2010) Cytokine-induced monocyte characteristics in SLE. Journal of biomedicine & biotechnology 2010: 507475.
24. Zhang Z, Song L, Maurer K, Bagashev A, Sullivan KE (2011) Monocyte polarization: the relationship of genome-wide changes in H4 acetylation with polarization. Genes Immun 12: 445–456.
25. Zhang Z, Song L, Maurer K, Petri MA, Sullivan KE (2010) Global H4 acetylation analysis by ChIP-chip in systemic lupus erythematosus monocytes. Genes Immun 11: 124–133.
26. Chauhan SK, Singh VV, Rai R, Rai M, Rai G (2013) Distinct autoantibody profiles in systemic lupus erythematosus patients are selectively associated with TLR7 and TLR9 upregulation. Journal of Clinical Immunology 33: 954–964.
27. Csiszar A, Nagy G, Gergely P, Pozsonyi T, Pocsik E (2000) Increased interferon-gamma (IFN-gamma), IL-10 and decreased IL-4 mRNA expression in peripheral blood mononuclear cells (PBMC) from patients with systemic lupus erythematosus (SLE). Clinical and Experimental Immunology 122: 464–470.
28. Eggleton P, Harries LW, Alberigo G, Wordsworth P, Viner N, et al. (2010) Changes in apoptotic gene expression in lymphocytes from rheumatoid arthritis and systemic lupus erythematosus patients compared with healthy lymphocytes. Journal of Clinical Immunology 30: 649–658.
29. Trapnell C, Roberts A, Goff L, Pertea G, Kim D, et al. (2012) Differential gene and transcript expression analysis of RNA-seq experiments with TopHat and Cufflinks. Nature protocols 7: 562–578.
30. Dennis G Jr, Sherman BT, Hosack DA, Yang J, Gao W, et al. (2003) DAVID: Database for Annotation, Visualization, and Integrated Discovery. Genome Biol 4: P3.
31. Zhang H, Hu J, Recce M, Tian B (2005) PolyA_DB: a database for mammalian mRNA polyadenylation. Nucleic Acids Research 33: D116–120.
32. Djebali S, Davis CA, Merkel A, Dobin A, Lassmann T, et al. (2012) Landscape of transcription in human cells. Nature 489: 101–108.
33. Robinson MD, McCarthy DJ, Smyth GK (2010) edgeR: a Bioconductor package for differential expression analysis of digital gene expression data. Bioinformatics 26: 139–140.
34. Kondrashov A, Meijer HA, Barthet-Barateig A, Parker HN, Khurshid A, et al. (2012) Inhibition of polyadenylation reduces inflammatory gene induction. Rna 18: 2236–2250.
35. Chipumuro E, Henriksen MA (2012) The ubiquitin hydrolase USP22 contributes to 3′-end processing of JAK-STAT-inducible genes. FASEB journal : official publication of the Federation of American Societies for Experimental Biology 26: 842–854.
36. Nagaike T, Logan C, Hotta I, Rozenblatt-Rosen O, Meyerson M, et al. (2011) Transcriptional activators enhance polyadenylation of mRNA precursors. Molecular Cell 41: 409–418.
37. Flavell SW, Kim TK, Gray JM, Harmin DA, Hemberg M, et al. (2008) Genome-wide analysis of MEF2 transcriptional program reveals synaptic target genes and neuronal activity-dependent polyadenylation site selection. Neuron 60: 1022–1038.
38. Mayr C, Bartel DP (2009) Widespread shortening of 3′UTRs by alternative cleavage and polyadenylation activates oncogenes in cancer cells. Cell 138: 673–684.
39. Lianoglou S, Garg V, Yang JL, Leslie CS, Mayr C (2013) Ubiquitously transcribed genes use alternative polyadenylation to achieve tissue-specific expression. Genes & Development 27: 2380–2396.
40. Tranter M, Helsley RN, Paulding WR, McGuinness M, Brokamp C, et al. (2011) Coordinated post-transcriptional regulation of Hsp70.3 gene expression by microRNA and alternative polyadenylation. The Journal of Biological Chemistry 286: 29828–29837.
41. Xu Z, Wei W, Gagneur J, Clauder-Munster S, Smolik M, et al. (2011) Antisense expression increases gene expression variability and locus interdependency. Molecular systems biology 7: 468.
42. Iliopoulos D, Rotem A, Struhl K (2011) Inhibition of miR-193a expression by Max and RXRalpha activates K-Ras and PLAU to mediate distinct aspects of cellular transformation. Cancer Research 71: 5144–5153.
43. Incoronato M, Garofalo M, Urso L, Romano G, Quintavalle C, et al. (2010) miR-212 increases tumor necrosis factor-related apoptosis-inducing ligand sensitivity in non-small cell lung cancer by targeting the antiapoptotic protein PED. Cancer Research 70: 3638–3646.
44. Mevorach D, Mascarenhas JO, Gershov D, Elkon KB (1998) Complement-dependent clearance of apoptotic cells by human macrophages. Journal of Experimental Medicine 188: 2313–2320.
45. Shoshan Y, Shapira I, Toubi E, Frolkis I, Yaron M, et al. (2001) Accelerated Fas-mediated apoptosis of monocytes and maturing macrophages from patients with systemic lupus erythematosus: relevance to in vitro impairment of interaction with iC3b-opsonized apoptotic cells. Journal of Immunology 167: 5963–5969.
46. Gibbert K, Joedicke JJ, Meryk A, Trilling M, Francois S, et al. (2012) Interferon-alpha Subtype 11 Activates NK Cells and Enables Control of Retroviral Infection. PLoS Pathog 8: e1002868.
47. Petersen T, Moller-Larsen A, Thiel S, Brudek T, Hansen TK, et al. (2009) Effects of interferon-beta therapy on innate and adaptive immune responses to the human endogenous retroviruses HERV-H and HERV-W, cytokine production, and the lectin complement activation pathway in multiple sclerosis. J Neuroimmunol 215: 108–116.
48. Weckerle CE, Mangale D, Franek BS, Kelly JA, Kumabe M, et al. (2012) Large-scale analysis of tumor necrosis factor alpha levels in systemic lupus erythematosus. Arthritis and Rheumatism 64: 2947–2952.
49. Zhang Z, Maurer K, Perin JC, Song L, Sullivan KE (2010) Cytokine-induced monocyte characteristics in SLE. J Biomed Biotechnol 2010: 507475.
50. Zhang Z, Song L, Maurer K, Bagashev A, Sullivan KE (2011) Monocyte polarization: the relationship of genome-wide changes in H4 acetylation with polarization. Genes Immun.
51. Goutieres F, Aicardi J, Barth PG, Lebon P (1998) Aicardi-Goutieres syndrome: an update and results of interferon-alpha studies. Annals of neurology 44: 900–907.
52. Kuijpers TW (2002) Aicardi-Goutieres syndrome: immunophenotyping in relation to interferon-alpha. European journal of paediatric neurology : EJPN : official journal of the European Paediatric Neurology Society 6 Suppl A: A59–64; discussion A65-56, A77-86.
53. Lebon P, Meritet JF, Krivine A, Rozenberg F (2002) Interferon and Aicardi-Goutieres syndrome. European journal of paediatric neurology : EJPN : official journal of the European Paediatric Neurology Society 6 Suppl A: A47–53; discussion A55-48, A77-86.
54. Ghazizadeh S, Carroll JM, Taichman LB (1997) Repression of retrovirus-mediated transgene expression by interferons: implications for gene therapy. Journal of Virology 71: 9163–9169.
55. Papewalis C, Jacobs B, Wuttke M, Ullrich E, Baehring T, et al. (2008) IFN-alpha skews monocytes into CD56+-expressing dendritic cells with potent functional activities in vitro and in vivo. J Immunol 180: 1462–1470.
56. Steinbach F, Henke F, Krause B, Thiele B, Burmester GR, et al. (2000) Monocytes from systemic lupus erythematous patients are severely altered in phenotype and lineage flexibility. Annals of the Rheumatic Diseases 59: 283–288.
57. Phillips R, Lomnitzer R, Wadee AA, Rabson AR (1985) Defective monocyte function in patients with systemic lupus erythematosus. Clinical Immunology and Immunopathology 34: 69–76.
58. Blanco P, Palucka AK, Gill M, Pascual V, Banchereau J (2001) Induction of dendritic cell differentiation by IFN-alpha in systemic lupus erythematosus. Science 294: 1540–1543.
59. Banchereau J, Pascual V (2006) Type I interferon in systemic lupus erythematosus and other autoimmune diseases. Immunity 25: 383–392.
60. Koscec M, Koren E, Wolfson-Reichlin M, Fugate RD, Trieu E, et al. (1997) Autoantibodies to ribosomal P proteins penetrate into live hepatocytes and cause cellular dysfunction in culture. Journal of Immunology 159: 2033–2041.

61. Moulton VR, Tsokos GC (2010) Alternative splicing factor/splicing factor 2 regulates the expression of the zeta subunit of the human T cell receptor-associated CD3 complex. The Journal of Biological Chemistry 285: 12490–12496.
62. Moulton VR, Grammatikos AP, Fitzgerald LM, Tsokos GC (2013) Splicing factor SF2/ASF rescues IL-2 production in T cells from systemic lupus erythematosus patients by activating IL-2 transcription. Proceedings of the National Academy of Sciences of the United States of America 110: 1845–1850.
63. Molad Y, Amit-Vasina M, Bloch O, Yona E, Rapoport MJ (2010) Increased ERK and JNK activities correlate with disease activity in patients with systemic lupus erythematosus. Annals of the Rheumatic Diseases 69: 175–180.
64. Rapoport MJ, Amit M, Aharoni D, Weiss M, Weissgarten J, et al. (2002) Constitutive up-regulated activity of MAP kinase is associated with down-regulated early p21Ras pathway in lymphocytes of SLE patients. Journal of Autoimmunity 19: 63–70.
65. Gorjestani S, Rider V, Kimler BF, Greenwell C, Abdou NI (2008) Extracellular signal-regulated kinase 1/2 signalling in SLE T cells is influenced by oestrogen and disease activity. Lupus 17: 548–554.
66. Zheng L, Sinniah R, Hsu SI (2008) Pathogenic role of NF-kappaB activation in tubulointerstitial inflammatory lesions in human lupus nephritis. The journal of histochemistry and cytochemistry : official journal of the Histochemistry Society 56: 517–529.
67. Takase O, Hirahashi J, Takayanagi A, Chikaraishi A, Marumo T, et al. (2003) Gene transfer of truncated IkappaBalpha prevents tubulointerstitial injury. Kidney International 63: 501–513.
68. Enzler T, Bonizzi G, Silverman GJ, Otero DC, Widhopf GF, et al. (2006) Alternative and classical NF-kappa B signaling retain autoreactive B cells in the splenic marginal zone and result in lupus-like disease. Immunity 25: 403–415.
69. Feroze U, Kalantar-Zadeh K, Sterling KA, Molnar MZ, Noori N, et al. (2012) Examining associations of circulating endotoxin with nutritional status, inflammation, and mortality in hemodialysis patients. Journal of renal nutrition : the official journal of the Council on Renal Nutrition of the National Kidney Foundation 22: 317–326.
70. del Campo R, Martinez E, del Fresno C, Alenda R, Gomez-Pina V, et al. (2011) Translocated LPS might cause endotoxin tolerance in circulating monocytes of cystic fibrosis patients. PLoS ONE 6: e29577.
71. Miller MA, McTernan PG, Harte AL, Silva NF, Strazzullo P, et al. (2009) Ethnic and sex differences in circulating endotoxin levels: A novel marker of atherosclerotic and cardiovascular risk in a British multi-ethnic population. Atherosclerosis 203: 494–502.
72. Zhang R, Miller RG, Gascon R, Champion S, Katz J, et al. (2009) Circulating endotoxin and systemic immune activation in sporadic amyotrophic lateral sclerosis (sALS). J Neuroimmunol 206: 121–124.
73. Miller JC, Meier E, Weatherly JN (2009) Assessing the reliability of the Gambling Functional Assessment. Journal of gambling studies/co-sponsored by the National Council on Problem Gambling and Institute for the Study of Gambling and Commercial Gaming 25: 121–129.
74. Sharma R, Bolger AP, Li W, Davlouros PA, Volk HD, et al. (2003) Elevated circulating levels of inflammatory cytokines and bacterial endotoxin in adults with congenital heart disease. Am J Cardiol 92: 188–193.
75. De Beaux AC, Fearon KC (1996) Circulating endotoxin, tumour necrosis factor-alpha, and their natural antagonists in the pathophysiology of acute pancreatitis. Scandinavian journal of gastroenterology Supplement 219: 43–46.
76. Casey WF, Hauser GJ, Hannallah RS, Midgley FM, Khan WN (1992) Circulating endotoxin and tumor necrosis factor during pediatric cardiac surgery. Critical care medicine 20: 1090–1096.
77. Lester RT, Yao XD, Ball TB, McKinnon LR, Omange WR, et al. (2009) HIV-1 RNA dysregulates the natural TLR response to subclinical endotoxemia in Kenyan female sex-workers. PLoS ONE 4: e5644.
78. Nowroozalizadeh S, Mansson F, da Silva Z, Repits J, Dabo B, et al. (2010) Microbial translocation correlates with the severity of both HIV-1 and HIV-2 infections. J Infect Dis 201: 1150–1154.

3

Incidence and Prevalence of Major Central Nervous System Involvement in Systemic Lupus Erythematosus: A 3-Year Prospective Study of 370 Patients

Eleni I. Kampylafka[1], Haralampos Alexopoulos[1], Michalis L. Kosmidis[1], Demosthenes B. Panagiotakos[2], Panayiotis G. Vlachoyiannopoulos[1], Marinos C. Dalakas[1], Haralampos M. Moutsopoulos[1], Athanasios G. Tzioufas[1]*

1 Department of Pathophysiology, School of Medicine, National and Kapodistrian University of Athens, Athens, Greece, **2** Department of Nutrition and Dietetics, Harokopio University, Athens, Greece

Abstract

Background: The incidence and prevalence of CNS involvement in SLE remains unclear owing to conflicting results in the published studies. The aim of the study was to evaluate the incidence and prevalence of major definite CNS events in SLE patients.

Methods: 370 SLE patients with no previous history of CNS involvement were prospectively evaluated in a tertiary hospital referral center for 3 years. Major CNS manifestations were codified according to ACR definitions, including chorea, aseptic meningitis, psychosis, seizures, myelopathy, demyelinating syndrome, acute confusional state and strokes. Minor CNS events were excluded. ECLAM and SLEDAI-SELENA Modification scores were used to evaluate disease activity and SLICC/ACR Damage Index was used to assess accumulated damage.

Results: 16/370 (4.3%) patients presented with a total of 23 major CNS events. These included seizures (35%), strokes (26%), myelopathy (22%), optic neuritis (8.7%), aseptic meningitis (4.3%) and acute psychosis (4.3%). Incidence was 7.8/100 person years. Among hospitalizations for SLE, 13% were due to CNS manifestations. Epileptic seizures were associated with high disease activity, while myelopathy correlated with lower disease activity and NMO-IgG antibodies *($P \leq 0.05$)*. Stroke incidence correlated with APS coexistence *($P = 0.06$)*. Overall, CNS involvement correlated with high ECLAM and SLEDAI scores *($P < 0.001$)*.

Conclusions: Clinically severe CNS involvement is rare in SLE patients, accounting for 7.8/100 person years. CNS involvement correlates with high disease activity and coexistence of specific features that define the respective CNS syndromes.

Editor: Fernando de Castro, Hospital Nacional de Parapléjicos - SESCAM, Spain

Funding: The present study has been co-financed by the European Social Fund (ESF) and Greek National funds through the Operational Program "Education and Lifelong Learning" of the National Strategic Reference Framework (NSRF) Research Funding Program: Heracleitus II. http://www.elke.uoa.gr. The funders had no role in study design, data collection and analysis, decision to publish, or preparation of the manuscript.

Competing Interests: The authors have declared that no competing interests exist.

* E-mail: agtzi@med.uoa.gr

Introduction

Systemic Lupus Erythematosus (SLE) is an autoimmune systemic disease which has a prevalence of 52.2/100.000 in the United States [1]. Neurological involvement in the morbidity and mortality of SLE is considered significant [2–4] and many studies have tried to determine the incidence and prevalence of neurologic manifestations. Major obstacles have been the often non-specific nature of these manifestations and the scarcity of specific laboratory tests. In addition, the need to differentiate Central Nervous System (CNS) involvement attributed to SLE from existing co-morbidities, drug adverse reactions or infections [5,6] had generated further diagnostic dilemmas [7]. In 1999, the American College of Rheumatology (ACR) formulated a nomenclature system which provided case definitions for 19 neuropsychiatric SLE syndromes[8].

Despite these advances, the reported frequency of neurologic involvement in SLE continues to vary greatly, ranging from 12% to 95% [9–12]. This discrepancy can be attributed to factors such as study design, diagnostic approach and patients' baseline characteristics [10,12]. Still, the main reason has been the inclusion of non-specific, minor symptoms including headaches, mild cognitive dysfunction and depression, which may occur in several chronic autoimmune diseases, treated with steroids and immunosuppressants [3,13,14].

The aim of the present study was to evaluate the prevalence, annual incidence and the clinical factors associated with definite organic CNS manifestations, in a cohort of SLE patients.

Materials and Methods

Study's Sample

The study was conducted between July 1st 2008 and July 31st 2011 in the Department of Pathophysiology, University of Athens. 370 SLE patients (32±14 years, 88% females) with no history of CNS involvement attributed to SLE were consecutively included. All patients fulfilled the 1997 ACR classification criteria for SLE [15] and diagnosis was upon recognition of ≥4 ACR criteria.

Patients were informed about the scope and procedures of the study and provided written informed consent. The study was approved by the Scientific Council of "Laikon" University Hospital and by the Ethical Committee of the Medical School.

Definition of the Organic CNS Involvement

Among the 19 ACR case definitions [8], we selected 8 objective major CNS manifestations. These were chorea, aseptic meningitis, psychosis, seizures, myelopathy, demyelinating syndrome, acute confusional state and strokes. Diagnosis was based on neurological examination, laboratory and imaging studies, and the exclusions and associations proposed in the ACR glossary [8]. CNS manifestations occurring in patients with recent cancer diagnosis (<5 years), non-controlled hypo- or hyperthyroidism, active CNS or systemic infection, HBV or HCV infection, and in patients who had received medications with potential neurological adverse reactions prior to the onset of the CNS manifestations, were excluded.

All cases of Peripheral Nervous System (PNS) involvement were excluded. Anxiety, headaches, subclinical cognitive dysfunction and mild depression were also excluded, as they lack SLE specificity [3,13,16]. Subclinical cognitive dysfunction is not an uncommon finding among SLE patients with or without overt CNS manifestations [17,18] and also appears in the Antiphospholipid Syndrome (APS) [19]. Searching for non self-reported cognitive deficits was beyond the scope of our study. Therefore, no detailed neuropsychological battery was applied. The Mini Mental Scale Examination (MMSE) [20,21] was performed in all patients with self-reported cognitive deficits during neurological examination, and overt cognitive dysfunction was defined as a MMSE score of <25.

Clinical and Laboratory Assessment

All major CNS manifestations attributed to SLE that occurred during the study period were recorded. Upon first visit, patients gave a medical history and underwent clinical and neurological examination, including routine laboratory and immunological testing. Demographic data were recorded. European Consensus Lupus Activity Measurement score (ECLAM) [22] and Systemic Lupus Erythematosus Disease Activity Index (SLEDAI) - SELENA Modification [23], were used to evaluate disease activity. The SLICC/ACR Damage Index (SDI) [24] was used to assess accumulated damage due to the disease. As ECLAM, SLEDAI and SDI scores include neurological variables they were also calculated after removing these variables. The indexes without neurological variables are referred to as modified ECLAM, SLEDAI and SDI (m-ECLAM, m-SLEDAI and m-SDI, respectively). The types of glomerulonephritis were classified according to the 2003 International Society of Nephrology/Renal Pathology Society (ISN/RPS) classification [25]. Secondary APS was diagnosed according to the 2006 update of the 1999 ACR criteria [26]. Patients were evaluated every 4 to 8 months or every time a disease relapse or complication occurred. Hospitalizations, irrespective of the overriding symptom, were recorded. A clinical and neurological examination by the same expert neurologist and CSF examinations/Magnetic Resonance Imaging (MRI)/Electroencephalogram (EEG) were conducted whenever a CNS event occurred. The presence of Antinuclear Antibodies (ANA) and anti-Ribosomal P antibodies [27] was detected by Indirect Immunofluorescence (IIF) on Hep-2 cells, while NMO-IgG/anti-AQP4 antibodies were detected by IIF on mouse brain tissue and a cell based assay [28,29]. ECLAM, SLEDAI and SDI scores were calculated at the occurrence of every new CNS event.

Statistical Analysis

Continuous variables are presented as mean ± SD when normally distributed, or as median and quartiles when skewed. Categorical variables are presented as frequencies. Normality was graphically tested using P-P plots. The chi-square test (categorical variables) and the Mann-Whitney test (quantitative variables) were used to evaluate associations between subgroups of patients with CNS involvement. Incidence was evaluated among newly diagnosed SLE patients using the person years of observation. Binary logistic regression models were applied to evaluate associations of patients' characteristics with CNS involvement. Results are presented as odds ratios and the corresponding 95% confidence intervals. Hosmer-Lemeshow statistics were used to evaluate all models' goodness of fit. The level of statistical significance was $P \leq 0.05$. SPSS statistical software was used for analyses (SPSS Hellas Inc., Athens, Greece).

Results

Prevalence and Incidence

A total of 370 SLE patients with no prior CNS manifestations were enrolled. Patients were predominantly female (88%), with a mean age of 32±14 and mean disease duration of 9±7.8 years. Demographic and clinical characteristics are presented in *Table 1*. After excluding the non-specific minor CNS complaints (n = 76 patients), the prevalence of major CNS events among SLE patients was 4.3%; 16/370 patients presented a total of 23 CNS events. The 23 CNS events were: seizures (n = 8, 35%), strokes (n = 6, 26%), myelopathy (n = 5, 22%), optic neuritis (n = 2, 8.7%), aseptic meningitis (n = 1, 4.3%) and acute psychosis (n = 1, 4.3%). All seizures were generalized tonic–clonic, while 3 patients evolved to *status epilepticus*. All strokes were ischemic. Two patients had 2 or more, small ischemic lesions, 2 patients had a large infarct due to thrombosis of a central artery, while one patient manifested multiple transient ischemic attacks in the course of days. Optic neuritis presented as part of Neuromyelitis Optica. Chorea, acute demyelinating disease and acute confusional state were not observed during the 3-year observation period. Finally, no patients were defined as having overt cognitive deficits (MMSE <25).

Seven out of 16 patients had CNS involvement upon diagnosis (44%), while 4 patients (25%) had a relapse of their initial CNS manifestations within the 3-year period. Two out of 16 patients (13%) had concurrent CNS manifestations; one presented with myelitis and optic neuritis, and the other with aseptic meningitis and psychosis. No death occurred in patients with CNS involvement. The all-cause mortality rate of the entire cohort ($n = 370$) during the follow up period was 0.5%. Demographic and clinical characteristics of SLE patients with CNS involvement are presented in *Table 1*.

Finally, the annual incidence of major CNS events among newly diagnosed SLE patients was 7.8 events/100 person-years (i.e., 8 cases out of 55 SLE patients).

Table 1. Demographic and clinical characteristics of the SLE patients.

Patient Characteristics	All SLE patients (n = 370)	Patients with CNS Involvement (n = 16)
Age at diagnosis *(m ± SD)*	32±14	30±12
Sex		
Male, *n (%)*	43 (12%)	1 (6.3%)
Female, *n (%)*	327 (88%)	15 (94%)
Disease duration in years *(m ± SD)*	9±7.8	5.7±8.2
ECLAM score *(m ± SD)*†	1.6±1.8	4.6±3
ECLAM score at end of follow up *(m ± SD)*	*NA*	0.4±0.7
SLEDAI score *(m ± SD)*†	3.6±5.5	18.1±9.9
SLEDAI score at end of follow up *(m ± SD)*	*NA*	0.9±1.4
SDI score at CNS Onset *(m ± SD)*	*NA*	1.4±0.8
SDI score at end of follow up *(m ± SD)*	*NA*	2.1±1.2
Secondary APS, *n (%)*	47 (13%)	4 (25%)
Individual Disease Manifestations**		
Serositis, *n (%)*	96 (26%)	6 (38%)
Pleurisy, *n (%)*	41 (11%)	5 (31%)
Pericarditis, *n (%)*	40 (11%)	5 (31%)
Arthritis, *n (%)*	174 (47%)	16 (100%)
Glomerulonephritis, *n (%)*	164 (44%)	7 (44%)
Class I, *n (%)*	5 (1.4%)	0 (0%)
Class II, *n (%)*	42 (11%)	2 (13%)
Class III, *n (%)*	63 (17%)	2 (13%)
Class IV, *n (%)*	37 (10%)	1 (6.3%)
Class V, *n (%)*	42 (11%)	3 (19%)
Class VI, *n (%)*	4 (1.1%)	0 (0%)
CNS involvement, *n (%)*	16 (4.3%)	16 (100%)
Hematologic disorder, *n (%)*	368 (66%)	10 (63%)
Serological Manifestations**		
ANA, *n (%)*	361(96%)	15 (94%)
Anti-dsDNA antibodies, *n (%)*	345 (70%)	11 (69%)
acL antibodies, *n (%)*	314 (40%)	8 (50%)
Anti-Rib P antibodies, *n (%)*	*Not determined*	2 (13%)
NMO-IgG antibodies, *n (%)*	*Not determined*	2 (13%)
Neurological Manifestations**		
Epileptic Seizures, *n (%)*	6 (1.6%)	6 (38%)
Strokes, *n (%)*	5 (1.4%)	5 (31%)
Myelopathy, *n (%)*	4 (1.1%)	4 (25%)
Optic Neuritis, *n (%)*	1 (0.3%)	1 (6.3%)
Psychosis, *n (%)*	1 (0.3%)	1 (6.3%)
Aseptic Meningitis, *n (%)*	1 (0.3%)	1 (6.3%)
1st CNS episode at SLE diagnosis, *n (%)*	*NA*	7 (44%)
Patients with relapsing CNS episodes, *n (%)*	*NA*	4 (25%)
Patients with >1 simultaneous CNS events, *n (%)*	*NA*	2 (13%)
Disease Manifestations Concurrent to CNS Onset		
Serositis, *n (%)*	*NA*	3 (19%)
Arthritis, *n (%)*	*NA*	16 (100%)
Glomerulonephritis, *n (%)*	*NA*	5 (31%)
Hematologic disorder, *n (%)*	*NA*	10 (63%)
Medications**		
Corticosteroids, *n (%)*	339 (92%)	16 (100%)

Table 1. Cont.

Patient Characteristics	All SLE patients (n = 370)	Patients with CNS Involvement (n = 16)
Azathioprine, *n (%)*	131 (35%)	4 (25%)
Hydroxychloroquine, *n (%)*	231 (62%)	7 (44%)
Methotrexate, *n (%)*	64 (17%)	2 (13%)
Cyclophosphamide, *n (%)*	123 (33%)	11 (69%)
Mycophenolate Mofetil, *n (%)*	119 (32%)	8 (50%)
Rituximab, *n (%)*	35 (9.5%)	5 (31%)

Hospitalization Rates

Eighty-seven out of the 370 SLE patients were admitted to the hospital 141 times during the 3-year follow-up period. 29 patients were hospitalized more than once. The most common hospitalization cause was a lupus flare (59%), while the second more frequent cause was an infection (20%). No CNS infections occurred. Flares included glomerulonephritis (27%), cytopenias (15%), CNS involvement (13%), musculoskeletal symptoms (8.5%), serositis (5.7%), hepatosplenomegaly and lymph node enlargement (4.3%), pneumonitis (3.5%), pancreatitis, colitis and myocarditis (<1%). Nearly one third (33%) of disease flares presented with more than one overlapping SLE manifestations. Overall, 16 SLE patients were admitted 18 times for neurological manifestations *(Table 2)*.

Clinical Associations

We evaluated clinical and serological associations with specific neurological manifestations for the 16 SLE patients with CNS involvement. Epileptic seizures were associated with high ECLAM disease activity score *(P = 0.02)*, late onset during the disease course *(P = 0.03)*, previous history of serositis *(P<0.01)*, and glomerulonephritis *(P = 0.03)*. Glomerulonephritis also tended to occur concurrently to the CNS events *(P = 0.03)*, though no correlations with any specific types of glomerulonephritis were found *(all P-values >0.10)*. Further, two clinical associations were of interest; epileptic seizures tended to associate with high SLEDAI score *(P = 0.07)* and younger age at disease onset *(P = 0.08)*.

Myelopathy correlated with lower disease activity scores, low complement and NMO-IgG antibodies *(all P-values <0.05)*. Two patients with myelitis (2/4, 50%) were NMO-IgG/anti-AQP4 positive; the first had Neuromyelitis Optica (NMO) [30], while the other had Longitudinal Extensive Transverse Myelitis (LETM), which belongs to the NMO spectrum of disorders [31]. Presence of strokes tended to associate with secondary APS *(P = 0.06)* and was associated with higher SDI scores *(P = 0.03)*. One patient with acute psychosis was positive only for anti-ribosomal P antibodies *(Figure 1)*.

Analysis was repeated after removing neurological variables from ECLAM, SLEDAI and SDI scores. All associations previously observed with ECLAM remained significant *(P<0.05)* after modification (m-ECLAM). The m-SLEDAI score tended to inversely correlate with myelitis *(P = 0.08)* but did not correlate with epileptic seizures *(P = 0.23)*. m-SDI did not correlate with strokes *(P = 0.21)*.

Table 2. Hospitalization causes of SLE patients during the 3 year follow up period.

Cause of Hospitalization	Hospitalizations (n)	Percentage (%)
Relapse**	83	59%
Glomerulonephritis	38	27%
Hematological	21	15%
CNS	18	13%
Musculosceletal	12	8.5%
Serositis	8	5.7%
Hepatosplenomegaly & Lymph Node Enlargement	6	4.3%
Pneumonitis	5	3.5%
Pancreatitis	3	<1%
Colitis	3	<1%
Myocarditis	1	<1%
Infection	28	20%
Other	30	21%
(Chronic Renal Insufficiency, Cancer, Budd-Chiari Syndrome, alveolar hemorrhage, pulmonary hypertension)		*(All less than 1%)*
Total	**141**	**100%**

**Relapse manifestations can coexist during the same hospitalization.

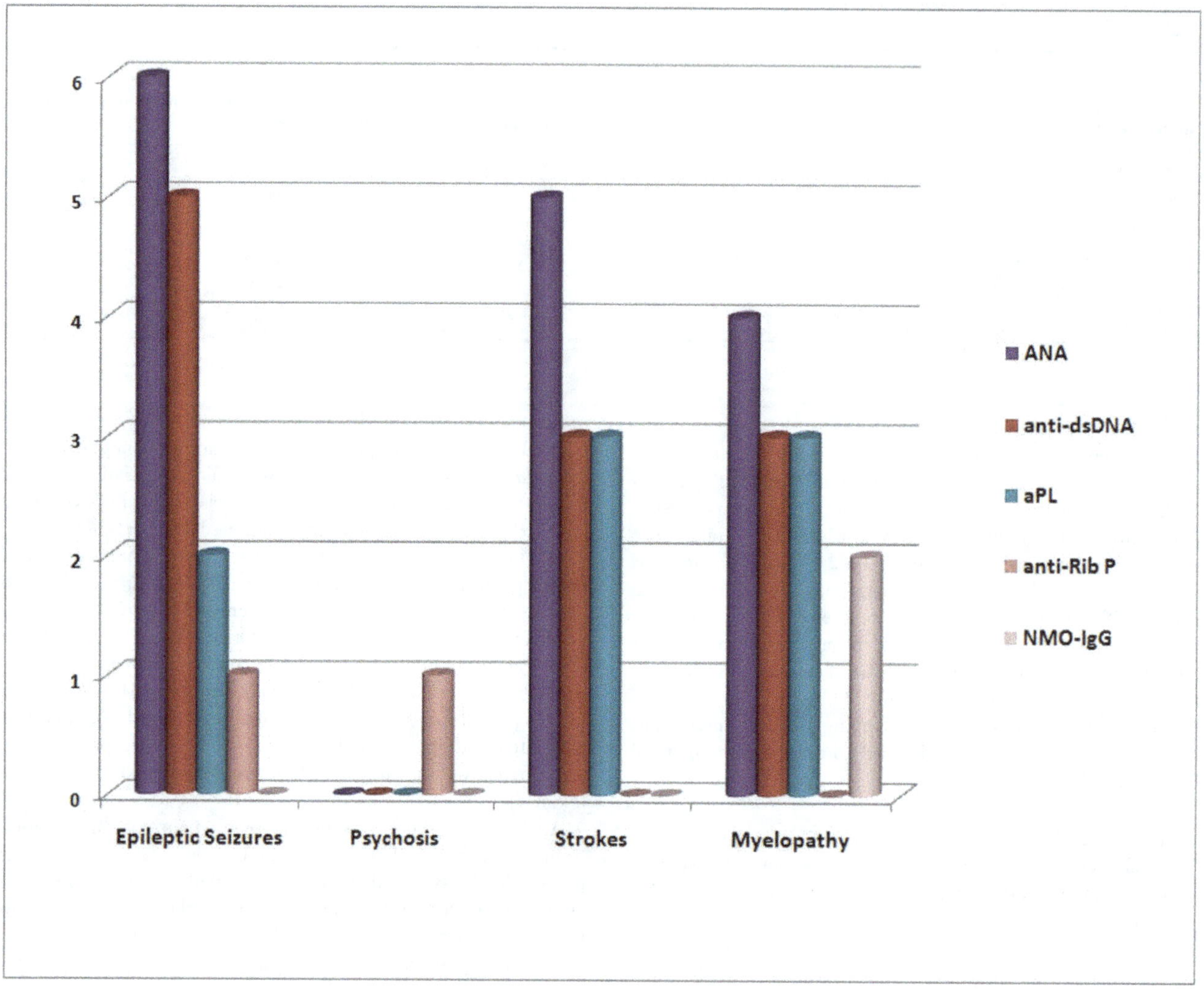

Figure 1. Numbers of patients with the respective antibodies within each CNS subgroup. Each column group refers to the respective CNS subgroup. Each column represents a discrete autoantibody, while Y axes displays the number of patients presenting with the respective autoantibody.

The 16 patients with CNS involvement were compared to the remaining 354 SLE patients without neurologic manifestations. The results from univariate analyses calculating the association of demographic and clinical characteristics with CNS involvement are presented in *Table 3*. Since residual confounding may exist, multiple logistic regression analysis was used to calculate the association of ECLAM and SLEDAI scores, modified ECLAM and SLEDAI scores, aCL antibodies, secondary APS, arthritis, serositis and glomerulonephritis coexistence with CNS involvement, after adjusting for age, sex, and disease duration. ECLAM and SLEDAI scores were mutually replaced in the model due to high inter-correlation. The same mutual replacement was conducted regarding m-ECLAM and m-SLEDAI, as well as APS coexistence and aCL antibodies. Arthritis and glomerulonephritis were excluded from the SLEDAI models, due to high inter-correlation. Both unmodified and modified ECLAM and SLEDAI scores were positively associated with increased likelihood of CNS involvement *(Odds ratio per 1 unit increase in* ECLAM = *2.077, 95%CI 1.55–2.79, Odds ratio per 1 unit increase in* SLEDAI = *1.39, 95%CI 1.24–1.56, Odds ratio per 1 unit increase in m-*ECLAM = *1.56, 95%CI 1.19–2.05, Odds ratio per 1 unit increase in m-*SLEDAI = *1.26, 95%CI 1.16–1.41)*, after adjusting for APS coexistence and the other factors mentioned above. Similar results were revealed when aCL antibodies replaced APS coexistence in the previous models (data not shown). Moreover, in the models that SLEDAI score was included, APS coexistence was associated with higher likelihood of CNS involvement *(Odds ratio per 1 unit increase in* SLEDAI = *0.16, 95%CI 0.03–0.87, Odds ratio per 1 unit increase in m-*SLEDAI = *0.26, 95%CI 0.07–1.04)*, a finding that was not confirmed in models that included the ECLAM score instead of SLEDAI.

Discussion

This work was focused on the distinction of major CNS manifestations in SLE and studied their prevalence and incidence in a cohort of unselected SLE patients. It was shown, that severe CNS involvement is rather uncommon with a prevalence of 4.3% and an incidence rate of 7.8/100 person years. Moreover, ECLAM and SLEDAI scores and APS coexistence were positively associated with increased likelihood of CNS involvement. Despite the limitations of the present work, mainly due to the relatively small sample size, the aforementioned findings deserve further

Table 3. Demographic and clinical characteristics of $n = 370$ SLE patients by CNS involvement group.

Variables	SLE patients with CNS Involvement ($n = 16$)	SLE patients without CNS Involvement ($n = 354$)	P
Age at Disease Onset	30±12	32±14	*0.48*
Sex			*0.70*
Male	1 (6.3%)	42 (12%)	
Female	15 (94%)	312 (88%)	
Disease Duration (yrs)	5.7±8.2	9.2±7.8	*0.009*
aCL antibodies	8 (50%)	140 (40%)	*0.60*
Secondary APS‡	4 (25%)	43 (12%)	*0.13*
ECLAM score	4.6±3	1.4±1.5	*<0.01*
m-ECLAM score†	3.3±2.5	1.4±1.5	*0.01*
SLEDAI score	18±9.9	3.1±4.1	*<0.01*
m-SLEDAI score†	12±8.1	3.1±4.1	*<0.01*
Arthritis	16 (100%)	170 (48%)	*0.07*
Glomerulonephritis	7 (44%)	157 (44%)	*1.00*
Serositis	6 (38%)	90 (25%)	*0.38*

P-values derived through chi-square test for the comparisons of sex, existence of aCL antibodies, secondary APS, arthritis, glomerulonephritis and serositis, and through Mann-Whitney U-test for the comparisons of age at disease onset, disease duration, ECLAM, SLEDAI, m-ECLAM and m- SLEDAI scores. †m-ECLAM and m-SLEDAI are the modified scores after exclusion of the neurological variables ‡APS, Antiphospholipid Syndrome.

attention since they highlight the importance and rarity of major CNS events that can occur in the context of SLE.

CNS involvement can influence both damage accrual and mortality in SLE [32,33]. This is mostly attributed to the major CNS manifestations of the disease, including seizures, myelopathy and strokes [2,32,34]. Furthermore, neurological involvement appears to be an independent risk factor for hospitalizations in SLE [35]. Our study reinforces these conclusions, as 13% (18/141) of SLE hospitalizations in our cohort were due to major CNS manifestations. An additional clinical observation is that 2 out of these 141 hospitalizations were in the Intensive Care Unit (ICU). Both were due to CNS involvement. The aforementioned findings underline the necessity for rapid diagnosis and treatment in patients presenting with major CNS manifestations.

The true incidence and prevalence of severe CNS involvement in SLE is often overshadowed by the inclusion of minor non-specific symptoms with no direct pathogenetic correlation with SLE, such as mild cognitive dysfunction, headache, mild depression, anxiety and paresthesias with negative electroneuromyography [9,13]. In the present prospective study, PNS symptoms and all the aforementioned minor events [9], were excluded and stringent criteria to include only CNS manifestations directly attributed to SLE were applied. Moreover, in a 2004 meta-analysis it was shown that prevalence of all types of headaches in SLE patents was not different from that of healthy controls [36], while another study has shown that SLE patients without neurological manifestations exhibit a decline in attention, memory, and reasoning [17].

Eight major CNS syndromes namely epileptic seizures, strokes, myelopathy, psychosis, aseptic meningitis, acute confusional state, chorea and demyelinating syndrome, were included. Although optic neuritis is categorized by the ACR [8] within the PNS syndromes, in our study it was included as a CNS event since it occurred in the context of Neuromyelitis Optica.

The estimated prevalence of definite CNS involvement in SLE in our cohort was 4.3%, much lower compared to previous prospective studies in which minor events and PNS symptoms were included, where the prevalence ranged from 13% to 46% [4,9,16].

Unlike prevalence, incidence has not been previously calculated, although a recent review proposed a cumulative incidence of approximately 30–40% [10]. In our study, incidence was calculated among newly diagnosed SLE patients (n = 55) during the 3-year follow-up period, and was 7.8/100 person years. In published series, most neurologic events tend to accumulate early during the disease[4,7,10]. CNS involvement was also an early event in our cohort, as 44% of our patients manifested their CNS events simultaneously with disease onset.

Roughly 13% of hospitalizations during the 3-year period were due to SLE-related CNS manifestations, making them the third more common lupus associated cause for patient admission. Evidently, even though rare, severe CNS manifestations account for a notable percentage of hospital admissions in SLE patients.

A statistically significant correlation was found between high disease activity and CNS manifestations *($P<0.001$)*, in line with other studies [10,37,38]. This conclusion was reinforced after evaluating our SLE patients using two different disease activity scores (ECLAM and SLEDAI) and repeating the analysis with the exclusion of neurological factors from the scores. Moreover, a statistically significant correlation was observed between secondary APS and CNS involvement *($P = 0.03$)*. Other studies have also proposed a correlation between neurological manifestations in SLE and secondary APS [37,39,40].

In our cohort, two discrete clinical phenotypes were identified. The first was the diffuse phenotype that included epileptic seizures and psychosis. The second was focal and included myelopathy and strokes. The correlation of discrete neurological syndromes with other clinical and serological features of the disease revealed that epileptic seizures appeared in patients with higher disease activity scores ($P = 0.02$ and $P = 0.07$, for ECLAM and SLEDAI scores respectively), when compared to other neurological manifestations. Furthermore, patients with epileptic seizures were younger at disease onset *($P = 0.08$)*, in agreement with previous studies [41], and expressed the seizures later during the disease *($P = 0.03$)*, unlike other studies where seizures appeared near the onset of the disease [42]. Glomerulonephritis was present more often in these patients and occurred concurrently to the onset of epileptic seizures *(P = 0.03)*. This observation is in line with a previous study, where epileptic seizures were a frequent manifestation in patients with lupus nephritis [43].

Three out of 6 patients who manifested epileptic seizures had characteristic features in their MRIs; two had Posterior Reversible Encephalopathy Syndrome (PRES) [44] and 1 had vasculitic-like lesions. All 3 patients had common clinical features; very high disease activity, active glomerulonephritis presenting as nephrotic syndrome, and symptom amelioration following immunosuppression and antiepileptic treatment. According to previous reports, two types of PRES in SLE are thought to exist; "hypertensive PRES," being reversible with antihypertensive and anticonvulsive treatment concomitant with inactive SLE, and PRES requiring immunosuppressive therapy that could be considered a neurological manifestation of active SLE [44]. Finally, as seizures preceded the onset of the nephrotic syndrome, it is unlikely that they were due to nephrotic encephalopathy.

Myelopathy correlated with lower disease activity scores and the presence of NMO-IgG/anti-AQP4 antibodies ($P \leq 0.05$). Patients with both myelopathy and NMO-IgG antibodies (2/4) had NMO spectrum symptoms [31]. The first had Neuromyelitis Optica and the second had LETM. These entities have been previously found in the context of systemic diseases [45]. A recent study [46] described two discrete subtypes of lupus myelitis. The first appeared with gray matter dysfunction, irreversible paraplegia, higher SLE activity and a CSF profile resembling that of bacterial meningitis. The second subtype involved patients with white matter dysfunction and lower SLE activity, who were more likely to meet criteria for NMO. In our study, patients fell into the second myelitis subtype.

Strokes appeared more frequently in patients with secondary APS *(P = 0.06)* and a worse SDI *(P = 0.03)*. m-SDI did not correlate to strokes, leading to the assumption that strokes themselves could aggravate disease damage.

CNS involvement in SLE is due to multiple mechanisms, including microvasculopathy, autoantibody-mediated injury or intrathecal production of cytokines that enhance the blood-brain barrier permeability, thus allowing leukocytes and antibodies to enter the CNS [10]. Autoantibodies with strong clinical correlation to neurological disease in SLE are the aPL (observed in our study in 8/16 patients), the anti-ribosomal P antibodies (2/16 patients), and the NMO-IgG/anti-AQP4 antibodies that appeared in 2 out of 4 patients with myelopathy [10,31,47].

Conclusions

Our study, despite certain limitations (single center, relatively short follow-up), focused on severe CNS involvement, attributed with certainty to SLE. Clinically severe CNS involvement appears to be relatively rare in SLE patients, correlates with disease activity and manifests with specific features, according to the respective CNS syndromes. Our work also highlights the necessity for speedy recognition and intensive treatment of such major events, due to their significant impact on SLE damage accrual and mortality. Multicenter and long-term follow up studies could be helpful to strengthen our conclusions.

Author Contributions

Conceived and designed the experiments: EIK HA AGT. Performed the experiments: EIK HA MLK. Analyzed the data: EIK DBP. Contributed reagents/materials/analysis tools: HA PGV HMM MCD. Wrote the paper: EIK HA DBP PGV MCD HMM AGT.

References

1. D'Cruz DP, Khamashta MA, Hughes GR (2007) Systemic lupus erythematosus. Lancet 369: 587–596.
2. Bernatsky S, Clarke A, Gladman DD, Urowitz M, Fortin PR, et al. (2006) Mortality related to cerebrovascular disease in systemic lupus erythematosus. Lupus 15: 835–839.
3. Hanly JG, Urowitz MB, Sanchez-Guerrero J, Bae SC, Gordon C, et al. (2007) Neuropsychiatric events at the time of diagnosis of systemic lupus erythematosus: an international inception cohort study. Arthritis Rheum 56: 265–273.
4. Hanly JG, Urowitz MB, Su L, Bae SC, Gordon C, et al. (2010) Prospective analysis of neuropsychiatric events in an international disease inception cohort of patients with systemic lupus erythematosus. Ann Rheum Dis 69: 529–535.
5. Bosnic D, Cerovec M, Anic B, Mayer M, Sentic M, et al. (2008) [Cryptococcal meningitis as a diagnostic problem in a patient with SLE-case report]. Lijec Vjesn 130: 136–140.
6. McCaffrey LM, Petelin A, Cunha BA (2011) Systemic lupus erythematosus (SLE) cerebritis versus Listeria monocytogenes meningoencephalitis in a patient with systemic lupus erythematosus on chronic corticosteroid therapy: The diagnostic importance of cerebrospinal fluid (CSF) of lactic acid levels. Heart Lung.
7. Bertsias GK, Ioannidis JP, Aringer M, Bollen E, Bombardieri S, et al. (2010) EULAR recommendations for the management of systemic lupus erythematosus with neuropsychiatric manifestations: report of a task force of the EULAR standing committee for clinical affairs. Ann Rheum Dis 69: 2074–2082.
8. The American College of Rheumatology (1999) The American College of Rheumatology nomenclature and case definitions for neuropsychiatric lupus syndromes, Appendix A. Arthritis Rheum 42: 599–608.
9. Ainiala H, Loukkola J, Peltola J, Korpela M, Hietaharju A (2001) The prevalence of neuropsychiatric syndromes in systemic lupus erythematosus. Neurology 57: 496–500.
10. Bertsias GK, Boumpas DT (2010) Pathogenesis, diagnosis and management of neuropsychiatric SLE manifestations. Nat Rev Rheumatol 6: 358–367.
11. Brey RL, Holliday SL, Saklad AR, Navarrete MG, Hermosillo-Romo D, et al. (2002) Neuropsychiatric syndromes in lupus: prevalence using standardized definitions. Neurology 58: 1214–1220.
12. Unterman A, Nolte JE, Boaz M, Abady M, Shoenfeld Y, et al. (2011) Neuropsychiatric syndromes in systemic lupus erythematosus: a meta-analysis. Semin Arthritis Rheum 41: 1–11.
13. Ainiala H, Hietaharju A, Loukkola J, Peltola J, Korpela M, et al. (2001) Validity of the new American College of Rheumatology criteria for neuropsychiatric lupus syndromes: a population-based evaluation. Arthritis Rheum 45: 419–423.
14. Sfikakis PP, Mitsikostas DD, Manoussakis MN, Foukaneli D, Moutsopoulos HM (1998) Headache in systemic lupus erythematosus: a controlled study. Br J Rheumatol 37: 300–303.
15. Hochberg MC (1997) Updating the American College of Rheumatology revised criteria for the classification of systemic lupus erythematosus. Arthritis Rheum 40: 1725.
16. Hanly JG, McCurdy G, Fougere L, Douglas JA, Thompson K (2004) Neuropsychiatric events in systemic lupus erythematosus: attribution and clinical significance. J Rheumatol 31: 2156–2162.
17. Kozora E, Arciniegas DB, Filley CM, West SG, Brown M, et al. (2008) Cognitive and neurologic status in patients with systemic lupus erythematosus without major neuropsychiatric syndromes. Arthritis Rheum 59: 1639–1646.
18. Petri M, Naqibuddin M, Carson KA, Sampedro M, Wallace DJ, et al. (2008) Cognitive function in a systemic lupus erythematosus inception cohort. J Rheumatol 35: 1776–1781.
19. Tektonidou MG, Varsou N, Kotoulas G, Antoniou A, Moutsopoulos HM (2006) Cognitive deficits in patients with antiphospholipid syndrome: association with clinical, laboratory, and brain magnetic resonance imaging findings. Arch Intern Med 166: 2278–2284.
20. Folstein MF, Folstein SE, McHugh PR (1975) "Mini-mental state". A practical method for grading the cognitive state of patients for the clinician. J Psychiatr Res 12: 189–198.
21. Carlomagno S, Migliaresi S, Ambrosone L, Sannino M, Sanges G, et al. (2000) Cognitive impairment in systemic lupus erythematosus: a follow-up study. J Neurol 247: 273–279.
22. Mosca M, Bencivelli W, Vitali C, Carrai P, Neri R, et al. (2000) The validity of the ECLAM index for the retrospective evaluation of disease activity in systemic lupus erythematosus. Lupus 9: 445–450.
23. Petri M, Kim MY, Kalunian KC, Grossman J, Hahn BH, et al. (2005) Combined oral contraceptives in women with systemic lupus erythematosus. N Engl J Med 353: 2550–2558.
24. Gladman D, Ginzler E, Goldsmith C, Fortin P, Liang M, et al. (1996) The development and initial validation of the Systemic Lupus International

Collaborating Clinics/American College of Rheumatology damage index for systemic lupus erythematosus. Arthritis Rheum 39: 363–369.
25. Weening JJ, D'Agati VD, Schwartz MM, Seshan SV, Alpers CE, et al. (2004) The classification of glomerulonephritis in systemic lupus erythematosus revisited. J Am Soc Nephrol 15: 241–250.
26. Miyakis S, Lockshin MD, Atsumi T, Branch DW, Brey RL, et al. (2006) International consensus statement on an update of the classification criteria for definite antiphospholipid syndrome (APS). J Thromb Haemost 4: 295–306.
27. Miyachi K, Tan EM (1979) Antibodies reacting with ribosomal ribonucleoprotein in connective tissue diseases. Arthritis Rheum 22: 87–93.
28. Lennon VA, Kryzer TJ, Pittock SJ, Verkman AS, Hinson SR (2005) IgG marker of optic-spinal multiple sclerosis binds to the aquaporin-4 water channel. J Exp Med 202: 473–477.
29. Lennon VA, Wingerchuk DM, Kryzer TJ, Pittock SJ, Lucchinetti CF, et al. (2004) A serum autoantibody marker of neuromyelitis optica: distinction from multiple sclerosis. Lancet 364: 2106–2112.
30. Wingerchuk DM, Lennon VA, Pittock SJ, Lucchinetti CF, Weinshenker BG (2006) Revised diagnostic criteria for neuromyelitis optica. Neurology 66: 1485–1489.
31. Wingerchuk DM, Lennon VA, Lucchinetti CF, Pittock SJ, Weinshenker BG (2007) The spectrum of neuromyelitis optica. Lancet Neurol 6: 805–815.
32. Chambers SA, Allen E, Rahman A, Isenberg D (2009) Damage and mortality in a group of British patients with systemic lupus erythematosus followed up for over 10 years. Rheumatology (Oxford) 48: 673–675.
33. Kasitanon N, Louthrenoo W, Sukitawut W, Vichainun R (2002) Causes of death and prognostic factors in Thai patients with systemic lupus erythematosus. Asian Pac J Allergy Immunol 20: 85–91.
34. Andrade RM, Alarcon GS, Gonzalez LA, Fernandez M, Apte M, et al. (2008) Seizures in patients with systemic lupus erythematosus: data from LUMINA, a multiethnic cohort (LUMINA LIV). Ann Rheum Dis 67: 829–834.
35. Petri M, Genovese M (1992) Incidence of and risk factors for hospitalizations in systemic lupus erythematosus: a prospective study of the Hopkins Lupus Cohort. J Rheumatol 19: 1559–1565.
36. Mitsikostas DD, Sfikakis PP, Goadsby PJ (2004) A meta-analysis for headache in systemic lupus erythematosus: the evidence and the myth. Brain 127: 1200–1209.
37. Govoni M, Bombardieri S, Bortoluzzi A, Caniatti L, Casu C, et al. (2011) Factors and comorbidities associated with first neuropsychiatric event in systemic lupus erythematosus: does a risk profile exist? A large multicentre retrospective cross-sectional study on 959 Italian patients. Rheumatology (Oxford).
38. Mikdashi J, Handwerger B (2004) Predictors of neuropsychiatric damage in systemic lupus erythematosus: data from the Maryland lupus cohort. Rheumatology (Oxford) 43: 1555–1560.
39. Karassa FB, Ioannidis JP, Touloumi G, Boki KA, Moutsopoulos HM (2000) Risk factors for central nervous system involvement in systemic lupus erythematosus. QJM 93: 169–174.
40. Padovan M, Castellino G, Bortoluzzi A, Caniatti L, Trotta F, et al. (2010) Factors and comorbidities associated with central nervous system involvement in systemic lupus erythematosus: a retrospective cross-sectional case-control study from a single center. Rheumatol Int.
41. Costallat LT, Coimbra AM (1994) Systemic lupus erythematosus: clinical and laboratory aspects related to age at disease onset. Clin Exp Rheumatol 12: 603–607.
42. Joseph FG, Lammie GA, Scolding NJ (2007) CNS lupus: a study of 41 patients. Neurology 69: 644–654.
43. Valentinov Monov S, Valentinova Monova D (2007) Neuropsychiatric lupus in patients with lupus glomerulonephritis. Med Pregl 60 Suppl 2: 70–73.
44. Fujieda Y, Kataoka H, Odani T, Otomo K, Kato M, et al. (2011) Clinical features of reversible posterior leukoencephalopathy syndrome in patients with systemic lupus erythematosus. Mod Rheumatol 21: 276–281.
45. Pittock SJ, Lennon VA, de Seze J, Vermersch P, Homburger HA, et al. (2008) Neuromyelitis optica and non organ-specific autoimmunity. Arch Neurol 65: 78–83.
46. Birnbaum J, Petri M, Thompson R, Izbudak I, Kerr D (2009) Distinct subtypes of myelitis in systemic lupus erythematosus. Arthritis Rheum 60: 3378–3387.
47. Tzioufas AG, Tzortzakis NG, Panou-Pomonis E, Boki KA, Sakarellos-Daitsiotis M, et al. (2000) The clinical relevance of antibodies to ribosomal-P common epitope in two targeted systemic lupus erythematosus populations: a large cohort of consecutive patients and patients with active central nervous system disease. Ann Rheum Dis 59: 99–104.

4

Common and Distinct Clinical Features in Adult Patients with Anti-Aminoacyl-tRNA Synthetase Antibodies: Heterogeneity within the Syndrome

Yasuhito Hamaguchi[1], Manabu Fujimoto[1]*, Takashi Matsushita[1], Kenzo Kaji[1], Kazuhiro Komura[1], Minoru Hasegawa[1], Masanari Kodera[2], Eiji Muroi[3], Keita Fujikawa[4], Mariko Seishima[5], Hidehiro Yamada[6], Ryo Yamada[7], Shinichi Sato[8], Kazuhiko Takehara[1], Masataka Kuwana[9]

1 Department of Dermatology, Kanazawa University Graduate School of Medical Science, Kanazawa, Japan, **2** Department of Dermatology, Social Insurance Chukyo Hospital, Nagoya, Japan, **3** Department of Dermatology, Nagasaki University Graduate School of Biomedical Sciences, Nagasaki, Japan, **4** Unit of Translational Medicine, Department of Immunology and Rheumatology, Nagasaki University Graduate School of Biomedical Sciences, Nagasaki, Japan, **5** Department of Dermatology, Ogaki Municipal Hospital, Ogaki, Japan, **6** Division of Rheumatology, Department of Internal Medicine, and Allergy, St. Marianna University, Kawasaki, Japan, **7** Center for Genomic Medicine, Graduate School of Medicine, Kyoto University, Kyoto, Japan, **8** Department of Dermatology, Faculty of Medicine, University of Tokyo, Tokyo, Japan, **9** Division of Rheumatology, Department of Internal Medicine, Keio University School of Medicine, Tokyo, Japan

Abstract

Objective: To identify similarities and differences in the clinical features of adult Japanese patients with individual anti-aminoacyl-tRNA synthetase antibodies (anti-ARS Abs).

Methods: This was a retrospective analysis of 166 adult Japanese patients with anti-ARS Abs detected by immunoprecipitation assays. These patients had visited Kanazawa University Hospital or collaborating medical centers from 2003 to 2009.

Results: Anti-ARS Ab specificity included anti-Jo-1 (36%), anti-EJ (23%), anti-PL-7 (18%), anti-PL-12 (11%), anti-KS (8%), and anti-OJ (5%). These anti-ARS Abs were mutually exclusive, except for one serum Ab that had both anti-PL-7 and PL-12 reactivity. Myositis was closely associated with anti-Jo-1, anti-EJ, and anti-PL-7, while interstitial lung disease (ILD) was correlated with all 6 anti-ARS Abs. Dermatomyositis (DM)-specific skin manifestations (heliotrope rash and Gottron's sign) were frequently observed in patients with anti-Jo-1, anti-EJ, anti-PL-7, and anti-PL-12. Therefore, most clinical diagnoses were polymyositis or DM for anti-Jo-1, anti-EJ, and anti-PL-7; clinically amyopathic DM or ILD for anti-PL-12; and ILD for anti-KS and anti-OJ. Patients with anti-Jo-1, anti-EJ, and anti-PL-7 developed myositis later if they had ILD alone at the time of disease onset, and most patients with anti-ARS Abs eventually developed ILD if they did not have ILD at disease onset.

Conclusion: Patients with anti-ARS Abs are relatively homogeneous. However, the distribution and timing of myositis, ILD, and rashes differ among patients with individual anti-ARS Abs. Thus, identification of individual anti-ARS Abs is beneficial to define this rather homogeneous subset and to predict clinical outcomes within the "anti-synthetase syndrome."

Editor: Frederick Miller, National Institutes of Health, United States of America

Funding: This work was supported by a research grant on intractable diseases from the Ministry of Health, Labor and Welfare of Japan (to Manabu Fujimoto). The funders had no role in study design, data collection and analysis, decision to publish, or preparation of the manuscript.

Competing Interests: The authors have declared that no competing interests exist.

* E-mail: fujimoto-m@umin.ac.jp

Introduction

The presence of autoantibodies (Abs) is one of the hallmarks of connective tissue diseases, such as systemic lupus erythematosus (SLE), systemic sclerosis (SSc), and idiopathic inflammatory myopathy. In particular, a variety of serum Abs is found in patients with idiopathic inflammatory myopathies, including polymyositis (PM) and dermatomyositis (DM) [1,2]. It is clinically of considerable importance to identify Abs in patients with PM/DM, because each Ab is closely associated with certain clinical features [3]. For example, anti-Mi-2 is associated with classic DM without interstitial lung disease (ILD) or malignancy and with good response to treatment [4–6]; anti-155/140 is associated with malignancy-associated or juvenile DM [7–10]; and anti-CADM-140/MDA5 is associated with clinically amyopathic DM (CADM) and rapidly progressive-ILD (RP-ILD) that results in poor prognosis [11,12]. Abs reactive with aminoacyl-tRNA synthetases (ARS) are also representative Abs that are detected in patients with PM/DM. Eight anti-ARS Abs have been described: anti-histidyl (anti-Jo-1), anti-threonyl (anti-PL-7), anti-alanyl (anti-PL-12), anti-glycyl (anti-EJ), anti-isoleucyl (anti-OJ), anti-asparaginyl (anti-KS), anti-phenylalanyl (anti-Zo), and anti-tyrosyl (anti-Ha) tRNAs [13–20]. Based on a unique combination of clinical features commonly observed in patients with anti-ARS Abs, Targoff proposed a disease entity termed "anti-synthetase syndrome," which is characterized by myositis, ILD, fever, Raynaud's phenomenon, arthritis, and mechanic's hands [21]. Although anti-synthetase syndrome has common clinical manifestations, further observations have distinguished some differences in clinical features associated with individual anti-ARS Abs [22]. For example, it has been reported that anti-Jo-1 Abs are closely associated with myositis [14,17], whereas patients with anti-KS are more likely to have ILD without clinical evidence of myositis [18,23]. On the other hand, Sato *et al* previously reported that the presence of anti-PL-7 is closely associated with PM/DM-SSc overlap as well as ILD in Japanese patients [24].

This is a large comprehensive study to focus on the clinical and laboratory features in adult patients with anti-ARS Abs for the investigation of similarities and differences in these anti-ARS Abs. The results of this study indicate that anti-ARS Abs share several clinical features, but also have some considerable differences. Thus, identification of each anti-ARS Ab is beneficial to define this rather homogeneous subset of patients and to predict clinical outcomes.

Patients and Methods

Ethics Statement

Ethical approval for the study was obtained from the individual institutional review boards (Kanazawa University, Keio University, Nagasaki University, St. Marianna University, Social Insurance Chukyo Hospital, and Ogaki Municipal Hospital) and all sera were collected after the subjects gave their written informed consent.

Patients and Sera

Serum samples were obtained from Japanese patients with autoimmune diseases or related disorders who had visited Kanazawa University Hospital or collaborating medical centers from 2003 to 2009. In total, 3164 samples (from 478 patients with DM/PM, 498 with SSc, 183 with ILD alone, 376 with SLE, 102 with mixed connective tissue disease, 398 with Sjogren's syndrome, and 1129 with rheumatoid arthritis) were screened by immunoprecipitation (IP) assay for the detection of antinuclear or anticytoplasmic antibodies. These patients were referred mainly by rheumatologists, dermatologists, or pulmonologists. PM and classic DM were defined by fulfillment of the Bohan and Peter criteria for definite or probable diagnoses [25]. DM was distinguished from PM based on the presence of heliotrope rash or Gottron's lesions (Gottron's papules and/or Gottron's sign). The diagnosis of CADM was based on the criteria proposed by Sontheimer [26], as follows: clinical skin manifestations typical of DM but minimal or no clinical features of myositis for >2 years after the onset of skin manifestations. All patients with SLE or SSc fulfilled the American College of Rheumatology criteria [27,28]. PM/DM-overlap was diagnosed by the coexistence of SLE and/or SSc in addition to PM or DM. "ILD alone" was defined by the presence of ILD without fulfillment of any of the criteria for PM, DM, CADM, SLE, or SSc. Patients with ILD alone were examined for potential coexistence of myositis by evaluating muscle weakness and serum muscle enzyme levels including creatine kinase (CK) and aldolase during follow-up, while those without ILD were examined for potential coexistence of ILD by examining dyspneic symptoms and chest radiograph and/or high-resolution computed tomography (HRCT) at every 3 to 6 months.

Clinical information was collected retrospectively for all patients with anti-ARS Abs by reviewing their clinical charts. Initial manifestations were defined as the clinical presentation at the first clinic visit. Patients who had at least one of the following symptoms: symmetrical proximal muscle weakness, muscle pain, or elevated levels of myogenic enzymes, underwent electromyogram, MRI, and/or muscle biopsy for confirmation of the presence of myositis. Patients were diagnosed with myositis if at least one of these confirmatory examinations showed findings compatible with inflammatory myopathy: a myogenic pattern on electromyogram [25], muscular edema on T2-weighted images with fat suppression on MRI [29], or necrosis, regeneration, and some atrophy of muscle fibers and inflammatory cell infiltration on muscle biopsy [25]. Patients were diagnosed as having ILD according to the images on chest HRCT. RP-ILD was defined as progressive dyspnea and progressive hypoxemia with a worsening of interstitial changes on the chest images within 1 month from the onset of respiratory manifestations [11]. Internal and hematologic malignancies in anti-ARS-positive patients was defined if the malignant disease was diagnosed concurrently with or within 3 years after diagnosis of anti-synthetase syndrome or if a preceding malignant disease occurred within 3 years before diagnosis of anti-synthetase syndrome [4]. Sjögren's syndrome was defined in accordance with the revised European criteria [30].

IP Assays

Protein IP assays were carried out with extracts of the leukemia cell line, K562 [11]. A total of 10 µl of the patient's serum was bound to 2 mg protein-A Sepharose beads (Amersham Biosciences, Piscataway, NJ) in 500 µl of IP buffer (10 mM Tris-HCl, pH 8.0, 50 mM NaCl, 0.1% Nonidet P-40), incubated for 2 h at 4°C, and then washed five times with IP buffer. Ab-coated Sepharose beads were mixed with 100 µl ^{35}S-methionine-labelled K562 cell extracts derived from 10^6 cells and rotated at 4°C for 2 h. After five washes, the beads were resuspended in sodium dodecyl sulphate (SDS) sample buffer and the polypeptides were fractionated by 7.5% SDS-polyacrylamide gel electrophoresis (PAGE) followed by autoradiography. For the analysis of RNA, immunoprecipitated RNA was detected in 8% urea-PAGE from a cell extract obtained from 3×10^6 non-radiolabeled K562 cells by phenol/chloroform, visualized by silver staining [31]. Each anti-ARS Ab was considered positive if serum samples produced precipitin lines with immunological identity to reference sera by both protein and RNA IP [32]. Anti-Ro Ab and anti-La Ab were detected by IP assays as well. Serum was considered positive for anti-Ro Ab if at least one of the Y1–Y5 RNAs was detected by RNA IP and the 60 kDa protein was detected by protein IP; serum was considered positive for anti-La Ab if RNAs contained in the 7S and 5.8S lesions were detected by RNA IP and the 48 kDa protein was detected by protein IP.

Immunofluorescence

Indirect immunofluorescence tests were carried out with slides of monolayer HEp-2 cells (Medical & Biological Laboratories [MBL], Nagoya, Japan) as substrate [33]. Anticentromere antibody was considered positive if serum diluted at 1:40 produced a characteristic staining pattern on HEp-2 cells as well as on commercially prepared HeLa cell chromosomal spreads (MBL) [34].

Statistical Analysis

Frequencies among all six anti-ARS-positive subgroups were compared with a chi-square test. If the overall P value was less than 0.05, pairwise comparisons were performed with a chi-square test with Yates' correction where appropriate. Continuous variables confirmed to be normally distributed were shown as mean and SD, and their comparisons among groups were carried out with an ANOVA. All statistical analyses were performed with StatView software.

Results

Detection of Anti-ARS Abs

Of 3164 samples screened by IP assays, anti-ARS Abs were detected in 166 patients (5.2%) (Figure 1). As shown in Figure 2, 6 anti-ARS specificities, including anti-Jo-1, anti-EJ, anti-PL-7, anti-PL-12, anti-KS, anti-OJ, were easily detectable and distinguishable by IP assays. Of 166 patients with anti-ARS Abs, anti-Jo-1 was found in 59 (36%) patients, anti-EJ was found in 38 (23%) patients, anti-PL-7 was found in 30 (18%) patients, anti-PL-12 was found in 19 (11%) patients, anti-KS was found in 13 (8%) patients, and anti-OJ was found in 8 (5%) patients. One patient with classic DM had antibodies reactive to both PL-7 and PL-12, and was excluded from the following analyses for clinical associations.

Coexistence of anti-ARS Abs and other autoimmune connective tissue disease-related Abs was examined (Table 1). Antibodies against Mi-2, 155/140, CADM-140/MDA5, MJ/NXP-2, topoisomerase I, centromere, U1RNP, Th/To, U3RNP, Sm and La/SS-B were rarely found in patients with anti-ARS Abs. In contrast, anti-Ro/SS-A Abs were found in 31 (19%) patients. These results were principally consistent with previous findings that myositis-specific Abs are relatively mutually exclusive, while myositis-associated Abs coexist with myositis-specific Abs [13,35].

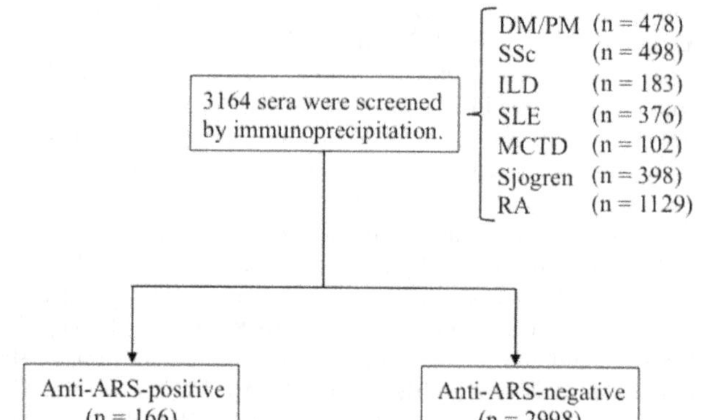

Figure 1. Enrollment and selection of patients. DM; dermatomyositis, PM; polymyositis, SSc; systemic sclerosis, ILD; interstitial lung disease, SLE; systemic lupus erythematosus, MCTD; mixed connective tissue disease, Sjogren; Sjogren's syndrome, RA; rheumatoid arthritis.

Associations between Clinical Diagnoses and Anti-ARS Abs

The distributions of classic DM, CADM, PM, PM/DM-overlap, SLE, SSc, and ILD alone in patients with individual anti-ARS Abs are shown in Figure 3. More than half of the patients with anti-Jo-1, anti-EJ, or anti-PL-7 had apparent myositis, including classic DM, PM, and PM/DM-overlap. The proportion with ILD alone was different among patients with various anti-ARS Abs. In particular, 10 of 13 (77%) patients with anti-KS and 5 of 8 (63%) patients with anti-OJ were diagnosed with ILD alone. Some patients with anti-ARS Abs were diagnosed with SSc or SLE, but the frequency was relatively low. Thus, most patients with anti-ARS Abs were diagnosed as having classic DM, CADM, PM, PM/DM-overlap, or ILD alone, while the proportion of these diagnoses was different among the subgroups of each anti-ARS Ab.

Comparison of Clinical Features among Patients with Anti-ARS Abs

A total of 95 patients with anti-ARS Abs had myositis and were diagnosed as having classic DM, PM, or PM/DM-overlap. We first compared clinical features between patients with myositis in the presence and absence of anti-ARS Ab (n = 95 and 152, respectively). Anti-ARS-positive patients with myositis had higher frequencies of Raynaud's phenomenon ($P = 0.034$), ILD ($P < 0.0001$), and polyarthritis ($P = 0.0015$) compared with anti-ARS-negative patients with myositis. There was no difference in the frequency of fever between the two groups ($P = 0.87$).

Then, we compared the demographic features among anti-ARS-based subgroups, as shown in Table 2. No differences were found in age of onset or sex. We next compared muscle weakness and ILD among individual anti-ARS subgroups, both at the initial visit and during the entire follow-up period. Muscle weakness was found in 71 (43%) patients at the initial visit and 95 (58%) during the entire follow-up period, but the frequencies varied among anti-ARS-based subgroups (overall $P = 0.0011$ and $P < 0.0001$, respectively). Patients with anti-Jo-1, anti-EJ, and anti-PL-7 had a higher frequency of muscle weakness (59%, 39%, and 52%, respectively, at the initial visit and 78%, 55%, and 76%, respectively during the entire follow-up period) than those with anti-PL-12 (17% for both), anti-KS (7% for both), and anti-OJ (25% for both). In contrast, most patients had ILD at the initial visit, and almost all patients eventually suffered from ILD. While most of them had the chronic type of ILD, a total of 13 patients (8 with anti-Jo-1, 4 with anti-EJ, and 1 with anti-PL-7) developed RP-ILD at their first visit or during their clinical course. Thus, the frequency of muscle weakness varied among anti-ARS subgroups, while ILD was observed at equally high frequencies among these subgroups.

Fever, Raynaud's phenomenon, polyarthritis, and mechanic's hands during the entire follow-up period were compared among anti-ARS subgroups. The frequency of fever varied among anti-ARS-based subgroups (8–44%), but there was no statistical difference. Raynaud's phenomenon was found in 40 of 165 (24%) patients with anti-ARS Abs and more frequently observed in patients with anti-PL-12 and anti-PL-7 (overall $P = 0.044$). Polyarthritis was most common in patients with anti-Jo-1 (58%) and infrequently observed in patients with anti-OJ (13%) (overall $P = 0.0029$). Mechanic's hands, which are the representative skin manifestation in anti-synthetase syndrome, were observed in all anti-ARS Ab-based subgroups, but the frequency was highest in patients with anti-Jo-1 (56%) (overall $P = 0.031$). Collectively, Raynaud's phenomenon, polyarthritis, and mechanic's hands were

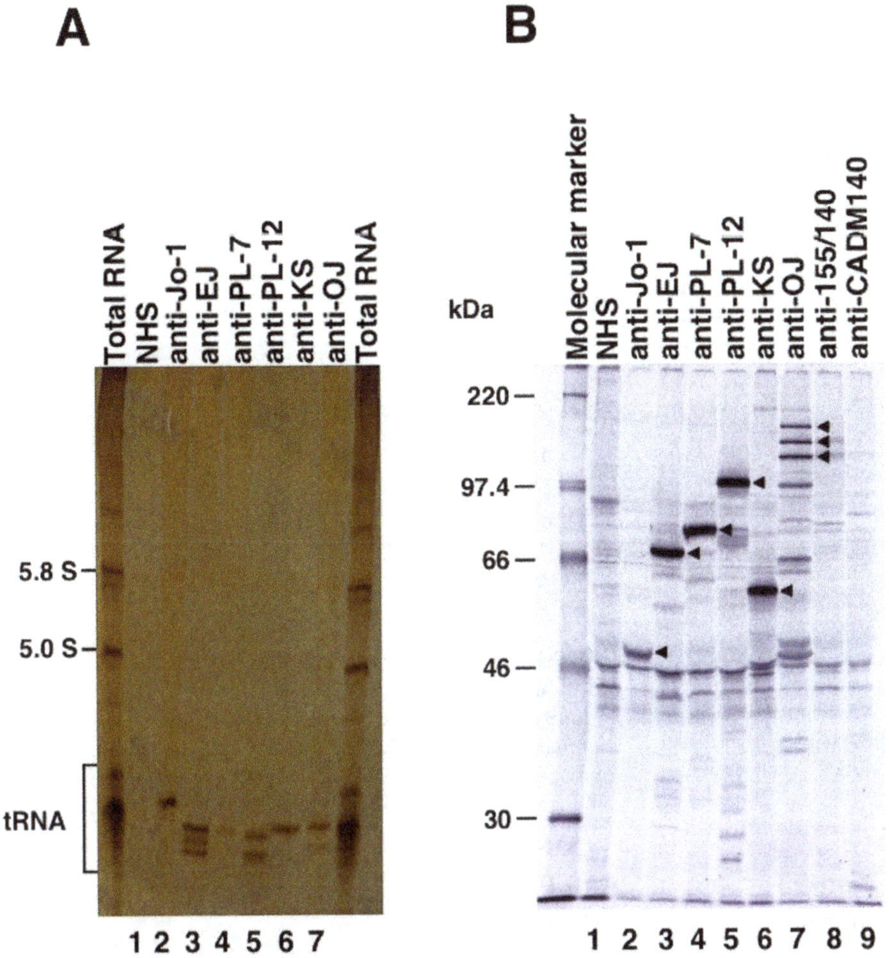

Figure 2. Representative immunoprecipitation assay for RNA with anti-aminoacyl-tRNA synthetase (anti-ARS) sera. A, Immunoprecipitation of histidyl-tRNA synthetase, glycyl-tRNA synthetase, threonyl-tRNA synthetase, alanyl-tRNA synthetase, asparaginyl-tRNA, and isoleucyl-tRNA synthetase by sera. K562 cell extracts were immunoprecipitated with sera, and RNA was extracted, electrophoresed on 8% urea-polyacrylamide gels, and visualized by silver staining. Total RNA, with the 5.8 and 5.0 S small ribosomal RNAs and the tRNA region indicated; Lane 1, normal health serum (NHS) indicated; Lanes 2–7: anti-ARS sera indicated, with antibodies to Jo-1 (histidyl-tRNA synthetase), EJ (glycyl-tRNA synthetase), PL-7 (threonyl-tRNA synthetase), PL-12 (alanyl-tRNA synthetase), KS (asparaginyl-tRNA synthetase), and OJ (isoleucyl-tRNA synthetase). **B,** Immunoprecipitation of ^{35}S-methionine-labeled K562 cell extracts was performed on anti-ARS sera and NHS, separated on 10% SDS-PAGE, and analyzed by autoradiography. Molecular weight markers include protein bands corresponding to 220, 97.4, 66, 46, and 30 kDa.

observed in each anti-ARS Ab subgroup, but the frequencies were rather heterogeneous.

We then compared heliotrope rash and Gottron's signs, which are the representative skin manifestations in DM. Heliotrope rash was found in 26 of 165 (16%) patients with anti-ARS Abs (overall $P = 0.0019$) and Gottron's sign (elbow and/or knee) was found in 51 (31%) (overall $P = 0.043$). These manifestations were predominantly found in patients with anti-EJ, anti-PL-7, and anti-PL-12.

With regard to laboratory findings, CK levels were lower in patients with anti-PL-12 and anti-KS (overall $P = 0.024$), and lactate dehydrogenase (LDH) was lowest in patients with anti-KS (overall $P = 0.019$). It is likely that these results were associated with the frequencies of muscle involvement. KL-6 and pulmonary surfactant protein D (SP-D) levels are associated with the activity and severity of ILD [36,37]. While elevations of both KL-6 and SP-D were observed in all anti-ARS-based subgroups, no significant differences were observed in serum KL-6 and SP-D levels.

As an association of malignancy with PM/DM has been reported, we examined the frequency of malignancies in patients with anti-ARS Abs (Table 2). Malignancies were observed in 19 (12%) of 165 patients with anti-ARS Abs, and 1 of those had a double malignancy. A summary of the malignancies is listed in Table 3. There were 4 patients with colon cancer, 4 with gastric cancer or carcinoid, 3 with breast cancer, 3 with lung cancer, and single cases of prostate cancer, nasopharyngeal cancer, uterine corpus cancer, thyroid cancer, ovarian cancer, and non-Hodgkin lymphoma. There was no trend in the prevalence of malignancy or the type of malignancy among anti-ARS-based subgroups. Seven of 19 patients with malignancy simultaneously developed PM/DM or ILD, while 7 of 19 had malignancy prior to the development of PM/DM or ILD, and 5 of 19 developed malignancy after the diagnosis of PM/DM or ILD.

Table 1. Coexistence of other autoantibodies in patients with anti-aminoacyl-tRNA synthetase antibodies.*

	Anti-Jo-1 (n = 59)	Anti-EJ (n = 38)	Anti-PL-7 (n = 29)	Anti-PL-12 (n = 18)	Anti-KS (n = 13)	Anti-OJ (n = 8)	Anti-PL-7/ PL-12 (n = 1)
Anti-Mi-2	0	0	0	0	0	0	0
Anti-155/140	0	0	0	0	0	0	0
Anti-CADM-140/MDA5	0	0	0	0	0	0	0
Anti-MJ/NXP-2	0	0	0	0	0	0	0
Anti-topoisomerase I	0	1	0	0	0	0	0
Anti-centromere	1	0	0	1	2	0	0
Anti-U1RNP	0	0	1	1	0	0	0
Anti-Th/To	0	0	0	1	0	0	0
Anti-U3RNP	1	0	0	0	0	0	0
Anti-Sm	0	0	1	0	0	0	0
Anti-Ro/SS-A	9	9	8	4	1	0	0
Anti-La/SS-B	0	2	2	0	0	0	0

*Values are the number of patients.

Causes of Death

Sixteen (10%) of 165 anti-ARS-positive patients died during the follow-up period (Table 4). Causes of death included ILD in 8, malignancy in 3, infection in 2, and one each of myocardial infarction, rupture of an abdominal aortic aneurysm, and hypertrophic cardiomyopathy.

Timing of Development of ILD and Myositis in Patients with Anti-ARS Abs

Initial manifestations in patients with anti-ARS Abs are summarized in Table 5. At initial presentation, the combination of manifestations, including DM rashes, myositis, and ILD, varied among patients with anti-ARS Abs. The frequency of ILD alone at

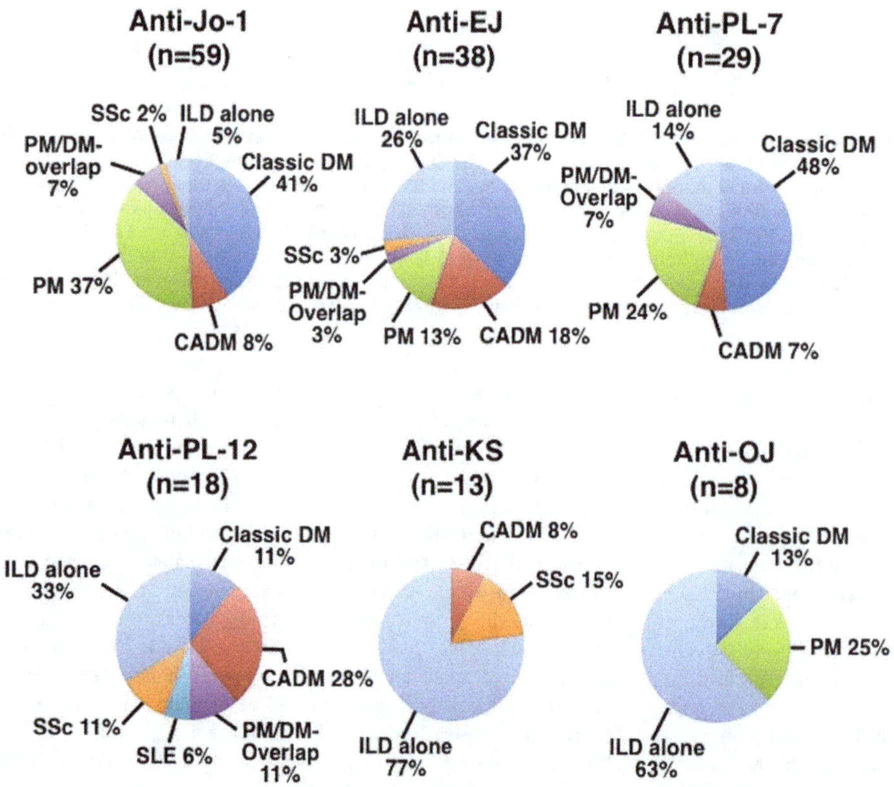

Figure 3. Prevalence of dermatomyositis (DM), clinically amyopathic DM (CADM), polymyositis (PM), PM/DM-overlap, systemic lupus erythematosus (SLE), systemic sclerosis (SSc), and interstitial lung disease (ILD) alone, in each subgroup of anti-synthetase syndrome.

Table 2. Comparison of clinical features in 165 adult Japanese patients with anti-aminoacyl-tRNA synthetase antibodies.*

	Anti-Jo-1 (n = 59)	Anti-EJ (n = 38)	Anti-PL-7 (n = 29)	Anti-PL-12 (n = 18)	Anti-KS (n = 13)	Anti-OJ (n = 8)	Overall P
Age at onset, median (range), y	53 (22–76)	53 (18–78)	53 (25–79)	48 (20–75)	54 (39–67)	57 (32–79)	0.61
No. of females/no. of males	43/16	32/6	26/3	16/2	7/6	6/2	0.077
Clinical features (at initial visit)							
Interstitial lung disease	71	84	76	89	100	100	0.077
Muscle weakness	59	39	52	17	7	25	0.0011[a]
Clinical features (entire follow-up period)							
Fever	27	39	34	44	8	13	0.16
Raynaud's phenomenon	19	13	38	44	31	13	0.044[b]
Interstitial lung disease	90	97	93	94	100	100	0.56
Muscle weakness	78	55	76	17	7	25	<0.0001[c]
Polyarthritis	58	24	31	22	31	13	0.0029[d]
Erosive arthritis	12	5	0	17	23	0	0.16
Malignancy	15	3	7	17	15	25	0.22
Sjögren's syndrome	7	16	14	0	8	0	0.32
Skin manifestations							
Heliotrope rash	7	21	38	17	0	0	0.0019[e]
Gottron's sign (hand)	44	45	41	33	8	13	0.10
Gottron's sign (elbow and/or knee)	27	39	45	33	0	13	0.043[f]
Mechanic's hands	56	29	45	22	23	38	0.031[g]
Laboratory findings							
CK, IU/L, mean ± SD	2213±3168	1681±2967	1768±2096	250±306	143±84	881±1129	0.024[h]
LDH, IU/L, mean ± SD	595±5961	427±223	565±406	346±187	215±77	355±197	0.019[i]
KL-6, U/mL, mean ± SD	1335±2067 (n = 54)	1425±1030	1374±1444	1630±1650	1527±1404 (n = 12)	1307±877	0.99
SP-D, ng/mL, mean ± SD	206±229 (n = 39)	318±626 (n = 36)	229±275 (n = 25)	250±170 (n = 15)	185±129	123±53 (n = 6)	0.74

*Unless noted otherwise, values are percentages of patients. NS: not significant; CK: creatine kinase; LDH: lactate dehydrogenase. One patient with DM who had antibodies reactive to both PL-7 and PL-12 was excluded from the analysis. Significant differences (overall $P<0.05$) were further analyzed by pairwise comparisons.
[a]$P<0.05$ between anti-PL-7 and anti-PL-12; $P<0.01$ between anti-Jo-1 and anti-PL-12, and between anti-KS and anti-Jo-1 or anti-PL-7;
[b]$P<0.05$ between anti-Jo-1 and anti-PL-7 or anti-PL-12, and between anti-EJ and anti-PL-7; $P<0.01$ between anti-EJ and anti-PL-12.
[c]$P<0.05$ between anti-EJ and anti-PL-12; $P<0.01$ between anti-Jo-1 and anti-PL-12, anti-KS or anti-OJ, between anti-EJ and anti-KS, and between anti-PL-7 and anti-PL-12, anti-KS or anti-OJ.
[d]$P<0.05$ between anti-Jo-1 and anti-PL-7, anti-KS or anti-OJ; $P<0.01$ between anti-Jo-1 and anti-EJ or anti-PL-12.
[e]$P<0.05$ between anti-Jo-1 and anti-EJ; $P<0.01$ between anti-PL-7 and anti-Jo-1 or anti-KS.
[f]$P<0.05$ between anti-KS and anti-EJ or anti-PL-12; $P<0.01$ between anti-PL-7 and anti-KS.
[g]$P<0.05$ between anti-Jo-1 and anti-PL-12 or anti-KS; $P<0.01$ between anti-Jo-1 and anti-EJ.
[h]$P<0.05$ between anti-EJ and anti-PL-12 or anti-KS; $P<0.01$ between anti-Jo-1 and anti-PL-12 or anti-KS, and between anti-PL-7 and anti-PL-12 or anti-KS.
[i]$P<0.05$ between anti-PL-7 and anti-PL-12; $P<0.01$ between anti-Jo-1 and anti-PL-12, and between anti-KS and anti-Jo-1, anti-EJ or anti-PL-7.

presentation was different among groups stratified by anti-ARS Abs (overall $P = 0.0001$). While some patients with anti-ARS Abs had 2 or more manifestations at initial diagnosis, others sequentially developed different manifestations, even when they were receiving therapy. Thus, we analyzed the timing of development of ILD and myositis. Figure 4A includes patients with ILD alone and DM rashes and ILD, and Figure 4B includes those with myositis alone and DM rashes and myositis at initial presentation. Patients with DM rashes alone, myositis and ILD, DM rashes, myositis, and ILD, and none of DM rashes, myositis, and ILD were excluded from this analysis. We assessed whether patients who had ILD alone at presentation developed myositis during follow-up (Figure 4A). As a result, 39%, 29%, and 64% of patients with anti-Jo-1, anti-EJ, and anti-PL-7, respectively, subsequently developed myositis. In contrast, none of the patients with anti-PL-12, anti-KS, and anti-OJ who had ILD alone at presentation developed myositis later in the course of the disease. The distribution of the frequencies for developing myositis among anti-ARS-based subgroups was statistically significant (overall $P = 0.0008$). In contrast, when patients who had myositis without ILD at presentation were selected, nearly all of them developed ILD later in the course of the disease (Figure 4B). There was no difference in observation period among the 6 groups (Jo-1, 62±24; EJ, 56±27; PL-7, 50±27; PL-12, 53±27; KS, 70±20; and OJ, 62±32 months). In addition, there was no difference in initial treatment regimen among the 6 groups stratified by anti-ARS Abs (Table 6), although 38% of patients with anti-KS did not receive immunosuppressive therapy and this frequency was highest among the 6 groups (overall $P = 0.0070$). Almost all patients with anti-ARS Abs who had ILD or myositis received immunosuppressive treatment, including corticosteroids alone or in combination with immunosuppressants. Accordingly, patients with anti-PL-12, anti-

Table 3. Summary of malignancy in patients with anti-aminoacyl-tRNA synthetase antibodies.

Anti-ARS	Age, y	Sex	Diagnosis	ILD	Type of malignancy	Onset
Anti-Jo-1	54	M	PM	−	Lung cancer	At same time
Anti-Jo-1	59	F	DM	+	Gastric cancer	Before DM
Anti-Jo-1	38	F	DM	+	Ovarian cancer	At same time
Anti-Jo-1	54	M	PM	+	Colon cancer	After PM
Anti-Jo-1	74	M	DM	+	Colon cancer	Before DM
Anti-Jo-1	42	F	DM	+	Breast cancer	Before DM
Anti-Jo-1	67	F	DM	+	Non-Hodgkin lymphoma	At same time
Anti-Jo-1	62	M	PM	−	Gastric cancer	After PM
Anti-Jo-1	57	F	DM	+	Thyroid cancer	At same time
Anti-EJ	43	F	DM	+	Nasopharyngeal cancer	At same time
Anti-PL-7	70	F	DM	+	Breast cancer	Before DM
Anti-PL-7	79	M	ILD	+	Gastric cancer	After ILD
Anti-PL-12	53	F	ILD	+	Lung+uterine corpus cancer	Before ILD
Anti-PL-12	66	M	ILD	+	Colon cancer	After ILD
Anti-PL-12	59	F	DM	+	Breast cancer	Before DM
Anti-KS	59	M	ILD	+	Lung cancer	After ILD
Anti-KS	66	M	ILD	+	Prostate cancer	Before ILD
Anti-OJ	71	F	DM	+	Gastric carcinoid	At same time
Anti-OJ	77	M	PM	+	Colon cancer	At same time

ILD: interstitial lung disease; PM: polymyositis; DM: dermatomyositis.

Table 4. Cause of death in patients with anti-aminoacyl-tRNA synthetase antibodies.

Anti-ARS	Age, y	Sex	Diagnosis	ILD	Cause of death	Time after diagnosis (y)
Anti-Jo-1	64	F	DM	+	ILD	0.3
Anti-Jo-1	38	F	DM	+	Infection	3
Anti-Jo-1	36	F	DM	+	ILD	5.5
Anti-Jo-1	62	M	PM	−	Gastric cancer	5
Anti-EJ	65	F	DM	+	ILD	2.5
Anti-EJ	55	F	ILD	+	ILD	0.6
Anti-EJ	55	F	DM	+	ILD	4.25
Anti-EJ	53	F	SSc	+	Infection	6
Anti-EJ	50	F	DM	+	Myocardial infarction	5.25
Anti-PL-7	63	F	DM	+	ILD	1.8
Anti-PL-7	71	F	DM	+	ILD	3
Anti-PL-7	75	M	ILD	+	ILD	0.3
Anti-PL-12	53	F	ILD	+	Lung cancer	3
Anti-PL-12	74	F	DM	+	Rupture of an abdominal aortic aneurysm	0.6
Anti-PL-12	75	F	ILD	+	Hypertrophic cardiomyopathy	2
Anti-KS	59	M	ILD	+	Lung cancer	1.5

ILD: interstitial lung disease; DM: dermatomyositis; PM: polymyositis; SSc: systemic sclerosis.

Table 5. Initial manifestations in patients with anti-aminoacyl-tRNA synthetase antibodies.*

	Anti-Jo-1 (n = 59)	Anti-EJ (n = 38)	Anti-PL-7 (n = 29)	Anti-PL-12 (n = 18)	Anti-KS (n = 13)	Anti-OJ (n = 8)	Overall *P*
DM rashes alone	2	0	14	11	8	0	0.14
Myositis alone	14	11	21	0	0	0	0.14
ILD alone	29	39	28	56	92	63	0.0001[a]
DM rashes and Myositis	10	5	4	6	0	0	0.45
DM rashes and ILD	19	16	10	11	0	0	0.46
Myositis and ILD	7	13	7	0	0	25	0.24
DM rashes, Myositis, and ILD	10	16	17	11	0	13	0.75
No DM rashes, Myositis, or ILD**	10	0	0	6	0	0	0.11

*Values are percentages of patients.
**These patients had polyarthritis at presentation. Significant differences (overall $P<0.05$) were further analyzed by pairwise comparisons.
[a]$P<0.05$ between anti-PL-12 and anti-Jo-1 or anti-KS; $P<0.01$ between anti-KS and anti-Jo-1, anti-EJ or anti-PL-7.

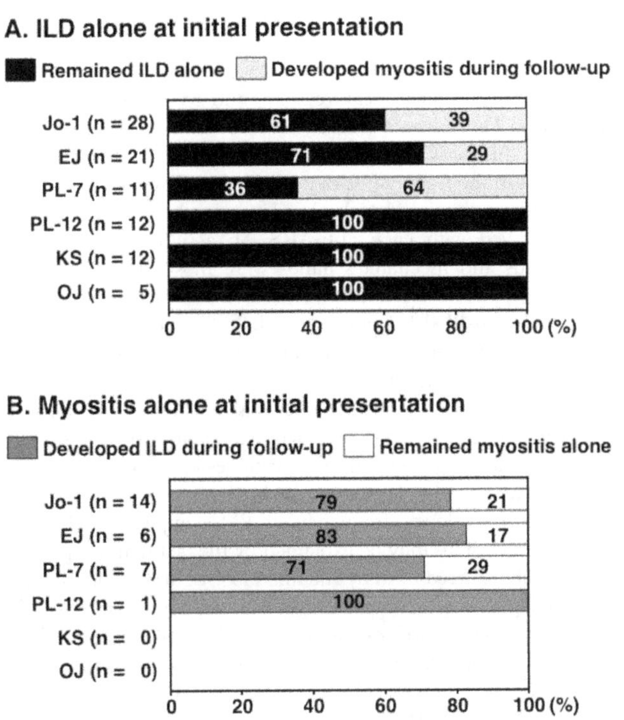

Figure 4. The clinical course of anti-synthetase syndrome patients who developed myositis or interstitial lung disease (ILD) with or without skin manifestations at disease onset. According to the clinical course, patients were classified into four types: remained with ILD alone, developed myositis during follow-up, developed ILD during follow-up, and remained with myositis alone. The clinical course of those who had ILD with or without skin manifestations, but without muscle involvement at their first assessment (A), and the clinical course of those who had myositis with or without skin manifestations, but without ILD at their first assessment (B).

KS, or anti-OJ were less likely to develop myositis during follow-up than those with anti-Jo-1, anti-EJ, or anti-PL-7.

Discussion

This comprehensive report aimed to compare clinical features among anti-ARS-based subgroups on a large scale. As reported previously, more than one anti-ARS Ab did not coexist in general. While this study confirmed that ILD, myositis, Raynaud's phenomenon, polyarthritis, and mechanic's hands were common manifestations in anti-synthetase syndrome, the frequencies of each manifestation varied. That is, myositis was well associated with anti-Jo-1, anti-EJ, and anti-PL-7. Additionally, a substantial number of patients positive for anti-EJ or anti-PL-12 had CADM. Therefore, most of the clinical diagnoses were PM or DM for anti-Jo-1, anti-EJ, and anti-PL-7; CADM or ILD for anti-PL-12; and ILD for anti-KS and anti-OJ. Although patients with anti-ARS Abs share several common manifestations, it is likely that each of these Abs defines a clinically distinct phenotype and may serve as a predictor for clinical complications.

Since nearly all patients with anti-ARS Abs had ILD, this study confirms previous findings that anti-ARS Abs are a marker for ILD [38–42]. Most of the clinical diagnoses in patients with anti-ARS Abs were classic DM, CADM, PM or ILD alone in this study. This finding was also in accordance with previous reports that anti-ARS Abs were highly specific for a proportion of patients with PM, DM, or ILD [4,38,43–45]. However, classic DM, CADM, or PM was found predominantly in patient subgroups with anti-Jo-1, anti-EJ, and anti-PL-7, whereas two-thirds of patients with anti-PL-12 were diagnosed with CADM or ILD. In contrast, anti-KS and anti-OJ were associated with ILD alone. Therefore, it is likely that the clinical diagnosis varies among anti-ARS-based subgroups.

Regarding myositis, it appears that anti-ARS Abs are divided into myositis-related and non-myositis-related subgroups. Anti-Jo-1, anti-EJ, and anti-PL-7 belong to the myositis-related subgroup, since myositis was found in at least half of the patients with these anti-ARS Abs. These findings agreed with previous reports describing a relationship of myositis with anit-Jo-1 [46], anti-EJ [13,17,47,48], and anti-PL-7 [24,49]. In contrast, anti-PL-12, anti-KS, and anti-OJ were not well related to myositis in this study. These results also paralleled those of former reports that anti-KS is highly associated with ILD [32,48]. However, rates of myositis in anti-PL-12 and anti-OJ appear to be different from previous

Table 6. Initial treatment in patients with anti-aminoacyltransfer RNA synthetase antibodies.*

	Anti-Jo-1 (n = 59)	Anti-EJ (n = 38)	Anti-PL-7 (n = 29)	Anti-PL-12 (n = 18)	Anti-KS (n = 13)	Anti-OJ (n = 8)	Overall *P*
No immunosuppressive therapy	7 (4)	5 (2)	3 (1)	11 (2)	38 (5)	13 (1)	0.0070[a]
Initial treatment							
CS oral only	68 (40)	68 (26)	59 (17)	67 (12)	46 (6)	88 (7)	0.45
CS pulse+oral	8 (5)	16 (6)	21 (6)	6 (1)	8 (1)	0 (0)	0.36
CS (pulse and/or oral)+CsA	10 (6)	3 (1)	3 (1)	11 (2)	0 (0)	0 (0)	0.41
CS (pulse and/or oral)+Tac	2 (1)	0 (0)	3 (1)	0 (0)	0 (0)	0 (0)	0.81
CS (pulse and/or oral)+CY (oral and/or iv)	3 (3)	0 (1)	0 (0)	0 (0)	0 (0)	0 (0)	0.82
CS (pulse and/or oral)+CsA or Tac+CY (oral and/or iv)	0 (0)	0 (0)	7 (2)	6 (1)	0 (0)	0 (0)	0.17
CS (pulse and/or oral)+MZR	0 (0)	3 (1)	3 (1)	0 (0)	0 (0)	0 (0)	0.69
CS (pulse and/or oral)+Buc	0 (0)	3 (1)	0 (0)	0 (0)	8 (1)	0 (0)	0.25

*Values are percentages of patients. Patient numbers are given in parenthesis. CS: corticosteroid; CsA: cyclosporine A; Tac: tacrolimus; CY: cyclophosphamide; iv: intravenous administration; MZR: mizoribine; Buc: bucillamine. Significant differences (overall $P<0.05$) were further analyzed by pairwise comparisons.
[a]$P<0.01$ between anti-KS and anti-Jo-1, anti-EJ or anti-PL-7.

reports. Of a total of 47 cases with anti-PL-12, muscle weakness was observed in 27 (57%) patients [16,23,50]. Sato *et al* reported 7 Japanese patients with anti-OJ, in which muscle weakness was seen in 4 patients [51]. Thus, whether anti-PL-12 and anti-OJ are related to myositis remains controversial. Collectively, patients with anti-ARS Abs form a basically homogenous clinical entity, as previously reported; mutual comparisons in this study elucidated certain differences in clinical features among patients with specific anti-ARS Abs.

Regarding skin manifestations, this study revealed an interesting observation. The main clinical diagnoses in anti-Jo-1, anti-EJ, anti-PL-7, and anti-PL-12 were classic DM or CADM. This resulted from the higher frequencies of DM-specific skin manifestations in these patients, which included heliotrope rash and Gottron's signs. However, the distribution of skin manifestations varied among anti-ARS Abs. Only less than 10% of patients with anti-Jo-1 had heliotrope rash, while approximately 20–30% of those with anti-EJ, anti-PL-7, and anti-PL12 had this eruption. On the other hand, the frequency of anti-Jo-1-positive patients who had Gottron's sign was similar compared to those with anti-EJ, anti-PL-7, and anti-PL-12. Thus, the prevalence of DM-specific skin manifestations is not identical among different anti-ARS Abs, even though the main diagnosis is classic DM or CADM.

With respect to the onset of evident manifestations of myositis and ILD, these patients were divided into three groups: i) patients with myositis preceding ILD; ii) patients with ILD preceding myositis; and iii) patients with simultaneous onset of both conditions. We reported previously that the onset of anti-synthetase syndrome is acute, but that the development of myositis may lag behind the onset of ILD in anti-ARS-positive DM patients [38]. A similar finding was described in another report [44]. In this study, most patients with anti-ARS Abs who had myositis without ILD at the onset of disease developed ILD later. On the other hand, the rate of subsequent occurrence of myositis differed among the subsets of anti-ARS Abs when the patients had ILD without myositis as their initial manifestation. Thus, screening and identification of anti-ARS Abs is found to be beneficial in predicting the onset of ILD.

Other than ILD and myositis, previous reports described that arthritis, Raynaud's phenomenon, fever, and mechanic's hands are common clinical features in anti-synthetase syndrome [21,40,44]. There was no significant difference in the frequency of fever in this study. On the other hand, this study revealed some differences in the frequencies of polyarthritis, Raynaud's phenomenon, and mechanic's hands. While these three manifestations were observed with each anti-ARS Ab at a comparable rate, polyarthritis and mechanic's hands were most frequently found with anti-Jo-1, and Raynaud's phenomenon was most frequently found with anti-PL-12. Nonetheless, the differences in frequencies of these manifestations among anti-ARS subgroups were less evident than that with myositis.

We acknowledge several limitations of this study. First, it included a relatively small number of patients with anti-PL-12, anti-KS, or anti-OJ. Second, most facilities enrolled in this study were referral centers. This study had a higher frequency of DM and a relatively lower frequency of PM compared with other similar studies. This may be explained by the fact that our patients were mainly referred to us by rheumatologists, dermatologists, and pulmonologists, and only a few of them were referred by neurologists. Therefore, we cannot exclude selection bias. Third, the possibility cannot be ruled out that coexistence of anti-Ro/SS-A Abs influence the clinical feature of anti-ARS-positive patients with anti-Ro/SS-A Abs, as anti-Ro/SS-A Abs are considered as myositis-associated Abs and form the subgroup. In the analysis of clinical course, possibilities are raised that the short observation period and the differences in treatment potentially affected the results. Additionally, patients who visited to referral centers were examined for the existence of myositis and they were categorized by Bohan and Peter and Sontheimer criteria that are commonly used for diagnosis of myositis in a current condition. However, as clinical features of patients with anti-ARS Abs are largely heterogeneous, it appears difficult to stratify the patients by current criteria. It may be clinically useful to classify the anti-ARS-positive patients based on the type of anti-ARS Abs, not current criteria. It needs to consider the conformity of the classification of the patients with anti-ARS Abs with diagnosis criteria for myositis. Indeed, Connors *et al* have proposed the criteria for anti-ARS syndrome as follows [40]. First, patients must have positive serologic testing for anti-ARS Abs. Then, patients have one or more of the following conditions: Evidence of myositis by Bohan and Peter criteria, evidence of ILD by American Thoracic Society criteria, evidence of arthritis by clinical examination, radiographic findings, or patient self-report, unexplained, persistent fever, Raynaud's phenomenon, and mechanic's hands. Therefore, more studies are needed for a better general understanding of the clinical characteristics of patients with anti-ARS Abs.

In summary, although anti-ARS Abs share common clinical features, each anti-ARS Ab appears to form some distinct clinical subset. However, the identification of anti-ARS Abs (except for anti-Jo-1) is limited only to certain facilities, as it requires a complicated technique. Establishment of a system routinely available to screen all anti-ARS Abs specificities is needed.

Acknowledgments

We thank Ms. Masako Matsubara, Yuko Yamada, Tomoko Hayashi, and Natsuho Yoshifuji for technical assistance.

Author Contributions

Conceived and designed the experiments: YH MF. Performed the experiments: YH MF. Analyzed the data: YH RY MF. Contributed reagents/materials/analysis tools: YH MF TM K. Kaji K. Komura MH M. Kodera EM KF MS HY SS KT M. Kuwana. Wrote the paper: YH MF M. Kuwana.

References

1. Targoff IN (2002) Laboratory testing in the diagnosis and management of idiopathic inflammatory myopathies. Rheum Dis Clin North Am. 28: 859–890, viii.
2. Mammen AL (2010) Dermatomyositis and polymyositis: Clinical presentation, autoantibodies, and pathogenesis. Ann N Y Acad Sci. 1184: 134–153.
3. Hamaguchi Y, Kuwana M, Hoshino K, Hasegawa M, Kaji K, et al. (2011) Clinical correlations with dermatomyositis-specific autoantibodies in adult Japanese patients with dermatomyositis: a multicenter cross-sectional study. Arch Dermatol. 147: 391–398.
4. Love LA, Leff RL, Fraser DD, Targoff IN, Dalakas M, et al. (1991) A new approach to the classification of idiopathic inflammatory myopathy: myositis-specific autoantibodies define useful homogeneous patient groups. Medicine (Baltimore). 70: 360–374.
5. Mierau R, Dick T, Bartz-Bazzanella P, Keller E, Albert ED, et al. (1996) Strong association of dermatomyositis-specific Mi-2 autoantibodies with a tryptophan at position 9 of the HLA-DR beta chain. Arthritis Rheum. 39: 868–876.
6. Komura K, Fujimoto M, Matsushita T, Kaji K, Kondo M, et al. (2005) Prevalence and clinical characteristics of anti-Mi-2 antibodies in Japanese patients with dermatomyositis. J Dermatol Sci. 40: 215–217.
7. Kaji K, Fujimoto M, Hasegawa M, Kondo M, Saito Y, et al. (2007) Identification of a novel autoantibody reactive with 155 and 140 kDa nuclear proteins in patients with dermatomyositis: an association with malignancy. Rheumatology (Oxford). 46: 25–28.
8. Targoff IN, Mamyrova G, Trieu EP, Perurena O, Koneru B, et al. (2006) A novel autoantibody to a 155-kd protein is associated with dermatomyositis. Arthritis Rheum. 54: 3682–3689.
9. Gunawardena H, Wedderburn LR, North J, Betteridge Z, Dunphy J, et al. (2008) Clinical associations of autoantibodies to a p155/140 kDa doublet protein in juvenile dermatomyositis. Rheumatology (Oxford). 47: 324–328.
10. Fujimoto M, Hamaguchi Y, Kaji K, Matsushita T, Ichimura Y, et al. (2012) Myositis-specific anti-155/140 autoantibodies target transcription intermediary factor 1 family proteins. Arthritis Rheum. 64: 513–522.
11. Sato S, Hirakata M, Kuwana M, Suwa A, Inada S, et al. (2005) Autoantibodies to a 140-kd polypeptide, CADM-140, in Japanese patients with clinically amyopathic dermatomyositis. Arthritis Rheum. 52: 1571–1576.
12. Sato S, Hoshino K, Satoh T, Fujita T, Kawakami Y, et al. (2009) RNA helicase encoded by melanoma differentiation-associated gene 5 is a major autoantigen in patients with clinically amyopathic dermatomyositis: Association with rapidly progressive interstitial lung disease. Arthritis Rheum. 60: 2193–2200.
13. Hirakata M, Mimori T, Akizuki M, Craft J, Hardin JA, et al. (1992) Autoantibodies to small nuclear and cytoplasmic ribonucleoproteins in Japanese patients with inflammatory muscle disease. Arthritis Rheum. 35: 449–456.
14. Yoshida S, Akizuki M, Mimori T, Yamagata H, Inada S, et al. (1983) The precipitating antibody to an acidic nuclear protein antigen, the Jo-1, in connective tissue diseases. A marker for a subset of polymyositis with interstitial pulmonary fibrosis. Arthritis Rheum. 26: 604–611.
15. Mathews MB, Reichlin M, Hughes GR, Bernstein RM (1984) Anti-threonyl-tRNA synthetase, a second myositis-related autoantibody. J Exp Med. 160: 420–434.
16. Bunn CC, Bernstein RM, Mathews MB (1986) Autoantibodies against alanyl-tRNA synthetase and tRNAAla coexist and are associated with myositis. J Exp Med. 163: 1281–1291.
17. Targoff IN (1990) Autoantibodies to aminoacyl-transfer RNA synthetases for isoleucine and glycine. Two additional synthetases are antigenic in myositis. J Immunol. 144: 1737–1743.
18. Hirakata M, Suwa A, Nagai S, Kron MA, Trieu EP, et al. (1999) Anti-KS: identification of autoantibodies to asparaginyl-transfer RNA synthetase associated with interstitial lung disease. J Immunol. 162: 2315–2320.
19. Betteridge Z, Gunawardena H, North J, Slinn J, McHugh N (2007) Anti-synthetase syndrome: a new autoantibody to phenylalanyl transfer RNA synthetase (anti-Zo) associated with polymyositis and interstitial pneumonia. Rheumatology (Oxford). 46: 1005–1008.
20. Hashish L, Trieu EP, Sadanandan P, Targoff IN (2005) Identification of autoantibodies to tyrosyl-tRNA synthetase in dermatomyositis with features consistent with antisynthetase syndrome. Arthritis Rheum 52 Suppl 9: S312.
21. Targoff IN (1992) Autoantibodies in polymyositis. Rheum Dis Clin North Am. 18: 455–482.
22. Hervier B, Devilliers H, Stanciu R, Meyer A, Uzunhan Y, et al. (2012) Hierarchical cluster and survival analyses of antisynthetase syndrome: Phenotype and outcome are correlated with anti-tRNA synthetase antibody specificity. Autoimmun Rev. 12: 210–217.
23. Kalluri M, Sahn SA, Oddis CV, Gharib SL, Christopher-Stine L, et al. (2009) Clinical profile of anti-PL-12 autoantibody. Cohort study and review of the literature. Chest. 135: 1550–1556.
24. Sato S, Hirakata M, Kuwana M, Nakamura K, Suwa A, et al. (2005) Clinical characteristics of Japanese patients with anti-PL-7 (anti-threonyl-tRNA synthetase) autoantibodies. Clin Exp Rheumatol. 23: 609–615.
25. Bohan A, Peter JB (1975) Polymyositis and dermatomyositis (second of two parts). N Engl J Med. 292: 403–407.
26. Sontheimer RD (2002) Would a new name hasten the acceptance of amyopathic dermatomyositis (dermatomyositis sine myositis) as a distinctive subset within the idiopathic inflammatory dermatomyopathies spectrum of clinical illness? J Am Acad Dermatol. 46: 626–636.
27. Tan EM, Cohen AS, Fries JF, Masi AT, McShane DJ, et al. (1982) The 1982 revised criteria for the classification of systemic lupus erythematosus. Arthritis Rheum. 25: 1271–1277.
28. Anonymous (1980) Preliminary criteria for the classification of systemic sclerosis (scleroderma). Subcommittee for Scleroderma Criteria of the American Rheumatism Association Diagnostic and Therapeutic Criteria Committee. Arthritis Rheum. 23: 581–590.
29. Tomasova, Studynkova J, Charvat F, Jarosova K, Vencovsky J (2007) The role of MRI in the assessment of polymyositis and dermatomyositis. Rheumatology (Oxford). 46: 1174–1179.
30. Vitali C, Bombardieri S, Jonsson R, Moutsopoulos HM, Alexander EL, et al. (2002) Classification criteria for Sjogren's syndrome: a revised version of the European criteria proposed by the American-European Consensus Group. Ann Rheum Dis. 61: 554–558.
31. Hamaguchi Y, Hasegawa M, Fujimoto M, Matsushita T, Komura K, et al. (2008) The clinical relevance of serum antinuclear antibodies in Japanese patients with systemic sclerosis. Br J Dermatol. 158: 487–495.
32. Hirakata M, Suwa A, Takada T, Sato S, Nagai S, et al. (2007) Clinical and immunogenetic features of patients with autoantibodies to asparaginyl-transfer RNA synthetase. Arthritis Rheum. 56: 1295–1303.
33. Kuwana M, Kaburaki J, Mimori T, Tojo T, Homma M (1993) Antoantibody reactive with three classes of RNA polymerases in sera from patients with systemic sclerosis. J Clin Invest. 91: 1399–1404.
34. Moroi Y, Peebles C, Fritzler MJ, Steigerwald J, Tan EM (1980) Autoantibody to centromere (kinetochore) in scleroderma sera. Proc Natl Acad Sci U S A. 77: 1627–1631.
35. Vancsa A, Gergely L, Ponyi A, Lakos G, Nemeth J, et al. (2010) Myositis-specific and myositis-associated antibodies in overlap myositis in comparison to primary dermatopolymyositis: Relevance for clinical classification: retrospective study of 169 patients. Joint Bone Spine. 77: 125–130.
36. Bandoh S, Fujita J, Ohtsuki Y, Ueda Y, Hojo S, et al. (2000) Sequential changes of KL-6 in sera of patients with interstitial pneumonia associated with polymyositis/dermatomyositis. Ann Rheum Dis. 59: 257–262.
37. Honda Y, Kuroki Y, Matsuura E, Nagae H, Takahashi H, et al. (1995) Pulmonary surfactant protein D in sera and bronchoalveolar lavage fluids. Am J Respir Crit Care Med. 152: 1860–1866.
38. Matsushita T, Hasegawa M, Fujimoto M, Hamaguchi Y, Komura K, et al. (2007) Clinical evaluation of anti-aminoacyl tRNA synthetase antibodies in Japanese patients with dermatomyositis. J Rheumatol. 34: 1012–1018.
39. Mammen AL (2011) Autoimmune myopathies: autoantibodies, phenotypes and pathogenesis. Nat Rev Neurol. 7: 343–354.
40. Connors GR, Christopher-Stine L, Oddis CV, Danoff SK (2010) Interstitial lung disease associated with the idiopathic inflammatory myopathies: what progress has been made in the past 35 years? Chest. 138: 1464–1474.
41. Gunawardena H, Betteridge ZE, McHugh NJ (2009) Myositis-specific autoantibodies: their clinical and pathogenic significance in disease expression. Rheumatology (Oxford). 48: 607–612.

42. Zong M, Lundberg IE (2011) Pathogenesis, classification and treatment of inflammatory myopathies. Nat Rev Rheumatol. 7: 297–306.
43. Hirakata M, Nagai S (2000) Interstitial lung disease in polymyositis and dermatomyositis. Curr Opin Rheumatol. 12: 501–508.
44. Yoshifuji H, Fujii T, Kobayashi S, Imura Y, Fujita Y, et al. (2006) Anti-aminoacyl-tRNA synthetase antibodies in clinical course prediction of interstitial lung disease complicated with idiopathic inflammatory myopathies. Autoimmunity. 39: 233–241.
45. Katzap E, Barilla-LaBarca ML, Marder G (2011) Antisynthetase syndrome. Curr Rheumatol Rep. 13: 175–181.
46. Mimori T, Imura Y, Nakashima R, Yoshifuji H (2007) Autoantibodies in idiopathic inflammatory myopathy: an update on clinical and pathophysiological significance. Curr Opin Rheumatol. 19: 523–529.
47. Targoff IN, Trieu EP, Plotz PH, Miller FW (1992) Antibodies to glycyl-transfer RNA synthetase in patients with myositis and interstitial lung disease. Arthritis Rheum. 35: 821–830.
48. Watanabe K, Handa T, Tanizawa K, Hosono Y, Taguchi Y, et al. (2011) Detection of antisynthetase syndrome in patients with idiopathic interstitial pneumonias. Respir Med. 105: 1238–1247.
49. Yamasaki Y, Yamada H, Nozaki T, Akaogi J, Nichols C, et al. (2006) Unusually high frequency of autoantibodies to PL-7 associated with milder muscle disease in Japanese patients with polymyositis/dermatomyositis. Arthritis Rheum. 54: 2004–2009.
50. Targoff IN, Arnett FC (1990) Clinical manifestations in patients with antibody to PL-12 antigen (alanyl-tRNA synthetase). Am J Med. 88: 241–251.
51. Sato S, Kuwana M, Hirakata M (2007) Clinical characteristics of Japanese patients with anti-OJ (anti-isoleucyl-tRNA synthetase) autoantibodies. Rheumatology (Oxford). 46: 842–845.

5

T Follicular Helper Cells and Regulatory B Cells Dynamics in Systemic Lupus Erythematosus

Xue Yang[1,2,3], Ji Yang[4], Yiwei Chu[5], Yu Xue[1,2,3], Dandan Xuan[1,2,3], Shucong Zheng[1,2,3], Hejian Zou[1,2,3*]

1 Division of Rheumatology, Huashan Hospital, Fudan University, Shanghai, China, 2 Institute of Rheumatology,Immunology and Allergy, Fudan University, Shanghai, China, 3 Institute of Molecular and Translational Medicine, Huashan Hospital, Fudan University, 4 Department of Dermatology, Zhongshan Hospital, Fudan University, Shanghai, China, 5 Department of Immunology, Shanghai Medical College, Fudan University, Shanghai, China

Abstract

T follicular helper (Tfh) cells aid effector B cells, and augment autoimmunity, whereas the role of Tfh cells on regulatory B (Breg) cells in systemic lupus erythematosus (SLE) is not known. The aim of this study is to investigate the percentage of Breg cells in SLE, and the role of Tfh cells on Breg cells. First, we demonstrated the presence of Breg cells in SLE peripheral blood mononuclear cells and in involved skins. Both the percentage of circulating Breg cells and the ability to produce interleukin-10 (IL-10) were elevated in SLE patients. The percentage of Breg cells increased during SLE flares and decreased following disease remission. Second, Tfh cell expansion was not only related to autoantibody production but also correlated with the increased percentage of Breg cells. Third, in vitro studies revealed that Tfh cell-derived IL-21 could promote IL-10 production and Breg cell differentiation. In conclusions, these data imply that SLE flares may be linked to the expansion of Tfh cells and that Breg cells are increased in a regulatory feedback manner. Thus, SLE development may be associated with the complex regulation of Tfh cells and diverse B cell subsets.

Editor: Frederic Rieux-Laucat, Pavillon Kirmisson, France

Funding: This work was supported by grants from National Natural Science Foundation of China (No. 81373213, 81072463, 81000693), Program of Shanghai Subject Chief Scientist (No. 11XD1401100), and Medical Guide Project from Shanghai Science and Technology Committee (No. 134119a8400). The funders had no role in study design, data collection and analysis, decision to publish, or preparation of the manuscript.

Competing Interests: The authors have declared that no competing interests exist.

* E-mail: hejianzou@gmail.com

These authors contributed equally to this work.

Introduction

Systemic lupus erythematosus (SLE) is an autoimmune disease that involves multiple organ systems [1]. The pathogenic mechanisms that cause lupus are unclear; however, the immune balance between regulatory T or B lymphocytes and effector T and B lymphocytes may be disturbed, contributing to the autoimmune injuries in SLE [2,3,4,5].

Interleukin (IL)-10-producing regulatory B (Breg) cells have recently been identified. These cells, which represent 1~3% of adult mouse spleen B cells, predominantly represent a subset of $CD19^{+}CD5^{+}CD1d^{high}$ B cells and function to negatively regulate immune responses [3,6,7]. The absence or loss of Breg cells exacerbates disease symptoms in contact hypersensitivity, experimental autoimmune encephalomyelitis, chronic colitis, and collagen-induced arthritis models [8,9,10,11]. IL-10 is a key cytokine produced by Breg cells, and diminished disease severity was observed following administration of IL-10 in the NZM2410 mouse model of lupus [12], whereas more severe disease occurred in both MRL/lpr mice on a IL-10 KO background and in Breg cell-deficient NZB/W mice [13,14]. The finding that transfer of IL-10-secreting $CD21^{hi}CD23^{hi}$ B cells mitigates disease in MRL/lpr mice [15] further suggests that B cell-derived IL-10 limits disease activity. Although several studies showed that Breg cells were present in lupus-prone mice, including MRL/lpr and NZW mice [6,13,16], the dynamic change of Breg cells in SLE patients is not clear, and the mechanism of Breg cell differentiation in SLE patients is unknown.

T follicular helper (Tfh) cells, a subset of $CD4^{+}$ T cells found in germinal centers (GCs), express high levels of C-X-C chemokine receptor type 5 (CXCR5), programmed death-1 (PD-1), and inducible costimulatory molecule (ICOS) [17,18,19]. Recently, expanded circulating Tfh cells were characterized as $CD4^{+}CXCR5^{+}ICOS^{high}PD\text{-}1^{high}$ in peripheral blood mononuclear cells (PBMCs) from SLE patients [20]. In addition, production of the CXCR5 ligand CXCL13 was also found to be elevated in SLE patients [21]. IL-21 is a key cytokine produced by Tfh cells [18,19]. Our previous study demonstrated that the genotype and allele frequencies for copy number amplifications of IL-21 are significantly higher in SLE patients than in healthy controls [22]. Tfh cell-derived IL-21 is thought to drive the differentiation of B cells to produce antibodies, a process that serves as an important regulator of humoral immune responses [19,23]. Recent studies showed that IL-21 is a pleiotropic cytokine, at least under specific circumstances, IL-21 can also exert anti-inflammatory actions due to its ability to inhibit dendritic cell maturation and stimulate IL-10 production in T cells [24,25]. Our recent study proved that Tfh cell-derived IL-21 could promote the differentiation of Breg cells in lupus-prone MRL/lpr mice [16], however the relationship between Tfh and Breg cells in SLE patients is not known. Whether Tfh cell-derived IL-21 may also play a key role in the differentiation of Breg cells in SLE patients need be clarified.

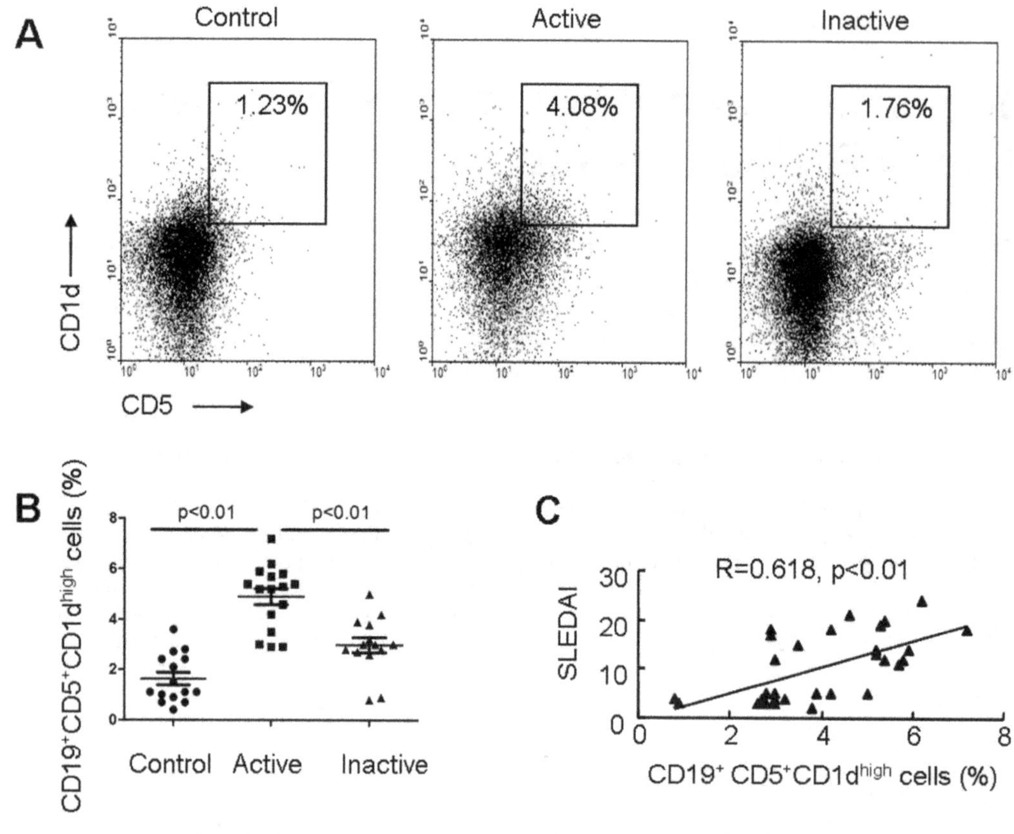

Figure 1. Expansion of circulating Breg cells in SLE patients. (A) Human PBMCs were labeled with lymphocyte-specific antibodies (CD19, CD5, and CD1d). The percentage of $CD5^+CD1d^{high}$ cells among a CD19 gate was determined by flow cytometry. (B) Results of flow cytometric analysis of Breg cells in patients with active SLE (n = 16), patients with inactive SLE (n = 14), and control subject (n = 15). (C) A positive correlation between the proportion of $CD5^+CD1d^{high}$ cells among $CD19^+$ B cells and the clinical severity of the flare as scored using the SLEDAI (n = 30) was observed.

Here, we provided evidence that Breg cells were present among PBMCs and involved skins in SLE patients. In detailed studies of Breg and Tfh cells from 30 SLE patients, we showed that Breg cells exhibited expansion rather than redistribution *in vivo*, and this expansion of Breg cells was related to disease activity. Further study demonstrated that expansion of Breg cells was related to Tfh cells in SLE. Tfh cell-derived IL-21 could promote IL-10 production and the differentiation of Breg cells. These data suggest that Tfh cell-derived IL-21 may induce the production of the anti-inflammatory cytokine IL-10 and result in expansion of Breg cells in SLE. Thus, the pathophysiology of SLE may be linked to a complex immune relationship between Tfh cells and diverse B subsets.

Results

Breg Cells are Expanded in SLE

Since $CD19^+CD5^+CD1d^{high}$ B cells with the capacity to negatively regulate immune responses have previously been named Breg cells [3,6,26,27], we investigated these lymphocyte subgroups in 30 patients with SLE, including 16 active SLE patients and 14 inactive SLE patients. 15 healthy individuals were also included. The percentages of circulating $CD19^+CD5^+CD1d^{high}$ B cells were measured by flow cytometry (Figure 1A). The percentage of circulating Breg cells was significantly increased in patients with active SLE (4.9±1.27%, n = 16) compared to inactive SLE (2.98±1.23%, n = 14) and healthy controls (1.63±0.99%, n = 15; Figure 1B). Furthermore, comparison of the percentage of Breg cells with the disease activity revealed a positive correlation between Breg cells and the SLEDAI value ($R = 0.618$, $p<0.01$, n = 30. Figure 1C). Although the absolute numbers of Breg cells were not significantly different between SLE patients and healthy controls, a positive correlation between absolute numbers of Breg cells and SLEDAI value was also detected (Figure S1A, B).

So far, other human Breg subsets have been described, namely $CD24^{high}CD27^{high}$ and $CD24^{high}CD38^{high}$ Breg cells in human and autoimmunity disease [28,29]. Paul A Blair, et al showed that the percentage of $CD24^{high}CD38^{high}$ Breg cells was expanded in SLE, but displayed similar numbers of $CD24^{high}CD38^{high}$ Breg cells compared with healthy controls [29]. In our study, we observed that the percentages of $CD19^+CD24^+CD38^+$ Breg cells were expanded in SLE patients than healthy controls, the absolute numbers were not significantly different between these two group (Figure S1C, D).

Breg cells with the capacity to produce IL-10 are also named B10 cells. To further investigate these B cell subgroups, we focused on the $IL\text{-}10^+$ B cells in involved skins. Using immunohistochemistry, we analyzed skins from 10 SLE patients. The SLE patient samples exhibited typical pathological changes of lupus that the cornified layer exhibits patchy follicular plugging, lymphocytic interface dermatitis is seen, associated with basal layer keratinocytes degeneration, superficial and deep perivascular and periadnexal lymphocytic infiltration (Figure 2A, upper panel), including a large number of infiltrating $CD20^+$ B cells (Figure 2A, middle panel). Examination of the $IL\text{-}10^+$ cells in consecutive levels obtained by serially section confirmed that IL-10^+ B cells were present (Figure 2A, lower panel, and Figure S2A). The presence of $CD20^+IL\text{-}10^+$ B cells in skin of SLE patient was further confirmed by immunofluorescence analysis (Figure S2B). These data indicate that Breg cells are present and expanded in SLE patients.

Breg Cells Produce more IL-10 in SLE

IL-10 is a key cytokine produced by Breg cells [3,9], our data showed that IL-10 mRNA was expressed at higher levels in PBMCs from active SLE patients than that in inactive SLE patients and healthy controls (Figure 3A). Furthermore, we confirmed that the secretion of IL-10 in sera from active SLE patients was significantly higher than that in sera from inactive patients and healthy controls (Figure 3B). Although our results implied that circulating Breg cells were expanded during the SLE disease process, multiple cell types can produce IL-10 [30], thus we further analyzed whether Breg cells in SLE patients have more ability of IL-10 production. We first proved that $CD19^+IL\text{-}10^+$ B cells were present in PBMCs of SLE patients by fluorescence microscopy (Figure S3A). Further study showed that the percentage of circulating $CD19^+IL\text{-}10^+$ B cells was expanded in patients with active SLE (3.44±0.69%, n = 6) than that of healthy controls (1.15±0.45%, n = 6, Figure 3C), while the absolute numbers of $CD19^+IL\text{-}10^+$ B cells were not significantly different between SLE patients and healthy controls (Figure S3B). Further examination revealed that IL-10 mRNA expression and protein secretion in sorted $CD19^+CD5^+CD1d^{high}$ Breg cells from SLE patient was higher than that in sorted Breg cells from healthy control (Figure 3D, E). All together, these data suggest that Breg cells form SLE patients have more potential to produce IL-10.

Tfh Cells are Related to the Expansion of Breg Cells in SLE

Tfh cells, a subset of $CD4^+$ T cells, are well described as $CXCR5^+PD\text{-}1^+$ and mainly produce IL-21 [17,18,31]. We first detected $CXCR5^+PD\text{-}1^+$ T cells in PBMCs of SLE patients by fluorescence microscopy (Figure S4A). The percentage of circulating Tfh cells in PBMCs of patients with SLE was determined by flow cytometry. Our data showed that the percentage of Tfh cells was significantly increased in active SLE patients (4.11±1.17%, n = 16) compared with inactive SLE patients (2.19±0.47%, $p<0.01$, n = 14) and healthy controls (1.49±0.48%, $p<0.01$, n = 15; Figure 4A). Furthermore, we also found a positive correlation between percentage of Tfh cells and the SLEDAI ($R = 0.894$, $p<0.01$, n = 30. Figure 4B). Interesting, a strong positive correlation between the proportion of Tfh cells and Breg cells in SLE patients was also found ($R = 0.630$, $p<0.01$, n = 30. Figure 4C). However the absolute numbers of Tfh cells were not significantly different between SLE patients and healthy controls (Figure S4B).

Our data confirmed that the secretion of IL-21 in sera from active SLE patients was significantly higher than that in sera from inactive SLE patients and healthy controls (Figure 4D). The ds-DNA titers in sera of SLE patients were checked by ELISA, and a positive correlation between serum IL-21 levels and ds-DNA titers in sera of SLE patients was detected (data not shown). In addition, a strong positive correlation between the IL-21 and IL-10 serum levels in SLE patients was observed ($R = 0.817$, $p<0.01$, n = 30. Figure 4E). These data indicate that Tfh cells are expanded in SLE patients and that Tfh cells may be involved in the expansion of Breg cells in SLE patients.

Tfh Cell-derived IL-21 Promotes IL-10 Production during the Differentiation of Breg Cells

Our data showed that IL-21 could promote IL-10 secretion during the differentiation of Breg cells (Figure 5A). Furthermore, IL-21 in concert with LPS and PIB promoted the differentiation of $CD19^+IL\text{-}10^+$ B cells (Figure 5B), which is consistent with the recently Nature published results that IL-21 is important for Breg cell expansion and IL-10 production [32]. To determine whether Tfh cell-derived IL-21 from SLE patients induces IL-10 production during the differentiation of Breg cells, $CD4^+CXCR5^+PD\text{-}1^+$ Tfh cells were first sorted from PBMCs of active SLE patients and

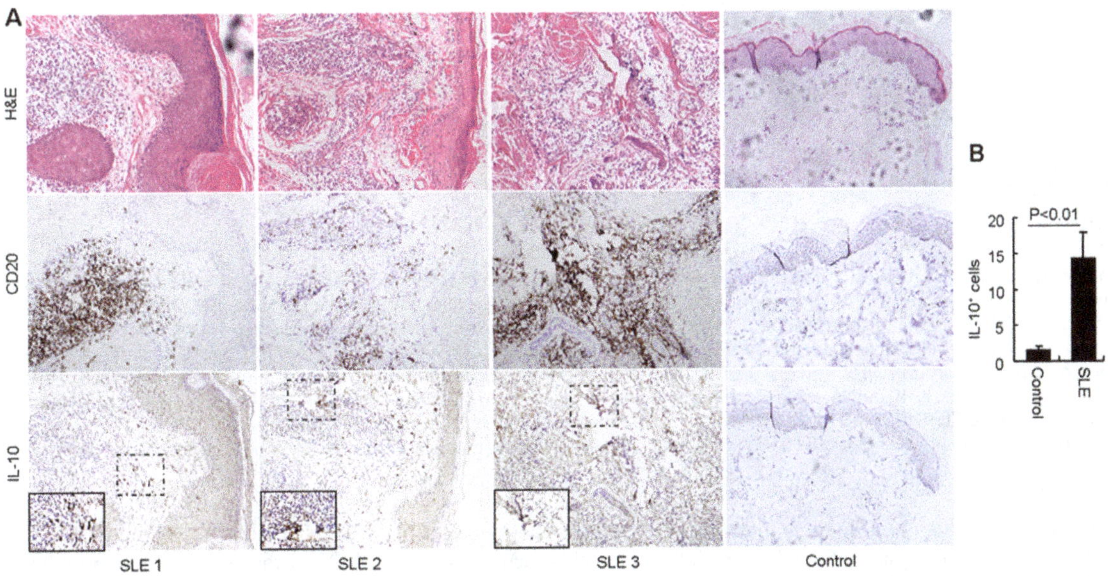

Figure 2. Infiltration of IL-10^+ B cells in involved skin of SLE patients. (A) Consecutive levels obtained by serially section showed typical pathological changes of lupus (upper panel), lymphocytes infiltration confirmed by CD20 (middle panel) and IL-10 (lower panel) immunohistochemical staining (× 100 magnification). Further magnification of the black-bordered box shows typical IL-10^+ lymphocytes (×400 magnification). (B) The counts of IL-10^+ lymphocytes in skins were showed in right (SLE patients n = 10, healthy controls n = 4).

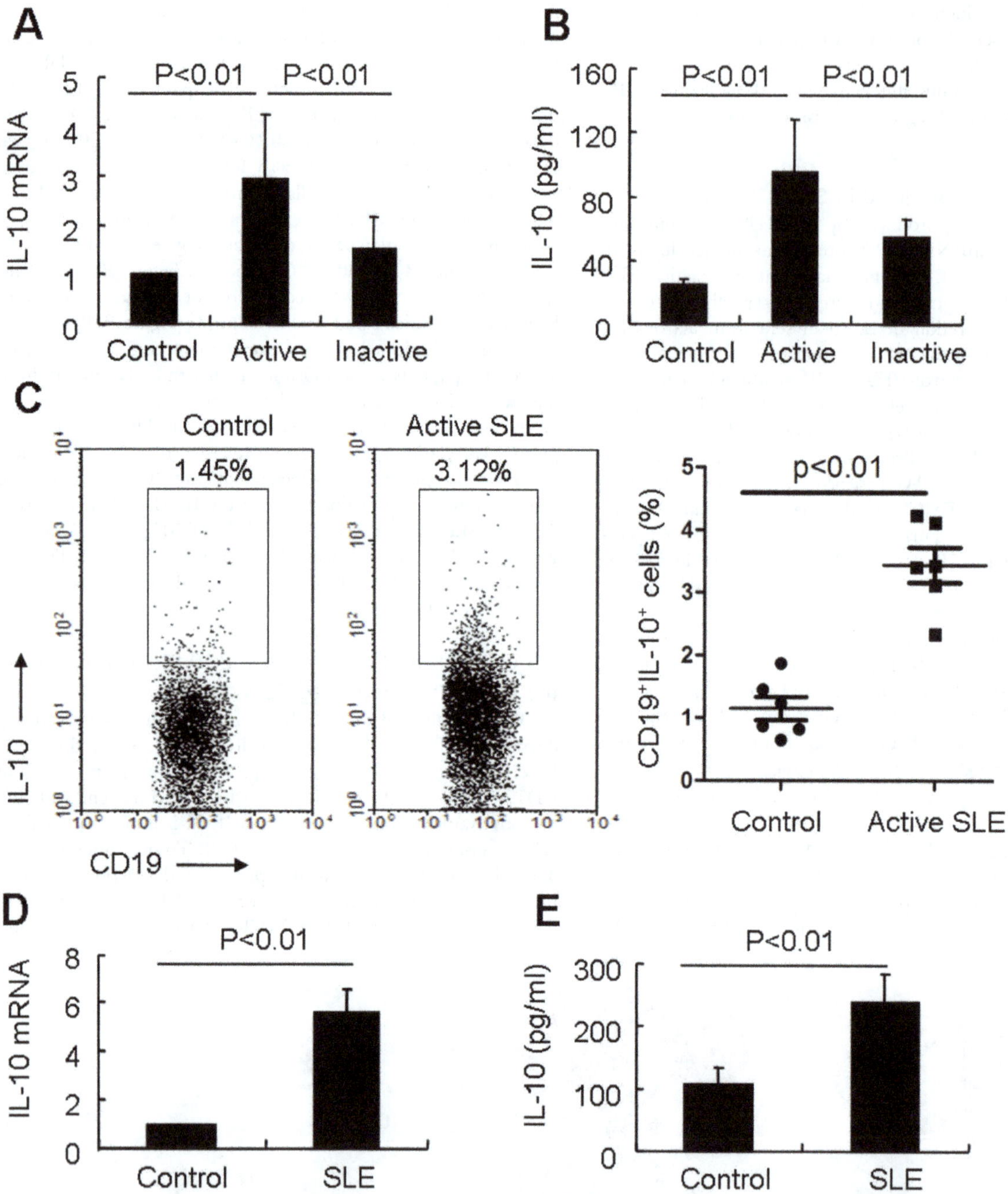

Figure 3. IL-10 production in Breg cells of SLE patients. (A) Real-time RT-PCR analysis of IL-10 mRNA expression in PBMCs from patients with active SLE (n = 16), patients with inactive SLE (n = 14), and control subject (n = 15). (B) Serum levels of IL-10 were detected in patients with active SLE (n = 16), patients with inactive SLE (n = 14), and control subject (n = 15) by ELISA. (C) PBMCs were isolated and stimulated with LPS for 24 hours and PIB for the final 5 hours. $CD19^+IL-10^+$ cells were detected by flow cytometry analysis in a CD19 gate (left). Results of flow cytometric analysis of $CD19^+IL-10^+$ cells (right, n = 6 for each group). (D) Sorted $CD19^+CD5^+CD1d^{high}$ B cells from SLE patients and healthy controls were stimulated with LPS for 24 hours and PIB for the last 5 hours. IL-10 mRNA expression was detected by real-time RT-PCR. Results shown are representative of at least three independent experiments. (E) Sorted $CD19^+CD5^+CD1d^{high}$ B cells from SLE patients and healthy controls were stimulated with LPS for 24 hours and PI for the last 5 hours. IL-10 in supernatants was detected by ELISA. Results shown are representative of at least three independent experiments.

healthy controls and stimulated with anti-CD3 and anti-CD28 for 48 hours. IL-21 secretion in the supernatants of the cultured Tfh cells from active SLE patients was significantly higher than that from Tfh cells from healthy controls ($p<0.01$. Figure 5C). We next examined the effects of the supernatants from cultured Tfh cells on IL-10 production during the differentiation of Breg cells. Supernatants from Tfh cells of SLE patients promoted IL-10 production during Breg cell differentiation (Figure 5D). More notably, neutralization of IL-21 in the culture medium inhibited IL-10 secretion by Breg cells (Figure 5D). Furthermore, the supernatants from Tfh cells of SLE patients promoted $CD19^+IL-10^+$ cell differentiation, and neutralization of IL-21 in the culture medium inhibited this differentiation of Breg cells (Figure 5E). The results were further confirmed that the supernatants from Tfh cells

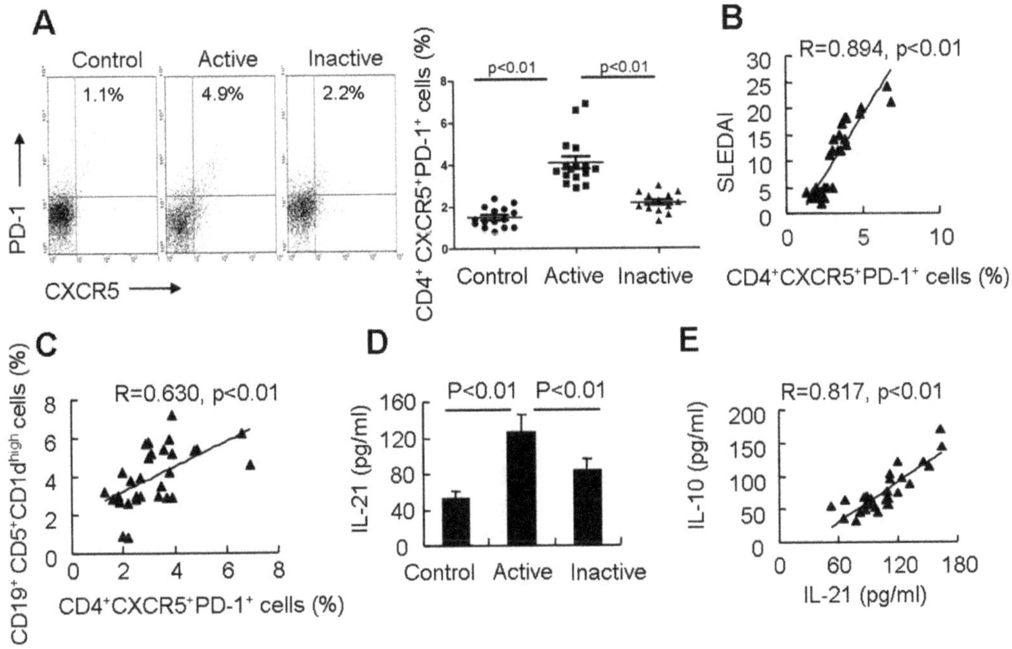

Figure 4. Tfh cells are associated with expansion of Breg cells in SLE patients. (A) Human PBMCs were labeled with lymphocyte-specific antibodies (CD4, CXCR5 and PD-1). The percentage of $CXCR5^+PD\text{-}1^+$ cells among $CD4^+$ T cells was analyzed by flow cytometry (left). Results of flow cytometric analysis of Tfh cells (right) in patients with active SLE (n = 16), patients with inactive SLE (n = 14), and control subject (n = 15). (B) A positive correlation between the proportion of $CXCR5^+PD\text{-}1^+$ cells among $CD4^+$ T cells and the clinical severity of the flare as scored using the SLEDAI (n = 30) was noted. (C) A positive correlation between the proportion of $CD4^+CXCR5^+PD\text{-}1^+$ T cells and $CD19^+CD5^+CD1d^{high}$ B cells in PBMCs from SLE patients (n = 30) was observed. (D) Serum IL-21 levels were detected in patients with active SLE (n = 16), patients with inactive SLE (n = 14), and control subject (n = 15) by ELISA. (E) A positive correlation between serum IL-10 levels and IL-21 levels in SLE patients (n = 30) was observed.

of SLE patients promoted part of $CD20^+CD27^-$ naïve B cells differentiate into IL-10^+ cells in the presence of LPS plus PIB (Figure S5). These data suggest that Breg cells are responsive to the stimulation by IL-21 that is produced by SLE patient-derived Tfh cells.

Taken together, these data confirmed that Tfh cells and Breg cells are expanded in SLE patients and that these cell subsets are correlated in these patients as well. Tfh cell-derived IL-21 may be involved in Breg cell expansion and IL-10 overproduction in SLE patients.

Discussion

The ability of B cells to negatively regulate cellular immune responses and inflammation has been described previously [7]. Most recently, $CD19^+CD5^+CD1d^{high}$ B cells with the capacity to produce IL-10 have been named Breg cells (B10) in mice [3,6,7]. Remarkably, Breg cells are potent negative regulators of inflammation and autoimmunity in mouse models of disease *in vivo* [10,11,33]. Recently, IL-10-producing $CD1d^{high}$, or $CD5^+$IL-10^+ Breg cells were identified in human [26,27,34], however little is known the dynamic changes of Breg cells in active or inactive SLE patient.

The balance between Breg cell negative regulation and B-cell positive contributions to immune responses are likely to vary in different diseases as well as during the course of disease. Breg cell numbers increase during some autoimmunity animal models like NZB/W mice [6,13], our recent data proved that Breg cells were expanded in MRL/lpr mice [16]. Here, we demonstrated that the percentage of peripheral blood $CD19^+CD5^+CD1d^{high}$ Breg cells was significantly increased in active SLE patients and was positively correlated with disease activity, Breg cells decreased during disease relief. Breg cells produced more IL-10 in active SLE patients than healthy control. In addition, more IL-10^+ B cells were detected in involved skin of SLE patients when compared with controls. In addition, the percentage of $CD19^+CD24^+CD38^+$ Breg cells was also expanded in SLE patients than heanlty control, which was consistent with previous results [29]. The absolute numbers of $CD19^+CD5^+CD1d^{high}$ cells, $CD19^+CD24^+CD38^+$ cells, and $CD19^+$IL-10^+ cells increased but not significantly in SLE patients when compared with healthy controls, which might be attributed to peripheral lymphopenia in SLE patients during flares.

The percentage of Breg cells was expanded in SLE patients and decreased following remission than in healthy controls, these data suggested that Breg cells are dynamic during the development of autoimmunity. Maintaining immunological balance involves the capacity of the immune system to upregulate immunosuppressive responses, which may limit deterioration by the autoimmune response. The upregulation of Breg cells in active SLE patients may reflect a regulatory feedback mechanism to restore cellular tolerance and ameliorate harmful autoimmune responses.

B10 cells were functionally identified by their ability to express cytoplasmic IL-10 after 5 hours of ex vivo stimulation, whereas progenitor B10 (B10pro) cells required 48 hours of in vitro stimulation before they acquired the ability to express IL-10. Recent study showed that the percentages of B10 cells in SLE patients were not significantly different from controls, but the percentages of B10+Bpro cells in SLE patients were significantly different from controls [28], these data implied that B cells in SLE have more potential to produce IL-10. In our study, modified methods were taken, the B cells were stimulated with LPS 24 hours and the last 5 hours of PIB stimulation, which was based on the previous reported methods [6]. Consistent with previous results

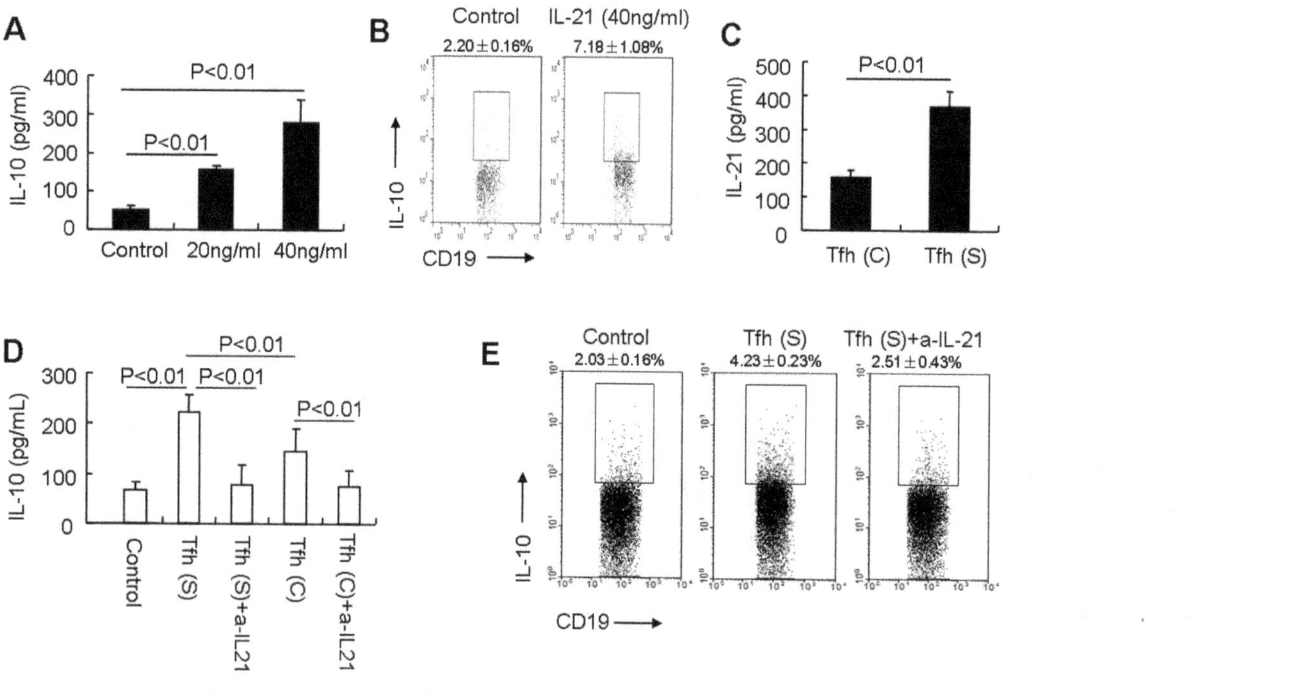

Figure 5. Tfh cell-derived IL-21 promotes IL-10 production during the differentiation of Breg cells. (A) Sorted B cells (CD43 depletion) from healthy controls were cultured in the presence of LPS and the indicated concentrations of IL-21 for 48 hours followed by stimulation with PI for the final 5 hours (Control: LPS+PIB). IL-10 in supernatants was detected by ELISA. Results shown are representative of at least three independent experiments. (B) Sorted B cells (CD43 depletion) from healthy controls were cultured in the presence of LPS with or without 40 ng/ml IL-21 for 48 hours followed by stimulation with PIB for the last 5 hours (Control: LPS+PIB). IL-10^+ cells were analyzed in a CD19 gate by flow cytometry. Results shown are representative of at least three independent experiments. (C) Sorted $CD4^+CXCR5^+PD\text{-}1^+$ T cells were cultured with anti-CD3 and anti-CD28 for 48 hours, IL-21 was detected in the supernatants by ELISA. Results shown are representative of at least three independent experiments (C: healthy controls; S: SLE patients). (D) Sorted B cells (CD43 depletion) were stimulated for 48 hours with LPS plus supernatants from cultures of Tfh cells of SLE patients with or without neutralization of IL-21. The cells were also stimulated with PI for the last 5 hours. Levels of IL-10 in the supernatants were determined by ELISA (Control: LPS+PI; Tfh (S): LPS+supernatants from Tfh cells of SLE patients+PI; Tfh (C): LPS+supernatants from Tfh cells of healthy controls+PI). Results shown are representative of at least three independent experiments. (E) Sorted B cells (CD43 depletion) were cultured for 48 hours in the presence of LPS plus supernatants from Tfh cells of SLE patients. These cells were cultured with or without neutralization of IL-21 and were stimulated with PIB for the last 5 hours (Control: LPS+PIB; Tfh (S): LPS+supernatants from Tfh cells of SLE patients+PIB). IL-10^+ cells were analyzed by flow cytometry with a CD19 gate. Results shown are representative of at least three independent experiments.

[28,35], our study confirmed that both IL-10 production and the percentage of $CD19^+IL\text{-}10^+$ B cells were increased in SLE patients; however, the reason behind this expansion of Breg cells in SLE was not addressed in the previous studies [28]. Our data showed that the absolute numbers of $CD4^+CXCR5^+PD\text{-}1^+$ Tfh cells were not significantly increased in SLE patients than in healthy controls, however the percentage of $CD4^+CXCR5^+PD\text{-}1^+$ Tfh cells were expanded in active SLE patients and that Tfh cell-derived IL-21 contributed to autoantibody production. Further analysis showed that the percentage of Tfh cells was positively related to disease activity in SLE, which suggested that Tfh cells may contribute to autoimmunity by helping B effector cells and inducing humoral immunity [19,36]. Secondly, we unexpectedly identified a strong positive correlation between Tfh cells and Breg cells in SLE patients, suggesting that Tfh cells may contribute to the expansion of Breg cells in SLE. Our *in vitro* data further revealed that SLE patient Tfh cell-derived IL-21 in synergy with LPS and PI promoted IL-10 production and the differentiation of Breg cells. This finding was verified as treatment of these cultures with an IL-21-neutralizing antibody inhibited IL-10 production and the generation of $CD19^+IL\text{-}10^+$ cells. IL-21 is a pleiotropic cytokine, and at least under certain circumstances, IL-21 can stimulate anti-inflammatory IL-10 production in T and B cells [24,25,32,37]. The generation of T and B subsets during autoimmune disease requires complex and reciprocal regulation; thus, micro-environmental cytokines or other factors may be involved in the development of pro-inflammatory or anti-inflammatory lymphocyte subsets. Our data suggest that Tfh cells facilitate immune homeostasis by increasing the number of regulatory B cells and the production of IL-10 via the stimulation of IL-21 in SLE patients.

All together, we define a novel role of Tfh cells in immune regulatory actions to promote production of the immunosuppressive cytokine IL-10, which extends the existing recognization that Tfh cells merely induce humoral responses and augment autoimmunity. Furthermore, IL-21 may serve as a potential upstream promoter for Breg cell differentiation and IL-10 production in SLE. These findings suggest that particular emphasis should be given to the regulatory function of Tfh cells and IL-21 in the treatment of SLE.

Materials and Methods

SLE Patients and Healthy Controls

This study was approved by the Ethical Committee of Huashan Hospital and Zhongshan Hospital, Fudan University (Shanghai, People's Republic of China). Thirty consecutive adult patients (28 women and 2 men, mean age 37.6±12.3 years) with a diagnosis of SLE, based on the American College of Rheumatology 1997 revised criteria [38], were included in the study. All patients enrolled in the study after giving informed and written consent. All SLE patients were referred to the Division of Rheumatology, Huashan Hospital or to the Department of Dermatology, Zhongshan Hospital, Fudan University, Shanghai, China. Disease activity was assessed by the SLE Disease Activity Index (SLEDAI). One group comprised subjects with active SLE (SLEDAI ≥6, n = 16, mean age 35.9±12.0 years, 15 women and 1 man), while the second group comprised subjects with inactive SLE (SLEDAI <6, n = 14, mean age 39.6±12.7 years, 13 women and 1 man) [2]. The following treatment was provided for the SLE group: prednisone, hydroxychloroquine+prednisone, or hydroxychloroquine +prednisone+cyclophosphamide. For the control group, 15 age and sex matched healthy individuals (mean age 36.2±12.7 years; 14 women and 1 man) were enrolled after giving informed consent. The ages, sex, and treatments of the patients are presented in Table 1.

Table 1. Patient characteristics.

Sex	Age, y	Disease duration, y	Treatment	SLEDAI score
F	41	3	HCQ	3
F	20	2	HCQ+Pred 10 mg/d	4
F	43	3	HCQ+Pred 15 mg/d	5
F	61	16	Pred 15 mg/d	4
M	45	7	Pred 20 mg/d	3
F	21	2	Pred 12.5 mg/d	4
F	36	10	Pred 7.5 mg/d	2
F	34	1.5	Pred 20 mg/d	4
F	44	3	HCQ+Pred 12.5 mg/d	5
F	36	11	Pred 12.5 mg/d	5
F	52	14	Pred 15 mg/d	5
F	61	10	None	3
F	32	1	Pred 10 mg/d	3
F	29	3	HCQ+Pred 15 mg/d	5
F	20	0.8	HCQ+Pred 35 mg/d	17
F	21	1	HCQ+Pred 50 mg/d	24
F	45	0.3	HCQ+Pred 25 mg/d	11
F	56	20	Pred 25 mg/d	13
F	44	7	Pred 20 mg/d	19
F	28	10	Pred 10 mg/d	12
M	38	0.5	Pred 15 mg/d	12
F	34	0.4	Pred 20 mg/d	18
F	43	15	None	21
F	23	2.5	Pred 20.25 mg/d	15
F	56	12	Pred 15 mg/d+CTX	18
F	27	0.5	HCQ+Pred 30 mg/d	12
F	28	0.9	Pred 15 mg/d	18
F	27	1	HCQ+Pred 50 mg/d	20
F	51	3	HCQ+Pred 15 mg/d	14
F	33	2	Pred 20 mg/d	14

HCQ = hydroxychloroquine; Pred = prednisone; CTX = cyclophosphamide.

B and T Cell Isolation, Culture Conditions, and Differentiation

Human B cells were purified from PBMCs of healthy donors (CD43 depletion) by negative selection following the manufacturer's instructions (Miltenyi Biotec, Bergisch Gladbach, Germany). For the differentiation of Breg cells, purified B cells (2×10^6 cells/ml) were cultured in 10 μg/ml lipopolysaccharide (LPS; Sigma-Aldrich, St. Louis, MO) for 24 or 48 hours and stimulated with PIB (50 ng/ml phorbol 12-myristate 13-acetate [PMA], Sigma-Aldrich; 500 ng/ml ionomycin [Sigma-Aldrich]; and 20 μg/ml brefeldin A [BFA], eBioscience, San Diego, CA) for the last 5 hours, as previously described [6,28]. Where indicated, cultures were supplemented with indicated doses of IL-21 (PeproTech, RockyHill, NJ) and LPS for 48 hours, and stimulated with PIB for the last 5 hours. In experiments to detect IL-10 in culture supernatants, BFA was not added. For some experiments, $CD20^+CD27^-$ naïve B cells (eBioscience) were sorted from PBMCs of healthy donors by flow cytometry, and cultured in certain conditions.

To determine the effects of Tfh cell-derived IL-21 on the activation of Breg cells, $CD4^+CXCR5^+PD\text{-}1^+$ Tfh cells from active SLE patients were first sorted by flow cytometry. The resultant Tfh cells (2×10^6 cells/ml) were stimulated with 2 μg/ml plate-bound anti-CD3 and 2 μg/ml soluble anti-CD28 (eBioscience) for 48 hours. Supernatants were collected for later use. Purified B cells or naïve B cells (2×10^6 cells/ml) from healthy donors were cultured with 10 μg/ml LPS (Sigma-Aldrich) in the presence or absence of 20% supernatants from the above-stimulated Tfh cells or 20 μg/ml anti-IL-21 neutralizing antibody (eBioscience) for 48 hours. Culture media with the same doses of anti-CD3 and anti-CD28 was used as a vehicle control. Cultures were stimulated with PIB for the last 5 hours. $IL\text{-}10^+$ cells were analyzed by flow cytometry with a CD19 gate. In experiments to detect IL-10 in culture supernatants by enzyme-linked immunosorbent assay (ELISA), BFA was not added. For some experiments, $CD19^+CD5^+CD1d^{high}$ Breg cells (4×10^5 cells) were obtained via cell sorting from PBMCs of SLE patients and healthy controls and were then cultured in the presence of LPS for 24 hours and PIB for the last 5 hours for the detection of IL-10 mRNA expression. For detecting IL-10 in culture supernatants, BFA was not added.

ELISA

Sera from SLE patients and healthy controls were collected and frozen at −80°C until needed. Concentrations of anti-double-stranded DNA (anti-dsDNA) were determined by ELISA (R&D, Minneapolis, MN). Serum levels of IL-21 and IL-10 in SLE patients were also detected by commercial ELISA (eBioscience). In some experiments, isolated B cells (5×10^5 cells) were cultured and stimulated with PMA and ionomycin (PI, Sigma-Aldrich) for the last 5 hours. IL-10 was detected in the supernatants by ELISA (eBioscience). Sorted $CD4^+CXCR5^+PD\text{-}1^+$ Tfh cells (5×10^5 cells) were stimulated with 2 μg/ml plate-bound anti-CD3 and 2 μg/ml soluble anti-CD28 (eBioscience) for 48 hours. IL-21 in supernatants was detected by ELISA (eBioscience).

Flow Cytometry

For detection of Tfh cells, human PBMCs were stained with Alexa Fluor 647-conjugated anti-CD4, Alexa Fluor 488-conjugated anti-CXCR5, and phycoerythrin (PE)-conjugated anti-PD-1 (all from BD Pharmingen, San Jose, CA). Cells were gated for $CD4^+$ T cells first and then for $CXCR5^+PD\text{-}1^+$ Tfh cells. For detection of Breg cells, PBMCs were stained with PerCP/Cy5.5-conjugated anti-CD19, fluorescein isothiocyanate (FITC)-conjugated anti-

CD5, and PE-conjugated anti-CD1d (eBioscience) for 15 minutes. $CD5^+CD1d^{high}$ cells were analyzed with a $CD19^+$ gate.

For intracellular IL-10 staining, PBMCs were incubated for 24 hours with 10 μg/ml LPS and stimulated with PIB for the last 5 hours. Surface staining with PerCP/Cy5.5-conjugated CD19 or FITC-conjugated anti-CD5 was first performed for 15 min, and cells were re-suspended in Fixation/Permeabilization solution (Invitrogen). Intracellular staining of PE-conjugated anti-IL-10 was performed according to the manufacturer's protocol (eBioscience). After staining, $IL\text{-}10^+$ cells were analyzed with a $CD19^+$ gate by flow cytometry. For some experiments, cells were stained with FITC-conjugated CD19 and PE-conjugated anti-IL-10 (eBioscience) and detected by immunofluorescence microscopy.

Immunohistochemistry

Skin biopsies from 10 SLE patients were obtained after informed consent, 4 normal skin biopsies (Three skin biopsies were from healthy donors after informed consent, one tissue was obtained from orthopedic surgery after informed consent) were used as controls. Tissues were processed and embedded in paraffin using routine methods. Tissue blocks were serially sectioned to obtain consecutive levels. Sections were stained with hematoxylin and eosin, and immunohistochemistry with the following antibodies was performed as previously described [2]. Antibodies to CD20 and IL-10 (Abcam, Cambridge, MA) were used. Immunohistochemical staining was assessed by two independent pathologists without knowledge of patient characteristics. The positive cells in per surface were counted under ×400 magnification, and five randomly selected independent microscopic fields were counted for each sample to ensure that the data were representative and homogeneous.

Analyses of Cytokine and Transcription Factor mRNA Expression

Total RNA was purified with the Trizol reagent (Invitrogen). cDNAs were synthesized using Primescript RT Master Mix Perfect Real-time Kit (TaKaRa, Tokyo, Japan), and mRNA expression was determined with the Bio-Rad iCycler 7500 Optical System (Bio-Rad, Richmond, CA) using a SYBR Premix EX Taq Real-time PCR Master Mix (TaKaRa). The $2^{-\Delta\Delta Ct}$ method was used to normalize transcription to β-actin and to calculate the fold induction relative to controls. The following primer pairs were used: Hum β-actin, forward ATCATGTTTGAGACCTTCAACA and reverse CATCTCTTGCTCGAAGTCCA and Hum IL-10, forward GAAGTGAAAACGAGACCAAGGT and reverse CTGCAAGTTAGATCCTCAGG.

Statistical Analyses

Results were expressed as means ± standard deviation. The statistical significance was determined by analysis of variance for comparisons of multiple means followed by the Bonferroni post hoc test, or the Student's *t*-test, and the Mann-Whitney U-test. Correlations were determined by Spearman's ranking.

Supporting Information

Figure S1 The absolute numbers of Breg cells in SLE patients. (A) The results of flow cytometric analysis of absolute numbers of $CD19^+CD5^+CD1d^{high}$ cells in patients with SLE (n = 30) and healthy controls (n = 15). (B) A positive correlation between the absolute numbers of $CD19^+$ $CD5^+CD1d^{high}$ cells and the clinical severity of the flare as scored using the SLEDAI (n = 30) was observed. (C) Human PBMCs were labeled with lymphocyte-specific antibodies (CD19, CD24, and CD38). The percentage of $CD24^+CD38^+$ cells among a CD19 gate was determined by flow cytometry (left). Results of flow cytometric analysis of percentage of $CD24^+CD38^+$ cells among a CD19 gate cells in patients with SLE and control subject (right, n = 7 for each group). (D) The results of flow cytometric analysis of absolute numbers of $CD19^+CD24^+CD38^+$ cells in patients with SLE and healthy controls (n = 7 for each group).

Figure S2 $IL\text{-}10^+$ cells in skins of SLE patients. (A) The skin tissues from SLE patient were serially sectioned to obtain consecutive levels. The sections were stained with antibodies to IL-10 and isotype control. (B) The skin tissues from SLE patient were stained with CD20 and IL-10, the $CD20^+IL\text{-}10^+$ cells were analyzed by immunofluorescence microscopy.

Figure S3 $IL\text{-}10^+$ cells in PBMCs of SLE patients. (A) PBMCs were isolated and stimulated with LPS for 24 hours and PIB for the final 5 hours. The presence of $CD19^+IL\text{-}10^+$ cells in PBMCs from active SLE patients was detected by immunofluorescence microscopy. The arrow indicates typical positive cells. (B) $CD19^+IL\text{-}10^+$ cells were detected by flow cytometry analysis in a CD19 gate (n = 6 for each group).

Figure S4 Tfh cells in PBMCs of SLE patients. (A) The presence of $CXCR5^+PD\text{-}1^+$ cells in PBMCs of active SLE patients was detected by immunofluorescence microscopy. The arrow indicates the typical positive cells. (B) The results of flow cytometric analysis of absolute numbers of $CD4^+CXCR5^+PD\text{-}1^+$ cells in patients with SLE (n = 30) and healthy controls (n = 15).

Figure S5 Tfh cell-derived IL-21 promotes the differentiation of Breg cells. Sorted $CD20^+CD27^-$ naïve B cells were cultured for 48 hours in the presence of LPS plus supernatants from Tfh cells of SLE patients. These cells were cultured with or without neutralization of IL-21 and were stimulated with PIB for the last 5 hours (Control: LPS+PIB; Tfh (S): LPS+supernatants from Tfh cells of SLE patients+PIB). $IL\text{-}10^+$ cells among the sorted B cells were analyzed by flow cytometry. Results shown are representative of at least three independent experiments.

Acknowledgments

We thank Prof. Xiao Kang Li, Prof. Liwei Lv and Song Guo Zheng for their precious suggestions and comments. We thank Huiming Ren, Weizhe Ma, Xiaoye Gu, Xiaoxia Zhu, Xue Xu, Minrui Liang, Haiyan Chen and Ning Kong for helpful discussions and experimental technique helps. We thank the patients, the healthy volunteer donors, and the doctors for their participation in this study.

Author Contributions

Conceived and designed the experiments: XY HZ. Performed the experiments: XY JY HZ. Analyzed the data: XY JY YC YX DX SZ HZ. Contributed reagents/materials/analysis tools: XY JY YC YX DX SZ HZ. Wrote the paper: XY JY HZ.

References

1. Arbuckle MR, McClain MT, Rubertone MV, Scofield RH, Dennis GJ, et al. (2003) Development of autoantibodies before the clinical onset of systemic lupus erythematosus. N Engl J Med 349: 1526–1533.
2. Yang J, Chu Y, Yang X, Gao D, Zhu L, et al. (2009) Th17 and natural Treg cell population dynamics in systemic lupus erythematosus. Arthritis Rheum 60: 1472–1483.
3. DiLillo DJ, Matsushita T, Tedder TF (2010) B10 cells and regulatory B cells balance immune responses during inflammation, autoimmunity, and cancer. Ann N Y Acad Sci 1183: 38–57
4. Herlands RA, Christensen SR, Sweet RA, Hershberg U, Shlomchik MJ (2008) T cell-independent and toll-like receptor-dependent antigen-driven activation of autoreactive B cells. Immunity 29: 249–260.
5. Yang J, Yang X, Zou H, Chu Y, Li M (2011) Recovery of the immune balance between Th17 and regulatory T cells as a treatment for systemic lupus erythematosus. Rheumatology (Oxford): 1366–1372.
6. Yanaba K, Bouaziz JD, Matsushita T, Tsubata T, Tedder TF (2009) The development and function of regulatory B cells expressing IL-10 (B10 cells) requires antigen receptor diversity and TLR signals. J Immunol 182: 7459–7472.
7. Yanaba K, Bouaziz JD, Haas KM, Poe JC, Fujimoto M, et al. (2008) A regulatory B cell subset with a unique CD1dhiCD5+ phenotype controls T cell-dependent inflammatory responses. Immunity 28: 639–650.
8. Mauri C, Gray D, Mushtaq N, Londei M (2003) Prevention of arthritis by interleukin 10-producing B cells. J Exp Med 197: 489–501.
9. Mauri C, Ehrenstein MR (2008) The 'short' history of regulatory B cells. Trends Immunol 29: 34–40.
10. Matsushita T, Yanaba K, Bouaziz JD, Fujimoto M, Tedder TF (2008) Regulatory B cells inhibit EAE initiation in mice while other B cells promote disease progression. J Clin Invest 118: 3420–3430.
11. Matsushita T, Horikawa M, Iwata Y, Tedder TF (2010) Regulatory B cells (B10 cells) and regulatory T cells have independent roles in controlling experimental autoimmune encephalomyelitis initiation and late-phase immunopathogenesis. J Immunol 185: 2240–2252.
12. Blenman KR, Duan B, Xu Z, Wan S, Atkinson MA, et al. (2006) IL-10 regulation of lupus in the NZM2410 murine model. Lab Invest 86: 1136–1148.
13. Watanabe R, Ishiura N, Nakashima H, Kuwano Y, Okochi H, et al. (2010) Regulatory B cells (B10 cells) have a suppressive role in murine lupus: CD19 and B10 cell deficiency exacerbates systemic autoimmunity. J Immunol 184: 4801–4809.
14. Yin Z, Bahtiyar G, Zhang N, Liu L, Zhu P, et al. (2002) IL-10 regulates murine lupus. J Immunol 169: 2148–2155.
15. Blair PA, Chavez-Rueda KA, Evans JG, Shlomchik MJ, Eddaoudi A, et al. (2009) Selective targeting of B cells with agonistic anti-CD40 is an efficacious strategy for the generation of induced regulatory T2-like B cells and for the suppression of lupus in MRL/lpr mice. J Immunol 182: 3492–3502.
16. Yang X, Yang J, Chu Y, Wang J, Guan M, et al. (2013) T Follicular Helper Cells Mediate Expansion of Regulatory B Cells via IL-21 in Lupus-Prone MRL/lpr Mice. PLoS One 8: e62855.
17. Nurieva RI, Chung Y, Hwang D, Yang XO, Kang HS, et al. (2008) Generation of T follicular helper cells is mediated by interleukin-21 but independent of T helper 1, 2, or 17 cell lineages. Immunity 29: 138–149.
18. Crotty S (2011) Follicular helper CD4 T cells (TFH). Annu Rev Immunol 29: 621–663.
19. King C, Tangye SG, Mackay CR (2008) T follicular helper (TFH) cells in normal and dysregulated immune responses. Annu Rev Immunol 26: 741–766.
20. Simpson N, Gatenby PA, Wilson A, Malik S, Fulcher DA, et al. (2010) Expansion of circulating T cells resembling follicular helper T cells is a fixed phenotype that identifies a subset of severe systemic lupus erythematosus. Arthritis Rheum 62: 234–244.
21. Wong CK, Wong PT, Tam LS, Li EK, Chen DP, et al. (2010) Elevated production of B cell chemokine CXCL13 is correlated with systemic lupus erythematosus disease activity. J Clin Immunol 30: 45–52.
22. Yu B, Guan M, Peng Y, Shao Y, Zhang C, et al. (2011) Copy number variations of interleukin-17F, interleukin-21, and interleukin-22 are associated with systemic lupus erythematosus. Arthritis Rheum 63: 3487–3492.
23. Zotos D, Coquet JM, Zhang Y, Light A, D'Costa K, et al. (2010) IL-21 regulates germinal center B cell differentiation and proliferation through a B cell-intrinsic mechanism. J Exp Med 207: 365–378.
24. Brandt K, Bulfone-Paus S, Foster DC, Ruckert R (2003) Interleukin-21 inhibits dendritic cell activation and maturation. Blood 102: 4090–4098.
25. Spolski R, Kim HP, Zhu W, Levy DE, Leonard WJ (2009) IL-21 mediates suppressive effects via its induction of IL-10. J Immunol 182: 2859–2867.
26. van der Vlugt LE, Labuda LA, Ozir-Fazalalikhan A, Lievers E, Gloudemans AK, et al. (2012) Schistosomes induce regulatory features in human and mouse CD1d(hi) B cells: inhibition of allergic inflammation by IL-10 and regulatory T cells. PLoS One 7: e30883.
27. Lee JH, Noh J, Noh G, Choi WS, Lee SS (2011) IL-10 is predominantly produced by CD19(low)CD5(+) regulatory B cell subpopulation: characterisation of CD19 (high) and CD19(low) subpopulations of CD5(+) B cells. Yonsei Med J 52: 851–855.
28. Iwata Y, Matsushita T, Horikawa M, Dilillo DJ, Yanaba K, et al. (2011) Characterization of a rare IL-10-competent B-cell subset in humans that parallels mouse regulatory B10 cells. Blood 117: 530–541.
29. Blair PA, Norena LY, Flores-Borja F, Rawlings DJ, Isenberg DA, et al. (2010) CD19(+)CD24(hi)CD38(hi) B cells exhibit regulatory capacity in healthy individuals but are functionally impaired in systemic Lupus Erythematosus patients. Immunity 32: 129–140.
30. Moore KW, de Waal Malefyt R, Coffman RL, O'Garra A (2001) Interleukin-10 and the interleukin-10 receptor. Annu Rev Immunol 19: 683–765.
31. Johnston RJ, Poholek AC, DiToro D, Yusuf I, Eto D, et al. (2009) Bcl6 and Blimp-1 are reciprocal and antagonistic regulators of T follicular helper cell differentiation. Science 325: 1006–1010.
32. Yoshizaki A, Miyagaki T, DiLillo DJ, Matsushita T, Horikawa M, et al. (2012) Regulatory B cells control T-cell autoimmunity through IL-21-dependent cognate interactions. Nature 491: 264–268.
33. Bouaziz JD, Yanaba K, Tedder TF (2008) Regulatory B cells as inhibitors of immune responses and inflammation. Immunol Rev 224: 201–214.
34. Sun F, Ladha SS, Yang L, Liu Q, Shi SX, et al. (2013) Interleukin-10 producing-B cells and their association with responsiveness to rituximab in myasthenia gravis. Muscle Nerve.
35. Amel Kashipaz MR, Huggins ML, Lanyon P, Robins A, Powell RJ, et al. (2003) Assessment of Be1 and Be2 cells in systemic lupus erythematosus indicates elevated interleukin-10 producing CD5+ B cells. Lupus 12: 356–363.
36. Dong W, Zhu P, Wang Y, Wang Z (2011) Follicular helper T cells in systemic lupus erythematosus: a potential therapeutic target. Autoimmun Rev 10: 299–304.
37. Good KL, Bryant VL, Tangye SG (2006) Kinetics of human B cell behavior and amplification of proliferative responses following stimulation with IL-21. J Immunol 177: 5236–5247.
38. Hochberg MC (1997) Updating the American College of Rheumatology revised criteria for the classification of systemic lupus erythematosus. Arthritis Rheum 40: 1725.

6

Functional Relevance for Associations between Genetic Variants and Systemic Lupus Erythematosus

Fei-Yan Deng[1], Shu-Feng Lei[1,2]*, Yong-Hong Zhang[1,2], Zeng-Li Zhang[1], Yu-Fan Guo[3]

1 Center for Genetic Epidemiology and Genomics, Soochow University, Suzhou, Jiangsu, P. R. China, **2** Department of Epidemiology, School of Public Health, Soochow University, Suzhou, Jiangsu, P. R. China, **3** Department of Rheumatology, the First Affiliated Hospital of Soochow University, Suzhou, Jiangsu, P. R. China

Abstract

Systemic lupus erythematosus (SLE) is a serious prototype autoimmune disease characterized by chronic inflammation, auto-antibody production and multi-organ damage. Recent association studies have identified a long list of loci that were associated with SLE with relatively high statistical power. However, most of them only established the statistical associations of genetic markers and SLE at the DNA level without supporting evidence of functional relevance. Here, using publically available datasets, we performed integrative analyses (gene relationship across implicated loci analysis, differential gene expression analysis and functional annotation clustering analysis) and combined with expression quantitative trait loci (eQTLs) results to dissect functional mechanisms underlying the associations for SLE. We found that 14 SNPs, which were significantly associated with SLE in previous studies, have cis-regulation effects on four eQTL genes (HLA-DQA1, HLA-DQB1, HLA-DQB2, and IRF5) that were also differentially expressed in SLE-related cell groups. The functional evidence, taken together, suggested the functional mechanisms underlying the associations of 14 SNPs and SLE. The study may serve as an example of mining publically available datasets and results in validation of significant disease-association results. Utilization of public data resources for integrative analyses may provide novel insights into the molecular genetic mechanisms underlying human diseases.

Editor: Massimo Pietropaolo, University of Michigan Medical School, United States of America

Funding: The study was supported by Natural Science Foundation of China (NSFC) (31271336, 31071097), NSFC-Canadian Institutes of Health Research (CIHR) Joint Health Research Initiative Proposal (30811120436), Startup Fund from Soochow University (Q41390112), and a Project of the Priority Academic Program Development of Jiangsu Higher Education Institutions. The funders had no role in study design, data collection and analysis, decision to publish, or preparation of the manuscript.

Competing Interests: The authors have declared that no competing interests exist.

* E-mail: leisf@suda.edu.cn

Introduction

Systemic lupus erythematosus (SLE) is a serious prototype autoimmune disease characterized by chronic inflammation, auto-antibody production and multi-organ damage. The estimated incidence of SLE ranges from 2.0–7.6 cases per 100,000 persons per year [1]. The overall prevalence of SLE in the United States ranges from 14.6–50 cases per 100,000 persons [1]. Heritable components play an important role in pathogenesis of SLE, as evidenced by up to 30 times higher risk for siblings of affected individuals than that for the general population and further increased risk for monozygotic twins [2–5].

Dissecting the genetic basis of SLE remains one of great challenges in human genetics, because of complex nature of genetic determination, including polygenic determinations, gene by gene and gene by environment interactions. Recently, there has been great progress in identification of genetic susceptibility in SLE [6–13]. A great number of genetic loci associated with SLE were identified with relatively high statistical power. However, most of these studies only established statistical associations of genetic markers and SLE at the DNA level without exploring functional mechanisms underlying the associations. Such established associations usually do not provide immediate insights into functions of genes or regulation of gene expression that bridges gene code information and SLE phenotype directly.

Currently, numerous public gene expression datasets (e.g., www.ncbi.nlm.nih.gov/geo) are available, which were used to identify genes relevant to SLE in the original studies [14]. These datasets will serve as important resources for further data mining to provide supplementary functional evidence to bridge the functional link between genetic markers and SLE.

Based on the publically available datasets and results, this study aims to dissect functional mechanisms underlying the associations identified in previous studies by performing integrative analyses (gene relationships among implicated loci (GRAIL), differential gene expression analysis and functional annotation clustering analysis) and by combining the findings with expression quantitative trait loci (eQTLs) analysis results.

Materials and Methods

Selection of SLE-Associated SNPs

GWAS Integrator [15] and Phenotype-Genotype Integrator (PheGenI) (www.ncbi.nlm.nih.gov/gap/PheGenI/) are two bioinformatics tools that provide robust lookup and analytic functionalities for published GWAS and meta-analysis studies. We used the phenotype "systemic lupus erythematosus" to search the two databases and found 135 interesting associations for 128 unique SNPs and SLE with $p<10^{-7}$ (**Table S1**) [6–13]. Seven SNPs have replicate associations in independent studies.

Gene Relationship across Implicated Loci (GRAIL)

In most situations, confidently significant SNP means at least one susceptible gene or functional locus is located within the nearby region of the SNP, which often contains multiple genes. A commonly used approach for identification of candidate gene is to select nearby genes physically located at two sides of each associated SNP as candidate genes for further functional studies. To increase chances of finding susceptible genes, we used the GRAIL [16] to prioritize and identify susceptible candidate genes near SLE-associated SNPs. This approach automatically assesses the degree of functional connectivity with the other candidate genes that were chosen for the analysis using 250,000 PubMed abstracts, then prioritizes and identifies the best candidate gene around associated SNP.

eQTL Analysis

As is commonly recognized, variants at the DNA level may lead to variations in quantifiable intermediate phenotypes (such as RNA level), which subsequently result in variations in end-point phenotypes, such as susceptibility to SLE. Several recent large-scale studies have identified thousands of putative eQTLs in multiple tissues or cells including liver, lymphoblastoid cell lines(LCLs), monocytes, T cells, brain and fibroblasts [17–23], which were summarized and archived in databases for quick and easy searching and comparison by web browsers (eQTL Browser: http://eqtl.uchicago.edu/cgi-bin/gbrowse/eqtl/; GTEx eQTL Browser: www.ncbi.nlm.nih.gov/gtex/GTEX2/gtex.cgi). To investigate the functional mechanisms underlying the above selected associations, we first searched the two databases for eQTLs to evaluate whether the above detected SNPs influence transcript levels of genes as cis-effect regulators (eSNP) in multiple SLE related cells (monocytes, LCLs and fibroblasts).

Differential Expression Analysis for SLE-Associated Genes

We performed differential expression analyses for the identified eQTL genes. First, we downloaded three publically available expression data sets from GEO Datasets (www.ncbi.nlm.nih.gov/geo) (GSE numbers: GSE37356, GSE20864). These studies were performed with original purposes of identifying genes underlying SLE using a design of SLE case and control in multiple tissues or cells, e.g., macrophages, mononuclear cells, and peripheral blood cells [14]. The experiment procedures and data analyses including normalization of raw data were detailed in the original publications [14]. By using the normalized data available on the public databases, T-tests were performed to identify differential expression genes (DEGs) by comparing means of the gene expression signals in SLE cases and controls.

Functional prediction for SNP

For the significant SNPs identified and other interesting SNPs, we utilized the FASTSNP program (http://fastsnp.ibms.sinica.edu.tw) to analyze and predict their functions. FASTSNP provides up-to-date information about known and potential functional effect of SNPs [24].

Functional annotation clustering analysis

Functional annotation clustering analyses were performed to explore functional similarity of the associated genes and to cluster them in particular biological GO terms and functional pathways as defined by the Gene Ontology (GO) project and KEGG database, respectively. The significantly associated genes were functionally annotated using the Database for Annotation, Visualization and Integrated Discovery (DAVID) integrated database query tools (http://david.abcc.ncifcrf.gov/) [25,26]. A P-value was calculated to determine whether GO term or pathway annotates a specified list of genes at a frequency greater than that would be expected by chance. Bonferroni correction was adopted for multiple testing.

Results

By searching the GWAS Integrator [15] and PheGenI (www.ncbi.nlm.nih.gov/gap/PheGenI/), we selected 135 robust genetic associations ($P<10^{-7}$) between SLE and 128 unique SNPs (**Table S1**). These association results come from 8 published SLE association studies [6–13]. Some of these studies have relatively large sample sizes, e.g., the study performed by Han et.al. [6] has 1,047 Chinese Han cases and 1,205 Chinese Han controls plus 3,152 Chinese Han cases and 7,050 Chinese Han controls in initial and replication analyses, respectively. As shown in Table S1, the majority of these associations (>100 associations) were mapped to the HLA region. These SLE-associated genetic variants in HLA region span ~6.4 M in length according to the physical location at chromosome 6p21.3.

As shown in **Table S1**, 7 SNPs have replication associations in multiple independent studies, e.g., rs7574865 in the intron region of STAT4 gene was significantly associated with SLE (P = 5.0E-42, and P = 2.0E-20) in two independent studies. The columns "Gene 1" and "Gene 2" listed the nearest genes physically located at two sides of the SNP, respectively. About 30 "susceptible" genes detected by GRAIL analysis, as listed in the column "implicated genes" of **Table S1**, are overlapped with the genes identified according to the physical positions (Columns "Gene 1" and "Gene 2"). The above two methods identified a total of 108 unique candidate genes, which were subject to further analyses.

EQTL analysis is an important approach in detection of functional mechanism underlying association by testing whether identified variants at the DNA level may lead to variations in mRNA expression of nearby genes. Among the 128 unique SNPs, we found that about 61 SNPs have potential eQTL effects either on the "identified" genes or on other genes (**Table 1** and **Table S2**). Fifty-five associations between 23 unique SNPs and expression of 11 "identified" genes from the list of **Table S1** (108 genes in total) were detected (**Table 1**) in monocytes and LCLs, which are two types of cells closely correlated with immune response. Among the 23 unique SNPs, only three were located at non-HLA regions. The entire 23 unique SNPs act as cis-effect regulators of the 11 "identified" genes. Especially, nine SNPs around HLA-DQB1 gene showed strong associations with expression level of HLA-DQB1 gene in two cell groups (LCLs and monocytes). Six SNPs (rs7192, rs9268832, rs9275224, rs2647012, rs9275572, and rs9275596), which extend more than 240 kb, were associated with the expression of HLA-DRA gene.

Furthermore, we performed differential expression analyses for the 11 identified eQTL genes in multiple SLE related cells: macrophages, mononuclear cells, and peripheral blood cells (**Table 2**). T-tests showed that four genes (HLA-DQA1, HLA-DQB1, HLA-DQB2, and IRF5) were differentially expressed in samples S1 or S3 (**Table 2**).

The above functional evidence, taken together, highlighted the significance of 14 SLE-associated SNPs, i.e., the first 14 SNPs listed in Table 1, as these SNPs serve as cis-effect regulators of four SLE-associated genes (HLA-DQA1, HLA-DQB1, HLA-DQB2, and IRF5), which also were differentially expressed in SLE-related cell groups. Functional analysis using FASTSNP program [24] found that the rs2187668 in the intron of HLA-DQA1 was possible transcriptional binding sites for intronic enhancers. Therefore, the SNP may regulate transcription by altering binding

Table 1. Expression quantitative trait locus (eQTL) analysis results between SNPs and the expressions of 11 genes from the 108 "identified" genes.

SNP ID	Chr.	Location	Allele	Role	Association P-value	Gene 1	Gene 2	Implicated Gene	eQTL gene	Effect	Score	Target	Ref.
rs4728142	chr7	128573967	A/G	unknown	8.00E-19	KCP	IRF5	IRF5	IRF5	eqtl	130.5	Monocytes	[18]
										eqtl	8.6	LCLs	[20]
rs1573649	chr6	32731258	C/T	5'utr	2.00E-10	HLA-DQB2	HLA-DQB2	HLA-DQB2	HLA-DQB2	PP-eqtl	0.1	LCLs	[19]
rs6903130	chr6	32732210	A/G	upstream	4.43E-10	HLA-DQB2	HLA-DQB2	HLA-DQB2	HLA-DQB2	PP-eqtl	0	LCLs	[19]
rs16898264	chr6	32677152	A/G	unknown	3.85E-09	HLA-DQB1	HLA-DQA2	HLA-DRA	HLA-DQB1	exonQTL	4.4	LCLs	[22]
										transcriptQTL	4	LCLs	[22]
rs2647012	chr6	32664458	A/G	unknown	1.27E-13	HLA-DQB1	HLA-DQA2	HLA-DRA	HLA-DQB1	exonQTL	6.9	LCLs	[22]
										transcriptQTL	5.6	LCLs	[22]
rs2647050	chr6	32669767	C/T	unknown	5.38E-09	HLA-DQB1	HLA-DQA2	HLA-DRA	HLA-DQB1	exonQTL	4.4	LCLs	[22]
										transcriptQTL	4	LCLs	[22]
rs2856717	chr6	32670308	C/T	unknown	1.03E-13	HLA-DQB1	HLA-DQA2	N/A	HLA-DQB1	eqtl	33.9	Monocytes	[18]
										exonQTL	6.3	LCLs	[22]
										transcriptQTL	4.8	LCLs	[22]
rs2856718	chr6	32670255	A/G	unknown	5.33E-09	HLA-DQB1	HLA-DQA2	HLA-DRA	HLA-DQB1	exonQTL	4.4	LCLs	[22]
										transcriptQTL	4.1	LCLs	[22]
rs2856725	chr6	32666738	A/G	unknown	1.11E-13	HLA-DQB1	HLA-DQA2	N/A	HLA-DQB1	exonQTL	6.4	LCLs	[22]
										transcriptQTL	4.9	LCLs	[22]
rs2858305	chr6	32670464	A/C	unknown	7.88E-14	HLA-DQB1	HLA-DQA2	N/A	HLA-DQB1	exonQTL	6.8	LCLs	[22]
										transcriptQTL	5.3	LCLs	[22]
rs9275572	chr6	32678999	A/G	unknown	6.41E-14	HLA-DQB1	HLA-DQA2	HLA-DRA	HLA-DQB1	eqtl	24.3	Monocytes	[18]
										exonQTL	7.1	LCLs	[22]
										transcriptQTL	5.7	LCLs	[22]
rs9275596	chr6	32681631	C/T	unknown	3.33E-16	HLA-DQB1	HLA-DQA2	HLA-DRA	HLA-DQB1	exonQTL	5.3	LCLs	[22]
										transcriptQTL	4.2	LCLs	[22]
rs2187668	chr6	32605884	A/G	intron	6.00E-28	HLA-DQA1	HLA-DQA1	HLA-DQB2	HLA-DQA1	eqtl	34.6	Monocytes	[18]
										exonQTL	4.3	LCLs	[22]
rs9271100	chr6	32576478	C/T	unknown	1.00E-12	HLA-DRB1	HLA-DQA1	N/A	HLA-DQA1	exonQTL	7.8	LCLs	[22]
										transcriptQTL	5.4	LCLs	[22]
rs3094061	chr6	30321189	G/T	unknown	1.24E-09	HLA-N	UBQLN1P1	IER3	HLA-H	eqtl	33.6	Monocytes	[18]
rs9271100	chr6	32576478	C/T	unknown	1.00E-12	HLA-DRB1	HLA-DQA1	N/A	HLA-DRB1	exonQTL	15.2	LCLs	[22]
										transcriptQTL	10.5	LCLs	[22]
rs2647012	chr6	32664458	A/G	unknown	1.27E-13	HLA-DQB1	HLA-DQA2	HLA-DRA	HLA-DRA	transcriptQTL	4.5	LCLs	[22]
rs7192	chr6	32411646	G/T	missense	2.02E-10	HLA-DRA	HLA-DRA	HLA-DRA	HLA-DRA	transcriptQTL	9	LCLs	[22]
rs9268832	chr6	32427789	C/T	unknown	1.53E-10	HLA-DRB9	HLA-DRB9	HLA-DRA	HLA-DRA	transcriptQTL	9.5	LCLs	[22]

Table 1. Cont.

SNP ID	Chr.	Location	Allele	Role	Association P-value	Gene 1	Gene 2	Implicated Gene	eQTL gene	Effect	Score	Target	Ref.
rs9275224	chr6	32659878	A/G	unknown	4.45E-12	HLA-DQB1	HLA-DQA2	HLA-DRA	HLA-DRA	transcriptQTL	4	LCLs	[22]
rs9275572	chr6	32678999	A/G	unknown	6.41E-14	HLA-DQB1	HLA-DQA2	HLA-DRA	HLA-DRA	eqtl	40.1	Monocytes	[18]
										transcriptQTL	5.1	LCLs	[22]
rs9275596	chr6	32681631	C/T	unknown	3.33E-16	HLA-DQB1	HLA-DQA2	HLA-DRA	HLA-DRA	transcriptQTL	4.7	LCLs	[22]
rs2647012	chr6	32664458	A/G	unknown	1.27E-13	HLA-DQB1	HLA-DQA2	HLA-DRA	HLA-DQA2	transcriptQTL	4.2	LCLs	[22]
rs2856725	chr6	32666738	A/G	unknown	1.11E-13	HLA-DQB1	HLA-DQA2	N/A	HLA-DQA2	transcriptQTL	4.2	LCLs	[22]
rs2858305	chr6	32670464	A/C	unknown	7.88E-14	HLA-DQB1	HLA-DQA2	N/A	HLA-DQA2	transcriptQTL	4.1	LCLs	[22]
rs9271100	chr6	32576478	C/T	unknown	1.00E-12	HLA-DRB1	HLA-DQA1	N/A	HLA-DRB1	eqtl	93	LCLs	Database#
rs13277113	chr8	11349186	A/G	unknown	1.00E-10	FAM167A	BLK	BLK	FAM167A	exonQTL	6.4	LCLs	[22]
										transcriptQTL	6.5	LCLs	[22]
rs12176317	chr6	26372786	A/G	intron	6.83E-10	BTN3A2	BTN3A2	TRIM38	BTN3A2	eqtl	21.4	LCLs	[19]
										exonQTL	4.8	LCLs	[22]
										PP-eqtl	0	LCLs	[19]
										transcriptQTL	10	LCLs	[22]
rs9379858	chr6	26367689	C/T	intron	6.21E-10	BTN3A2	BTN3A2	TRIM38	BTN3A2	eqtl	21.4	LCLs	20]
										PP-eqtl	0	LCLs	20]
rs9379859	chr6	26369549	C/T	intron	3.79E-10	BTN3A2	BTN3A2	TRIM38	BTN3A2	eqtl	21.4	LCLs	20]
										exonQTL	8.4	LCLs	[22]
										PP-eqtl	0	LCLs	20]
										transcriptQTL	10	LCLs	[22]
rs2618476	chr8	11352541	C/T	intron	2.00E-08	BLK	BLK	BLK	BLK	eqtl	57.1	LCLs	Database#

Note: N/A:not available; "Score": −log10 (P); LCLs: lymphoblastoid cell lines; transcript-QTL: transcript expression levels against SNPs; exon-QTL: quantified reads for known exons by RNA sequencing against SNPs; sQTL: splicing QTL; PP-eqtl: posterior probability-eqtl.
All the eqtls have cis-effects.
Database#: http://eqtl.uchicago.edu/cgi-bin/gbrowse/eqtl.
"Gene 1" and "Gene 2"are the nearby genes physically located at two sides of SNP.
"GRAIL P-value "and "Implicated gene" are the results from Gene Relationships Across Implicated Loci (GRAIL) analyses.

Table 2. Differential expression analyses for the detected eQTL genes in multiple SLE related cells.

Sample	**S1**			**S2**			**S3**		
Disease	SLE			SLE			SLE		
Target cells	Macrophages			Mononuclear cells			Peripheral blood cells		
Sample size	20:16			20:16			21:45		
Platform	Illumina HumanHT-12 V4.0 expression beadchip			Illumina HumanHT-12 V4.0 expression beadchip			Hitachisoft AceGene Human Oligo Chip 30K 1 Chip		
Ref.	Database#			Database#			[14]		
GSE NO.	GSE37356			GSE37356			GSE20864		
Gene symbol	**Probe ID**	**T-test P-value**	**SLE/control**	**Probe ID**	**T-test**	**SLE/control**	**Probe ID**	**T-test P-value**	**SLE/Control***
HLA-DQA1	ILMN_1808405	3.10E-01	1.04	ILMN_1808405	6.86E-01	1.01	AGhsA101413	4.88E-02	16.19048
HLA-DQB1	ILMN_1661266	6.99E-01	1.02	ILMN_1661266	9.83E-01	1	AGhsA030823	4.77E-02	6.2/5.08
HLA-DQB2	ILMN_1741648	2.49E-02	1.01	ILMN_1741648	6.25E-02	0.99	N/A	N/A	N/A
IRF5	ILMN_1670576	5.67E-01	0.98	ILMN_1670576	5.68E-01	0.98	AGhsB110506	1.62E-02	8.89/5.95

Note: Sample size: SLE cases: controls; N/A: Not available;
*:ratio of mean expression values of log2(sample/reference).
GSE NO: Gene Expression Omnibus Number, www.ncbi.nlm.nih.gov/geo/.
Database#: The data downloaded from the database (www.ncbi.nlm.nih.gov/geo/) according to GSE number.
We only listed the most significant expression results of probes if one gene has multiple detected probes.

sites for transcription factors or by increasing or decreasing the affinity of binding for transcription factors. Functions for the other 13 SNPs are unknown yet.

To test the probability of our "identified" genes clustering into a particular biological pathway and GO term, we performed a functional annotation clustering analysis using functional annotation tool of DAVID database. We found significant GO terms and KEGG pathways even after Bonferroni correction. The "identified" genes tend to enrich in immune-related pathways (such as "autoimmune thyroid disease", "Intestinal immune network for IgA production", and "immune response") (data not shown). Especially, we found a significant clustering (Bonferroni correction P = 8.00E-06) of 8 genes (HLA-DQB1, TNF, HLA-DRB1, HIST1H2AH, HLA-DOB, HLA-DQA2, HLA-DQA1, HLA-DRA) directly involved in SLE. Among the 11 identified eQTL genes, five genes (HLA-DQB1, HLA-DRB1, HLA-DQA2, HLA-DQA1, and HLA-DRA) were significantly clustered in multiple immune related KEGG pathways or GO terms (**Table S3**).

Discussion

By using publically available datasets, this study performed integrative analyses and combined with eQTL results to detect functional mechanisms underlying the associations for SLE. We discovered 23 SNPs acting as cis-effect regulators on 11 "identified" genes. Four eQTL genes have differential expression signals in the SLE-associated cells or tissues. The "identified" genes tend to enrich in KEGG Pathways (autoimmune thyroid disease, intestinal immune network for IgA production, and immune response), which are very closely relevant to SLE.

In biologic systems, genetic information carried by DNA is passed on to RNA molecules via transcription and then to protein molecules through translation. Sequence variants at the DNA level represent a class of heritable molecules and contribute to variability of complex traits in the population. The functional mechanisms underlying associations between variants at the DNA level and SLE may be that DNA sequence variants lead to variation in quantifiable intermediate phenotypes (such as RNA level), which subsequently lead to variation of susceptibility to SLE. Therefore, integrating substantial evidences from multiple levels (i.e., DNA, RNA) could ascertain potential functioning mechanism of genes and their contribution to variation in susceptibility to SLE.

Recent association studies have identified a long list of loci that were associated with SLE with relatively high statistical power. A majority of these associations (>100 associations) were mapped to the HLA region. It is well-known that there is strong linkage disequilibrium (LD) at HLA region. It is reasonable to infer that the significant signals for some of the genetic markers may be due to their strong LD with true functional variants within the HLA region. As shown in Results section, multiple SNPs, extending a relatively long distance (240 kb), were consistently associated with the expression of HLA-DRA. Strong LD at HLA region may partially contribute to this observation.

HLA-DQA1, HLA-DQB1, and HLA-DQB2 are HLA class II genes involved in immune response. Class II molecules are heterodimers consisting of an alpha (DQA) and a beta chain (DQB), both anchored to the membrane, which play a central role in the immune system by presenting peptides derived from extracellular proteins. These genes have been found to consistently associate with SLE in several populations [7,8] at DNA level, though functions for these genes and mechanism for the observed associations were not studied. The functional evidence from this study, taken together, suggested potential regulatory mechanisms underlying the associations between SLE and the associated SNPs. Briefly, different genotypes of the SNPs, by regulating differential mRNA transcriptions of functional genes (HLA-DQA1, HLA-DQB1, and HLA-DQB2) and thus differential protein expression and enzyme activity, consequently effect on variation of susceptibility to SLE in the population.

Interferon (IFN) regulatory factor 5 (IRF5) is a pivotal transcription factor in the type I IFN pathway, which regulates inflammatory cytokines, expression of IFN-dependent genes, and genes involved in apoptosis. Previous studies identified IRF5 as one of the most strongly and consistently SLE-associated loci outside the HLA region. Four functional variants in IRF5 were identified in multiple ethnic groups: a 5 bp indel (insertion–deletion) near the 5′ untranslated region (UTR), rs2004640 in the first intron, a 30 bp indel in the sixth exon, and rs10954213 in the 3′ UTR [27–35] . In addition, a SNP, rs4728142, located 10 kb downstream of IRF5 gene, was highly strongly associated with SLE (P = 8.00E-19) [6]. In the eQTL analysis, this SNP was consistently and highly associated with expression of IRF5 gene in both monocytes (P<E-130) [18] and lymphoblastoid cell lines (P<E-08) [30]. Compared with GG genotype at rs4728142, AA genotype individuals tend to have higher IRF5 expression levels. The combined evidence from association analyses, eQTL analyses, and differential expression analyses suggested that the rs4728142 or other nearby genetic variant contribute significant to variation of susceptibility to SLE in the population.

To be noted, failure to find functional evidence underlying the selected associations through mining publically available data and results does not necessarily exclude the importance of the associations with SLE, given that (1) absence of association between SLE-associated SNP and mRNA expression may result from limited statistical power due to small sample size or small effect of the SNP; (2) the associated genes may exert effects on SLE through other tissues or cells not studied herein; (3) sequence variant in a gene may lead to SLE by other mechanisms (e.g., epigenetic regulation) instead of regulating gene expression. In-depth functional studies are required, which may provide novel insights into mechanisms underlying the associations detected at DNA level.

In addition, this exploratory pilot study has two potential limitations. First, although we gained some functional evidence for the associations between SLE and 14 SNPs, based on the current available evidence, it is very challenging to discriminate causal variants with nearby SNPs with potential functional effects, especially for SNPs at the HLA region where there is strong LD. Second, although we used two methods to select the potential genes involved in associations (gene selection according to the physical location and GRAIL analysis based on previous literature), this study does not exclude the possibility that other genes around the SNPs are also directly involved in the association around SNPs.

In summary, the functional evidence gained in this study, taken together, supports and highlights the significance of 14 SLE-associated SNPs. These SNPs act as cis-effect regulators to regulate expression of genes that were found differentially expressed between SLE patients and controls. The above evidence laid a supporting clue for us to pursue in-depth validation studies to dissect their involvements and molecular functional mechanisms in SLE. This study sets an example of mining publically available datasets and results to validate significant disease-association results. Utilization of public data resources for integrative analyses may provide novel insights into the molecular genetic mechanisms underlying human diseases.

Supporting Information

Table S1 The selected association results (p<10-7) from previous 8 published studies. Note: N/A: not available; PMID: PubMed ID. "Gene 1" and "Gene 2" are the nearby genes physically located at two sides of SNP. "GRAIL p-value" and "Implicated gene" are the results from Gene Relationships Across Implicated Loci (GRAIL) analyses. * associated with anti-dsDNA negative SLE; #associated with anti-dsDNA positive SLE.
(XLS)

Table S2 Results of eQTL analyses for the selected significant SLE-associated SNPs that have eQTL effects not on the corresponding "identified" genes but on other genes. Note: N/A:not available;"Score": −log10 (P); LCLs: lymphoblastoid cell lines; transcript-QTL: transcript expression levels against SNPs; exon-QTL: quantified reads for known exons by RNA sequencing against SNPs; sQTL: splicing QTL; PP-eqtl: posterior probability-eqtl; Database#: http://eqtl.uchicago.edu/cgi-bin/gbrowse/eqtl; PMID for eQTL: PubMed ID for eQTL results. "Gene 1" and "Gene 2"are the nearby genes physically located at two sides of SNP. "GRAIL p-value "and "Implicated gene" are the results from Gene Relationships Across Implicated Loci (GRAIL) analyses.

Table S3 Functional annotation clustering analysis for the eQTL genes. Note: Functional annotation clustering analysis was performed using functional annotation tool of DAVID database.

Author Contributions

Conceived and designed the experiments: SFL FYD. Analyzed the data: FYD YHZ. Wrote the paper: FYD ZLZ YFG SFL.

References

1. Jimenez S, Cervera R, Font J, Ingelmo M (2003) The epidemiology of systemic lupus erythematosus. Clin Rev Allergy Immunol 25: 3–12.
2. Sestak AL, Shaver TS, Moser KL, Neas BR, Harley JB (1999) Familial aggregation of lupus and autoimmunity in an unusual multiplex pedigree. J Rheumatol 26: 1495–1499.
3. Ramos-Niembro F, Alarcon-Segovia D (1978) Familial aspects of mixed connective tissue disease (MCTD). I. Occurrence of systemic lupus erythematosus in another member in two families and aggregation of MCTD in another family. J Rheumatol 5: 433–440.
4. Arnett FC, Shulman LE (1976) Studies in familial systemic lupus erythematosus. Medicine (Baltimore) 55: 313–322.
5. Deapen D, Escalante A, Weinrib L, Horwitz D, Bachman B, et al. (1992) A revised estimate of twin concordance in systemic lupus erythematosus. Arthritis Rheum 35: 311–318.
6. Han JW, Zheng HF, Cui Y, Sun LD, Ye DQ, et al. (2009) Genome-wide association study in a Chinese Han population identifies nine new susceptibility loci for systemic lupus erythematosus. Nat Genet 41: 1234–1237.
7. Hom G, Graham RR, Modrek B, Taylor KE, Ortmann W, et al. (2008) Association of systemic lupus erythematosus with C8orf13-BLK and ITGAM-ITGAX. N Engl J Med 358: 900–909.
8. Chung SA, Taylor KE, Graham RR, Nititham J, Lee AT, et al. (2011) Differential genetic associations for systemic lupus erythematosus based on anti-dsDNA autoantibody production. PLoS Genet 7: e1001323.
9. Kozyrev SV, Abelson AK, Wojcik J, Zaghlool A, Linga Reddy MV, et al. (2008) Functional variants in the B-cell gene BANK1 are associated with systemic lupus erythematosus. Nat Genet 40: 211–216.
10. Yang W, Shen N, Ye DQ, Liu Q, Zhang Y, et al. (2010) Genome-wide association study in Asian populations identifies variants in ETS1 and WDFY4 associated with systemic lupus erythematosus. PLoS Genet 6: e1000841.
11. Harley JB, Alarcon-Riquelme ME, Criswell LA, Jacob CO, Kimberly RP, et al. (2008) Genome-wide association scan in women with systemic lupus erythematosus identifies susceptibility variants in ITGAM, PXK, KIAA1542 and other loci. Nat Genet 40: 204–210.
12. Graham RR, Cotsapas C, Davies L, Hackett R, Lessard CJ, et al. (2008) Genetic variants near TNFAIP3 on 6q23 are associated with systemic lupus erythematosus. Nat Genet 40: 1059–1061.
13. Yang J, Yang W, Hirankarn N, Ye DQ, Zhang Y, et al. (2011) ELF1 is associated with systemic lupus erythematosus in Asian populations. Hum Mol Genet 20: 601–607.
14. Lee HM, Sugino H, Aoki C, Nishimoto N (2011) Underexpression of mitochondrial-DNA encoded ATP synthesis-related genes and DNA repair genes in systemic lupus erythematosus. Arthritis Res Ther 13: R63.
15. Yu W, Yesupriya A, Wulf A, Hindorff LA, Dowling N, et al. (2011) GWAS Integrator: a bioinformatics tool to explore human genetic associations reported in published genome-wide association studies. Eur J Hum Genet 19: 1095–1099.
16. Raychaudhuri S, Plenge RM, Rossin EJ, Ng AC, Purcell SM, et al. (2009) Identifying relationships among genomic disease regions: predicting genes at pathogenic SNP associations and rare deletions. PLoS Genet 5: e1000534.
17. Schadt EE, Molony C, Chudin E, Hao K, Yang X, et al. (2008) Mapping the genetic architecture of gene expression in human liver. PLoS Biol 6: e107.
18. Zeller T, Wild P, Szymczak S, Rotival M, Schillert A, et al. (2010) Genetics and beyond–the transcriptome of human monocytes and disease susceptibility. PLoS One 5: e10693.
19. Veyrieras JB, Kudaravalli S, Kim SY, Dermitzakis ET, Gilad Y, et al. (2008) High-resolution mapping of expression-QTLs yields insight into human gene regulation. PLoS Genet 4: e1000214.
20. Stranger BE, Nica AC, Forrest MS, Dimas A, Bird CP, et al. (2007) Population genomics of human gene expression. Nat Genet 39: 1217–1224.
21. Dimas AS, Deutsch S, Stranger BE, Montgomery SB, Borel C, et al. (2009) Common regulatory variation impacts gene expression in a cell type-dependent manner. Science 325: 1246–1250.
22. Montgomery SB, Sammeth M, Gutierrez-Arcelus M, Lach RP, Ingle C, et al. (2010) Transcriptome genetics using second generation sequencing in a Caucasian population. Nature 464: 773–777.
23. Pickrell JK, Marioni JC, Pai AA, Degner JF, Engelhardt BE, et al. (2010) Understanding mechanisms underlying human gene expression variation with RNA sequencing. Nature 464: 768–772.
24. Yuan HY, Chiou JJ, Tseng WH, Liu CH, Liu CK, et al. (2006) FASTSNP: an always up-to-date and extendable service for SNP function analysis and prioritization. Nucleic Acids Res 34: W635–641.
25. Huang da W, Sherman BT, Lempicki RA (2009) Systematic and integrative analysis of large gene lists using DAVID bioinformatics resources. Nat Protoc 4: 44–57.
26. Huang da W, Sherman BT, Lempicki RA (2009) Bioinformatics enrichment tools: paths toward the comprehensive functional analysis of large gene lists. Nucleic Acids Res 37: 1–13.
27. Graham RR, Kozyrev SV, Baechler EC, Reddy MV, Plenge RM, et al. (2006) A common haplotype of interferon regulatory factor 5 (IRF5) regulates splicing and expression and is associated with increased risk of systemic lupus erythematosus. Nat Genet 38: 550–555.
28. Graham RR, Kyogoku C, Sigurdsson S, Vlasova IA, Davies LR, et al. (2007) Three functional variants of IFN regulatory factor 5 (IRF5) define risk and protective haplotypes for human lupus. Proc Natl Acad Sci U S A 104: 6758–6763.
29. Sigurdsson S, Goring HH, Kristjansdottir G, Milani L, Nordmark G, et al. (2008) Comprehensive evaluation of the genetic variants of interferon regulatory factor 5 (IRF5) reveals a novel 5 bp length polymorphism as strong risk factor for systemic lupus erythematosus. Hum Mol Genet 17: 872–881.
30. Demirci FY, Manzi S, Ramsey-Goldman R, Minster RL, Kenney M, et al. (2007) Association of a common interferon regulatory factor 5 (IRF5) variant with increased risk of systemic lupus erythematosus (SLE). Ann Hum Genet 71: 308–311.
31. Shin HD, Sung YK, Choi CB, Lee SO, Lee HW, et al. (2007) Replication of the genetic effects of IFN regulatory factor 5 (IRF5) on systemic lupus erythematosus in a Korean population. Arthritis Res Ther 9: R32.
32. Kawasaki A, Kyogoku C, Ohashi J, Miyashita R, Hikami K, et al. (2008) Association of IRF5 polymorphisms with systemic lupus erythematosus in a Japanese population: support for a crucial role of intron 1 polymorphisms. Arthritis Rheum 58: 826–834.
33. Siu HO, Yang W, Lau CS, Chan TM, Wong RW, et al. (2008) Association of a haplotype of IRF5 gene with systemic lupus erythematosus in Chinese. J Rheumatol 35: 360–362.
34. Kelly JA, Kelley JM, Kaufman KM, Kilpatrick J, Bruner GR, et al. (2008) Interferon regulatory factor-5 is genetically associated with systemic lupus erythematosus in African Americans. Genes Immun 9: 187–194.
35. Lofgren SE, Yin H, Delgado-Vega AM, Sanchez E, Lewen S, et al. (2010) Promoter insertion/deletion in the IRF5 gene is highly associated with susceptibility to systemic lupus erythematosus in distinct populations, but exerts a modest effect on gene expression in peripheral blood mononuclear cells. J Rheumatol 37: 574–578.

7

Increased Arterial Stiffness in Systemic Lupus Erythematosus (SLE) Patients at Low Risk for Cardiovascular Disease

Karim Sacre[1,2,3]*, Brigitte Escoubet[4], Blandine Pasquet[5], Marie-Paule Chauveheid[1], Maria-Christina Zennaro[6], Florence Tubach[5], Thomas Papo[1,2,3]

1 Département de Médecine Interne, Hôpital Bichat, Université Paris Diderot, PRES Sorbonne Paris Cité, Assistance Publique Hôpitaux de Paris, Paris, France, **2** INSERM U1149, Paris, France, **3** Département Hospitalo-Universitaire FIRE (Fibrosis, Inflammation and Remodelling in Renal and Respiratory Diseases), Paris, France, **4** Département de Physiologie, Hôpital Bichat, Université Paris Diderot, PRES Sorbonne Paris Cité, Assistance Publique Hôpitaux de Paris, INSERM U1138, Paris, France, **5** Département d'Epidémiologie et Recherche Clinique, Hôpital Bichat, Université Paris Diderot, PRES Sorbonne Paris Cité, Assistance Publique Hôpitaux de Paris, INSERM CIE 801, Paris, France, **6** Département de Cardiologie, Hôpital Européen Georges Pompidou, Université Paris Descartes, PRES Sorbonne Paris Cité, Assistance Publique-Hôpitaux de Paris, INSERM, UMRS 970, Paris, France

Abstract

Cardiovascular disease (CVD) is a major cause of death in systemic lupus erythematosus (SLE) patients. Although the risk for cardiovascular events in patients with SLE is significant, the absolute number of events per year in any given cohort remains small. Thus, CVD risks stratification in patients with SLE focuses on surrogate markers for atherosclerosis at an early stage, such as reduced elasticity of arteries. Our study was designed to determine whether arterial stiffness is increased in SLE patients at low risk for CVD and analyze the role for traditional and non-traditional CVD risk factors on arterial stiffness in SLE. Carotid-femoral pulse wave velocity (PWV) was prospectively assessed as a measure of arterial stiffness in 41 SLE patients and 35 controls (CTL). Adjustment on age or Framingham score was performed using a logistic regression model. Factors associated with PWV were identified separately in SLE patients and in controls using Pearson's correlation coefficient for univariate analysis and multiple linear regression for multivariate analysis. SLE patients and controls displayed a low 10-year risk for CVD according to Framingham score (1.8±3.6% in SLE vs 1.6±2.8% in CTL, $p = 0.46$). Pulse wave velocity was, however, higher in SLE patients (7.1±1.6 m/s) as compared to controls (6.3±0.8 m/s; $p = 0.01$, after Framingham score adjustment) and correlated with internal carotid wall thickness ($p = 0.0017$). In multivariable analysis, only systolic blood pressure ($p = 0.0005$) and cumulative dose of glucocorticoids ($p = 0.01$) were associated with PWV in SLE patients. Interestingly, the link between systolic blood pressure (SBP) and arterial stiffness was also confirmed in SLE patients with normal systolic blood pressure. In conclusion, arterial stiffness is increased in SLE patients despite a low risk for CVD according to Framingham score and is associated with systolic blood pressure and glucocorticoid therapy.

Editor: Gualtiero I. Colombo, Centro Cardiologico Monzino IRCCS, Italy

Funding: The authors have no support or funding to report.

Competing Interests: The authors have declared that no competing interests exist.

* E-mail: karim.sacre@bch.aphp.fr

Introduction

Accelerated atherosclerosis accounts for premature mortality among systemic lupus erythematosus (SLE) patients. Most specialists now consider SLE as an independent risk factor for the development of cardiovascular disease (CVD) [1–9].

Although the risk for cardiovascular events in patients with SLE is significant, the absolute number of events per year in any given cohort remains small. Thus, CVD risks stratification in patients with SLE focuses on biological or imaging surrogate markers of subclinical atherosclerosis in attempt to identify atherosclerosis at the earliest stage.

Arterial stiffness reflects changes in mechanical wall properties that occur early at onset of vascular disease and predispose to major cardiovascular disease. Besides peripheral pulse pressure (computed as the difference between systolic and diastolic blood pressure), arterial stiffness is commonly assessed with aortic pulse wave velocity (PWV) measurement [10]. Factors associated with increased PWV include age and long-term effects of traditional cardiovascular risk factors such as blood pressure. In addition, most studies indicate a predictive value of PWV for cardiovascular events and mortality, that is additive to traditional risk factors [11]. Arterial stiffness may be a reliable surrogate marker of cardiovascular risk in patients with SLE [12,13].

To date, two major studies have evaluated arterial stiffness in SLE patients. The first study concluded that PWV was related to both SLE-related and traditional cardiovascular risk factors. This study however lacked a control population [14]. The second study included SLE or rheumatoid arthritis (RA) patients that were analyzed as a whole [15]. More recently, 2 studies have shown an association between PWV and metabolic syndrome (MetS) in SLE patients [16,17]. Our study was designed to determine whether carotid-femoral PWV as a measure of arterial stiffness is increased in SLE patients asymptomatic for cardiovascular disease and at low risk for CVD, in comparison to healthy controls and to determine the role for traditional and non-traditional CVD risk factors on arterial stiffness in SLE.

Patients and Methods

Study participants

Forty-one consecutive patients with systemic lupus erythematosus (SLE) followed in the department of Internal Medicine, Bichat Hospital, Paris-Diderot University, Paris were enrolled between February and October 2012. All subjects fulfilled at least four of the American College of Rheumatology criteria for SLE [18]. At enrolment, patients were treated with prednisone at a stable dose for at least 3 months. Exclusion criteria consisted of known coronary disease or symptoms suggestive of CVD (angina, arrhythmia, congestive heart failure, stroke, and peripheral arterial disease).

Controls were healthy non-carrier relatives of pseudohypoaldosteronism type 1 patients from a clinical study that aimed to evaluate cardiovascular disease with similar tools (Assistance Publique-Hôpitaux de Paris, NCT00646828). All controls had undergone vascular ultrasound imaging between 2008 and 2011 and none had coronary disease or symptoms suggestive of CVD. The first patient with SLE was considered with respect to age and sex. The clinical trial database was examined to find the first control patient of the same age ±3 years and sex. Matches within the range were found for 35 SLE participants.

Extensive screening for conventional cardiovascular risk factors (age, sex, smoking status, family history of coronary artery disease, body-mass index, waist circumference, hypertension, diabetes mellitus, Framingham score for 10-year risk of heart attack) was undertaken in all cases.

SLE-related data were also analyzed: nephritis, thrombosis, central nervous system involvement, Raynaud's phenomenon, cardiac valvulopathy, pulmonary hypertension and medication including hormonal contraception, statins, hydroxychloroquine, steroid and immunosuppressive treatment.

A family history of coronary artery disease was defined when a first-degree relative had suffered a myocardial infarction or stroke before the age of 55 years in males or before the age of 65 years in females [19]. Height and weight were measured, and the body-mass index was calculated as the weight in kilograms divided by the square of the height in meters. Subjects were considered to have hypertension if they repeatedly had a systolic blood pressure (SBP) of at least 140 mm Hg or a diastolic blood pressure of at least 90 mm Hg. Diabetes mellitus was defined by a persistent finding of fasting hyperglycemia and the need for antidiabetic drug therapy [20]. The risk for cardiovascular events was calculated as the absolute risk within the next 10 years using the Framingham risk equation, which includes age, sex, total cholesterol level, high-density lipoprotein cholesterol level, smoking history, and SBP [19].

Systemic lupus erythematosus disease activity was assessed using the SELENA-SLEDAI score [21,22].

The diagnosis of antiphospholipid syndrome (APS) was based on a history of venous and/or arterial thromboses or recurrent miscarriages in the presence of aPL antibodies in accordance with published criteria [23].

Blood tests included complete blood count, creatinine, total cholesterol, high-density lipoprotein cholesterol, low-density lipoprotein cholesterol, triglycerides, glycated hemoglobin, homocysteine, 25(OH)-D3 vitamin, lupus serology (anti-DNA antibodies, complement) and antiphospholipid antibodies (anticardiolipin and anti-β2GP1 antibodies, lupus anticoagulant). Urine sample was assayed for creatinine, red blood cells and proteins.

Vascular assessment

Vascular ultrasound study was performed in the context of care, in a temperature-controlled room after a 15 min rest (Vivid 7, General Electric, Horten, Norway). All subjects had fastened for at least 12 hours before PWV evaluation. A single investigator conducted vascular measurements in controls and SLE patients. All data were analysed offline (EchoPAC, General Electric Ultrasound). Aortic pulse wave velocity (PWV) was measured by the carotid to femoral method [24]. The time delay between ECG R wave and the Doppler flow onset was measured at right common carotid artery and common femoral artery and the difference was computed (t). D is the body surface distance between the 2 measurement points minus the distance from the suprasternal notch to the carotid measurement point. PWV was computed as D/t. Internal carotid wall thickness (ICWT) was measured at the carotid bulb level at end diastole, as gated on ECG. Right and left values were averaged for each patient. Carotid plaques were defined as thickness greater than 2 mm.

Statistical analysis

Continuous variables are expressed as mean (SD) or median (IQR). Categorical variables are expressed as frequencies and percentages. Data were compared between SLE patients and controls using Chi2 test (or Fisher) for dichotomous variables and Student test (or Wilcoxon non-normally distributed) for continuous variables. The two-way ANOVA test was performed when specified. Arterial stiffness was compared between SLE patients and controls using the Wilcoxon rank-sum test. Adjustment on age or Framingham score was performed with a logistic regression model. Factors associated to PWV were identified separately in SLE patients and in controls by use of the Pearson's correlation coefficient (univariate analysis) and multiple linear regression (multivariate analysis). Variables correlated to PWV in univariate analysis with a p-value below 10% were considered for the multivariate model. Variable selection relied on the AIC index.

Ethics statement

Our study is a human non-interventional study where 1-subjects were not assigned to treatment, 2-subjects were assigned to a diagnosis strategy within current practice (i.e. vascular ultrasound), 3-study involved products with a marketing authorization that are prescribed in the usual manner and used in accordance with French agencies authorizations (i.e. vascular ultrasound), 4-epidemiological methods were used to analyze the data, and 5-information used in the study were collected for clinical care.

According to the Public Health French Law (art L 1121-1-1, art L 1121-1-2), approval from institutional review board and written consent are not required for human non-interventional studies. For ethical consideration, patients were however informed that data that was collected in medical records might be used for research study in accordance to privacy rule. Written informed consent was obtained from each patient and the study protocol conforms to the ethical guidelines of the 1975 Declaration of Helsinki. Our study involves personal health data and has been authorized by the Commission nationale de l'informatique et des libertés (CNIL) (declaration number 1685680 v 0)

Table 1. Characteristics of SLE (systemic lupus erythematosus) and controls subjects.

	SLE patients (n = 41)	Controls (n = 35)	p
Female Sex, n (%)	34 (82.9)	28 (80)	0.77
Age, years	39 (±10) (21–62)	37 (±8) (23–59)	0.21
Familial History of CAD, n (%)	1 (2.4)	NA	
Smoker current, n (%)	14 (34.1)	12 (34.3)	1
Hypertension, n (%)	12 (29.2)	8 (22.9)	0.61
Diabetes, n (%)	1 (2.4)	1 (2.8)	1
BMI, kg/m^2	25.5 (±5.4) (18–44)	26.7 (±6.6) (19–41)	0.69
Waist circumference, cm	93.4 (±15) (72–150)	94.9 (±15.5) (78–131)	0.63
Systolic Blood Pressure, mmHg	130+18 (96–169)	127+11 (115–150)	0.37
LDL-Cholesterol, g/l	0.92 (±0.3) (0.36–1.53)	1.2 (±0.3) (0.62–1.73)	0.001
HbA1c, %	5.4 (±0.5) (4.4–6.7)	5.4 (±0.4) (4.7–6.1)	0.39
10-year risk of heart attack, %	1.8 (±3.6) (0.5–23)	1.6 (±2.8) (0.5–16)	0.53
Homocysteine/creatinine ratio	0.18 (±0.07) (0.06–0.42)		
25(OH)-D3 vitamin, ng/ml	23.4 (±11.5) (5–41.7)		
GFR, ml/mn/1.73 m^2	84.9 (±34.6) (16.3–168.4)	102 (±21) (63–164)	0.002
Proteinuria/Creatininuria, mg/mmol	85.4 (±215) (5–1188)		
Lymphocytes, G/l	1.4 (±0.6) (0.3–3.4)		
Duration of SLE disease, y	13 (±7.3) (1–37)		
SELENA SLEDAI score	2.1 (±2.8) (0–13)		
Lupus nephritis, n (%)	27 (65.8)		
LA antibodies, n (%)	7 (17)		
aCL antibodies, n (%)	12 (29.3)		
anti-B2GP1 antibodies, n (%)	2 (4.9)		
APS, n (%)	5 (12.2)		
Cumulative years of steroid treatment	10.5 (±7) (0–26)		
Cumulative dose of steroid treatment, g	42.3 (±29.2) (0–132)		
Antiplatelet treatment, n (%)	7 (17.1)		
Anticoagulant treatment, n (%)	6 (14.6)		
Hormonal contraception, n (%)	12/34 (35.3)		
Statin, n (%)	10 (24.4)	1 (2.8)	0.009
Hydroxychloroquine, n (%)	41 (100)		
Other therapy, n (%)	28 (68.3)		

CAD, coronary artery disease; BMI, body mass index; SELENA, safety of estrogens in lupus erythematosus national assessment; SLEDAI, systemic lupus erythematosus disease activity index; LA, lupus anticoagulant; aCL, anti-cardiolipin antibody; β2GP1, β2-Glycoprotein 1; APS, antiphospholipid syndrome.
10-year risk of heart attack was calculated using the Framingham equation.
Normal value for homocysteine/creatinine ratio was below 0.17.
Normal value for 25(OH)-D3 vitamin was above 30 ng/ml (nanogram per liter)
GRF, glomerular rate filtration, calculated with the Modification of Diet in Renal Disease (MDRD) equation and expressed in milliliters per minute per 1.73 square meters of body surface area
Hormonal contraception was progestin-only pill in all cases.
Other therapy included cyclophosphamide (n = 24), azathioprine (n = 14), mycophenolatemofetil (n = 11), methotrexate (n = 3), rituximab (n = 1), or intravenous immunoglobulin (n = 1)
cm, centimeter; g/l, gram per liter; g, gram; millimeter of mercure, mmHg
Results are shown as mean and (SD), and (range)

Results

Characteristics of SLE patients and controls

Forty-one SLE patients and 35 controls (CTL) were studied. The mean age of SLE subjects was 39±10 years (37±8 in controls) and 34 (82.9%) were female (80% in controls). Forty patients (97.5%) received long-term glucocorticoids and 27 (65.9%) still used prednisone at a mean daily dose of 9±3 mg (range: 5–17) at study time. Twenty-eight (68.3%) had received immunosuppressive or immunomodulatory drugs at some point during follow-up. SLE patients were treated with angiotensin converting enzyme inhibitor or angiotensin receptor antagonist (n = 18), beta blocker (n = 3) or calcium channel blocker (n = 1). No control subject was receiving anti-hypertensive drugs at PWV measurement.

Age, sex, tobacco use, hypertension, diabetes, BMI, LDL-cholesterol level, or absolute risk of cardiovascular events occurring within the next 10 years according to the Framingham score were not statistically different between SLE patients and

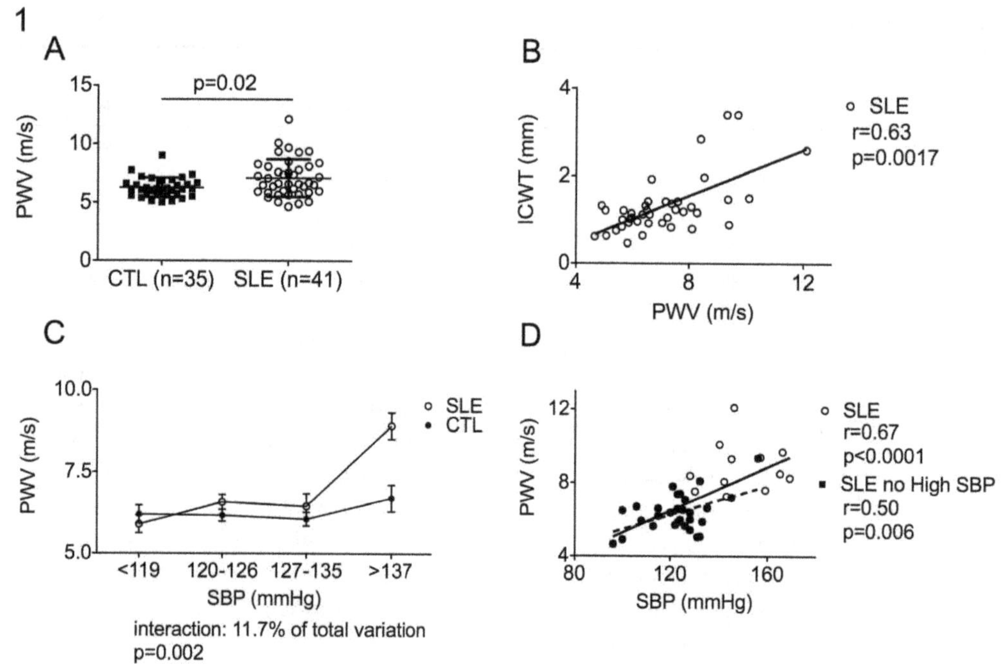

Figure 1. Pulse Wave Velocity (PWV) is high in SLE patients and correlates with systolic blood pressure. (A) Pulse wave velocity (PWV) are higher in SLE patients (SLE, n = 41, right) as compared to controls (CTL, n = 35, left) and (B) correlated with internal carotid wall thickness (ICWT). (C) SLE patients and controls were stratified according to systolic blood pressure quartiles (SBP <119; 120–126, >127–135, >137 mmHg). Two-ways ANOVA showed a significant independent interaction of SBP and group (SLE, CTL) on PWV. (D) PWV correlated with systolic blood pressure (SBP) in SLE subjects with (white circles) and without (black circles) high systolic blood pressure. Plain and dashed lines represented linear regression in SLE subjects with and without high systolic blood pressure (SBP), respectively. p was calculated after age adjustment. m/s refers to meter per second; mm, to millimeter; r, to linear correlation coefficient

controls. LDL-cholesterol level was lower in SLE patients as compared to controls (0.92±0.3 vs 1.2±0.3 g/l, p = 0.001). Only one SLE subject (2.4%) had a family history of CVD.

Among non-traditional CVD risk factors in SLE patients, waist circumference was above 88 cm (ranging from 90 to 150 cm) in 64.7% (22/34) of women and above 102 cm in 14.3% (1/7) of men. Sixteen (39%) patients had a blood homocysteine/creatinine ratio above the normal value of 0.17 (range: 0.18 to 0.42). Twenty-four (61%) had a vitamin D deficiency assessed by a blood level of 25(OH)-D3 vitamin below 30 ng/ml (range: 5 to 28.1).

Clinical characteristics of SLE patients and controls are shown in detail in Table 1.

Arterial stiffness and carotid wall thickness are higher in SLE patients

Pulse wave velocity (PWV) was higher in SLE patients as compared to controls as shown in Figure 1A (7.1±1.6 vs 6.3±0.8 m/s; p = 0.02 after age adjustment; p = 0.01 after Framingham score adjustment). In the same line, internal carotid wall thickness (ICWT) was higher in SLE patients (ICWT: 1.31±0.67 vs 0.93±0.25 mm; p = 0.007 after age adjustment; p = 0.003 after Framingham score adjustment) and eight (19.5%) SLE patients, but only one control (2.8%) (p = 0.03), displayed a carotid atherosclerotic plaque as defined as a local wall thickening greater than 2 mm. Moreover in SLE patients, PWV significantly correlated with ICWT (r = 0.63, 95% CI: 0.4–0.79, p = 0.0017 after age adjustement) (Figure 1B).

Risk factors for arterial stiffness: univariate analysis

In SLE patients, PWV was shown to correlate positively with age, systolic blood pressure (SBP), cumulative dose of glucocorticoids and glomerular filtration rate (GFR). No statistical relationship was found between PWV and Framingham score, BMI, blood levels of LDL-cholesterol, homocystein, 25(OH)-D3 vitamin, lymphocytes count, anti-dsDNA antibodies level, current dose of steroids, C3 level, anti-β2GP1 or anticardiolipine antibodies levels and SELENA SLEDAI score. Correlations between PWV and glycated hemoglobin or duration of SLE disease failed to reach statistical significance (Table 2). In controls, PWV only correlated with age and Framingham score (Table 3).

The frequency of subjects with high blood pressure (29.2% of SLE patients vs 22.9% of controls, p = 0.61) and the mean SBP at study time (130±18 in SLE vs 127±11 in CTL, p = 0.37) did not significantly differ between groups. Interestingly, after stratification according to SBP quartiles, the correlation between SBP and PWV for a given level of SBP appeared to be higher in SLE patients as compared to controls. Indeed the interaction between SBP and SLE status was accounting for 11.7% of the observed variance (p = 0.002) (Figure 1C). Moreover, the correlation between PWV and SBP was observed even in SLE patients without high systolic blood pressure (r = 0.50, p = 0.006) (Figure 1D).

The proportion of SLE patients with high blood pressure and the mean SBP at study time did not significantly differ between patients that were currently receiving or not glucocorticoid (33.3% (9/27) vs 35.7% (5/14), p = 1.00 and 130±17 (range: 96–169) vs 132±19 (108–165) mmHg, p = 0.67; respectively).

Table 2. Univariate analysis of risk factors for arterial stiffness in SLE subjects.

	Number of subjects	Mean PWV (SD)	Median PWV (IQR)	p
Sex				0.60
Male	7	4.9 (9.3)	6.8 (1.5)	
Female	34	4.7 (12.1)	7.2 (1.6)	
Smoker current				0.54
No	27	4.7 (10.1)	7.0 (1.5)	
Yes	14	4.9 (12.1)	7.3 (1.9)	
Diabetes				0.78
No	40	4.7 (12.1)	7.1 (1.6)	
Yes	1	7.5 (7.5)	7.5 (.)	
High blood pressure				<0.0001
No	29	4.7 (9.4)	6.4 (1.0)	
Yes	12	5.7 (12.1)	8.5 (1.6)	
Statin				0.85
No	31	4.7 (12.1)	7.1 (1.5)	
Yes	10	4.9 (10.1)	7.0 (1.9)	
Lupus Nephritis				0.40
No	14	4.9 (10.1)	6.8 (1.5)	
Yes	27	4.7 (12.1)	7.2 (1.7)	
Familial History of CAD				0.66
No	40	4.7 (12.1)	7.1 (1.6)	
Yes	1	7.8 (7.8)	7.8 (.)	
APS				0.54
No	36	4.7 (10.1)	7.0 (1.4)	
Yes	5	4.9 (12.1)	8.0 (2.8)	
	Linear correlation coefficient		**95% CI**	**P**
Age	0.49		0.21 to 0.69	0.001
Systolic blood pressure	0.67		0.44 to 0.81	<0.0001
GFR	−0.52		−0.71 to −0.25	0.0003
BMI	0.13		−0.18 to 0.42	0.41
10-year risk of heart attack	0.23		−0.08 to 0.5	0.14
LDL-Cholesterol	0.12		−0.20 to 0.41	0.47
Waist circumference	0.08		−0.24 to 0.38	0.62
HbA1c	0.26		−0.05 to 0.52	0.10
Cumulative steroid dose	0.38		0.07 to 0.61	0.01
Homocysteine/creatinine ratio	−0.23		−0.5 to 0.09	0.16
25(OH)-D3 vitamin	0.03		−0.29 to 0.34	0.84
Duration of SLE disease	0.26		−0.05 to 0.53	0.10
Proteinuria/Creatininuria	0.15		−0.17 to 0.44	0.37
SELENA SLEDAI score	−0.18		−0.46 to 0.14	0.27
C3	0.24		−0.04 to 0.50	0.09

CAD, coronary artery disease; BMI, body mass index; SELENA, safety of estrogens in lupus erythematosus national assessment; SLEDAI, systemic lupus erythematosus disease activity index; APS, antiphospholipid syndrome.
10-year risk of heart attack was calculated using the Framingham equation.
Normal value for homocysteine/creatinine ratio was below 0.17.
Normal value for 25(OH)-D3 vitamin was above 30 ng/ml (nanogram per liter)
GRF, glomerular rate filtration, calculated with the Modification of Diet in Renal Disease (MDRD) equation and expressed in milliliters per minute per 1.73 square meters of body surface area
PWV, pulse wave velocity is expressed in meter per second
IQR, interquartile range
SD, standard deviation

Table 3. Univariate analysis of risk factors for arterial stiffness in Control subjects.

	Number of subjects	Mean PWV (SD)	Median PWV (IQR)	p
Sex				0.73
Male	7	5.5 (7.7)	6.4 (0.8)	
Female	28	5.0/9.0	6.2 (0.9)	
Smoker current				0.51
No	23	5.0/9.0	6.3 (0.8)	
Yes	12	5.1/7.7	6.1 (0.8)	
Diabetes				0.69
No	1	6.6/6.6	6.6 (.)	
Yes	34	5.0/9.0	6.3 (0.8)	
High blood pressure				0.33
No	27	5.0/7.7	6.2 (0.7)	
Yes	8	5.5/9.0	6.5 (1.1)	
	Linear correlation coefficient		**95% CI**	**p**
Age	0.48		0.17 to 0.70	0.003
Systolic blood pressure	0.17		−0.17 to 0.48	0.32
GFR	−0.15		−0.46 to 0.19	0.38
BMI	0.04		−0.30 to 0.37	0.82
10-year risk of heart attack	0.37		0.03 to 0.62	0.03
LDL-Cholesterol	0.30		−0.04 to 0.57	0.08
Waist circumference	0.04		−0.30 to 0.37	0.82
HbA1c	0.05		−0.29 to 0.38	0.78

BMI, body mass index;
10-year risk of heart attack was calculated using the Framingham equation
GRF, glomerular rate filtration, calculated with the Modification of Diet in Renal Disease (MDRD) equation and expressed in milliliters per minute per 1.73 square meters of body surface area
PWV, pulse wave velocity is expressed in meter per second
IQR, interquartile range
SD, standard deviation

Twenty-seven (65.8%) SLE patients had experienced lupus nephritis in the past, mostly (20/27, 74%) class IV diffuse nephritis according to International Society of Nephrology/Renal Pathology Society (ISN/RPS) classification of lupus nephritis [25]. No SLE patient displayed active lupus nephritis at study time. No history of renal disease was reported in controls. The glomerular filtration rate (GFR), calculated with the Modification of Diet in Renal Disease (MDRD) equation, was below 60 ml/mn/1.73 m^2 (range: 16.3 to 55.6) in 8 (19.5%) SLE patients. All control subjects displayed a GFR above 60 ml/mn/1.73 m^2 ($p=0.01$, as com-

Table 4. Multivariate analysis of risk factors for arterial stiffness.

SLE subjects				
	Linear correlation coefficient	**Unstandardized betas**	**95% CI**	**p**
Age	0.49	0.03	0.21 to 0.69	0.08
Systolic blood pressure	0.67	0.04	0.44 to 0.81	0.0005
GFR	0.52	−0.008	0.71 to 0.25	0.17
Cumulative steroid dose	0.38	0.015	0.07 to 0.61	0.01
Controls				
	Linear correlation coefficient	**Unstandardized betas**	**95% CI**	**p**
Age	0.48	0.04	0.17 to 0.70	0.005
LDL-Cholesterol	0.30	0.69	0.04 to 0.57	0.10

GRF, glomerular rate filtration, calculated with the Modification of Diet in Renal Disease (MDRD) equation and expressed in milliliters per minute per 1.73 square meters of body surface area pared to SLE). Moreover, the mean GFR was significantly higher in controls (102 ± 21 ml/mn/1.73 m^2) as compared to SLE patients (84.9 ± 34.6, $p<0.05$), especially as compared to SLE subjects with history of lupus nephritis (74.5 ± 30.6, $p<0.005$).

The mean protein urinary output, assessed by measuring the morning urinary protein/creatinine ratio, was 84.5 (±215) mg/mmol in SLE patients and 13 (31%) patients had a ratio above 30 mg/mmol (range: 41.3 to 1188). No correlation was found between PWV and urinary protein/creatinine ratio in SLE patients ($p=0.36$).

Risk factors for arterial stiffness: multivariate analysis

In the multivariate analysis (Table 4), both systolic blood pressure ($p=0.0005$) and cumulative prednisone intake ($p=0.01$) were associated with arterial stiffness in SLE patients. The association between age and PWV failed to reach statistical significance ($p=0.08$). In controls, only age was associated with PWV ($p=0.005$)

Discussion

Cardiovascular diseases (CVD) are a major cause of morbidity and mortality in systemic lupus erythematosus (SLE) [1–6]. The pathogenesis of CVD associated with SLE is unknown. Our study shows that, despite a low cardiovascular risk according to Framingham score, SLE patients display increased arterial stiffness as compared to controls. Systolic blood pressure (SBP) and glucorticoid treatment are the main contributors to this phenomenon. Moreover we observe that, in SLE patients, increased arterial stiffness parallels with subclinical atherosclerosis assessed by internal carotid wall thickness (ICWT) measurement.

Arterial stiffness is a consequence of arterial wall thickening and early changes in mechanical properties of the vascular wall. Previous research has found a strong association between hypertension and arterial stiffness in general population [26,27]. Moreover, hypertension was shown to be associated with an increased frequency of cardiovascular events (CVE) in SLE patients [28]. Interestingly, in our study, SBP correlated with arterial stiffness even in SLE patients with normal blood pressure. Moreover, at a given level of SBP, the correlation between systolic blood pressure and arterial stiffness, was stronger in SLE patients as compared to controls.

Hypercholesterolemia was reported to be the best predictor of CVE in SLE patients [28]. We did not confirm such correlation between hypercholesterolemia and arterial stiffness in SLE patients. However, treatment with statins was started when the LDL-cholesterol was >1 g/l according to current guidelines in our SLE patients [29]. Statin treatment explains the fact that level of LDL-cholesterol is lower in SLE patients as compared to controls.

In previous studies, SLE-specific variables appeared to be independently associated with increased PWV [14,17]. Although we may argue that the cumulative dose of steroid taken is related to a more severe SLE disease, we do not observe significant association between SLE-related variables - such as disease activity score or duration of SLE disease - and arterial stiffness.

Among non traditional risk factors for atherosclerosis in SLE patients, the role played by glucocorticoids, a first line treatment for lupus, remains a matter of debate. The estimated 2-year coronary risk for a patient treated with an average dosage of 30 mg/day of prednisone for 1 year, is approximately 60% higher than it would be for a patient with the same SLE activity level and similar risk factors receiving no steroids [30]. On the other hand, since inflammation is implicated in atherosclerosis, low dose corticosteroids may exert a beneficial anti-inflammatory action [31]. Subclinical atherosclerosis in SLE has indeed been correlated with both a low dose of corticosteroids and less immunosuppressive drugs [5]. In contrast, our study suggests that, even in subjects at low risk for CVD according to Framingham score, cumulative prednisone treatment contributes to arterial stiffness and may play a role in accelerated atherosclerosis in SLE. An association between PWV and metabolic syndrome has recently been shown in two cross-sectional studies in SLE patients [16,17]. Consistent with our data, metabolic syndrome in SLE patients was also associated with a higher daily prednisolone dose [32].

Our study has several limitations. First, sample size is small and our work may lack statistical power to show the effect of SLE-specific factors on arterial stiffness. Second, causation cannot be concluded from a cross-sectional study. Eventually, biases cannot be excluded in the selection of healthy controls.

In conclusion, our results support the fact that both systolic blood pressure and glucocorticoid therapy are major contributors to premature arterial stiffness in SLE patients.

Acknowledgments

We are thankful to C. François and M.C. Vanderhaegen for help with study organization.

Author Contributions

Conceived and designed the experiments: KS TP. Performed the experiments: KS BE. Analyzed the data: KS BE BP FT TP. Contributed reagents/materials/analysis tools: MPC MCZ BP FT. Wrote the paper: KS TP.

References

1. Esdaile JM, Abrahamowicz M, Grodzicky T, Li Y, Panaritis C, et al. (2001) Traditional Framingham risk factors fail to fully account for accelerated atherosclerosis in systemic lupus erythematosus. Arthritis and Rheumatism 44: 2331–2337.
2. Aranow C, Ginzler EM (2000) Epidemiology of cardiovascular disease in systemic lupus erythematosus. Lupus 9: 166–169.
3. Bjornadal L, Yin L, Granath F, Klareskog L, Ekbom A (2004) Cardiovascular disease a hazard despite improved prognosis in patients with systemic lupus erythematosus: results from a Swedish population based study 1964-95. The Journal of Rheumatology 31: 713–719.
4. Manzi S, Meilahn EN, Rairie JE, Conte CG, Medsger TA Jr, et al. (1997) Age-specific incidence rates of myocardial infarction and angina in women with systemic lupus erythematosus: comparison with the Framingham Study. American Journal of Epidemiology 145: 408–415.
5. Roman MJ, Shanker BA, Davis A, Lockshin MD, Sammaritano L, et al. (2003) Prevalence and correlates of accelerated atherosclerosis in systemic lupus erythematosus. The New England Journal of Medicine 349: 2399–2406.
6. Ward MM (1999) Premature morbidity from cardiovascular and cerebrovascular diseases in women with systemic lupus erythematosus. Arthritis and Rheumatism 42: 338–346.
7. Svenungsson E, Jensen-Urstad K, Heimburger M, Silveira A, Hamsten A, et al. (2001) Risk factors for cardiovascular disease in systemic lupus erythematosus. Circulation 104: 1887–1893.
8. Doria A, Shoenfeld Y, Wu R, Gambari PF, Puato M, et al. (2003) Risk factors for subclinical atherosclerosis in a prospective cohort of patients with systemic lupus erythematosus. Annals of the Rheumatic Diseases 62: 1071–1077.
9. Goldberg RJ, Urowitz MB, Ibanez D, Nikpour M, Gladman DD (2009) Risk factors for development of coronary artery disease in women with systemic lupus erythematosus. The Journal of Rheumatology 36: 2454–2461.
10. Kullo IJ, Malik AR (2007) Arterial ultrasonography and tonometry as adjuncts to cardiovascular risk stratification. Journal of the American College of Cardiology 49: 1413–1426.
11. Greenland P, Alpert JS, Beller GA, Benjamin EJ, Budoff MJ, et al. (2010) 2010 ACCF/AHA guideline for assessment of cardiovascular risk in asymptomatic adults: a report of the American College of Cardiology Foundation/American

Heart Association Task Force on Practice Guidelines. Journal of the American College of Cardiology 56: e50–103.
12. Cacciapaglia F, Zardi EM, Coppolino G, Buzzulini F, Margiotta D, et al. (2009) Stiffness parameters, intima-media thickness and early atherosclerosis in systemic lupus erythematosus patients. Lupus 18: 249–256.
13. Chin CW, Tan RS, Thumboo J (2012) Endothelial function and arterial stiffness assessment as early surrogate markers of vascular risk in patients with systemic lupus erythematosus. Clinical and Experimental Rheumatology 31: 295–301.
14. Selzer F, Sutton-Tyrrell K, Fitzgerald S, Tracy R, Kuller L, et al. (2001) Vascular stiffness in women with systemic lupus erythematosus. Hypertension 37: 1075–1082.
15. Roman MJ, Devereux RB, Schwartz JE, Lockshin MD, Paget SA, et al. (2005) Arterial stiffness in chronic inflammatory diseases. Hypertension 46: 194–199.
16. Sabio JM, Vargas-Hitos J, Zamora-Pasadas M, Mediavilla JD, Navarrete N, et al. (2009) Metabolic syndrome is associated with increased arterial stiffness and biomarkers of subclinical atherosclerosis in patients with systemic lupus erythematosus. The Journal of Rheumatology 36: 2204–2211.
17. Valero-Gonzalez S, Castejon R, Jimenez-Ortiz C, Rosado S, Tutor-Ureta P, et al. (2013) Increased arterial stiffness is independently associated with metabolic syndrome and damage index in systemic lupus erythematosus patients. Scandinavian Journal of Rheumatology. DOI: 10.3109/03009742.2013.803150
18. Hochberg MC (1997) Updating the American College of Rheumatology revised criteria for the classification of systemic lupus erythematosus. Arthritis and Rheumatism 40: 1725.
19. Expert Panel on Detection, Evaluation, and Treatment of High Blood Cholesterol in Adults (2001) Executive Summary of The Third Report of The National Cholesterol Education Program (NCEP) Expert Panel on Detection, Evaluation, And Treatment of High Blood Cholesterol In Adults (Adult Treatment Panel III). JAMA: The Journal of the American Medical Association 285: 2486–2497.
20. (1979) Classification and diagnosis of diabetes mellitus and other categories of glucose intolerance. National Diabetes Data Group. Diabetes 28: 1039–1057.
21. Bombardier C, Gladman DD, Urowitz MB, Caron D, Chang CH (1992) Derivation of the SLEDAI. A disease activity index for lupus patients. The Committee on Prognosis Studies in SLE. Arthritis and Rheumatism 35: 630–640.
22. Buyon JP, Petri MA, Kim MY, Kalunian KC, Grossman J, et al. (2005) The effect of combined estrogen and progesterone hormone replacement therapy on disease activity in systemic lupus erythematosus: a randomized trial. Annals of Internal Medicine 142: 953–962.
23. Miyakis S, Lockshin MD, Atsumi T, Branch DW, Brey RL, et al. (2006) International consensus statement on an update of the classification criteria for definite antiphospholipid syndrome (APS). Journal of Thrombosis and Haemostasis: JTH 4: 295–306.
24. Blacher J, Guerin AP, Pannier B, Marchais SJ, Safar ME, et al. (1999) Impact of aortic stiffness on survival in end-stage renal disease. Circulation 99: 2434–2439.
25. Weening JJ, D'Agati VD, Schwartz MM, Seshan SV, Alpers CE, et al. (2004) The classification of glomerulonephritis in systemic lupus erythematosus revisited. Journal of the American Society of Nephrology: JASN 15: 241–250.
26. Asmar R, Benetos A, Topouchian J, Laurent P, Pannier B, et al. (1995) Assessment of arterial distensibility by automatic pulse wave velocity measurement. Validation and clinical application studies. Hypertension 26: 485–490.
27. Taquet A, Bonithon-Kopp C, Simon A, Levenson J, Scarabin Y, et al. (1993) Relations of cardiovascular risk factors to aortic pulse wave velocity in asymptomatic middle-aged women. European Journal of Epidemiology 9: 298–306.
28. Rahman P, Aguero S, Gladman DD, Hallett D, Urowitz MB (2000) Vascular events in hypertensive patients with systemic lupus erythematosus. Lupus 9: 672–675.
29. Peters MJ, Symmons DP, McCarey D, Dijkmans BA, Nicola P, et al. (2010) EULAR evidence-based recommendations for cardiovascular risk management in patients with rheumatoid arthritis and other forms of inflammatory arthritis. Annals of the Rheumatic Diseases 69: 325–331.
30. Karp I, Abrahamowicz M, Fortin PR, Pilote L, Neville C, et al. (2008) Recent corticosteroid use and recent disease activity: independent determinants of coronary heart disease risk factors in systemic lupus erythematosus? Arthritis and Rheumatism 59: 169–175.
31. Ruyssen-Witrand A, Fautrel B, Saraux A, Le Loet X, Pham T (2011) Cardiovascular risk induced by low-dose corticosteroids in rheumatoid arthritis: a systematic literature review. Joint, Bone, Spine: revue du rhumatisme 78: 23–30.
32. Parker B, Urowitz MB, Gladman DD, Lunt M, Bae SC, et al. (2013) Clinical associations of the metabolic syndrome in systemic lupus erythematosus: data from an international inception cohort. Annals of the Rheumatic Diseases 72: 1308–1314.

8

The Effect of Mycophenolate Mofetil on Disease Development in the *gld.apoE*$^{-/-}$ Mouse Model of Accelerated Atherosclerosis and Systemic Lupus Erythematosus

Christophe Richez[1,2,3], Rocco J. Richards[3], Pierre Duffau[2,4], Zachary Weitzner[3], Christopher D. Andry[5], Ian R. Rifkin[3], Tamar Aprahamian[3]*

1 Service de Rhumatologie, Hôpital Pellegrin, CHU de Bordeaux, Bordeaux, France, **2** UMR-CNRS 5164, Université Victor Segalen Bordeaux 2, Bordeaux, France, **3** Department of Medicine-Renal Section, Boston University School of Medicine, Boston, Massachusetts, United States of America, **4** Service de Médecine Interne, Hôpital Saint André, CHU de Bordeaux, Bordeaux, France, **5** Department of Medicine-Pathology, Boston University School of Medicine, Boston, Massachusetts, United States of America

Abstract

Systemic lupus erythematosus (SLE) is a systemic autoimmune disease that is characterized by autoantibody production and inflammatory disease involving multiple organs. Premature atherosclerosis is a common complication of SLE and results in substantial morbidity and mortality from cardiovascular disease (CVD). The reasons for the premature atherosclerosis in SLE are incompletely understood, although chronic inflammation is thought to play an important role. There is currently no known preventative treatment of premature atherosclerosis in SLE. Mycophenolate mofetil (MMF) is an immunosuppressive agent that is commonly used for treatment of patients with SLE. In order to study the impact of this drug on murine lupus disease including premature atherosclerosis development, we treated *gld.apoE*$^{-/-}$ mice, a model of SLE and accelerated atherosclerosis, with MMF. We maintained seven-week old *gld.apoE*$^{-/-}$ mice on a high cholesterol Western diet with or without MMF. After 12 weeks on diet, mice receiving MMF showed decreased atherosclerotic lesion area compared to the control group. MMF treatment also improved the lupus phenotype, indicated by a significant decrease circulating autoantibody levels and ameliorating lupus nephritis associated with this model. This data suggests that the effects of MMF on the immune system may not only be beneficial for lupus, but also for inflammation driving lupus-associated atherosclerosis.

Editor: Christine Beeton, Baylor College of Medicine, United States of America

Funding: This work was supported in part by a research grant from Aspreva Pharmaceuticals to I.R.; and by grant: K01 AR055965-02 from NIAMS/NIH to T.A. Its contents are solely the responsibility of the authors and do not necessarily represent the official views of the NIAMS or NIH. The funders had no role in study design, data collection and analysis, decision to publish, or preparation of the manuscript.

Competing Interests: This study was funded in part by Aspreva Pharmaceuticals.

* E-mail: aprahami@bu.edu

Introduction

Systemic lupus erythematosus (SLE) is a complex systemic autoimmune disease involving multiple organs that is characterized by autoantibody production and chronic inflammation [1]. Over time, management of SLE patients has improved and life expectancy of these patients has increased to reach a 10-year survival rate about 70% [2]. However, several studies have revealed that atherosclerosis-attributed vascular events are significantly more frequent in these surviving lupus patients, compared to age-related individuals without SLE [3,4].

Atherosclerosis is characterized by a chronic inflammatory state where immune cell activity is linked to plaque formation and remodeling [5]. A plaque is formed within the lumen of medium- and large-sized arteries due to physiological imbalances caused by chronic inflammation; the plaque is described as a progressive accumulation of lipid, inflammatory cells, smooth muscle cells, and connective tissue within the intima of arteries [6]. It has become widely accepted that atherosclerosis is an inflammatory disease, and that the immune system plays a pivotal role in disease development. Therefore, it is reasonable to suggest that the chronic inflammatory condition encountered in SLE and the activation of immune cells may predispose patients to an increased risk of premature atherosclerosis leading to cardiovascular disease (CVD). For these reasons, immunomodulatory therapy might be of benefit in ameliorating atherosclerosis in patients with SLE. However, with the exception of hydroxychloroquine [7] and some statins [8], the availability of beneficial treatments to decrease CVD risk in SLE is limited.

Mycophenolate mofetil (MMF) is an immunosuppressive drug used in the treatment of patients with SLE, particularly those with nephritis [9]. It is also approved to prevent transplant rejection, especially in heart and kidney transplantation. MMF is an ester pro-drug which is metabolized in the body to the active compound mycophenolic acid (MPA). MPA is a noncompetitive inhibitor of a rate-limiting purine biosynthetic enzyme, inosine-5′-monophosphate dehydrogenase (IMPDH). IMPDH is involved in *de novo* synthesis of purines, and lymphocytes rely exclusively on this *de novo* pathway for nucleotide synthesis [10,11]. Therefore, MMF selectively targets lymphocyte proliferation. Importantly, MMF has been shown to reduce immune-mediated vascular injury in transplantation-associated atherosclerosis (known as coronary allograft vasculopathy) [12] and to attenuate plaque inflammation in patients with symptomatic carotid artery stenosis [13]. These findings further suggest a potential role for MMF in the treatment of atherosclerosis.

In the study presented here, we utilized a mouse model that displays synergy between lupus and atherosclerosis [14]. The *gld.apoE−/−* mouse model incorporates the *gld* inactivating mutation in Fas ligand (FasL) which develops lupus-like autoimmunity together with splenomegaly and lymphadenopathy; and the *apoE−/−* strain which spontaneously displays increased plasma levels of cholesterol and triglycerides and the development of atherosclerosis, particularly when mice are given a high cholesterol "Western diet". In the study presented here, we used the *gld.apoE*$^{-/-}$ mouse model to reflect the accelerated atherosclerosis that occurs in patients with immune disorders to determine if MMF is effective in the treatment of lupus-associated atherosclerosis.

Methods

Animals and Study Protocol

The *gld.apoE*$^{-/-}$ mice used in this study were obtained by crossing *gld* and *apoE*$^{-/-}$ mice as previously described [14]. Starting at 7 weeks of age, the mice were maintained on Adjusted Calories Western diet (21% fat) (#88137, Harlan-Teklad) for 12 weeks, supplemented with 200 mg/kg/day mycophenolate mofetil (MMF) (n = 8) or not supplemented (control) (n = 8). The concentration was chosen based on an equivalent mouse dosage value converted from a human dosage of 2000 mg/day, using equations presented by Ng [15]. MMF was incorporated into our experimental Western diet by Harlan-Teklad Special Diets using CellCept® Oral Suspension (Roche Laboratories) and the conversion ratios we provided. This study was carried out in accordance with the recommendations in the Guide for the Care and Use of Laboratory Animals of the National Institutes of Health. The protocol was approved by the Institutional Animal Care and Use Committee of Boston University School of Medicine (Protocol number: AN-14843). All efforts were made to minimize suffering.

Calculation of Drug Dosage in Experimental Groups

The amount of drug incorporated into the diet of each experimental group was based on established dosages of MMF used in human lupus patients. An average dose is 2000–3000 mg MMF/day, therefore for the studies presented here, we chose 2000 mg. The human dosage was converted into an equivalent dosage appropriate for mice, as metabolism of drugs differs greatly between humans and mice. Equations presented by Ng [15] were used to convert drug dosages among species of the same Class (in this case, placental mammals). First, the minimum energy cost (MEC) was established for the murine model according to the equation: $MEC_{mouse} = K(BW_{kg}^{0.75})$; where K is a constant of 70 (for placental mammals), and BW is the body weight of the model animal (average mouse body weight is 0.025 kg). Therefore, the MEC_{mouse} value was calculated to be 4.4. Next, the MEC_{mouse} value was converted into a corresponding drug dosage. The next conversion step is to calculate a Universal MEC (UMEC) based on the MEC of a human (1694, a value established in many pharmocokinetic studies [16]) and the established human dose of 2000 mg/day. The equation to calculate this is: $MEC_{human}(UMEC) = dose(mg/day)_{human}$; where MEC_{human} is 1694 and the drug dose is 2000 mg/day, yielding a UMEC value of 1.18. An appropriate murine dosage equivalent to the 2000 mg/day human dosage may be calculated, by using the same equation to calculate UMEC, instead using the MEC value of a mouse: $MEC_{mouse}(UMEC) = dose(mg/day)_{mouse}$; where MEC_{mouse} is 4.4 and the UMEC is 1.18, giving a murine drug dosage of 5.2 mg/day. By incorporating mouse body weight (0.025 kg) into this calculation, a value of 208 mg/kg/day is obtained. This dosage is equivalent to the 2000 mg/day human dosage (28.57 mg/kg/day, assuming a 70 kg human). According to the manufacturer's product insert, there are 35 g of pure drug in the 110 g CellCept® oral suspension powder. Assuming that mice eat 5 g of chow per day and that the average body weight of a mouse is 0.025 kg, a ratio of CellCept® oral suspension powder that should be incorporated into each kilogram of Harlan Teklad Western diet was calculated using a pharmacokinetic equation provided by Sedgwick [16] and Gibson [12].

Analysis of Atherosclerosis, Splenomegaly, Lymphadenopathy, and Body Weight

After 12 weeks of Western diet, the final body weights were recorded, the mice were euthanized, and the spleen and submandibular lymph nodes were removed and weighed. The heart containing the aortic root, was frozen in OCT. Frozen sections of aortic root were stained with Oil Red O solution and microphotographs were taken and values of total atherosclerotic lesion area were analyzed using Adobe Photoshop 7.0.

Kidney Histology

Paraffin embedded tissue was sectioned (5 μm) and slides were stained with hematoxylin and eosin. Cross-sectional areas of at least 25 glomeruli were measured in each animal using computer-assisted pixel counting (Photoshop CS3; Adobe).

Serum Measurements

Circulating anti-nuclear antibodies (ANA) were measured by immunofluorescence using HEp-2 coated slides (The Binding Site Inc., San Diego, California). Slides were incubated for 1 h with serial log-scale dilutions (1:100 to 1:90000; as previously described by Komori, et al.) [17] of mouse serum, washed in PBS, and then incubated with FITC-labeled goat anti-mouse IgG (whole molecule; Sigma-Aldrich, St. Louis, Missouri). Slides were viewed using fluorescent microscopy. Serum cholesterol levels were determined using a total cholesterol microtiter procedure according to the manufacturers instructions (Wako Diagnostics, Richmond VA).

Statistical Analysis

The significant differences between mean values of atherosclerotic lesion area, spleen weight, and lymph node weight were assessed by a Mann Whitney test; a p-value <0.05 was considered significant.

Results

Body Weight and Food Intake

MMF has an excellent oral bioavailability. However, this treatment frequently induces gastrointestinal symptoms in humans [18], which could decrease drug intake. In order to ensure that the mice in each experimental group were ingesting similar amounts of food, the amount of food ingested was recorded weekly over the course of the experiment, and total ingestion of each group is presented in Figure 1A. Total body weights of the mice were also measured at intervals throughout the experiment (Figure 1B). There was no difference between the mice treated with MMF and control mice with regard to total food intake or body weight.

The Development of Splenomegaly, Lymphadenopathy and Autoantibodies are Inhibited by MMF Treatment

After 12 weeks treatment, the spleen and submandibular lymph nodes of the *gld.apoE*$^{-/-}$ mice were removed and weighed. The mice receiving MMF had a significantly smaller spleen weight compared to mice not receiving MMF (control): 0.41±0.08 g versus 0.63±0.05 g in the MMF group (p = 0.02, using Mann Whitney test) (Figure 2A), as well as a lower, but not significant, lymph node weight compared to control (mean ± SEM): 0.23±0.02 g versus 0.44±0.09 g, respectively (p = 0.09) (Figure 2B). To determine if MMF effects were due to a modification of lymphocyte population, we performed immunohistochemical staining for T-cells and B-cells in lymph node sections from treated and untreated mice. Similar to a previous report [19], no significant effect was observed in the appearance or distribution of T- or B-cells within the lymph nodes regardless of treatment (data not shown). We then examined the effect of MMF dose on autoantibody production. In humans, a decrease in autoantibody titers has been shown during the course of MMF therapy [9]. We found a similar result in our lupus-associated

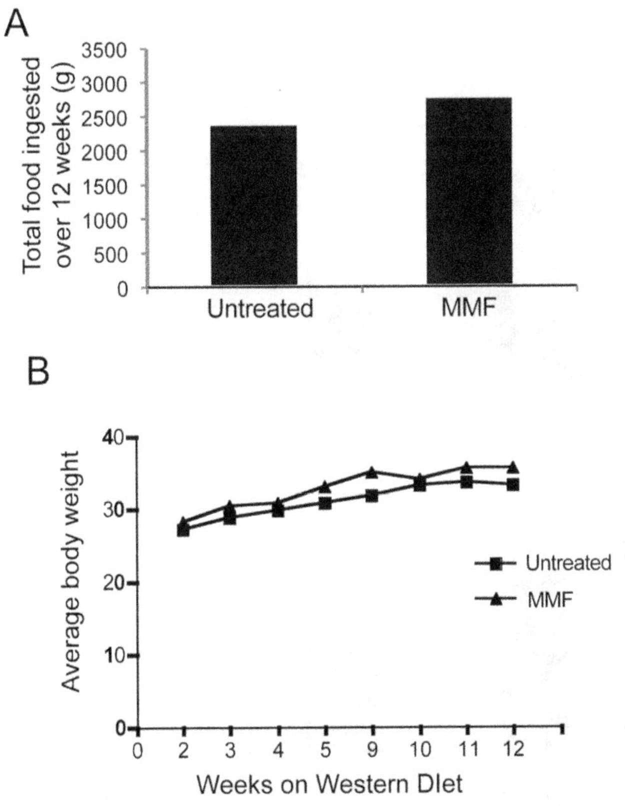

Figure 1. Total food intake and average body weights. *A*, Food was weighed weekly and total amount ingested was recorded for each group (control, n = 8; MMF, n = 9). *B*, Evolution of body weight as weighed weekly during the course of the experiment.

atherosclerosis mouse model with a significant decrease of anti-nuclear antibody (ANA) titer in the MMF group compared to the controls (median [IQR]): 1.5 [1.5–2] versus 4 [4–5.5], respectively (p = 0,001) (Figure 2C).

Improvement of Nephritis in gld.apoE$^{-/-}$ Mice Receiving MMF

MMF is currently used as induction therapy, maintenance therapy, or both for patients with lupus nephritis [9,20,21,22,23]. Although B6 mice deficient in Fas (*lpr*) or FasL (*gld*) display mild or no kidney disease [24], the lack of apoE associated with the *gld* mutation induces significant kidney disease [14]. We assessed the extent of renal damage associated with the lupus phenotype, in control versus the MMF treated experimental *gld.apoE*$^{-/-}$ group. Glomerular tuft size and cell count were significantly decreased in *gld.apoE*$^{-/-}$ after treatment with MMF (respectively, p = 0.002 and p = 0.004) (Figure 3A–C). Of note, infiltration of inflammatory cells as well as modest crescent formation was observed in control mice, but not in MMF treated mice. Our findings demonstrate the efficacy of MMF on lupus parameters in our mouse model, as previously described in human SLE and other mouse models.

MMF Decreases the Severity of Atherosclerosis in gld.apoE$^{-/-}$ Mice

To determine the effect of MMF on atherosclerotic parameters, the aortic root of each mouse was stained with Oil red O to reveal areas of atherosclerotic lesion after 12 weeks on Western diet (WD), (Figure 4A). A significant decrease in lesion area was observed in the MMF-treated mice compared to control (Figure 4B) (p = 0.02). Serum levels of total cholesterol were also examined to determine whether the protective effects of MMF on atherosclerosis severity could be explained by differences in serum cholesterol levels. However, there was no detectable difference between mice treated with MMF compared to control: 716±63 mg/dl versus 669±32 mg/dl, respectively (p = 0.38) (Figure 4C).

Discussion

The purpose of this experiment was to investigate the effects of mycophenolate mofetil (MMF), on development of premature atherosclerosis in a murine mouse model of accelerated atherosclerosis and systemic lupus erythematosus (SLE). The *gld.apoE*$^{-/-}$ model is ideal to use for this experiment based on previous findings of synergistic disease presentation of both SLE and atherosclerosis in mice [14]. Our study investigated the effect of a physiologically relevant dose of MMF on disease development. The 200 mg/kg/day concentration of MMF in mouse diet is roughly equivalent to the 2000 mg/day dose of MMF approved for use in human renal transplant prophylaxis and commonly used for the treatment of human SLE. Severity of cardiovascular disease was assessed by quantifying the atherosclerotic lesion area in the aortic root. To assess the hallmarks of SLE associated with the *gld.apoE*$^{-/-}$ model, spleen and submandibular lymph node were weighed. As such, the data show that the dosage of 200 mg/kg/day yields a significant ameliorating effect on atherosclerosis, splenomegaly and lymphadenopathy presentation. These data suggest that MMF treatment of patients with SLE could not only be beneficial to lupus, but also decrease the risk of cardiovascular disease.

With advances in medical care, the quality of life has improved and survival rate has increased for patients with SLE [2]. However, with this increased survival rate, there is also a correlated increase in CVD. Chronic inflammation has been implicated as

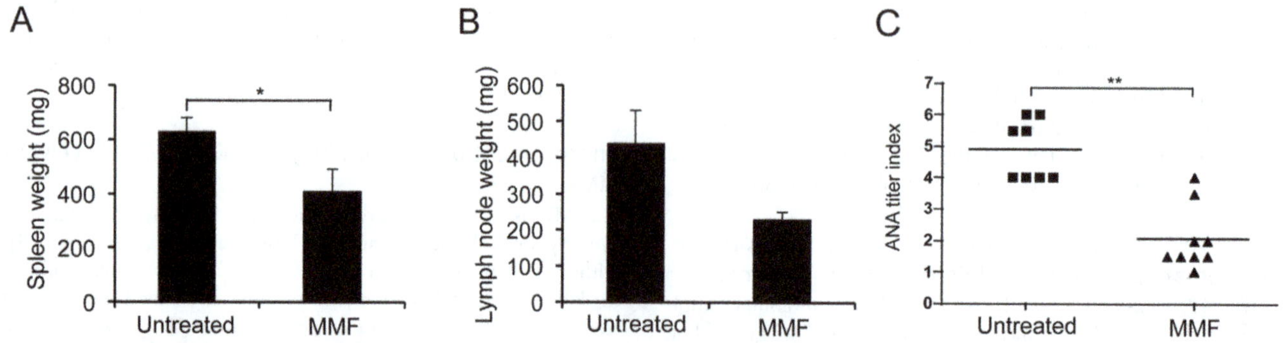

Figure 2. MMF treatment decreases the autoimmune phenotype in *gld.apoE−/−* mice. *A*, Spleen from mice, treated with 200 mg/kg/day MMF or untreated, was harvested and weighed (*, $p<0.05$). *B*, The lymph nodes were also harvested and weighed. *C*, ANA titer was determined from serum samples using HEp-2-coated slides and scored using the value of the last positive dilution (**, $p = 0.001$). Data are expressed as means ± SEM.

a contributing factor for the development of premature atherosclerosis in SLE patients [3,25,26,27]. Therefore, there is an interest in using anti-inflammatory or immunomodulatory therapies for this condition. MMF, an immunosuppressive agent, is currently used for the treatment of SLE patients, particularly those with kidney involvement, as well as for the prevention of rejection in transplant patients.

MMF was first demonstrated to inhibit T-cell function, however, MMF also exerts inhibitory effects on other immune cells and effectors, including downregulation of cell adhesion molecules and attenuation of monocyte and macrophage responses [28]. MMF has also been shown to suppress a number of the inflammatory events that are involved in the development of atherosclerosis. T-lymphocyte infiltration to atherosclerotic plaque and circulation to sites of inflammation is abrogated by MMF treatment [28]. MMF has been shown to reduce the expression of vascular adhesion molecules in atherosclerosis by inhibiting the nuclear factor NFκB which is required for their transcriptional upregulation [29]. Raisanen *et al* [30] showed that MMF treatment reduces the appearance and proliferation of smooth muscle cells in the intima, which normally contribute to atherosclerotic plaque formation by recruitment of extracellular matrix and self-proliferation. Thus, MMF has properties that could be considered anti-atherogenic: inhibiting T-cells, blocking leukocyte adhesion and inhibiting proliferation of smooth muscle

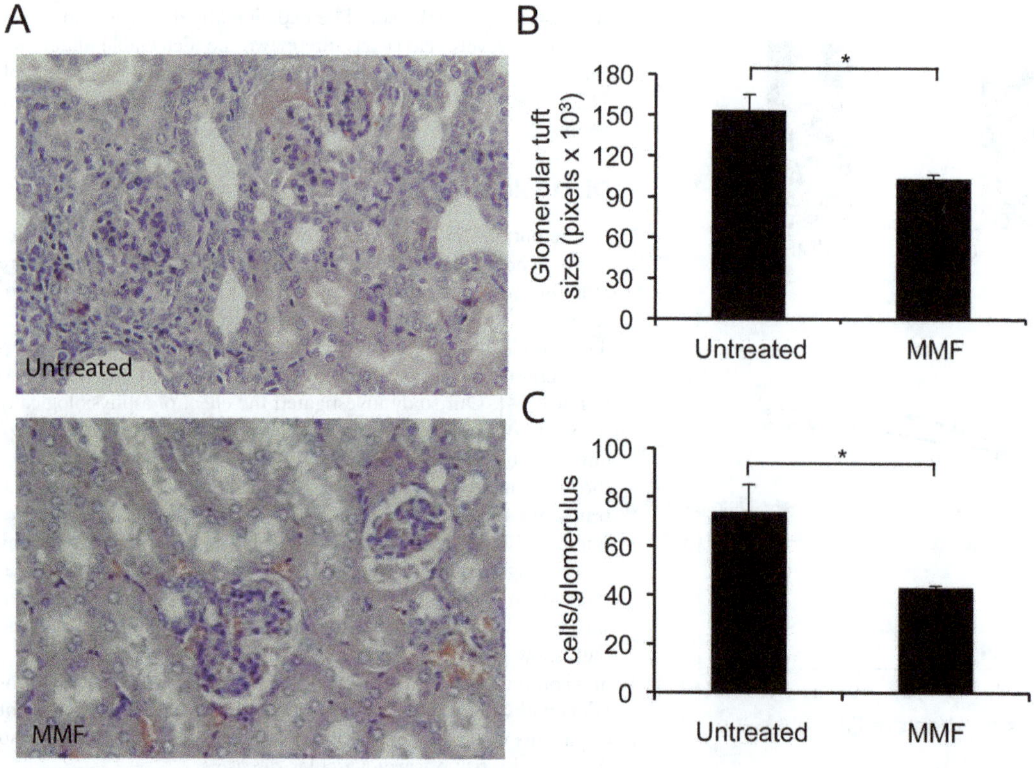

Figure 3. Renal disease is ameliorated in *gld.apoE−/−* mice after MMF treatment. The mice were treated with MMF or control for 12 wk. *A*, Representative H&E-stained sections of kidney in both groups. Glomerular tuft size (*B*) (*, $p = 0.002$) and cell count (*C*) (**, $p = 0.004$) were measured by computer-assisted pixel counting. Values shown are the mean ± SEM.

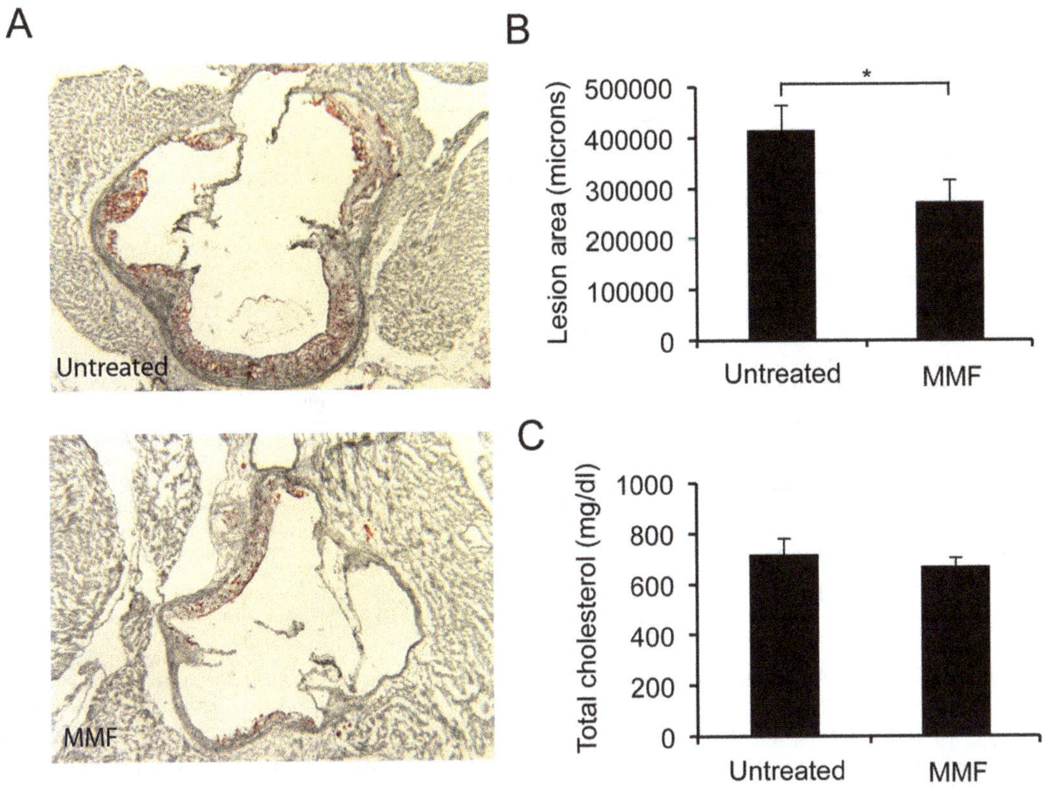

Figure 4. Decreased atherosclerosis in *gld.apoE−/−* mice treated with MMF. Aortic root atherosclerotic lesion area in MMF-treated or control mice. *A*, Representative photographs of aortic root stained with Oil Red O from mice maintained on Western diet for 12 wk and treated with 200 mg/kg/day MMF or untreated. *B*, Atherosclerotic lesion area of Oil Red O-stained aortae was quantified in both groups (*, $p = 0.02$). *C*, Total serum cholesterol was quantified in control mice and mice treated with 200 mg/kg/day MMF.

cells; therefore making it a potentially valuable drug to prevent the development of atherosclerosis in patients with SLE.

A recent publication examined the effect of MMF on atherosclerosis development by using bone marrow transplantation to generate a mouse model of lupus with associated atherosclerosis [31]. van Leuven et al. report that the LDLr−/−. Sle mouse shows decreased atherosclerosis after MMF treatment, although lesion area does not decrease with atorvastatin treatment alone. However, despite the beneficial effects to atherosclerosis, there are no discernable differences in circulating autoantibody levels or kidney pathology. While it is known that B6 mice deficient in Fas (*lpr*) or FasL (*gld*) display mild or no kidney disease, the *gld.apoE*$^{-/-}$ model develops glomerular tuft enlargement and significant inflammatory cell infiltrate to the kidney [14]. The results presented in the current study show a decrease in both lupus-disease and cardiovascular disease. It is reasonable to suggest that differences in the disease models utilized (*Ldlr−/−* versus *apoE−/−*, respectively; and *Sle1.2.3* versus *gld*, respectively) or the dosage (40 mg/kg/day versus 200 mg/kg/day) could have contributed to the contrasting results.

Substantial evidence exists to support a critical role of inflammation in the pathology of both SLE and CVD caused by atherosclerosis. The chronic inflammation associated with SLE correlates to the increased risk in CVD seen in patients [25,26,27]. The current study suggests that MMF, in addition to this well-known efficacy on lupus nephritis, might be a promising agent for the prevention of atherosclerosis in SLE. A more extensive analysis of atherosclerosis and SLE in these MMF-treated *gld.apoE*$^{-/-}$ mice will need to be performed to fully determine how MMF impacts the accelerated atherosclerosis of our lupus mouse model and potentially bring a better understanding of the link between atherogenesis and autoimmune disease.

Author Contributions

Conceived and designed the experiments: IRR CDA TA. Performed the experiments: CR RR TA ZW. Analyzed the data: CR PD. Wrote the paper: IRR CR TA.

References

1. Tsokos GC (2011) Systemic lupus erythematosus. N Engl J Med 365: 2110–2121.
2. Pons-Estel GJ, Alarcon GS, Scofield L, Reinlib L, Cooper GS (2010) Understanding the epidemiology and progression of systemic lupus erythematosus. Semin Arthritis Rheum 39: 257–268.
3. Westerweel PE, Luyten RK, Koomans HA, Derksen RH, Verhaar MC (2007) Premature atherosclerotic cardiovascular disease in systemic lupus erythematosus. Arthritis Rheum 56: 1384–1396.
4. Urowitz MB, Gladman D, Ibanez D, Bae SC, Sanchez-Guerrero J, et al. (2010) Atherosclerotic vascular events in a multinational inception cohort of systemic lupus erythematosus. Arthritis Care Res (Hoboken) 62: 881–887.
5. Galkina E, Ley K (2009) Immune and inflammatory mechanisms of atherosclerosis. Annu Rev Immunol 27: 165–197.
6. Ross R (1999) Atherosclerosis–an inflammatory disease. N Engl J Med 340: 115–126.

7. Jung H, Bobba R, Su J, Shariati-Sarabi Z, Gladman DD, et al. (2010) The protective effect of antimalarial drugs on thrombovascular events in systemic lupus erythematosus. Arthritis Rheum 62: 863–868.
8. Ferreira GA, Navarro TP, Telles RW, Andrade LE, Sato EI (2007) Atorvastatin therapy improves endothelial-dependent vasodilation in patients with systemic lupus erythematosus: an 8 weeks controlled trial. Rheumatology (Oxford) 46: 1560–1565.
9. Dooley MA, Jayne D, Ginzler EM, Isenberg D, Olsen NJ, et al. (2011) Mycophenolate versus azathioprine as maintenance therapy for lupus nephritis. N Engl J Med 365: 1886–1895.
10. Allison AC, Eugui EM (1993) Immunosuppressive and other effects of mycophenolic acid and an ester prodrug, mycophenolate mofetil. Immunol Rev 136: 5–28.
11. Franklin TJ, Cook JM (1969) The inhibition of nucleic acid synthesis by mycophenolic acid. Biochem J 113: 515–524.
12. Gibson WT, Hayden MR (2007) Mycophenolate mofetil and atherosclerosis: results of animal and human studies. Ann N Y Acad Sci 1110: 209–221.
13. van Leuven SI, van Wijk DF, Volger OL, de Vries JP, van der Loos CM, et al. (2010) Mycophenolate mofetil attenuates plaque inflammation in patients with symptomatic carotid artery stenosis. Atherosclerosis 211: 231–236.
14. Aprahamian T, Rifkin I, Bonegio R, Hugel B, Freyssinet JM, et al. (2004) Impaired clearance of apoptotic cells promotes synergy between atherogenesis and autoimmune disease. J Exp Med 199: 1121–1131.
15. Ng R (2004) Drugs development and preclinical studies. In: Sons JW, editor. Drugs: From Discovery to Approval. 107–138.
16. Sedgwick C, Pokras MA (1988) Extrapolating rational drug doses and treatment periods by allometric scaling. Proceedings of the 55th Annual Meeting of the American Animal Hospital Association. Washington, D.C. 156–157.
17. Komori H, Furukawa H, Mori S, Ito MR, Terada M, et al. (2006) A signal adaptor SLAM-associated protein regulates spontaneous autoimmunity and Fas-dependent lymphoproliferation in MRL-Faslpr lupus mice. J Immunol 176: 395–400.
18. Epinette WW, Parker CM, Jones EL, Greist MC (1987) Mycophenolic acid for psoriasis. A review of pharmacology, long-term efficacy, and safety. J Am Acad Dermatol 17: 962–971.
19. Van Bruggen MC, Walgreen B, Rijke TP, Berden JH (1998) Attenuation of murine lupus nephritis by mycophenolate mofetil. J Am Soc Nephrol 9: 1407–1415.
20. Appel GB, Contreras G, Dooley MA, Ginzler EM, Isenberg D, et al. (2009) Mycophenolate mofetil versus cyclophosphamide for induction treatment of lupus nephritis. J Am Soc Nephrol 20: 1103–1112.
21. Chan TM, Li FK, Tang CS, Wong RW, Fang GX, et al. (2000) Efficacy of mycophenolate mofetil in patients with diffuse proliferative lupus nephritis. Hong Kong-Guangzhou Nephrology Study Group. N Engl J Med 343: 1156–1162.
22. Ginzler EM, Dooley MA, Aranow C, Kim MY, Buyon J, et al. (2005) Mycophenolate mofetil or intravenous cyclophosphamide for lupus nephritis. N Engl J Med 353: 2219–2228.
23. Ong LM, Hooi LS, Lim TO, Goh BL, Ahmad G, et al. (2005) Randomized controlled trial of pulse intravenous cyclophosphamide versus mycophenolate mofetil in the induction therapy of proliferative lupus nephritis. Nephrology (Carlton) 10: 504–510.
24. Kelley VE, Roths JB (1985) Interaction of mutant lpr gene with background strain influences renal disease. Clin Immunol Immunopathol 37: 220–229.
25. Lockshin MD, Salmon JE, Roman MJ (2001) Atherosclerosis and lupus: a work in progress. Arthritis Rheum 44: 2215–2217.
26. Manzi S, Meilahn EN, Rairie JE, Conte CG, Medsger TA, Jr., et al. (1997) Age-specific incidence rates of myocardial infarction and angina in women with systemic lupus erythematosus: comparison with the Framingham Study. Am J Epidemiol 145: 408–415.
27. Riboldi P, Gerosa M, Luzzana C, Catelli L (2002) Cardiac involvement in systemic autoimmune diseases. Clin Rev Allergy Immunol 23: 247–261.
28. van Leuven SI, Kastelein JJ, Allison AC, Hayden MR, Stroes ES (2006) Mycophenolate mofetil (MMF): firing at the atherosclerotic plaque from different angles? Cardiovasc Res 69: 341–347.
29. Huang HD, Liu ZH, Zhu XJ, Chen ZH, Li LS (2002) Inhibition of mycophenolic acid on NF-kappaB activity in human endothelial cells. Acta Pharmacol Sin 23: 649–653.
30. Raisanen-Sokolowski A, Vuoristo P, Myllarniemi M, Yilmaz S, Kallio E, et al. (1995) Mycophenolate mofetil (MMF, RS-61443) inhibits inflammation and smooth muscle cell proliferation in rat aortic allografts. Transpl Immunol 3: 342–351.
31. van Leuven SI, Mendez-Fernandez YV, Wilhelm AJ, Wade NS, Gabriel CL, et al. (2012) Mycophenolate mofetil but not atorvastatin attenuates atherosclerosis in lupus-prone LDLr(−/−) mice. Ann Rheum Dis 71: 408–414.

9

Lexis Diagram and Illness-Death Model: Simulating Populations in Chronic Disease Epidemiology

Ralph Brinks[1,2]*, Sandra Landwehr[1,3], Rebecca Fischer-Betz[2], Matthias Schneider[2], Guido Giani[3]

1 German Diabetes Center, Institute of Biometry and Epidemiology, Duesseldorf, Germany, **2** University Hospital, Polyclinics for Rheumatology, Duesseldorf, Germany, **3** Heinrich-Heine-University, Institute for Statistics in Medicine, Duesseldorf, Germany

Abstract

Chronic diseases impose a tremendous global health problem of the 21st century. Epidemiological and public health models help to gain insight into the distribution and burden of chronic diseases. Moreover, the models may help to plan appropriate interventions against risk factors. To provide accurate results, models often need to take into account three different time-scales: calendar time, age, and duration since the onset of the disease. Incidence and mortality often change with age and calendar time. In many diseases such as, for example, diabetes and dementia, the mortality of the diseased persons additionally depends on the duration of the disease. The aim of this work is to describe an algorithm and a flexible software framework for the simulation of populations moving in an illness-death model that describes the epidemiology of a chronic disease in the face of the different times-scales. We set up a discrete event simulation in continuous time involving competing risks using the freely available statistical software R. Relevant events are birth, the onset (or diagnosis) of the disease and death with or without the disease. The Lexis diagram keeps track of the different time-scales. Input data are birth rates, incidence and mortality rates, which can be given as numerical values on a grid. The algorithm manages the complex interplay between the rates and the different time-scales. As a result, for each subject in the simulated population, the algorithm provides the calendar time of birth, the age of onset of the disease (if the subject contracts the disease) and the age at death. By this means, the impact of interventions may be estimated and compared.

Editor: Catalin Buiu, Politehnica University of Bucharest, Romania

Funding: Financial support for this study was provided by a grant from the Hiller Foundation, Erkrath, Germany. The funder had no role in study design, data collection, analysis and interpretation, decision to publish, or preparation of the manuscript.

Competing Interests: The authors have declared that no competing interests exist.

* Email: ralph.brinks@ddz.uni-duesseldorf.de

Introduction

Chronic diseases impose a tremendous global health problem of the 21st century. The World Health Organization estimates that 63% of all deaths in 2008 were caused by chronic diseases [1]. Besides taking measures in politics and society, research efforts are needed to oppose this threat. In studying the characteristics of chronic diseases from a public health perspective, it is often important to consider different time-scales [2]. The age of the subjects in a population is a risk factor for many diseases. Changes in life-style and medical care influence the risk of contracting and dying from the disease on a secular scale. Thus, the incidence rate of the chronic disease as well as the mortality rates (with and without the disease) depend on the calendar time. Moreover, the mortality of people with the disease often depends on the duration since its onset. Examples are diabetes [3,4], dementia [5], depression [6], and systemic lupus erythematosus [7]. For decision-makers all time-scales may be important.

As a hypothetical example, consider the question which health programme to choose from two possibilities A and B if the outcome of interest is the gain of life-years. Possibility A is known to decrease the incidence of the disease by 15%, and possibility B lowers the mortality of those having the disease for more than ten years by 50%. The decision depends on several factors. If, on the one hand, the incidence rate is non-zero for children only and the birth rate in the population is low, possibility A may have little effect with respect to the gain of life-years. If, on the other hand, the chronic disease has very few people reaching ten-year survival after onset, programme B can be nearly useless. In problems similar to the example, the decision-maker may face a complex interplay of epidemiological and demographical considerations.

The aim of this work is to describe an algorithm and a flexible software framework for simulation of populations moving in a multi-state model (illness-death model) that describes a chronic disease. The simulation takes into account the different time-scales: calendar time, age, and duration of the disease. Although simulations using multi-state models are subject to recent textbooks [8], to our knowledge no algorithm has been described that incorporates the effects of all the different time-scales.

Methods

A popular framework for studying irreversible diseases is the illness-death model (IDM) consisting of the three states *Normal*, *Disease* and *Death*, [9–11]. The associated transition rates, synonymously *densities* (in units "per person-time", not to be confused with risks or probabilities [12]), are the incidence i, and the mortality rates m_0 and m_1 (Figure 1). In general, these rates

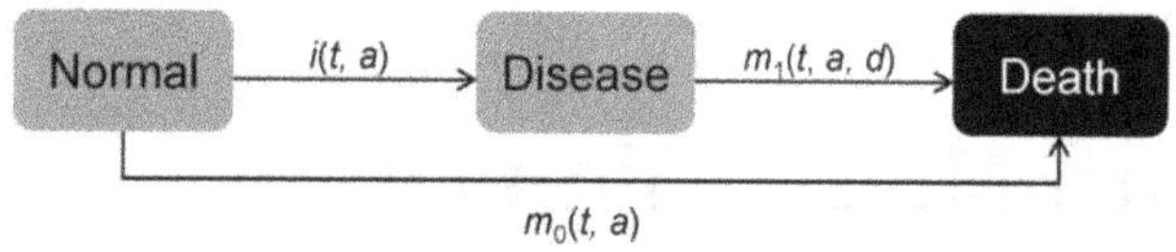

Figure 1. Three states model of normal (healthy), diseased and dead subjects. The transition rates may depend on calender time t, age a, and in case of m_1 also on the duration d of the disease.

depend on calendar time (t), age (a) and in case of m_1 on the duration of the disease (d).

This article presents a method for simulating populations moving in the IDM. The motivation for the algorithms comes from analytical epidemiology where relations between common epidemiological measures are studied. Examples for those measures are the prevalence, the duration of a disease, the age of onset (or diagnosis), and lost life-years (due to the disease). A typical question may be: what is the mean age of diagnosis of subjects born in a certain time period? What is their mean age at death? Another interesting aim is the estimation of the incidence rate i from cross-sectional information. At a specific point in time t', each of the subjects $j=1,\ldots,n$, has a unique "status". Neglecting those who are unborn or dead at t', the status in the IDM is either *normal* (non-diseased) or *diseased*. Thus, the status can be seen as a binary random variable, and data of this kind are typically called *current status data* [13]. The current status is closely linked with the incidence i and the mortalities m_0 and m_1 before t'. Estimating the incidence from current status data, for example, has been a topic in research for decades [14]. The framework presented here may be useful in this field.

Overview of the simulation algorithm

The simulation is a microsimulation, i.e., it treats each person in the population as an autonomous unit. For each person, indexed $j, j=1,\ldots,n$, the relevant events *diagnosis* and *death* are simulated. This is accomplished in two steps:

1. Contracting the disease or dying without the disease is modelled as competing risk [11]. Given the time $t_0^{(j)}$ of birth of person j, the cumulative distribution function $F_1^{(j)}$ of the *first failure time* $T_1^{(j)}$ is

$$F_1^{(j)}(t)=1-\exp\left(-\int_0^t i\left(t_0^{(j)}+\tau,\tau\right)+m_0\left(t_0^{(j)}+\tau,\tau\right)\mathrm{d}\tau\right). \quad (1)$$

The term *first failure time* $T_1^{(j)}$ refers to the time of diagnosis or death without disease and is measured in time units after birth of person j. Thus, $T_1^{(j)}$ is the age at which the first transition from the state *Normal* occurs. Given that a transition occurs at $T_1^{(j)}$ for person j, then the odds of moving into state *Disease* versus moving into state *Death* is

$$\frac{i\left(t_0^{(j)}+T_1^{(j)},T_1^{(j)}\right)}{m_0\left(t_0^{(j)}+T_1^{(j)},T_1^{(j)}\right)}.$$

2. If the event at $T_1^{(j)}$ is the death (without the disease), the simulation for person j is finished. If, however, the event is the diagnosis of the disease, the "second failure time" $T_2^{(j)}$ to death (with disease) has the distribution function $F_2^{(j)}$:

$$F_2^{(j)}\left(t|T_1^{(j)}\right)=1-\exp\left(-\int_0^t m_1\left(t_0^{(j)}+T_1^{(j)}+\tau,T_1^{(j)}+\tau,\tau\right)\mathrm{d}\tau\right). (2)$$

The next section describes in detail how the integrals in Equations (1) and (2) may be calculated in the simulation. After calculating the integrals, the question arises how the times T_1 and T_2 can be obtained from F_1 and F_2. This is done by the *inverse transform sampling method*: Let F be a cumulative distribution function and $u\in(0,1)$. For $F^{-1}(u) := \inf\{x|F(x)\geq u\}$ it holds: If U is a uniform random variable on (0,1), then $F^{-1}(U)$ follows the distribution F. Thus, the simulation of T_1 and T_2 is easy, if a random number generator for U such as `runif` in R is available.

For each of the n persons in the population we store four pieces of data:

1. a unique identifier j,
2. the date $t_0^{(j)}$ of birth (`dob`) of person j,
3. the age at diagnosis (`adi`) of person j, and
4. the age at death (`ade`) of person j.

If the person j does not contract the disease, the age at diagnosis `adi` is set to `NA` (missing). In summary, we get the Algorithm 1.

Algorithm 1 Simulation of populations moving in the IDM

for $j=1$ **to** n **do**
  `dob` $\leftarrow t_0^{(j)}$
  calculate event time $T_1^{(j)}$ according to Equation (1)
  simulate type of event that has happened at $T_1^{(j)}$ by Equation (1)
  if event is diagnosis **then**
    `adi` $\leftarrow T_1^{(j)}$
    calculate time $T_2^{(j)}$ of death using Equation (2)
    `ade` $\leftarrow T_1^{(j)}+T_2^{(j)}$
  else
    `adi` $\leftarrow$ `NA`
    `ade` $\leftarrow T_1^{(j)}$
  end if
  write `j, dob, adi, ade` to file
end for

Calculating line integrals

In this section the calculation of the integrals in Equations (1) and (2) is described. The situation in which analytical expressions for these integrals exist, is straightforward. The first simulation in the next section is an example. However, in real world applications, analytical expressions for the integrals are rarely given. For convenience, mathematical functions (e.g., splines) may be fitted to the data and integration is accomplished with the fitted functions. Since the aim of this work is a flexible way of treating the incidence and mortality rates, we assume that the rates are given as numerical values on a regular grid. Here we focus on the most general case, which is characterized by:

1. None of the time-scales t,a, and d is negligible, and
2. the values of i,m_0,m_1 are given as data points only.

For many chronic diseases, we think this is the most relevant case: The mortality rates m_0 and m_1 depend on a and t. Since age is a risk factor for many diseases, the dependency on age is obvious. Healthier life-style and medical progress in many countries lead to secular trends in m_0 and m_1. In addition, disease duration d is likely to have an impact on m_1 in many chronic diseases. Thus, none of the time-scales is negligible, which is covered in the second and third example.

In the most general case, the integrands i, m_0, and m_1 are given by data points only. We assume that the numerical values are located on a regular grid. The grid is two-dimensional in case of i and m_0, which depend on two time-scales t and a; and the grid is three-dimensional in case of m_1 which depends on t, a, and d.

In event history analysis [2], a useful concept is the *Lexis diagram*, which is a co-ordinate system with axes calendar time t (abscissa) and age a (ordinate). The t-dimension sometimes is referred to as period. Each subject is represented by a line segment from time and age at entry to time and age at exit. Entry and exit may be birth and death, respectively, or entry and exit in a epidemiological study or clinical trial. There are excellent and extensive introductions about the theory of Lexis diagrams (see for example [9,15,16] and references therein), which allows us to be short here. In irreversible diseases, the common two-dimensional Lexis diagram with axes in t- and a-direction may be generalized to a three-dimensional co-ordinate system with disease duration d represented by the applicate (i.e., the z-axis). If a subject does not contract the disease during lifetime, the life line remains in the t-a-plane parallel to the line bisecting abscissa and ordinate. In other words, the life line for the time without disease is parallel to $e_1 := (1,1,0)$ (where the triple (t,a,d) denotes the co-ordinates in time, age and duration direction, respectively). However if at a certain point in time E the disease is diagnosed, the life line changes its direction, henceforth runs parallel to $e_2 := (1,1,1)$.

The situation is illustrated in Figure 2. The life lines of two subjects are shown in the three-dimensional Lexis space. At birth (denoted $B_\nu, \nu = 1,2$) both subjects are disease-free; both life lines are parallel to e_1. The first subject contracts the disease at E. Henceforth, the life line is parallel to e_2 until death at D_1. The second subject remains disease-free until death at D_2.

Having the concept of the Lexis diagram at hand, we observe that F_1 and F_2 in Equations (1) and (2) are line integrals in the Lexis space. We start with calculating the first failure times T_1. For subject j the associated life line starts at $(t,a) = (t_0^{(j)}, 0)$. We chose an age $\omega > 0$, when it is certain that a transition to one of the states *Disease* or *Death* has occurred, say $\omega = 150$ (years). For calculating $F_1^{(j)}$, we trace the hypothetical life line from $B_j := (t_0^{(j)}, 0)$ to $D_j := (t_0^{(j)} + \omega, \omega)$. Thus, the hypothetical life line has a representation

$$\mathcal{L}_j : B_j + \alpha \cdot (D_j - B_j), \alpha \in [0,1].$$

Following the life line is related to the method of ray-tracing in the field of computer graphics, where efficient algorithms for this purpose exist. In Siddon's algorithm [17], the key idea is to follow $\mathcal{L}_j$ by calculating intersections with volume elements (voxels), which form a regular partition of the Lexis space. Let

$$A_j^\star = \{\alpha^{(j)}(p) | p = 1, \ldots, P^{(j)}\}$$

with $0 = \alpha^{(j)}(1) < \ldots < \alpha^{(j)}(P^{(j)}) = 1$ be a parametrization of the points where $\mathcal{L}_j$ intersects the voxel faces plus the start and end points B_j and D_j. Details for the calculation of $A_j^\star$ are described in the supporting information to this article. The parametrization $A_j^\star$ is ideally suited for approximating the integral in Equation (1) by the trapezoidal rule [18]. The reason lies in the fact that in calculating $F_1^{(j)}(\omega)$ the values $F_1^{(j)}\left(t_0^{(j)} + \alpha^{(j)}(p)\omega\right), p = 1, \ldots, P^{(j)}$, are a by-product. Algorithm 2 shows the necessary steps.

Algorithm 2 Calculating F_1

for $j = 1$ **to** n **do**

  calculate $A_j^\star = \{\alpha^{(j)}(p) | p = 1, \ldots, P^{(j)}\}$

  $\ell_1 \leftarrow 0$

  $\tau_1 \leftarrow 0$

  $f_1 \leftarrow i\left(t_0^{(j)}, 0\right) + m_0\left(t_0^{(j)}, 0\right)$

  $F_1^{(j)}(\tau_1) \leftarrow 0$

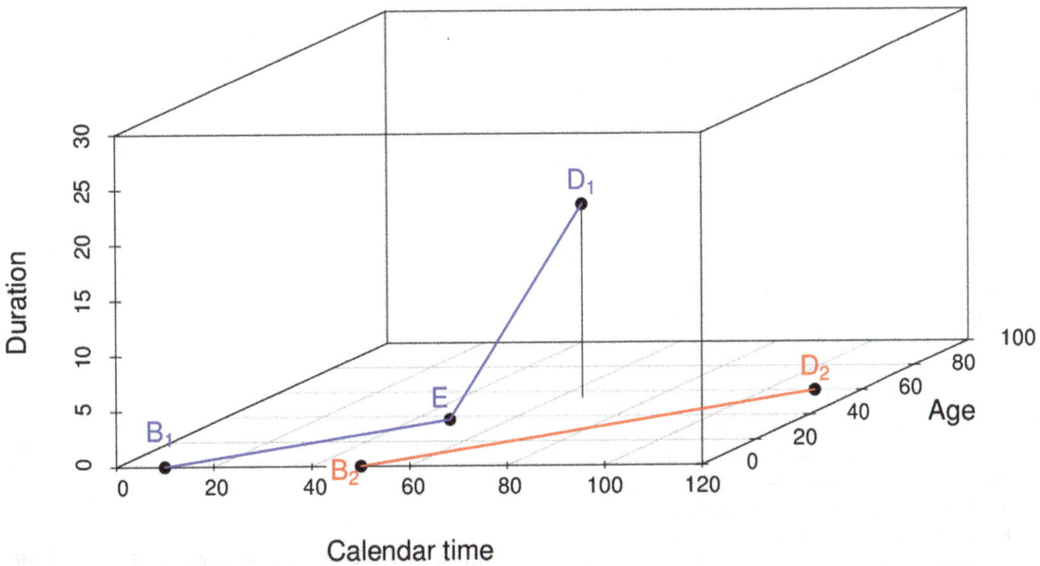

Figure 2. Three-dimensional Lexis diagram with two life lines. Abscissa, ordinate and applicate (z-axis) represent calendar time t, age a and duration d, respectively. The life lines start at birth B_ν and end at death $D_\nu, \nu = 1,2$. The first subject (blue line segments) contracts the disease at E. Then, the life line changes its direction. The second subject (red line segment) does not contract the disease, the life line remains in the t-a-plane.

for $p=2$ **to** $P^{(j)}$ **do**
 $\tau_p \leftarrow \alpha^{(j)}(p)\cdot\omega$
 $f_p \leftarrow i\left(t_0^{(j)}+\tau_p,\tau_p\right)+m_0\left(t_0^{(j)}+\tau_p,\tau_p\right)$
 $\ell_p \leftarrow \ell_{p-1}+\frac{1}{2}\cdot(\tau_p-\tau_{p-1})\cdot(f_p+f_{p-1})$
 $F_1^{(j)}\left(t_0^{(j)}+\tau_p\right)\leftarrow 1-\exp(-\ell_p)$
end for
end for

Since the values of i and m_0 are given on the voxel grid only, the calculation of $f_p, p=1,\ldots,P^{(j)}$, needs bilinear interpolation of the values of the adjacent voxels [19].

After preparing $F_1^{(j)}, j=1,\ldots,n$, the values of the times $T_1^{(j)}$ can be calculated by the inverse transform sampling method. Since we have $F_1^{(j)}$ calculated at points $\zeta_p := t_0^{(j)}+\tau_p, p=1,\ldots,P^{(j)}$, the inverse transform sampling would yield only those ζ_p. A better accuracy can be obtained by (linear) inverse interpolation [18]. For $t\in(\zeta_{p-1},\zeta_p), p=2,\ldots,P^{(j)}$, let $\xi := \frac{t-\zeta_{p-1}}{\zeta_p-\zeta_{p-1}}$. Then, it holds

$$F_1^{(j)}(t)\approx(1-\xi)\cdot F_1^{(j)}(\zeta_{p-1})+\xi\cdot F_1^{(j)}(\zeta_p).$$

Thus, for $u\in(0,1)$ drawn from a uniform distribution, we find the unique $p\in\{2,\ldots,P^{(j)}\}$, such that $F_1^{(j)}(\zeta_{p-1})\leq u<F_1^{(j)}(\zeta_p)$, and set

$$t=\zeta_{p-1}+\left(u-F_1^{(j)}(\zeta_{p-1})\right)\cdot\frac{\zeta_p-\zeta_{p-1}}{F_1^{(j)}(\zeta_p)-F_1^{(j)}(\zeta_{p-1})}$$

as the inverse $\left(F_1^{(j)}\right)^{-1}(u)$.

For those subjects j' who contract the disease, the associated $F_2^{(j')}(\cdot|T_1^{(j')})$ can be derived in a similar way as in Algorithm 2. The associated line segment starts at $(t,a,d)=(t_0^{(j')}+T_1^{(j')},T_1^{(j')},0)$. Again, a hypothetical maximal disease duration ω' is assumed, say $\omega'=80$ (years), such that the line segment ends at $(t,a,d)=(t_0^{(j')}+T_1^{(j')}+\omega',T_1^{(j')}+\omega',\omega')$. Thus, the line segment is parallel to $e_2=(1,1,1)$. The Siddon algorithm computes the corresponding set of intersections with the voxel grid accordingly. The ages $T_2^{(j')}$ at death with disease are obtained from Algorithm 2 mutatis mutandis. The interpolation of m_1 needs to be trilinear.

Examples

This section shows the results of different simulation settings. The associated R [20] code is provided with this article. The first simulation is about a hypothetical chronic disease with rates i,m_0,m_1 only depending on a. The corresponding age-specific prevalence can be calculated analytically, which allows cross-checking the results of the simulation. In the second example, another hypothetical disease is treated with mortality rates depending on t,a, and d. Here we use the ray-tracing approach in the Lexis diagram. Again, the outcomes of the simulation are compared with analytical results. The third simulation is about a relatively rare rheumatic disease. A hypothetical birth cohort of 100000 women is followed from birth to death and examined if the disease is diagnosed. Finally, the last simulation demonstrates applicability in the context of medical decision-making. Two interventions are compared with respect to the outcome *life-years gained*.

Simulation 1: Analytical example

In the first simulation, only one time-scale is involved. Assuming $m_0(a)=m_1(a)=\exp(-10+0.1\,a)$, and

$$i(a)=\begin{cases}0 & \text{for } a<20\\ \dfrac{0.005}{1-0.005\,(a-20)} & \text{for } a\geq 20,\end{cases}$$

one can show that the age-specific prevalence $p(a)$ is given by $p(a)=0.005(a-20)_+$ [21]. The notation x_+ means the positive part of $x: x_+=\max(0,x)$. The integrals of $i(a), m_0(a)$, and $m_1(a)$ can easily be expressed analytically. Figure 3 shows the age-specific prevalence in a simulated cohort with $n=200000$ subjects. For comparison, the true (analytical) prevalence is depicted as a solid line. The result of the simulation agrees very well with the analytical age profile of the prevalence, which indicates the correctness of the implemented R code.

Simulation 2: Mortality depends on duration

The second simulation is about a hypothetical disease with all time-scales t,a and d playing a role. We aim at calculating epidemiological measures that describe the population of the diseased. For example, age of onset, mean duration of the disease and age at death may be important to plan resource allocation (e.g., inpatient facilities).

In each of sixty consecutive years $t=0,\ldots,59$, 2000 persons are born and followed from birth to death. The incidence of a hypothetical chronic disease is assumed to be $i(t,a)=\frac{(a-30)_+}{3000}$, the age-specific mortality rate of the non-diseased is chosen to be $m_0(t,a)=\exp(-10.7+0.1a+t\ln(0.998))$ and the mortality of the diseased is $m_1(t,a,d)=m_0(t,a)\cdot(0.04(d-5)^2+1)$. In total, 42299 of the 120000 simulated persons contract the disease. The simulated data allows the derivation of important epidemiological measures. For example, the histograms of the age of onset and age at death are shown in Figure 4.

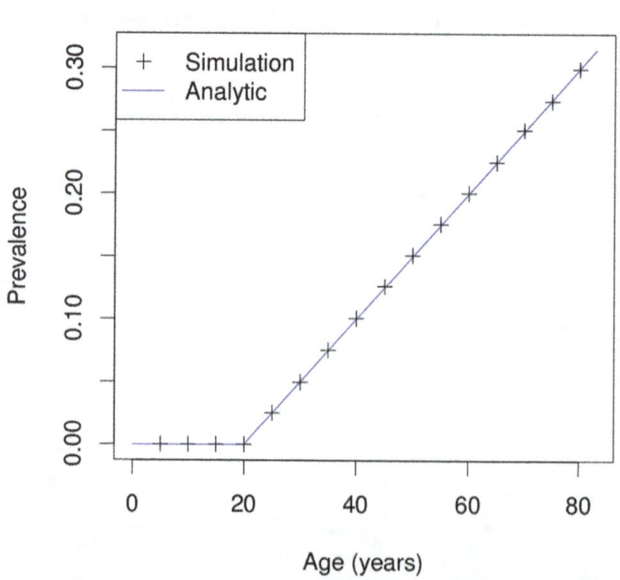

Figure 3. Theoretical and simulated age-specific prevalence. Simulation 1 comprises $n=200000$ persons. The resulting age-specific prevalence (black crosses) is compared to the analytically calculated prevalence (blue solid line). The example shows the very good agreement between the simulation and the theoretical results.

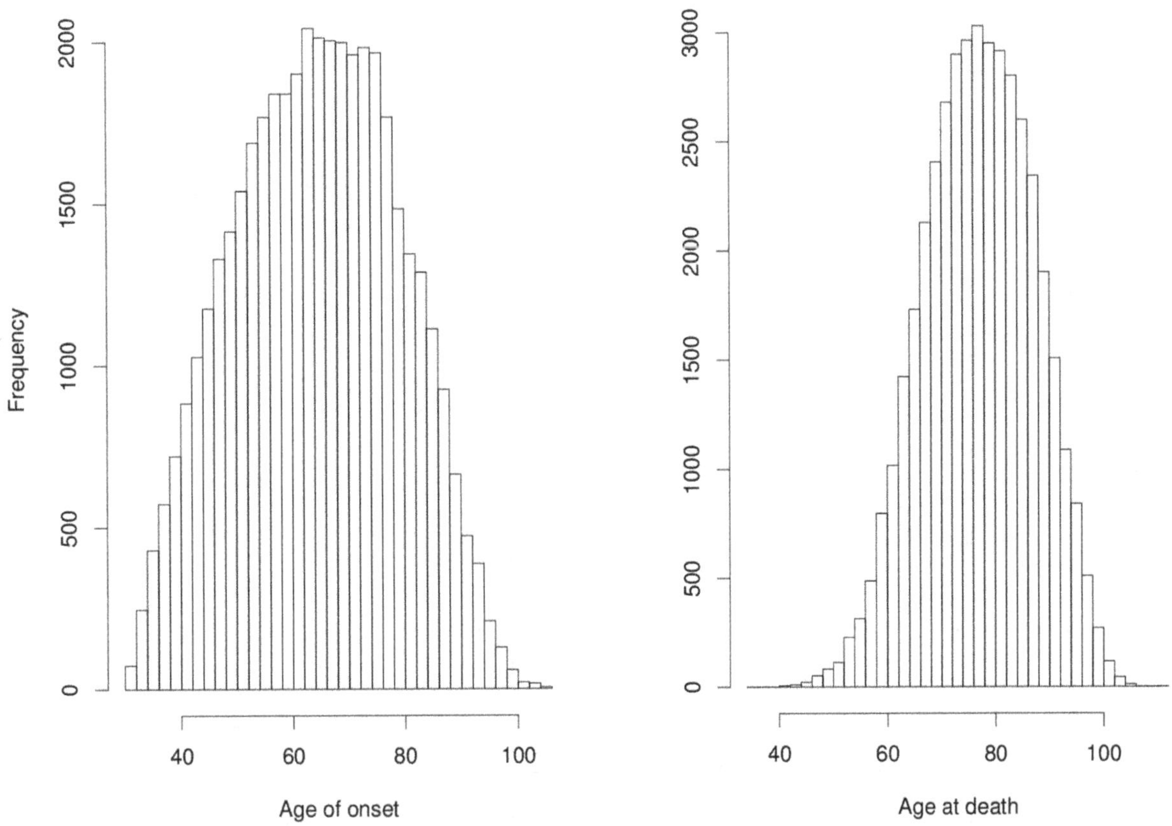

Figure 4. Histograms of the age of onset and age at death in a hypothetical chronic disease. In Simulation 2 the empirical distributions of the age of onset (left) and the age at death of the diseased persons (right) are estimated.

The median age at death of those who contracted the disease is 77.20 (years) whereas the median age at death of those without the disease is 79.67 (years). The median duration of the disease in the 42299 ill subjects is 12.69, the interquartile range is 7.46–17.60 (years).

Finally, we can cross-check the results of the simulation by comparison with an analytical calculation. In year $t = 100$, exactly 76548 persons are alive, 8802 of those having the hypothetical disease. Figure 5 shows the age-specific prevalence at $t = 100$. The black lines indicate the prevalence of several age groups together with 95% confidence bounds as given by the simulation. The blue line represents the prevalence calculated analytically by the exact formula in ([9], Section 7.2). The results agree quite well within the confidence bounds.

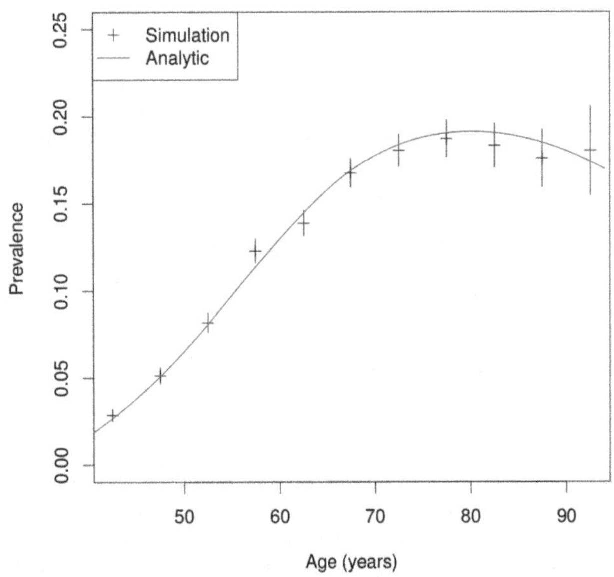

Figure 5. Calculated and simulated prevalence in Simulation 2. If we mimic a cross-sectional study at year $t = 100$, we obtain the age-specific prevalence as indicated by the black bars (with 95% confidence bounds). For comparison the analytically calculated age-specific prevalence is shown as blue line.

Simulation 3: Systemic lupus erythematosus in the UK

The third simulation is about a hypothetical cohort of 100000 women born in the United Kingdom in 1945. The disease under consideration is systemic lupus erythematosus (SLE), which is an autoimmune disorder with significant morbidity and increased mortality. Women are more often affected than men; in terms of age-standardized incidence, the ratio is 5:1 [22]. The peak of the age-specific incidence in British women is located at the age of about 50. Since Somers et al. could not find a significant secular trend in the age-standardized incidence in 1990–1999, we assume that the incidence does not depend on t, [22]. The aim of this example is to study the interplay between age of onset and the mortality of the diseased women in a realistic setting.

Mortality m_0 has been taken from the official life tables of the British Office for National Statistics [23]. The calendar time trend in m_0 has been simplified by assuming that the yearly decrease in mortality is 0.36% for all age groups. This is the geometric mean of the decrease in female mortality taken over all reported age groups in the past 60 years. Mortality m_1 of the women with SLE has been modelled according to [7], which takes into account several covariables: sex, age, duration of SLE, calendar time of diagnosis and geographical region. Unfortunately, an interaction analysis of these factors has not been reported, which forces us to make assumptions. We assume a multiplicative model of the impact of sex, age, region and SLE duration:

$$m_1(t,a,d) = c \cdot m_0(t,a) \cdot H_{\text{age}}(a) \cdot H_{\text{dur}}(d).$$

The constant c reflects the impact of sex and the region, H_{age} and H_{dur} are hazard ratios. The hazard ratio H_{dur} of SLE duration has been interpolated affine-linearly on a logarithmic scale from the published values and backtransformed. The age dependency of $H_{\text{age}}(a)$ has been treated similarly. Due to the weak (and possibly insignificant) effect, the impact of the calendar time of diagnosis has been neglected.

From the 100000 women in the simulation, 513 contract SLE. This corresponds to a lifetime risk of about 0.5%. For comparison, a recent publication about women in the US estimated 0.9% [24]. The study [24] included women with African ancestors, who are known to have a higher risk. The median age of onset in the simulation is 46.07 years, which is in nearly perfect agreement with the result of 46.1 years based on another simulation using the same data but a different method [25]. Table 1 shows the interplay between age of diagnosis and duration of SLE in the simulation.

From Table 1 it is apparent that ten-year survival is not easy to reach. Substantial loss of life time is also indicated by the age at death: Median age at death for the diseased and the non-diseased women is 61.4 and 77.1 (years), respectively. This indicates a considerable loss of lifetime in the population of the diseased compared to the non-diseased. Fortunately, this situation has changed in the last years with better medical care for SLE patients. Especially the introduction of optimized treatment regimes in the last decade lead to an enormous reduction of mortality [26]. These effects have not been included in the simulation.

Simulation 4: Effectiveness of two interventions

We take Simulation 2 as the basecase and compare the effectiveness of two hypothetical intervention programmes A and B with respect to the total gain of life-years. Assume that the primary prevention programme A gradually lowers the incidence rate for all $a \geq 30$ in the calendar years $t \in [0,10]$ by 15% and remains at the 85% level for $t > 10$. Programme B is assumed to reduce the mortality m_1 of the diseased people gradually by 50% starting after six years with the disease. B could be achieved, for example, by listing a new drug on the formulary. After running the simulation, we find that in total the 120000 simulated persons in the basecase, in intervention A, and intervention B, have 9275008, 9348941, and 9351338 life-years, respectively. Hence, intervention A and B yield about 73900 and 76300 life-years more than the basecase. With respect to the chosen outcome parameter, gain of life-years, programme B turns out to be superior to programme A. Thus, primary prevention by programme A, in this example, is less effective than lowering the mortality of the diseased. This result is

Table 1. Age at diagnosis and disease duration of 513 British women with SLE in a simulated cohort.

Age at		SLE duration (years)					
diagnosis		<1	1–2.4	2.5–4	5–9	10–24	≥25
5–34	(n = 134)	12.7%	9.0%	11.9%	14.9%	19.4%	32.1%
35–44	(n = 108)	15.7%	10.2%	14.8%	13.9%	19.4%	25.9%
45–59	(n = 149)	16.1%	14.1%	14.8%	13.4%	26.8%	14.8%
≥60	(n = 122)	29.5%	16.4%	21.3%	23.0%	9.0%	0.8%

Example how to read the table: 108 of the women are diagnosed in the age group 35–44, 13.9% of those die 5–9 years after diagnosis.

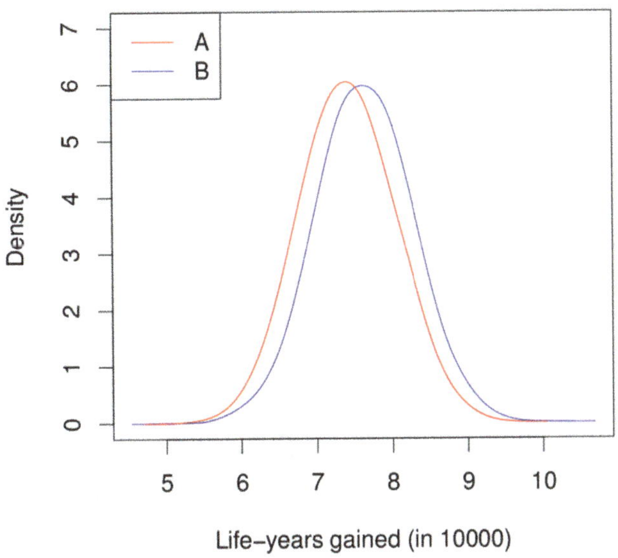

Figure 6. Esimtated densities of the gain in life-years in two intervention programmes. Simulation 4 compares two intervention programmes in a population of 120000 persons. The estimated densities of the total gain in life-years (compared to a basecase) are shown as red and blue curve for programmes A and B, respectively.

hardly predictable without a simulation and demonstrates the usefulness of our algorithm in decision making.

To obtain the empirical distributions of the total gain of life-years in both interventions, 5000 random samples of size 120000 have been drawn (with replacement from the simulated 120000 persons) [27]. Figure 6 shows the resulting densities and the superiority of programme B.

Conclusions

This article is about simulating populations in an illness-death model consisting of the three states *Normal, Disease*, and *Death*. The relevant events, diagnosis and death, in the most general case depend on three time-scales: calendar time, age and disease duration.

After birth of a subject in the population, two cases may occur:

1. the subject dies without the disease, or
2. the subject contracts the disease and dies with the disease.

Both situations can be represented in the Lexis space, a common tool in event history analysis. In the first case, the life line is solely located in the time-age-plane. In the second case, the life line changes its direction after onset of the disease, which allows to model the duration of the disease. In many diseases, the duration plays an important role for the mortality. Beside systemic lupus erythematosus as treated above, other diseases such as diabetes [3,4], depression [6] and dementia [5] may serve as examples.

In the most general case, the simulation requires to numerically solve line integrals. Therefore, a synthesis between a ray-tracing technique and numerical integration is exploited. The method provides a fast way to follow the individual life lines in the Lexis diagram. Computation time is an issue, because the number of simulated subjects in the population may be large (several thousands). For example, Simulation 4 takes almost nine minutes (525 seconds) on an Intel i3 personal computer with 3.3 GHz and 8 GB RAM. Simulations 1, 2, and 3 take 40, 170 and 85 seconds, respectively.

Beside the areas mentioned above, we think the method may be applicable in following the fields:

- In epidemiology, the simulation may be used to study the interplay between characteristics in chronic diseases: prevalence, mean disease duration, age of onset, age at death of the non-diseased and diseased population.
- The algorithms may serve as a test bench for estimation methods. For example, in [21] the age-specific incidence is derived from prevalence data. The simulation may be used to study the performance of this and related methods.
- In health economics, the result of our simulation allow the application of cost weights to each subject of the population. For example, in diabetes it is well-known that disease related costs depend on the duration since onset [28]. For each individual the disease related costs may be calculated at a specific point in time. By summing over all subjects, the total costs may be estimated easily.
- Similarly, for many chronic diseases, the health related quality of life depends on the duration of the disease [29]. By assigning utility weights to each individual and summing them up, the total quality-adjusted life-years (QALY) may be calculated.

The last two points are related to health economic modelling. We think that our algorithm may yield a contribution in that domain, because often health economic models are Markov models. Due to memoryless property of Markov models, the dependency of the relevant outcomes on the duration cannot be included directly ([30], Sec. 4.2.3). In the field of diabetes, for example, at least six out of ten important economic models are not capable to accurately account for diabetes duration [31]. This may not be necessary in every research question, but if highly accurate results are needed, modelling the disease duration should be considered.

Acknowledgments

We dedicate this work to the statistician and demographer Wilhelm Lexis on the 100th anniversary of his death.

Author Contributions

Contributed to the writing of the manuscript: RB. Developed the methods, drafted the text, and made the programming: RB. Critically revised the text, gave important intellectual contributions and final approval of the version to be published: RB SL RFB MS GG.

References

1. WHO (2011). Noncommunicable diseases country profiles. URL http://whqlibdoc.who.int/publications/2011/9789241502283eng.pdf. Last access: May 20st, 2014.
2. Keiding N (2006) Event history analysis and the cross-section. Statistics in Medicine 25: 2343–2364.

3. Carstenson B, Kristensen JK, Ottosen P, Borch-Johnsen K (2008) The Danish National Diabetes Register: Trends in Incidence, Prevalence and Mortality. Diabetologia 51: 2187–2196.
4. Fox C, Sullivan L, Sr RD, Wilson P (2004) The significant effect of diabetes duration on coronary heart disease mortality: the framingham heart study. Diabetes Care 27: 704–708.
5. Rait G, Walters K, Bottomley C, Petersen I, Iliffe S, et al. (2010) Survival of people with clinical diagnosis of dementia in primary care: cohort study. BMJ 341: c3584.
6. Geerlings S, Beekman A, Deeg D, Twisk J, Van Tilburg W (2002) Duration and severity of depression predict mortality in older adults in the community. Psychological Medicine 32: 609–618.
7. Bernatsky S, Boivin JF, Joseph L, Manzi S, Ginzler E, et al. (2006) Mortality in systemic lupus erythematosus. Arthritis and Rheumatism 54: 2550–2557.
8. Beyersmann J, Allignol A, Schumacher M (2011) Competing Risks and Multistate Models with R. Use R! Springer.
9. Keiding N (1991) Age-specific incidence and prevalence: a statistical perspective. Journal of the Royal Statistical Society A 154: 371–412.
10. Kalbfleisch J, Prentice R (2002) The Statistical Analysis of Failure Time Data. John Wiley & Sons, 2nd edition.
11. Aalen O, Borgan O, Gjessing H (2008) Survival and Event History Analysis. Springer-Verlag.
12. Vandenbroucke JP, Pearce N (2012) Incidence Rates in Dynamic Populations. International Journal of Epidemiology 41: 1472–1479.
13. Jewell NP, van der Laan M (2003) Current status data: Review, recent developments and open problems. In: Balakrishnan N, Rao C, editors, Advances in Survival Analysis, Elsevier, volume 23 of *Handbook of Statistics*. pp. 625–642. doi:10.1016/S0169-7161(03)23035-2. URL http://www.sciencedirect.com/science/article/pii/S0169716103230352.
14. Hens N, Aerts M, Faes C, Shkedy Z, Lejeune O, et al. (2010) Seventy-five Years of Estimating the Force of Infection from Current Status Data. Epidemiology of Infections 138: 802–812.
15. Keiding N (1990) Statistical interference in the lexis diagram. Philosophical Transactions of the Royal Society London A 332: 487–509.
16. Carstensen B (2006) Age-Period-Cohort Models for the Lexis Diagram. Statistics in Medicine 26: 3018–3045.
17. Siddon RL (1985) Fast Calculation of the Exact Radiological Path for a Three-Dimensional CT Array. Medical Physics 12: 252–255.
18. Dahlquist G, Björck Å (1974) Numerical Methods. Dover Books on Mathematics Series. Dover Publications.
19. Press WH, Flannery BP, Teukolsky SA, Vetterling WT (1988) Numerical Recipes in C. Cambridge University Press.
20. R Development Core Team (2012) R: A Language and Environment for Statistical Computing. R Foundation for Statistical Computing, Vienna, Austria. URL http://www.R-project.org.
21. Brinks R, Landwehr S, Icks A, Koch M, Giani G (2013) Deriving age-specific incidence from prevalence with an ordinary differential equation. Statistics in Medicine 32: 2070–2078.
22. Somers EC, Thomas SL, Smeeth L, Schoonen WM, Hall AJ (2007) Incidence of systemic lupus erythematosus in the united kingdom, 1990–1999. Arthritis Care & Research 57: 612–618.
23. ONS (2011). Office for national statistics: Population estimates quinary age groups for uk constituent countries. URL http://www.ons.gov.uk.
24. Crowson CS, Matteson EL, Myasoedova E, Michet CJ, Ernste FC, et al. (2011) The lifetime risk of adult-onset rheumatoid arthritis and other inflammatory autoimmune rheumatic diseases. Arthritis & Rheumatism 63: 633–639.
25. Brinks R, Fischer-Betz R, Landwehr S, Schneider M, Giani G (2013) Stochastic differential equation modeling the prevalence of rare chronic diseases with an application to systemic lupus erythematosus. Statistica Neerlandica 67: 202–210.
26. Chehab G, Fischer-Betz R, Schneider M (2011) Entwicklung von mortalitt und morbiditt beim systemischen lupus erythematodes. Zeitschrift fr Rheumatologie 70: 480–485.
27. Efron B, Tibshirani R (1993) An Introduction to the Bootstrap. Monographs on statistics and applied probabilities. Chapman & Hall/CRC.
28. Caro J, Ward A, O'Brien J (2002) Lifetime costs of complications resulting from type 2 diabetes in the u.s. Diabetes Care 25: 476–481.
29. Sparring V, Nyström L, Wahlström R, Jonsson PM, Östman J, et al. (2013) Diabetes duration and health-related quality of life in individuals with onset of diabetes in the age group 1534 years a swedish population-based study using eq-5d. BMC Public Health 13: 377.
30. Putter H, Fiocco M, Geskus RB (2007) Tutorial in biostatistics: competing risks and multi-state models. Statistics in Medicine 26: 2389–2430.
31. Yi Y, Philips Z, Bergman G, Burslem K (2010) Economic models in type 2 diabetes. Current Medical Research and Opinion 26: 2105–2118.

10

An Antibody-Based Leukocyte-Capture Microarray for the Diagnosis of Systemic Lupus Erythematosus

Ming-Wei Lin[1,2☯¤], Joshua W. K. Ho[3☯], Leonard C. Harrison[4], Cristobal G. dos Remedios[5], Stephen Adelstein[1,2*]

1 Department of Clinical Immunology, Royal Prince Alfred Hospital, Sydney, New South Wales, Australia, **2** Discipline of Medicine, Sydney Medical School, The University of Sydney, Sydney, New South Wales, Australia, **3** Division of Genetics, Department of Medicine, Brigham and Women's Hospital, Harvard Medical School, Boston, Massachusetts, United States of America, **4** The Walter and Eliza Hall Institute of Medical Research, Department of Clinical Immunology and Burnet Clinical Research Unit, The Royal Melbourne Hospital, Parkville, Victoria, Australia, **5** Discipline of Anatomy, Bosch Institute, The University of Sydney, Sydney, New South Wales, Australia

Abstract

The diagnosis of Systemic Lupus Erythematosus (SLE) is challenging due to its heterogeneous clinical presentation and the lack of robust biomarkers to distinguish it from other autoimmune diseases. Further, currently used laboratory tests do not readily distinguish active and inactive disease. Several groups have attempted to apply emerging high throughput profiling technologies to diagnose and monitor SLE. Despite showing promise, many are expensive and technically challenging for routine clinical use. The goal of this work is to develop a better diagnostic and monitoring tool for SLE. We report a highly customisable antibody microarray that consists of a duplicate arrangement of 82 antibodies directed against surface antigens on peripheral blood mononuclear cells (PMBCs). This high-throughput array was used to profile SLE patients (n = 60) with varying disease activity, compared to healthy controls (n = 24), patients with rheumatoid arthritis (n = 25), and other autoimmune diseases (n = 28). We used a computational algorithm to calculate a score from the entire microarray profile and correlated it with SLE disease activity. Our results demonstrate that leukocyte-capture microarray profiles can readily distinguish active SLE patients from healthy controls (AUROC = 0.84). When combined with the standard laboratory tests (serum anti-dsDNA, complements C3 and C4), the microarrays provide significantly increased discrimination. The antibody microarrays can be enhanced by the addition of other markers for potential application to the diagnosis and stratification of SLE, paving the way for the customised and accurate diagnosis and monitoring of SLE.

Editor: Frederic Rieux-Laucat, Pavillon Kirmisson, France

Funding: Studies were supported by the NWG Macintosh Memorial Fund of the Department of Anatomy & Histology, University of Sydney and the Special Purposes Trust Fund and generous donors to the Department of Clinical Immunology, Royal Prince Alfred Hospital. The funders had no role in study design, data collection and analysis, decision to publish, or preparation of the manuscript.

Competing Interests: The authors have declared that no competing interests exist.

* E-mail: stephen.adelstein@sydney.edu.au

☯ These authors contributed equally to this work.

¤ Current address: Department of Clinical Immunology, Westmead Hospital, New South Wales, Australia

Introduction

Systemic Lupus Erythematosus (SLE) is an immune-mediated, multisystem, inflammatory disease characterised by autoantibody production. Its diagnosis relies on identification of combinations of clinical features and laboratory tests to distinguish it from other autoimmune disorders [1]. This is often problematic in clinical practice as some of the features required to fulfill the diagnostic criteria may take years to develop and some individuals with pathognomonic features do not meet all the established criteria. The clinical course of the disease is typified by unpredictable flares manifest by the onset of new organ involvement, worsening of existing disease, and periods of remission. Although several laboratory measurements, such as serum complement C3 and C4 levels, anti-dsDNA antibody titers and erythrocyte sedimentation rate (ESR) are routinely used in the clinic to help with disease management, individually they are not diagnostic of SLE and do not on their own give an accurate indication of disease activity. Consequently, assessment of disease activity and response to therapy remains largely clinical. The development of reliable biomarkers would enable us to distinguish between SLE and other autoimmune or infective conditions with similar clinical presentations, and would assist in the diagnosis and management of the condition. Such markers would ideally stratify the condition, predict flares, determine disease severity and activity, and response to therapy, and thereby limit unnecessary investigation and exposure to the side effects of immunosuppressive agents.

By using gene transcripts grouped into modules, Chaussabel *et al.* [2] developed a bioinformatics system to monitor disease activity in SLE. Their results raise the possibility of more precise characterisation of disease activity based on the pathogenesis of the condition and its molecular expression. However, the high cost, need for batch analysis and the delays in acquisition of results of molecular analyses using current technology limits the clinical utility of this approach for individual patients.

Autoantibodies are the hallmark of many autoimmune diseases. To circumvent the limitations of the DNA gene array, many groups [3–6] have employed miniaturised formats of parallel detection of autoantibodies using antigen microarrays. Of particular interest, Robinson *et al.* [4] fabricated 1152-feature arrays containing 196 distinct biomolecules representing major autoantigens targeted by autoantibodies from patients with autoimmune rheumatic diseases and found them to be of comparable sensitivity and specificity to conventional assays. Fattal *et al.* [7] used an array to measure antibodies to 930 different antigens including viral proteins in 40 SLE patients and successfully identified particular combinations of markers specific for the disease at various levels of activity. They quoted a sensitivity of >93% and specificity of >88% in distinguishing SLE from normal controls.

Belov *et al.* demonstrated the utility of leukocyte-capture antibody microarrays in the diagnosis, monitoring and stratification of patients with lymphoproliferative diseases [8,9]. The concept was co-invented by one of the authors (CGdR) and has been successfully employed to identify different clonally expanded leukocytes populations that are characteristic of human leukaemias [8,9]. However, it soon became clear that these cell capture microarrays could also be used to detect more subtle changes in leukocyte populations, for example cell activation or inflammatory changes in patients with heart disease and other inflammatory diseases [10–15]. We postulated that inflammatory diseases such as SLE would also cause changes to the expression of leukocyte surface molecules that could be detected by the cell array. To demonstrate the potential utility of this microarray in the diagnosis and stratification of SLE, we conducted a study of patients with SLE and demonstrated that the leukocyte capture array profile of these patients is readily distinguishable from that of healthy controls. By generating an immunophenotypic fingerprint for each patient, the cell capture microarray can identify common patterns that permit identification of subgroups based on disease activity. Notably, we show that our microarray can on its own distinguish SLE from healthy controls and can complement standard laboratory tests to improve stratification of SLE patients based on disease activity. Further customisation with other antibodies, based on knowledge of leukocytes surface antigen expression related to pathogenesis of SEL, is likely to improve the sensitivity and specificity of the array.

Methods

Microarray construction

Antibody microarrays (DotScan^{TM}) were purchased from Medsaic Pty. Ltd., Sydney. The construction of the antibody microarray has been described previously [8]. It consists of a duplicate set of 82 mouse monoclonal antibodies directed against human cluster of differentiation (CD) antigens that are robotically placed on the surface of a nitrocellulose-coated glass slide (Schleicher and Schuell, FAST slides). The slides and the antibodies, including the appropriate isotype control antibodies, are listed in Figure S1. Unoccupied binding sites on the remaining surface of the slide are then blocked using powdered skim milk to minimise non-specific binding. A set of mouse isotype control antibodies is included, and the perimeter of the CD antibody array is marked by anti-CD44, a pan-leukocyte CD antibody, used to show that leukocytes are evenly distributed across the antibody area. Only 10 nL of each antibody is required for each spot, which, once deposited on the nitrocellulose surface, spreads to a diameter of 450–500 μm. This is large enough to accommodate up to 1500 leukocytes, providing an acceptable statistical sampling of the population of cells applied to the array surface. After 30 minutes any leukocytes that are not immobilized at the antibody dots are removed by gentle washing, the slide is scanned, and the attached cells are quantified by light scattering [8]. We previously reported a good correlation between the dot intensities on antibody microarrays and flow cytometry with the same antibodies [8], but both the production of the microarrays and the nitrocellulose slides have changed since this was published. Accordingly, we have included new data from the batch of antibody microarrays to those used in the experiments report in this paper. PBMCs from a healthy blood donor were stimulated by overnight exposure to anti-CD3 monoclonal antibody and then applied to microarrays and quantified by densitometry as described above and also monitored by flow cytometry. The microarray spot densities for four randomly selected expressed antigens (CD25, CD69, CD71 and HLA-DR) are well matched by the cell numbers determined by flow cytometry from the same sample (Figure S2).

Patients

Written informed consent was obtained from 117 subjects attending clinics of the Royal Prince Alfred Hospital. 137 assessments were performed: 60 on patients with SLE, 53 with other autoimmune diseases including rheumatoid arthritis (RA) (N = 25), vasculitis (N = 9), polymyositis (N = 1), seronegative arthritis (N = 8), scleroderma (N = 3), Sjogren's syndrome (N = 1), undifferentiated connective tissue diseases (N = 6), and 24 healthy controls. All SLE patients fulfilled at least four of the American College of Rheumatologists (ACR) criteria for the disease [1] and their disease activity was determined according to the SLE Disease Activity Index (SLEDAI) score [16]. We assigned patients into three disease activity groups according to their SLEDAI score with ≥8 defined as clinically active, 5–7 as intermediate (semi-active) activity and, ≤4 as inactive. The details of their immunosuppressive medications were recorded at the time of each clinic visit. Thirty three (55%) patients had inactive disease, 16 (27%) had intermediate disease activity, usually following treatment of a disease flare, and 11 (18%) were clinically active. There were no differences between the demographics of the patients in any of the clinical categories, their use of immunosuppressants at the time of study or the number of ACR criteria fulfilled during the course of their illness (Table 1). The results of anti-dsDNA antibodies (Farr assay, Trinity Biotech, Ireland) and serum complements C3 and C4 levels (Immage® 800, Beckman Coulter) were recorded at each visit. The project was approved by the Royal Prince Alfred Hospital Ethics Committee (Approval number X06-0089).

Blood processing and microarray profiling

Anticoagulated whole blood was collected in EDTA tubes from each participant and maintained at room temperature until use within 24 hours. Leukocytes from peripheral blood mainly consisting of peripheral blood mononuclear cells (PBMCs) were isolated using Histopaque (Sigma-Aldrich), washed in PBS, resuspended in PBS containing 1 mM EDTA to a density of 10^7 cells/ml, and incubated on the cell array for 30 min at room temperature; unbound cells were then gently washed off with PBS. Arrays were then fixed for at least one hour in PBS containing 1% (v/v) formaldehyde (Sigma-Aldrich) washed in PBS, scanned, and the light scattering by the attached cells recorded in an image file. The microarray data is accessible at National Center for Biotechnology Information (NCBI)'s Gene Expression Omnibus (Accession number: GSE27293).

Preprocessing of microarray expression data

The raw intensity light scatter values at each spot on the slide were scale-normalised such that the expression value for each CD antigen is between 0 and 10. This normalisation method has been

Table 1. Demographic and clinical characteristics of the patients.

	SLE active	SLE intermediate	SLE inactive
Number	11	16	33
Demographics			
Age, mean (range), years	43 (36–59)	36 (28–48)	47 (24–80)
Female (%)	10/11 (91%)	14/16 (88%)	29/33 (88%)
Caucasian	8 (73%)	11 (69%)	26 (79%)
Asian	3 (27%)	5 (31%)	7 (21%)
No of ACR criteria fulfilled	6	6	7
Laboratory criteria			
Anti dsDNA positive*	10(91%)	9 (56%)	8 (24%)
C4*	7 (64%)	7 (44%)	7 (21%)
C3*	7 (64%)	10 (63%)	8 (24%)
Medications			
No immunosuppressants	3(27%)	2 (13%)	10(30%)
Prednisone alone	1(9%)	3 (19%)	7 (21%)
Immunosuppressants alone	2(18%)	1 (6%)	3 (9%)
Prednisone+immunosuppressants	5(45%)	10 (63%)	13(39%)

*at time of assessment

shown to generate antigen expression levels that correlate linearly with corresponding cell counts by flow cytometry [11]. Further, we applied two filtering criteria to the data: Firstly, antigens that had low expression across all samples were excluded. An antigen was deemed to have low expression if its median expression value among the 20% most highly expressed samples was less than 1, since this is approximately the lower limit of the technology to reliably detect antigen binding [11]. Secondly, CD antigens that had a low signal-to-noise ratio (SNR) were rejected. The SNR of an antigen was defined as the ratio of the standard deviation of its mean expression value across all samples against the mean absolute difference between the two intra-slide replicate measurements across all samples. CD antigens with a SNR less than 1.2 were filtered out since this ratio appeared to be a conservative threshold that filtered out most of the negative control spots on the array.

Individual CD antigen biomarkers for SLE

To identify CD antigens that individually showed strong evidence of association with the class label (*e.g.*, SLE or control), we performed a linear model analysis using the R package, *limma* [17], which is a program specifically designed for microarray analysis. A p value was calculated using the moderated t statistics for each CD antigen to determine whether it was statistically significant. We also calculated the Area Under the Receiver Operating Characteristic (AUROC) curve for each CD antigen. This analysis was performed using the R package *ROCR* [18].

We tested whether the expression levels of each individual CD antigen were significantly associated with SLE activity using a moderated t test and AUROC. Six sets of comparisons were performed to assess whether each individual marker was good for diagnosis or stratification of SLE. A CD antigen qualified as a singleton biomarker if it had $p<0.05$ and AUROC>0.7 in any comparison.

Measurement of SLE activity based on the multiple biomarkers

We used an advanced classification algorithm, Support Vector Machine (SVM) [19,20] to create an SLE activity score from the entire antigen expression profile. We used the SVM implementation in the R package *e1071* with default parameters (kernel = - radial basis kernel, cost = 1). Briefly, a SVM uses labelled training examples to construct a non-linear decision rule (*i.e.*, a decision boundary) that can best distinguish the expression profiles of SLE patients from those of healthy controls. We assumed there is a linear trend in SLE disease activity; therefore we trained the SVM model using profiles from healthy controls and active SLE patients only. Once the SVM model was trained we calculated an SLE activity measure, which we refer to as an S-score, for every expression profile, x, based on the profile's distance, $f(x)$, from the decision boundary as determined by the SVM classifier. The S-score is calculated by the following formula:

$$Sscore = \exp(-f(x))$$

Cross-validation

We used a three-fold repeated sub-sampling cross-validation strategy to assess the performance of the SLE activity score. Briefly, we iteratively performed the following steps 100 times: randomly partitioned the samples into three equal portions and used two of these portions as the training set to build a SVM model. The remaining portion was a testing set to assess the model's sensitivity and specificity for each of the three SLE activity states. An ROC curve and an AUROC value were generated at each iteration and the mean and standard deviation of AUROC of the 100 iterations were recorded.

Table 2. A list of the CD antigens that exhibit statistically significant SLE-activity dependent expression patterns.

CD antigens	Category	Inactive vs. healthy		Semi-active vs. healthy		Active vs. healthy		Active vs. inactive		Semi-active vs. inactive		Active vs. semi-active	
		p	*AUROC*	*p*	*AUROC*	*p*	*AUROC*	*p*	*AUROC*	*p*	*AUROC*	*p*	*AUROC*
Down regulated in SLE													
TCR a/b	T cells	0.24	0.60	0.01	0.73	0.19	0.62	0.63	0.54	0.09	0.65	0.37	0.59
CD2	T cells	0.00	0.74	0.00	0.86	0.00	0.82	0.22	0.58	0.12	0.64	0.92	0.52
CD3	T cells	0.09	0.64	0.00	0.79	0.01	0.75	0.16	0.62	0.07	0.66	0.86	0.53
CD4	T cells	0.04	0.65	0.01	0.76	0.02	0.73	0.38	0.58	0.24	0.60	0.89	0.51
CD5	T cells	0.01	0.68	0.00	0.86	0.00	0.82	0.11	0.63	0.02	0.69	0.64	0.54
CD7	T cells	0.01	0.71	0.00	0.89	0.00	0.80	0.13	0.62	0.03	0.69	0.73	0.53
CD8	T cells	0.28	0.62	0.02	0.79	0.03	0.77	0.16	0.68	0.11	0.66	1.00	0.59
CD28	T cells	0.03	0.63	0.01	0.71	0.15	0.61	0.85	0.51	0.32	0.59	0.34	0.60
CD45RA	Naïve T and B cells	0.17	0.62	0.01	0.78	0.02	0.72	0.15	0.63	0.09	0.68	0.95	0.52
CD56	NK cells	0.00	0.67	0.00	0.78	0.01	0.75	0.57	0.58	0.26	0.59	0.71	0.50
CD57	NK cells	0.72	0.59	0.03	0.75	0.05	0.75	0.07	0.65	0.04	0.66	0.98	0.52
CD52	Membrane glycopeptide	0.01	0.70	0.00	0.82	0.06	0.67	0.99	0.51	0.35	0.58	0.48	0.59
kappa 1/4 IM	B cells	0.16	0.64	0.02	0.74	0.28	0.66	0.96	0.55	0.22	0.56	0.36	0.51
lambda 1/4 IM	B cells	0.22	0.63	0.05	0.68	0.15	0.70	0.58	0.56	0.30	0.57	0.76	0.50
Up regulated in SLE													
CD66c	Platelets	0.11	0.69	0.07	0.73	0.03	0.73	0.33	0.58	0.60	0.61	0.64	0.51
CD95	Granulocytes	0.30	0.59	0.76	0.52	0.04	0.70	0.16	0.64	0.22	0.61	0.03	0.74
Conventional laboratory tests													
dsDNA	dsDNA							0.01	0.80	0.12	0.70	0.22	0.62
C3	Complement C3							0.01	0.79	0.01	0.74	0.69	0.66
C4	Complement C4							0.54	0.65	0.11	0.69	0.49	0.57

Significant SLE-activity dependent expression patterns are determined based on moderated *t*-test and AUROC ($p<0.05$ and AUROC >0.7 in at least one comparison). All p-value less than 0.05 and AUROC value greater than 0.7 are highlighted in bold.

Results

Analysis of singleton biomarkers for SLE

After the normalisation and filtering steps, 57 antibody spots passed our quality filters and were used in subsequent analyses. The results demonstrate (Table 2) that many T and NK-cell surface markers are down-regulated in SLE. Another important observation was that, although many of these CD antigens have statistically significant associations with the disease, none are good biomarkers of SLE activity because the AUROC values are not sufficiently high (<0.85), and do not positively correlate with disease activity. This indicates that no CD antigen alone, as measured by our antibody microarray, can be used as a reliable biomarker for monitoring the activity of SLE. We performed the same moderated *t* test and ROC analysis for each of the conventional laboratory markers (anti-dsDNA, complement C3 and C4), and found that they can generally differentiate patients with inactive SLE from those with active forms of SLE, but cannot reliably distinguish semi-active patients and active ones (Table 2). In particular, anti-dsDNA and C3 show reasonable discriminatory ability that no single marker in the current version of the microarray can match.

The heat map in Figure 1A shows the expression pattern of singleton CD antigen biomarkers. Hierarchical clustering reveals two large clusters of profiles, one dominated by SLE patients (left hand side of Figure 1A), and one dominated by healthy subjects (right side of Figure 1A). Although the clustering analysis cannot perfectly separate the SLE patients from healthy controls, the results suggest that the antigen profiles contain useful discriminatory information for building a diagnostic test.

To investigate whether the set of CD biomarkers contained redundancy (by having multiple biomarkers with highly correlated expression patterns), we performed a Pearson's correlation coefficient among the expression profile of all singleton CD antigen biomarkers listed in Table 2. Figure 1B shows that there are several strongly co-expressed clusters of CD antigens among T cell (CD7, CD5, CD3, and CD2), NK cell (CD56, CD57) and B cell markers (kappa, lambda). Some of the CD antibodies that produced highly correlated antigen expression profiles can therefore be selectively removed from the microarray without decreasing its predictive value. It is well known in the machine learning literature that the best feature sets for classification are those that individually are strongly associated with the class label, but are unrelated to each other. The conventional serum biomarkers such as C3, C4 and anti-dsDNA measured in the patient cohort have little correlation with other CD biomarkers in the study, suggesting that they can provide complementary information in the assessment of SLE.

Leukocyte capture arrays can discriminate SLE from healthy subjects

Next we explored whether building a SLE classification rule based on the expression of multiple antigens can result in a more accurate and robust diagnostic assay. We built a multivariate classifier for our microarray profile using SVM, and validated the classification performance using rigorous cross-validation. We used this SVM classification approach to construct a SLE diagnostic score, called the S-score, using expression of all the 57 CD antigens measured, and assessed the quality of the S-score using cross-validation. The ROC plots in Figure 2A demonstrate that inactive SLE cannot be reliably separated from healthy controls, but semi-active and active SLE patients can (AUROC = 0.83 and 0.84 respectively). In addition, we also investigated whether the S-score is positively correlated with SLE disease activity. The average S-score of the samples belonging to the four classes (healthy, SLE inactive, SLE semi-active and SLE active) from the 100 rounds of cross-validation are summarised in Figure 2B, and demonstrate a positive correlation between the S-score and disease activity. This is a particularly encouraging finding since the SVM model was trained using samples from healthy subjects and active SLE patients only, but it correctly identified the relative disease activity of semi-active and inactive patients, which supports the robustness of this approach.

We also investigated whether the antibody array can distinguish SLE patients from patients with other autoimmune diseases. In this analysis, we independently built a two-class SVM classifier for each comparison (RA vs. healthy, RA vs. SLE inactive, RA vs. SLE semi-active and so on) as shown in Figure 2C. These analyses show that active and semi-active SLE can be reliably distinguished from healthy controls with an AUROC greater than 0.8 (black

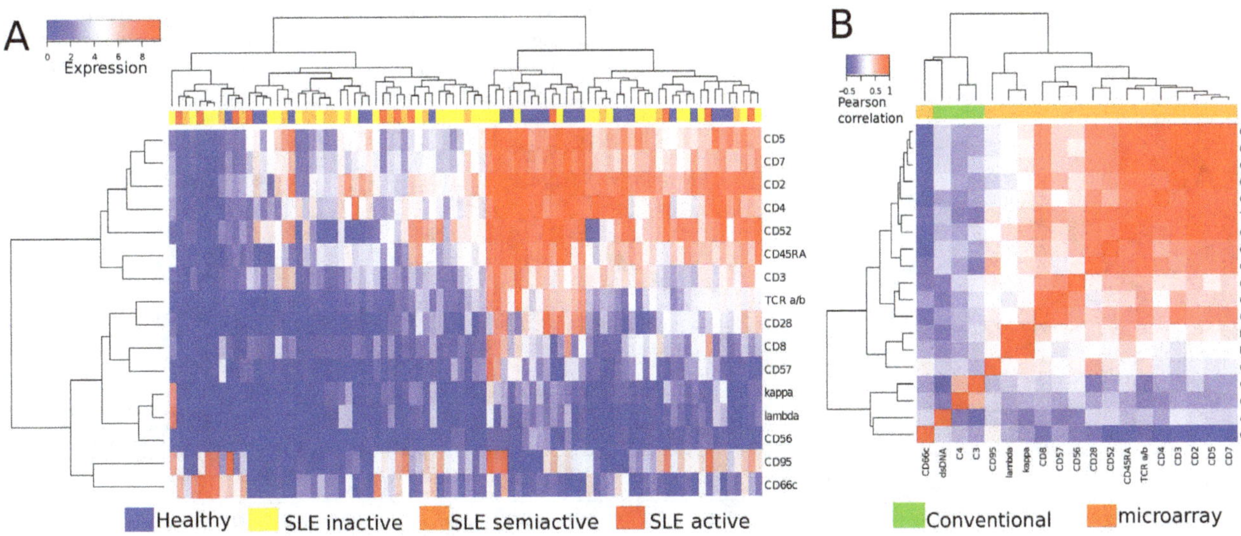

Figure 1. SLE singleton biomarker analysis. (A) Heat map of singleton CD biomarkers from SLE patients and healthy controls. (B) Heat map of Pearson's correlation coefficient between each pair of CD biomarkers and conventional laboratory biomarkers.

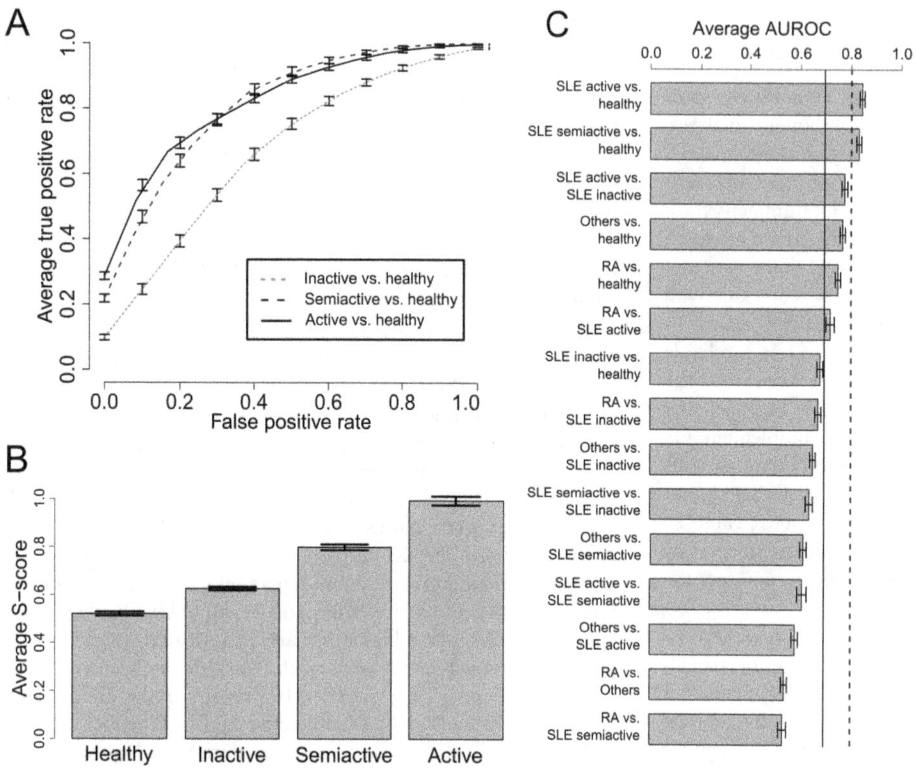

Figure 2. Cross-validation analysis of a SVM based classifier for diagnosis and stratification of SLE. (A) ROC analysis of the SLE classification measure. **(B)** The average S-score of test samples from 100 rounds of cross-validation (error bar represents S.E.M). **(C)** Average AUROC of comparisons between SLE, healthy controls, rheumatoid arthritis (RA) and other autoimmune diseases (others). The black dotted line at AUROC = 0.8 indicates a classifier that can readily separate the two classes, and a black solid line at AUROC = 0.7 indicates a classifier that is moderately effective for separating two classes (error bar represents S.E.M).

dotted line). Active SLE compared to inactive disease, other autoimmune diseases and RA compared to healthy subjects and RA compared to active SLE, have AUROC values between 0.7 and 0.8 (between the black solid and dotted lines) that indicate discrimination with less certainty, while the remainder of the diseases with AUROC values <0.7 (to the left of the solid black line (*e.g.*, RA and other autoimmune diseases vs. SLE inactive etc) cannot be reliably distinguished.

Leukocyte capture arrays improve the discriminative ability of conventional laboratory tests in SLE

Currently the assessment of SLE activity is based on a combination of clinical symptoms, signs, and laboratory tests. Since discriminating inactive SLE from more active forms of SLE (*i.e.*, semi-active or active) may be important in management, we evaluated the discriminatory ability of combination of tests including antibody arrays and the serological and immunochemical tests performed. For each of the datasets, we trained a classifier using the SVM approach, and its discriminatory ability was

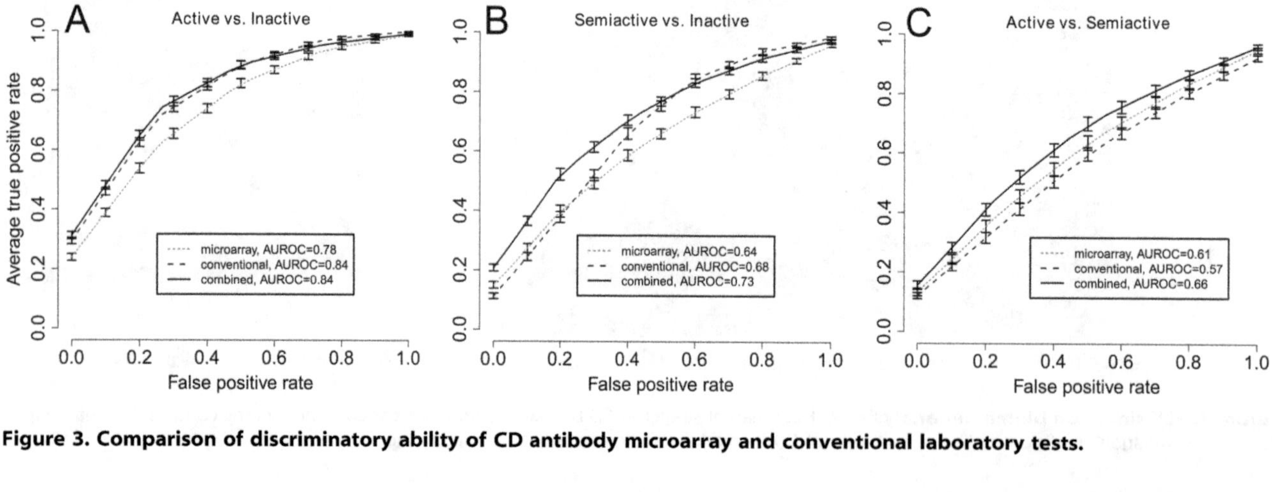

Figure 3. Comparison of discriminatory ability of CD antibody microarray and conventional laboratory tests.

evaluated with 100 rounds of three-fold cross validation (Figure 3). The serum tests, anti-dsDNA antibodies, C3, and C4 levels, are more discriminating than our antibody microarray (p<0.001, one-sided paired t test) in distinguishing semi-active and active SLE from inactive SLE (Figure 3A and B). However, our antibody microarray can better distinguish active from semi-active SLE (p<0.001). When we trained a SVM based on the results of both microarray and the serum tests, we achieved a significantly better separation of semi-active SLE from inactive and active SLE (p<0.001 for both classification tasks). Given the clinically heterogeneous presentation of SLE patients, it is particularly encouraging to note that the microarray can improve the discriminative ability of conventional laboratory tests for semi-active vs. inactive SLE. Taken together with the observation that nearly all singleton CD biomarkers have very low expression correlation with the measurements from the three conventional laboratory tests (Figure 1B), we believe that the leukocyte microarray does indeed provide additional information.

Discussion

This antibody microarray yields comparable diagnostic sensitivity and specificity to the DNA microarray system described by Chaussabel *et al.* [2]. The antibody microarray we described is, however, a potentially more practical platform for use in the diagnostic laboratory, since the analytical equipment required is less technically challenging and much less expensive (cost per microarray is ~US$90) than gene expression microarrays or flow cytometry for the same number of antibodies, and it can be performed rapidly on an *ad hoc* basis. Traditionally, cellular markers and populations (and more importantly the changes in these populations) are detected by flow cytometry. This is generally a technically challenging, slow and expensive method that, when performed in a sophisticated laboratory with large sample volumes of sera and reagents and skilled technicians, can analyze no more than 17 CD antigens in a single analysis. The cell capture microarrays, in contrast to flow cytometry, can be performed on the bench in any laboratory and can simultaneously determine the presence of more than 100 antigens expressed on the surface of leukocytes. Furthermore, the microarray provides a semi-quantitative method of monitoring the numbers of cells in a sample since the light scattering from the cells is proportional to the number of cells immobilized on the arrays [8,11]. In our experience, the method requires minimal training and uses only small volumes of antibodies and peripheral blood. In addition to the discriminatory ability demonstrated in this study, the technical simplicity of this profiling technology makes it attractive for clinical use.

The high-throughput nature of this microarray is also particularly attractive because it allows rapid identification of an immunophenotype for each patient based on the expression of multiple cell surface molecules that have been perturbed due to current or previous activation events in SLE. In principle, combinations of expressed surface membrane proteins (CD antigens and other membrane proteins) characterise functional subsets of leukocytes. One key idea of this study is that such leukocyte surface markers carry useful information about SLE activity. Our data represent a proof of concept only and will need to be validated using a much larger sample size before the microarray is applied in a clinical setting.

It is possible to turn our antibody microarray approach on its head, namely to immobilize the antigen and capture the antibodies as undertaken by Fattal *et al.* [7] and Robinson *et al.* [4]. Although these methods can distinguish SLE from healthy controls, their clinical performance in distinguishing SLE from other autoimmune and rheumatic has not been demonstrated and performance characteristics in the clinic are not yet reported. Our pilot study demonstrates that leukocyte surface markers contain information that may be used alone or in combination to other markers (such as anti-dsDNA) to distinguish SLE from normal controls, stratify disease activity, and may even distinguish SLE from other autoimmune and rheumatic conditions, although the later requires further study.

We show that a disease activity score can be constructed based on the entire antigen expression profile through a state-of-the-art machine learning technique. Similar supervised machine learning approaches for clinical diagnostic support using microarray technology have been reported extensively in the last decade, particularly in the field of cancer classification [21,22]. Unlike a traditional singleton biomarker, the calculation of our S-score depends on the size and quality of the training examples. Different SVM decision functions are generated by using different training samples. Therefore, we performed a cross-validation analysis to estimate the sensitivity and specificity of this classifier for SLE. This analysis indicates that our approach for generating the S-score is generally robust even when different subsets of the training samples are used.

We note that some CD antigens, including CD95 [23], CD86 [24,25], which have previously been reported to be associated with SLE, do not show statistical significance in our singleton biomarker analysis. This is surprising given their role in co-stimulation and cell activation. We suspect this may reflect the lack of specificity of the clone of antibodies used in this version of the microarray. From our experience, different clones of antibodies have different antigen-binding characteristics, and further experiments using different antibody clones will determine if alternative antibodies will contribute to the discriminatory ability of the array.

Although the discriminatory ability of the current version of the microarray on its own is no better than conventional tests, the fact that the microarray provides additional information for clinical assessment of SLE is an important finding. The expression values from about 40% of the antibody spots in the current version of the microarray were filtered out because of low expression or high variability in performance. This is not surprising as this version of microarray was originally designed for the diagnosis of lymphoproliferative diseases [8]. It is likely that a customised antibody microarray containing rationally selected antibodies that target CD antigens known to reflect the pathogenesis and activity of SLE will improve the sensitivity and specificity of the antibody microarray [26]. In particular, we propose that a customised SLE antibody microarray can be developed by retaining only those informative biomarkers in the current generation of the array, and augmenting the array with other antibodies directed to cell surface markers whose expression has been reported to be perturbed in patients with SLE. These could include antibodies related to innate immunity (CD1a, CD14, CD83), adaptive immunity (CD161), adhesion molecules (CD166 and CD6), other markers (CD279 and other chemokines *e.g.*, CCR6). These and other molecules have been shown to be potentially involved in the pathogenesis of SLE and may therefore also be useful markers of the disease and level of activity [26,27].

Conclusion

Our observations using a first-generation antibody microarray demonstrate that SLE patients can be distinguished from healthy controls based on the differential expression of CD markers on PBMCs. Our analysis indicates that the current version of PBMC

CD antibody microarray can be combined with current laboratories tests to provide superior discriminatory ability to stratify SLE patients according to disease activity. We postulate that the addition of rationally selected antibodies based on reports of their altered expression in SLE will result in an even higher discriminatory ability than currently used tests, with potential benefits both for diagnosis and monitoring of disease and tailoring of therapy.

Supporting Information

Figure S1 An image of the scanned microarray from a healthy control and SLE patients with different disease activity.

Figure S2 Validation of expressed microarray CD antigen markers using flow cytometry. (A) Unnormalized microarray spot intensity of four randomly selected expressed CD antigens in CD3 stimulated leukocytes. **(B)** Flow cytometry analysis of the same four antibodies in the same cell population, and also controls. All four measured expressed CD antigens detected by the microarray are also detected as being expressed by flow cytometry.

Acknowledgments

We thank members of the Department of Rheumatology at the Royal Prince Alfred Hospital for recruiting patients with rheumatoid arthritis for the study.

Author Contributions

Conceived and designed the experiments: SA CGdR. Performed the experiments: MWL LCH. Analyzed the data: JWKH. Wrote the paper: MWL JWKH CGdR SA.

References

1. Tan EM, Cohen AS, Fries JF, Masi AT, McShane DJ, et al. (1982) The 1982 revised criteria for the classification of systemic lupus erythematosus. Arthritis Rheum 25: 1271–1277.
2. Chaussabel D, Quinn C, Shen J, Patel P, Glaser C, et al. (2008) A modular analysis framework for blood genomics studies: application to systemic lupus erythematosus. Immunity 29: 150–164. doi:10.1016/j.immuni.2008.05.012.
3. Joos TO, Schrenk M, Höpfl P, Kröger K, Chowdhury U, et al. (2000) A microarray enzyme-linked immunosorbent assay for autoimmune diagnostics. Electrophoresis 21: 2641–2650. doi:10.1002/1522-2683(20000701)21:13<2641::AID-ELPS2641>3.0.CO;2-5.
4. Robinson WH, DiGennaro C, Hueber W, Haab BB, Kamachi M, et al. (2002) Autoantigen microarrays for multiplex characterization of autoantibody responses. Nat Med 8: 295–301. doi:10.1038/nm0302-295.
5. Huang RP, Huang R, Fan Y, Lin Y (2001) Simultaneous detection of multiple cytokines from conditioned media and patient's sera by an antibody-based protein array system. Anal Biochem 294: 55–62. doi:10.1006/abio.2001.5156.
6. Hueber W, Kidd BA, Tomooka BH, Lee BJ, Bruce B, et al. (2005) Antigen microarray profiling of autoantibodies in rheumatoid arthritis. Arthritis Rheum 52: 2645–2655. doi:10.1002/art.21269.
7. Fattal I, Shental N, Mevorach D, Anaya J-M, Livneh A, et al. (2010) An antibody profile of systemic lupus erythematosus detected by antigen microarray. Immunology 130: 337–343. doi:10.1111/j.1365-2567.2010.03245.x.
8. Belov L, Vega O de la, Remedios CG dos, Mulligan SP, Christopherson RI (2001) Immunophenotyping of Leukemias Using a Cluster of Differentiation Antibody Microarray. Cancer Res 61: 4483–4489.
9. Belov L, Mulligan SP, Barber N, Woolfson A, Scott M, et al. (2006) Analysis of human leukaemias and lymphomas using extensive immunophenotypes from an antibody microarray. Br J Haematol 135: 184–197. doi:10.1111/j.1365-2141.2006.06266.x.
10. Lal S, Lui R, Nguyen L, Macdonald P, Denyer G, et al. (2004) Increases in leukocyte cluster of differentiation antigen expression during cardiopulmonary bypass in patients undergoing heart transplantation. Proteomics 4: 1918–1926. doi:10.1002/pmic.200300756.
11. Brown A, Lattimore J-D, McGrady M, Sullivan D, Dyer W, et al. (2008) Stable and unstable angina: Identifying novel markers on circulating leukocytes. Proteomics Clin Appl 2: 90–98.
12. Lui R, Brown A, Wu B, Lin M-W, Thompson J, et al. (2008) Use of Antibody Microarrays in the Analysis of Inflammation, Autoimmunity, Viral Infection, and Cancer Metastases. In: Eyk JEV, Dunn MJ, editors. Clinical Proteomics. Wiley-VCH Verlag GmbH & Co. KGaA. pp. 571–592. Available:http://onlinelibrary.wiley.com/doi/10.1002/9783527622153.ch31/summary.Accessed 30 June 2012.
13. Lal S, Brown A, Nguyen L, Braet F, Dyer W, et al. (2009) Using antibody arrays to detect microparticles from acute coronary syndrome patients based on cluster of differentiation (CD) antigen expression. Mol Cell Proteomics 8: 799–804. doi:10.1074/mcp.M800335-MCP200.
14. Mohamed A, Lal S, Brown A, Lui R, Ho J, et al. (2010) How to Interrogate the cellular immune system in patients with ischemic heart disease. Myocardial Ischemia: Causes, Symptoms and Treatment. Nova Biomedical Press. pp. 195–216.
15. Ho JWK, Koundinya R, Caetano T, Remedios CG dos, Charleston MA (2008) Inferring differential leukocyte activity from antibody microarrays using a latent variable model. Genome Informatics 21: 126–137.
16. Bombardier C, Gladman DD, Urowitz MB, Caron D, Chang CH (1992) Derivation of the SLEDAI. A disease activity index for lupus patients. The Committee on Prognosis Studies in SLE. Arthritis Rheum 35: 630–640.
17. Smyth GK (2004) Linear models and empirical bayes methods for assessing differential expression in microarray experiments. Stat Appl Genet Mol Biol 3: Article3. doi:10.2202/1544-6115.1027.
18. Sing T, Sander O, Beerenwinkel N, Lengauer T (2005) ROCR: visualizing classifier performance in R. Bioinformatics 21: 3940–3941. doi:10.1093/bioinformatics/bti623.
19. Cortes C, Vapnik V (1995) Support-Vector Networks. Mach Learn 20: 273–297.
20. Cristianani N, Shawe-Taylor J (2000) An Introduction to Support Vector Machines: and other kernel-based learning methods. Cambridge University Press, UK.
21. Ramaswamy S, Tamayo P, Rifkin R, Sayan Mukherjee, Yeang C-H, et al. (2001) Multiclass cancer diagnosis using tumor gene expression signatures. Proc Natl Acad Sci USA 98: 15149–15154.
22. Golub TR, Slonim DK, Tamayo P, Huard C, Gaasenbeek M, et al. (1999) Molecular classification of cancer: Class discovery and class prediction by gene expression monitoring. Science 286: 531–537.
23. Bijl M, Horst G, Limburg PC, Kallenberg CG (2001) Fas expression on peripheral blood lymphocytes in systemic lupus erythematosus (SLE): relation to lymphocyte activation and disease activity. Lupus 10: 866–872.
24. Bijl M, Horst G, Limburg PC, Kallenberg CG (2001) Expression of costimulatory molecules on peripheral blood lymphocytes of patients with systemic lupus erythematosus. Ann Rheum Dis 60: 523–526.
25. Morris DL, Graham RR, Erwig L-P, Gaffney PM, Moser KL, et al. (2009) Variation in the upstream region of P-Selectin (SELP) is a risk factor for SLE. Genes Immun 10: 404–413. doi:10.1038/gene.2009.17.
26. Ho JWK, Lin M-W, Braet F, Su YY, Adelstein S, et al. (2010) Customising an antibody leukocyte capture microarray for systemic lupus erythematosus: beyond biomarker discovery. Proteomics Clin Appl 4: 179–189. doi:10.1002/prca.200900165.
27. Tsokos GC (2011) Systemic lupus erythematosus. N Engl J Med 365: 2110–2121. doi:10.1056/NEJMra1100359.

11

Inhibition of Aberrant Circulating Tfh Cell Proportions by Corticosteroids in Patients with Systemic Lupus Erythematosus

Xuebing Feng[1]*, Dandan Wang[1], Jingjing Chen[1], Lin Lu[1], Bingzhu Hua[1], Xia Li[1], Betty P. Tsao[2], Lingyun Sun[1]*

1 Department of Rheumatology, The Affiliated Drum Tower Hospital of Nanjing University Medical School, Nanjing, Jiangsu, China, **2** Division of Rheumatology, David Geffen School of Medicine at UCLA, Los Angeles, California, United States of America

Abstract

Objective: To observe the proportion of peripheral T follicular helper (Tfh) cells in patients with systemic lupus erythematosus (SLE) and to assess the role of steroids on Tfh cells from SLE patients.

Methods: Peripheral blood mononuclear cells (PBMCs) from 42 SLE patients and 22 matched healthy subjects were collected to assess proportions of circulating $CXCR5^+PD1^+/CD4^+$ T cells (Tfh), $CD4^+CCR6^+$ T cells (Th17-like) and $CD19^+CD138^+$ plasma cells by flow cytometry. 8 of the patients had their blood redrawn within one week after receiving methylprednisolone pulse treatment. Disease activity was evaluated by SLE disease activity index. To test the effect of IL-21 and corticosteroids on Tfh cells in vitro, PBMCs harvested from another 15 SLE patients were cultured with medium, IL-21, or IL-21+ dexamethasone for 24 hours and 72 hours. PBMCs from an independent 23 SLE patients were cultured with different concentrations of dexamethasone for 24 hours.

Results: Compared to normal controls, percentages of circulating Tfh cells, but not Th17 cells, were elevated in SLE patients and correlated with disease activity. Proportions of Tfh cells in SLE patients were positively correlated with those of plasma cells and serum levels of antinuclear antibodies. After methylprednisolone pulse treatment, both percentages and absolute numbers of circulating Tfh cells were significantly decreased. In vitro cultures showed an increase of Tfh cell proportion after IL-21 stimulation that was totally abolished by the addition of dexamethasone. Both 0.5 and 1 μM dexamethasone decreased Tfh cells dose dependently (overall $p = 0.013$).

Conclusions: We demonstrated that elevated circulating Tfh cell proportions in SLE patients correlated with their disease activities, and circulating levels of plasma cells and ANA. Corticosteroids treatment down-regulated aberrant circulating Tfh cell proportions both *in vivo* and *in vitro*, making Tfh cells a new treatment target for SLE patients.

Editor: Gernot Zissel, University Medical Center Freiburg, Germany

Funding: This work was supported by National Natural Science Foundation of China (grant number 30972735, 81172846), Jiangsu Province's Key Provincial Talents Program, "Six Talent Summit" Program and Nanjing Medical Science and Technique Development Foundation. B.P.T. was supported by RO1 43814 from the the NIAMS NIH. The funders had no role in study design, data collection and analysis, decision to publish, or preparation of the manuscript.

Competing Interests: The authors have declared that no competing interests exist.

* E-mail: fengxuebing@hotmail.com (XF); lingyunsun2001@yahoo.com.cn (LS)

These authors contributed equally to this work.

Introduction

Systemic lupus erythematosus (SLE) is a prototype autoimmune disease characterized by the production of multiple autoantibodies, particularly antinuclear antibodies (ANA). Both the B-cell and T-cell compartments exhibit functional abnormalities that could lead to the autoantibody production in SLE. Recently, much attention has focused on the role of the T follicular helper (Tfh) cell in supporting antibody production. This $CD4^+$ T subset helps the generation of germinal center (GC) responses where somatic hyper-mutation and affinity maturation take place leading to the generation of memory B cells and plasma cells [1].

Tfh cells can migrate to the germinal center through chemokine receptor CXCR5, while programmed death 1 (PD-1) signaling limits the number of Tfh cells and enhances their ability to promote interleukin (IL)-21 expressions [2]. It has been demonstrated that co-expressions of CXCR5 with ICOS and/or PD-1 are a useful phenotypic profile to distinguish this T helper cell subset, and circulating Tfh cells are in proportion to their GC counterparts [3–5]. Growing evidence has suggested that Tfh cell may have a crucial role in the pathogenesis of SLE, as the aberrant expressions of Tfh cell-associated molecules, such as ICOS, SAP, PD-1 and IL-21, are all linked to autoantibody production and/or lupus-like disease in murine models [6–9]. In SLE patients, expression of Tfh cell phenotypes by circulating peripheral blood cells has been shown to correlate with diversity and titers of autoantibodies and with disease severity [5].

IL-21, which is mainly expressed by Tfh cells, is crucial for Tfh cell development [10]. Previously we have shown there was a nearly perfect correlation between the extent of IL-21 and ANA production in vitro [11], strongly supporting a role of Tfh cell in the developing of SLE. However, it is still unclear how these cells are modulated in SLE. In this study, we explored the frequency of Tfh cells in peripheral blood from SLE patients, and examined the role of IL-21 and steroids on these cells. We found a high frequency of circulating Tfh cells in lupus patients, especially in those with active disease, which could be alleviated by corticosteroids both *in vivo* and *in vitro*.

Materials and Methods

Study Subjects

Study protocol and informed consent were reviewed and approved by the Ethics Committee of the Affiliated Drum Tower Hospital of Nanjing University Medical School and all participants provided their written informed consents to participate in this study. All the SLE patients fulfilled the 1997 updated revised criteria of the American College of Rheumatology (ACR) [12] and healthy volunteers were recruited as normal controls with an effort to match age and gender of SLE patients.

Forty-two SLE patients (35 women and 7 men, mean age 33.7±2.0 years) were enrolled for the measuring of circulating Tfh cells. Disease activity at the time of blood drawn was assessed by their rheumatologists and verified by two of the authors (DW and BH) using the SLE disease activity index (SLEDAI) [13]. Eight of the patients (7 women and 1 man, mean age 27.4±4.1 years) had their blood redrawn after high-dose steroid therapy. The demographics for these patients were shown in Table 1 and Table 2. Of the 42 SLE patients recruited, 29 was reassessed for ANA values, 24 for IgG antibodies to anti-dsDNA and 37 for anti-extractable nuclear antigen using reagents from Euroimmun AG (Lübeck, Germany). Values for ANA were calculated as described [11] and detection range for IgG anti-dsDNA antibody is 10~800 IU/ml.

As for in vivo studies, peripheral blood mononuclear cells (PBMCs) were obtained from 15 SLE patients (14 women and 1 man, mean age 34.7±3.1 years) and another 23 samples (21 women and 2 men, mean age 32.9±3.3 years) were collected to observe the dose effect of steroids.

Flow Cytometry

PBMCs were isolated by Ficoll-Paque Plus density gradient centrifugation (Burlington, Onlario, Canada). As described elsewhere [14], PBMCs at 10^6/tube were stained with fluorescein isothiocyanate (FITC)-conjugated anti-CD4, phycoerythrin (PE)-conjugated anti-PD1, phycoerythrin-Cy5 (PE-Cy5)-conjugated anti-CCR6 and Alexa Fluor 647-conjugated anti-CXCR5 (BD PharMingen San Diego, CA) or isotype-matched control IgG, according to the manufacturer's protocol. Flow data were determined in a FACSCalibur system (BD Biosciences, San Jose, CA), followed by analysis using Flowjo software (Tree Star, version 5.7.2). At least 50,000 events per sample were analyzed. Cells were gated on the forward scatter of living cells and then centered on $CD4^+$ T cells. As illustrated in Figure 1, the proportion of Tfh cells was analyzed as the percentage of $CXCR5^+$ $PD1^+$ cells within total $CD4^+$ T cells for each sample ($CXCR5^+$ $PD1^+/CD4^+$ T cells, using isotype control staining for CXCR5 and PD1 to set the threshold). To determine the absolute number of circulating Tfh cells, lymphocyte numbers per liter were obtained by automated complete blood cell counts at the same day blood drawn and then multiplied by percentages of $CD4^+$ and percentages of $CXCR5^+$ $PD1^+/CD4^+$ cells. $CD4^+$ $CCR6^+$ T cells proportion was defined as Th17-like cells as previously described [15]. For the detection of circulating plasma cells, PBMC were stained with APC-conjugated anti-CD19 and PE-conjugated anti-CD138, and gating on $CD19^+$ $CD138^+$ cells [16]. Data were reported as $CD19^+$ $CD138^+$ percentages of total PBMCs.

Table 1. Demographics of SLE patients and normal controls*.

	SLE patients (n = 42)	Normal controls (n = 22)
Age, years	33.7±2.0 (14–62)	34.1±2.2 (21–55)
Female gender	35 (83.3)	20 (90.9)
Disease duration, years	7.05±1.02 (0.25–33)	
SLEDAI score	8.26±0.55 (2–16)	
ANA positivity	100%	

*Values are shown by mean ± SEM (range) or number (percentage). There were no significant differences between patients with systemic lupus erythematosus (SLE) and normal controls or disease controls in terms of age and gender.

Table 2. Alteration of Tfh cells before and after MP treatment.

No	Age	Gender	Before MP treatment		After MP treatment	
			Tfh (%)	Tfh num (10^6/L)	Tfh (%)#	Tfh num (10^6/L)*
1	29	f	11.26%	56.3	5.48%	43.8
2	25	f	15.31%	275.6	8.25%	173.3
3	37	f	7.33%	161.3	9.51%	190.2
4	22	f	18.5%	166.5	8.62%	43.1
5	49	f	22.46%	202.1	14.16%	141.6
6	14	m	12.24%	195.8	7.67%	115.1
7	29	f	22.43%	314.0	15.29%	183.5
8	14	f	32.5%	617.5	28.83%	403.6

MP: methylprednisolone. Data were analyzed by paired t-test.
#$p<0.01$ vs Tfh cell percentage before MP treatment,
*$p<0.05$ vs absolute Tfh cell numbers before MP treatment.

Cell Culture

PBMCs were collected by Ficoll-Paque Plus density gradient, resuspended in RPMI 1640 medium, then distributed to 96-well plates (Corning, Tewksbury, MA) at $(0.5-1.5)\times10^6$ per well. Cells incubated at 37°C in a humidified atmosphere with 5% CO_2 were treated as follows: (a) in RPMI-1640 medium containing 10% FCS alone, (b) recombinant human IL-21 (200 ng/μL) (PeproTech, Rocky Hill, NJ) added, or (c) IL-21 and dexamethasone (1 μM, as described before [17]) (Jinlin pharmacy, China) added simultaneously. Experiments were carried out in duplicates and cell numbers were equal among the 3 groups for each patient. After 24 and 72 hours, all the cells in culture wells were harvested and then stained with FITC-conjugated anti-CD4, PE-conjugated anti-PD1 and Alexa Fluor 647-conjugated anti-CXCR5 for the detection of Tfh cell percentage by flow cytometry. To observe the role of dexamethasone on unstimulated Tfh cells, PBMCs were cultured in RPMI-1640 medium containing 10% FCS with or without different concentrations of dexamethasone (0.5 μM, 1 μM) for 24

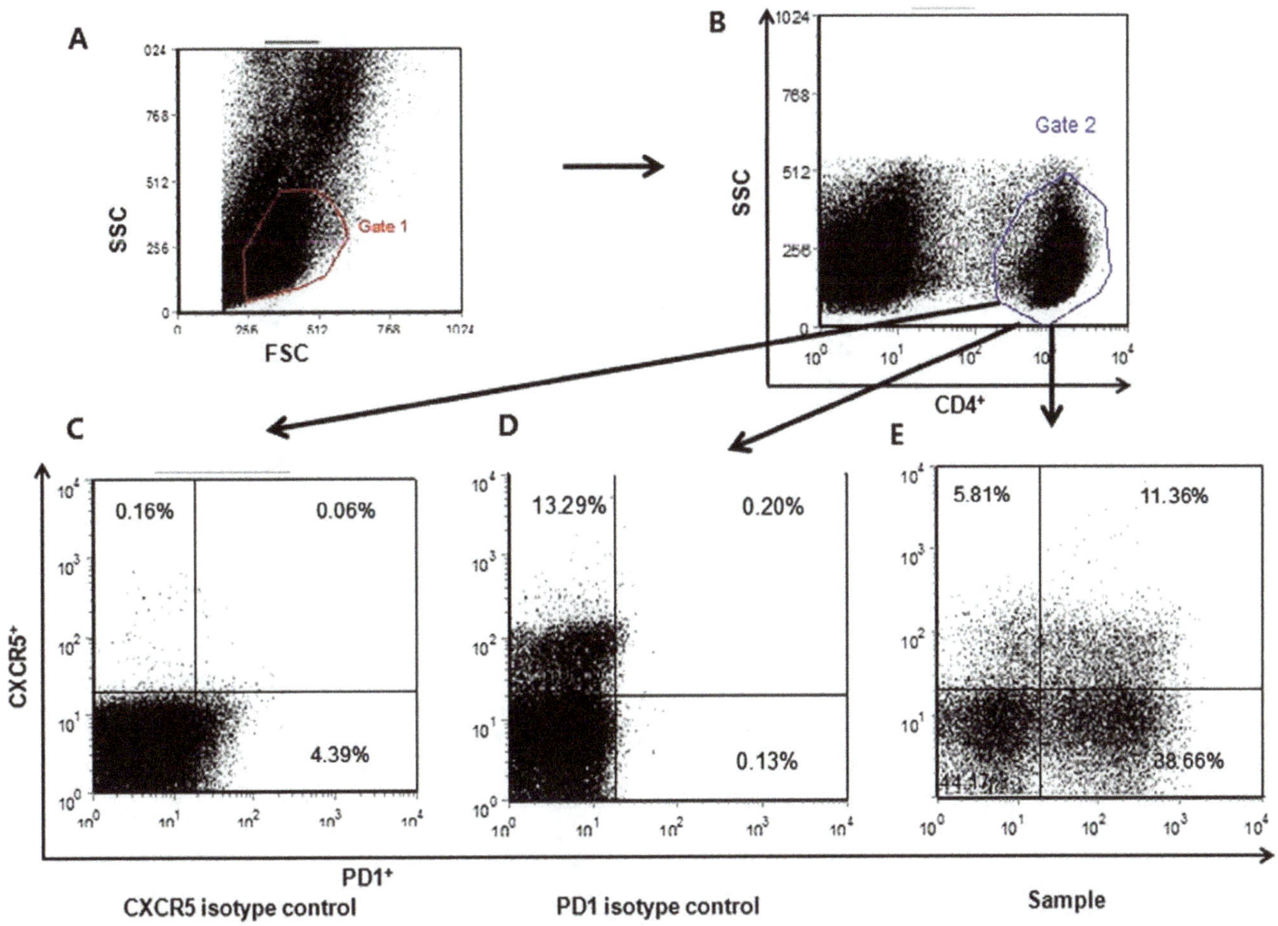

Figure 1. FACS analysis of Tfh cells. Three tubes from one sample, stained with 1) CD4, CXCR5 isotype control and PD1, 2) CD4, CXCR5 and PD1 isotype control, and 3) CD4, CXCR5 and PD1 separately, were analyzed at the same time. PBMCs are gated on the forward scatter of living cells and then centered on $CD4^+$ T cells (A,B). After setting the threshold using isotype control staining for CXCR5 (C) and PD1 (D), the proportion of Tfh cells is analyzed as the percentage of $CXCR5^+$ $PD1^+$ cells within total $CD4^+$ T cells (E).

hours. To analyze the status of cell apoptosis after dexamethasone treatment, cultured cells were harvested, stained with PE-conjugated anti-CD4, PE-Cy7-conjugated anti-PD1, APC-conjugated anti-CXCR5 and FITC-conjugated Annexin V, and then measured by FACS.

Statistical Analysis

To compare numeration data between two groups from *in vivo* studies, Mann-Whitney U test was conducted because some of the data were not normally distributed and values were shown as medians with 25th and 75th percentiles and interquartile range (IQRs), except that alterations of Tfh cells before and after methylprednisolone treatment were analyzed by paired t-test. Chi-square test or Fisher exact probability test was applied for quantitative data, and Pearson correlation was used to depict linear relationships between two factors. For our *in vitro* studies, paired t-test was applied to compare results between two groups and Kruskal-Wallis test was used to determine the difference among three groups. Data were analyzed using the Prism 3.0 program (GraphPad, La Jolla, CA, USA) and SPSS 16.0 software, and $p<0.05$ was considered significant.

Results

Percentages of Circulating $CXCR5^+$ $PD1^+/CD4^+$ T cells Increased in SLE Patients and Correlated with Disease Activity

Percentages of peripheral blood $CD4^+$ $CXCR5^+$ $PD1^+$ cells in $CD4^+$ T cells from 42 Chinese SLE patients and 22 normal controls were analyzed by flow cytometry. Compared with the normal controls, the SLE patients were not significantly different in terms of age and gender (Table 1). As shown in Figure 2A, percentages of $CXCR5^+$ $PD1^+/CD4^+$ cells were higher in peripheral blood samples from SLE patients compared with those from normal controls (median 10.94 (25th and 75th percentiles 8.11, 18.32) % vs. 8.17 (7.20, 9.93) %, $p<0.01$). To assess whether T helper type 17 (Th17) cells, another subset of $CD4^+$ T cells involved in IL-21 and subsequent antibody production, played a role in SLE, peripheral blood $CD4^+$ $CCR6^+$ cells from 26 SLE patients and 8 normal controls were measured concordantly. As shown in Figure 2B, the proportion of circulating $CD4^+$ $CCR6^+$ in $CD4^+$ T cells showed no difference between SLE patients (26.75 (19.33, 34.83) %) and healthy controls (24.15 (22.78, 27.53) %, $p>0.05$). Next we compared percentages of circulating $CXCR5^+$ $PD1^+/CD4^+$ cells in SLE patients with varying levels of disease activity, as assessed by the SLEDAI score at the time blood was

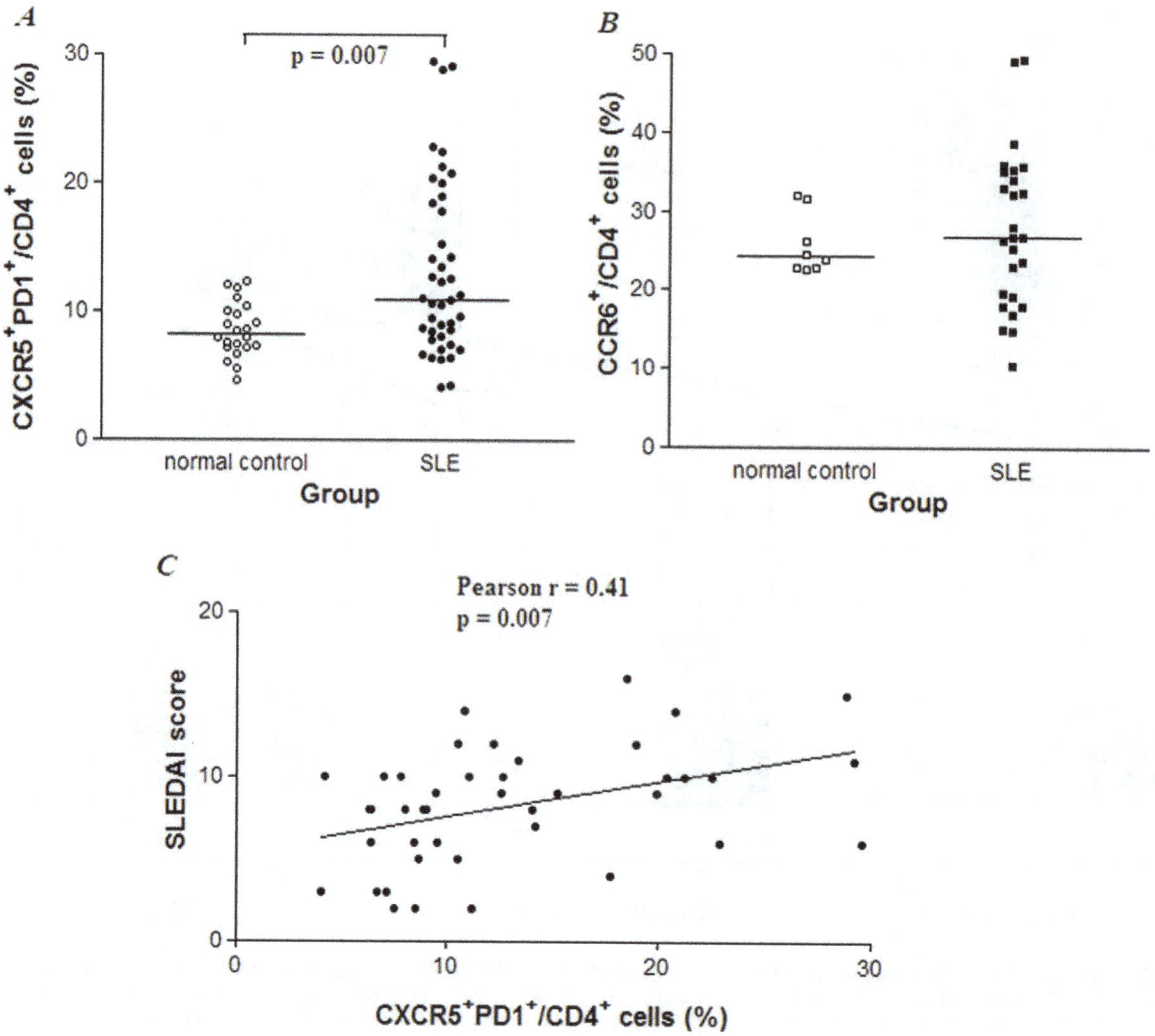

Figure 2. Aberrant circulating $CXCR5^+$ $PD1^+/CD4^+$ but not $CCR6^+/CD4^+$ T cells correlated with disease activity in SLE patients. A. Elevated circulating $CXCR5^+$ $PD1^+/CD4^+$ cells in SLE patients compared to normal controls. PBMCs were quantified by FACS, each symbol represented an individual sample and horizontal lines showed median values. Mann-Whitney U test was conducted to compare the data between two groups. B. Circulating $CCR6^+/CD4^+$ cell proportions enriched for Th17-like cells were compared between SLE patients and normal controls. C. Correlation between percentages of $CXCR5^+$ $PD1^+/CD4^+$ cells and disease activity of 42 SLE patients. Pearson correlation was applied to depict linear relationships.

obtained. A positive correlation between Tfh cells and SLEDAI scores was observed (Pearson $r = 0.41$, $p<0.01$) (Figure 2C).

Correlation of Tfh cell Proportions with Levels of Autoantibodies and Plasma Cell Proportions in SLE Patients

Within our 42 patients, all had a positive documented ANA. 29 of their samples were measured for ANA levels and 24 for anti-dsDNA levels by ELISA using serum collected at the time of blood draw. Percentages of $CXCR5^+$ $PD1^+/CD4^+$ cells were correlated with ANA levels in these patients (Pearson $r = 0.40$, $p = 0.032$) (Figure 3A), but not correlated with levels of IgG anti-dsDNA antibodies (Figure 3B). In 37 patients who were routinely checked for anti-extractable nuclear antigen (ENA) antibodies, only anti-SSA/SSB was associated with Tfh cell proportion as shown in Table 3 ($p<0.05$).

The link between Tfh cell and ANA prompted us to test the status of B cell activation in SLE patients. Flow cytometry analysis revealed a significant higher proportion of circulating $CD19^+$ $CD138^+$ plasma cells in 23 SLE patients (0.22 (0.12, 0.33) %) compared to those in 23 healthy controls (0.08 (0.05, 0.12) %, $p<0.0001$) (Figure 3C), and percentages of $CD19^+$ $CD138^+$ cells was positively correlated with percentages of $CXCR5^+$ $PD1^+/CD4^+$ cells in SLE patients (Pearson $r = 0.45$, $p = 0.031$) (Figure 3D).

Tfh cell and SLE Clinical Features

Renal involvement, serositis, leucopenia, thrombocytopenia, hypocomplementemia, and ongoing rash as well as oral ulcer contributed to SLEDAI scores in most of our SLE patients, and 3 of them had central nervous system (CNS) involvement. Patients were divided into high Tfh group ($n = 16$, defined as having a percentage of $CXCR5^+$ $PD1^+/CD4^+$ cells 2 standard deviations above the mean of normal controls) and normal Tfh group ($n = 26$). Based on our data (Table 3), all the manifestations listed above were not associated with percentages of Tfh cells.

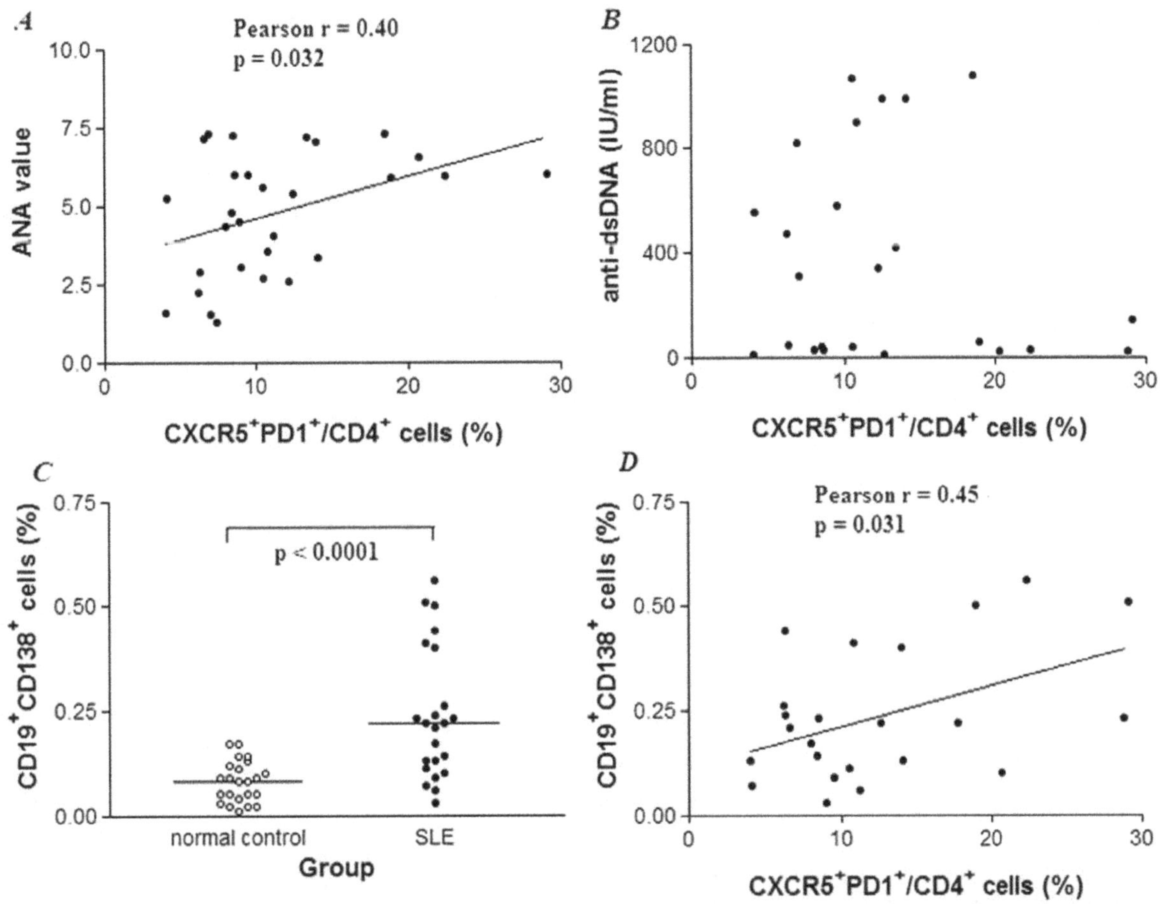

Figure 3. Positive correlation of CXCR5$^+$ PD1$^+$/CD4$^+$ cells with ANA and CD19$^+$ CD138$^+$ cells in SLE patients. A. Percentages of circulating CXCR5$^+$ PD1$^+$/CD4$^+$ cells were positively correlated with ANA values (Pearson r = 0.40, $p<0.05$) in 29 SLE patients. B. There were no association between percentages of CXCR5$^+$ PD1$^+$/CD4$^+$ cells and circulating levels of IgG anti-dsDNA by Pearson correlation test. However, in those patients having high levels of anti-dsDNA antibodies (~ 50%), a trend of correlation with CXCR5$^+$ PD1$^+$/CD4$^+$ cells was observed. C. Circulating CD19$^+$ CD138$^+$ cells were elevated in SLE patients as compared with normal controls. Each symbol represented an individual sample, horizontal lines showed median values, and Mann-Whitney U test was applied. D. Percentages of CXCR5$^+$ PD1$^+$/CD4$^+$ cells were positively correlated with percentages of CD19$^+$ CD138$^+$ cells in 23 SLE patients (Pearson r = 0.45, $p<0.05$).

Interestingly, there was a trend showing patients with high Tfh expression had elevated incidences of vasculitis (25% vs 3.8%, p = 0.06).

Decreased Proportion of Tfh cells after Methylprednisolone Pulse Treatment in SLE Patients

All recruited patients had been treated with different dose of corticosteroids (<60 mg of methylprednisolone per day) before blood drawn. Subsequently, 8 of them were given high dose of intravenous methylprednisolone (120–500 mg/day for 3–4 days) to control their active disease (including 2 CNS lupus, 5 lupus nephritis and 1 severe thrombocytopenia), which provided us an excellent opportunity to explore the role of corticosteroids in Tfh cell *in vivo*. To evaluate the alteration of circulating CXCR5$^+$ PD1$^+$/CD4$^+$ cells, blood was redrawn from these 8 patients within one week after the pulse treatment. As shown in Table 2, concomitantly with the amelioration of clinical manifestations, there was a significant reduction of circulating CXCR5$^+$ PD1$^+$/ CD4$^+$ cell proportion post-treatment ($p<0.01$). To exclude the influence of corticosteroids on total lymphocyte numbers, absolute numbers of Tfh cells pre- and post- treatments were enumerated. Our data showed that absolute number of CXCR5$^+$ PD1$^+$/CD4$^+$ cells was also decreased after the treatment ($p<0.05$, Table 2).

Inhibition of IL-21 Stimulated Tfh cell of by Dexamethasone in vitro

To further elucidate the role of IL-21 and steroids in Tfh cell production, PBMCs from another 15 randomly selected SLE patients were collected. Each sample was divided into 3 groups: medium control group, IL-21 stimulation group and IL-21+ dexamethasone group, cultured for 24 hours and harvested to measure CXCR5$^+$ PD1$^+$/CD4$^+$ cells by flow cytometry. We found percentages of CXCR5$^+$ PD1$^+$/CD4$^+$ cells significantly increased after IL-21 stimulation ($p<0.01$) which could be totally abolished by adding dexamethasone ($p<0.0001$) (Figure 4A). Similar results were observed after culturing these PBMCs for 72 hours ($p<0.05$) (Figure 4B).

Dose Dependent Effects of Dexamethasone on Tfh cell

PBMCs were collected from 23 SLE patients and each sample was divided into 3 parts to cultured with different concentrations of dexamethasone (0, 0.5 μM and 1 μM, defined as control, low dose and high dose) for 24 hours and then measured for CXCR5$^+$

Table 3. Correlation between clinical manifestations and Tfh cells in SLE patients*.

Clinical manifestations	Circulating Tfh cells		p
	High expression#	Low expression	
Mucocutaneous	5/16 (31.3)	9/26 (34.6)	0.82
Renal involvement$	12/16 (75.0)	17/26 (65.4)	0.73
Renal insufficiency	4/16 (25.0)	5/26 (19.2)	0.71
CNS lupus	1/16 (6.3)	2/26 (7.7)	1
Serositis	5/16 (31.3)	3/26 (11.5)	0.22
Vasculitis	4/16 (25.0)	1/26 (3.8)	0.061
Leucopenia	4/16 (25.0)	5/26 (19.2)	0.71
Thrombocytopenia	5/16 (31.3)	3/26 (11.5)	0.22
Hypocomplementemia	8/16 (50.0)	15/26 (57.7)	0.63
Autoantibodies			
Anti-RNP	3/13 (23.1)	10/24 (41.7)	0.31
Anti-SSA/SSB	9/13 (69.2)	8/24 (33.3)	0.047
Anti-Sm	3/13 (23.1)	7/24 (29.2)	1

*Values were the number of patients positive/total number tested (%) and Chi-square test or Fisher exact probability test was applied to compare results between two groups.
#Defined as having a percentage of CXCR5$^+$ PD1$^+$/CD4$^+$ cells 2 SD above the mean of normal controls.
$Defined as having proteinuria, hematuria or urinary casts.

PD1$^+$/CD4$^+$ cells. We found the percentages of CXCR5$^+$ PD1$^+$/CD4$^+$ cells significantly decreased after culturing with dexamethasone ($p<0.01$ for low dose group and $p<0.0001$ for high dose group as compared to control group, and overall p value among 3 groups were 0.013 by Kruskal-Wallis test). Percentages of CXCR5$^+$ PD1$^+$/CD4$^+$ cells were lower in the high dose group comparing to those in the low dose group ($p<0.05$), indicating a dose dependent effect of dexamethasone on Tfh cell (Figure 4C). To address whether the down-regulation of Tfh cells by dexamethasone was due to a concentration-related decrease in cell numbers, total cells in each group were counted and there was no difference among the groups ($p>0.05$, Figure 4D). Next we evaluated the status of cell apoptosis after dexamethasone treatment by using Annexin V staining. Our data showed that Annexin V$^+$ cells were increased both in CXCR5$^+$ PD1$^+$/CD4$^+$ group and in CXCR5$^-$PD1$^-$/CD4$^+$ group when treated with dexamethasone, especially for those using high dosage. However, the percentages of Annexin V$^+$ cells were much high in CXCR5$^+$ PD1$^+$/CD4$^+$ groups (Figure 4E).

Discussion

To our knowledge, this is the first paper to report the effect of corticosteroids in the aberrant expression of Tfh cells in SLE patients. Our study showed that proportions of the CXCR5$^+$ PD1$^+$/CD4$^+$ T (Tfh) cells in peripheral blood of SLE patients were elevated compared to those in normal subjects, exhibiting positively correlations with disease activity score, peripheral plasma cells as well as ANA titers (Figure 2 and 3). Tfh cell numbers dramatically reduced after the patients received methylprednisolone pulse treatment (Table 2). Adding IL-21 to PBMC cultures could increase Tfh cell numbers *in vitro*, which was down-regulated when cocultured with dexamethasone in a dose-dependently manner (Figure 4), suggesting that Tfh cells could be a new therapeutic target for autoimmune disease.

Consistent with ours [11], several studies have also provided evidences that the IL-21 pathway plays an important role in the pathogenesis of SLE [18,19]. The production of IL-21 is mainly restricted to two subsets of CD4$^+$ T cells, Th17 and Tfh. Th17 cells are associated with the production of inflammation mediators, and it has been observed by several groups that SLE patients have an enhanced Th17 cell response [20,21], which is different from our results showing that there is no elevation of CD4$^+$ CCR6$^+$ cell percentage in PBMCs from SLE patients as compared to that from normal controls. Because cell types other than Th17, such as Th22, could also express CCR6, we measured CD3$^+$ CD8$^-$ IL-17A$^+$ cells in PBMCs after stimulation by FACS and found no difference in their proportions between SLE patients and normal controls (data not shown). Since more than 90% of IL-17-secreting CD4$^+$ T cells were also CCR6$^+$ cells [22], it was reasonable to assume that CD4$^+$ CCR6$^+$ could represent Th17-like cells. Although the sample size in this study was not large enough to draw a conclusion, evidences have shown that increased Th17 cells in SLE patients were linked to the use of corticosteroids [23], implicating an abnormal Th17 response in SLE might be derived from treatments rather than the disease itself. Consistent with our findings, Dolff et al has shown percentages of IL-21$^+$ T cells were increased in SLE patients, while percentages of IL-17$^+$ T cells were not [18]. Recently, it has been shown that both CXCR5$^+$ CD4$^+$ T cells and CXCR5$^-$ CD4$^+$ T cells (Th17 related) producing IL-21 were increased in SLE patients. However, only the former cell subset was correlated with increased circulating germinal center B cells [24].

In addition to Th17 cells, another subset of CD4$^+$ T cells named Tfh cells could also produce massive IL-21 [25]. IL-21 has been considered as the master cytokine for the regulation of Tfh development and function in an autocrine fashion [26]. Here we found proportions of circulating Tfh cells were elevated in SLE patients and correlated with disease activity as measured by SLEDAI scores, suggesting Tfh cells but not Th17 cells might be the main producer of IL-21 in SLE that contribute to the disease processes. To support our results, frequencies of cells displaying Tfh phenotypes have been shown to increase in peripheral blood and spleens of human SLE patients and lupus-prone mice [5,27]. No association of Tfh cell expression with renal, CNS or hematological involvement was observed in our study. However, an increased tendency of vasculitis was suggested for those with high Tfh cell expression (Table 3).

The involvement of Tfh cells in pathogenic mechanisms of SLE remains to be demonstrated. Tfh cells express higher levels of co-stimulatory molecules like OX40, CD40L, ICOS and PD-1 as compared to other T cell subsets, thus could provide co-stimulation signal to activate antigen presenting B cells and consequently exuberance in the positive selection of somatically mutated B cells will lead to excessive autoantibody production [28,29]. In addition, Tfh cells are capable of secreting cytokines (such as IL-21 and IL-6) to drive B cell expansion and differentiation [3]. In this study, we showed significantly positive correlation of proportions of Tfh cells with long-lived plasma cells in SLE patients. Similar to that reported [5], proportion of Tfh cells was also associated with ANA and anti-SSA antibody production, supporting the notion that Tfh cells may interact with B cells to facilitate plasma cells differentiation and antibody production.

Our next question is whether Tfh cells could be modulated by current treatments. Corticosteroids are still the mainstay of treatment for SLE patients, which can decrease pro-inflammatory

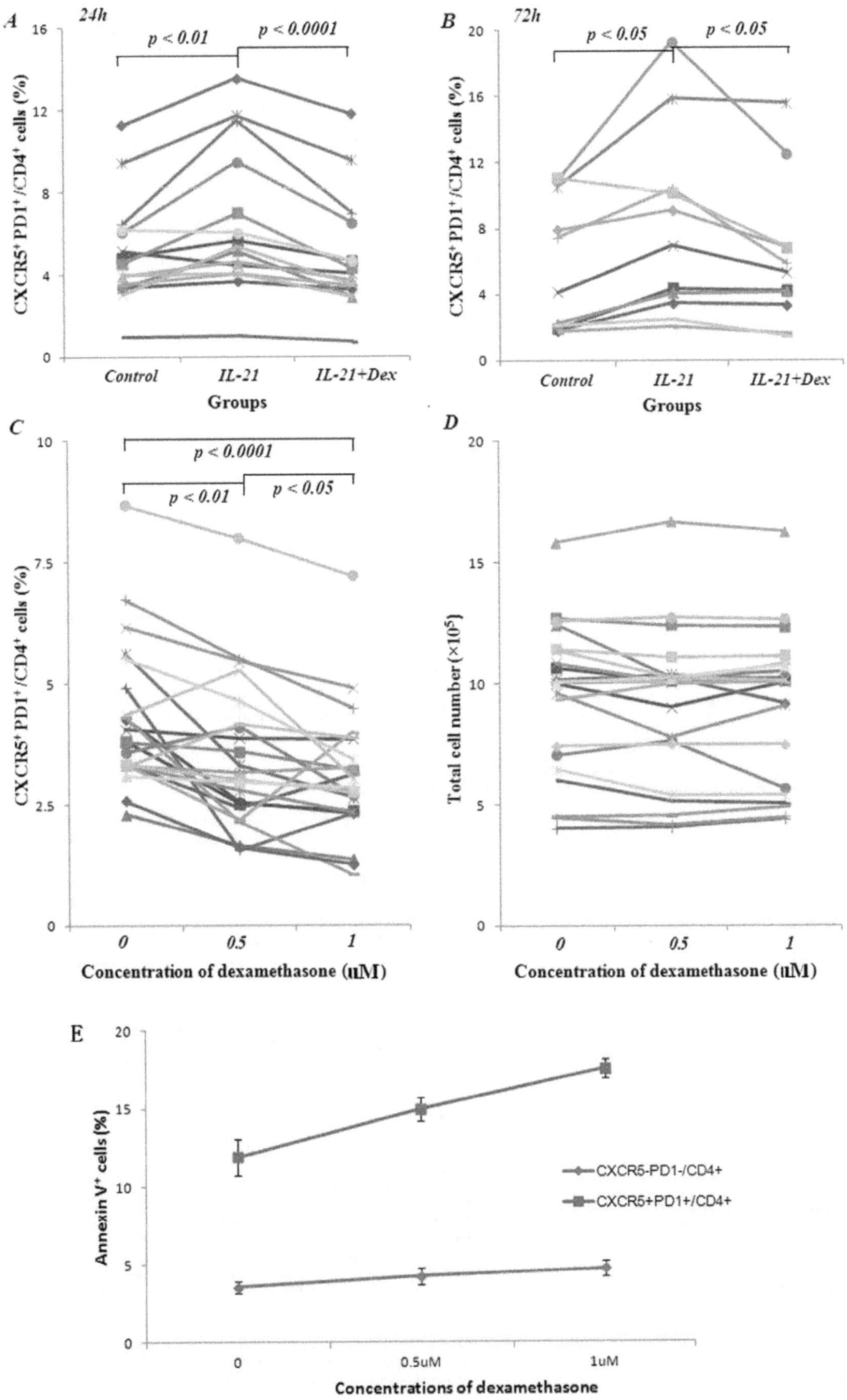
A
24h
p < 0.01
p < 0.0001
CXCR5+PD1+/CD4+ cells (%)
Control
IL-21
IL-21+Dex
Groups
B
72h
p < 0.05
p < 0.05
CXCR5+PD1+/CD4+ cells (%)
Control
IL-21
IL-21+Dex
Groups
C
p < 0.0001
p < 0.01
p < 0.05
CXCR5+PD1+/CD4+ cells (%)
Concentration of dexamethasone (uM)
D
Total cell number (×10^5)
Concentration of dexamethasone (uM)
E
Annexin V+ cells (%)
CXCR5-PD1-/CD4+
CXCR5+PD1+/CD4+
0
0.5uM
1uM
Concentrations of dexamethasone

Figure 4. Decreased CXCR5$^+$ PD1$^+$/CD4$^+$ cell production by dexamethasone. A. Dexamethasone (Dex) reduced the proportion of IL-21 stimulated CXCR5$^+$ PD1$^+$/CD4$^+$ cell. Each line represented the alterations of CXCR5$^+$ PD1$^+$/CD4$^+$ cell percentages of an individual sample when cultured with medium control, IL-21 or IL-21+ Dex for 24 hours in vitro. Paired t-test was applied to compare results between two groups and Kruskal-Wallis test was used to determine the difference among three groups. Compared with control group, CXCR5$^+$ PD1$^+$/CD4$^+$ cells were increased when cultured with IL-21 ($p<0.01$). Adding dexamethasone to IL-21 culture system significantly inhibited the production of CXCR5$^+$ PD1$^+$/CD4$^+$ cells ($p<0.0001$). B. A similar tendency was observed when cells were cultured for 72 hours. Each line represented the alterations of CXCR5$^+$ PD1$^+$/CD4$^+$ cell percentages of an individual sample. C. Dexamethasone reduced the proportion of CXCR5$^+$ PD1$^+$/CD4$^+$ cell in a dose-dependent manner. Each line represented the changes of CXCR5$^+$ PD1$^+$/CD4$^+$ cell percentages of an individual sample when cultured with different concentrations of dexamethasone for 24 hours in vitro and paired t-test was applied to compare results between two groups. D. Downregulation of CXCR5$^+$ PD1$^+$/CD4$^+$ cell by dexamethasone was not a consequence of the decline in total cell numbers. Cells were equally divided into 3 groups to culture with different concentrations of dexamethasone. After 24 hours culturing, all the cells were harvested and counted by flow cytometry. There were no differences of total cell numbers among the groups ($p>0.05$). E. Increased cell apoptosis after dexamethasone treatment. PBMCs from 6 SLE patients were collected and cultured in the presence or absence of dexamethasone for 24 hours. Then cells were harvested and quantified by FACS. Data were shown as mean $\pm$ SEM. The percentages of Annexin V$^+$ cells are much higher in CXCR5$^+$ PD1$^+$/CD4$^+$ groups, especially for those treated with high dose dexamethasone.

cytokine synthesis, T-cell function, and Fc receptor expression, thereby controlling inflammation and resolving lupus activity [30,31]. For those patients with severe organ involvement (for example, cardiopulmonary, renal or CNS involvement), usually high-dose of corticosteroids are given to control disease activity. Previously it has been shown the expansion of Tfh cells in peripheral blood is a fixed phenotype and not related to immunosuppressive therapy [5]. Here we observed a significant reduction in the Tfh cells after methylprednisolone pulse treatment. Considering there was a slight decline of total lymphocyte numbers after corticosteroid treatment (data not shown), absolute Tfh cell numbers were calculated and a similar result was shown. To confirm this finding, *in vitro* studies were performed and we found Tfh proportions were significantly decreased when dexamethasone added to the culture system.

The underlying mechanisms for corticosteroid in modulating Tfh cells and its relation to IL-21 are still unclear. As reported, Tfh cells could be differentiated or transformed from other T cell types under suitable conditions, and IL-21 was a key cytokine to induce Tfh production [10]. In this paper, we have shown that IL-21 stimulation did increase Tfh cell proportion, but the effect diminished when dexamethasone was added to the culture system. To interpret this phenomenon, cell apoptosis after *in vitro* culturing was measured by using Annexin V staining. Our data showed that Annexin V$^+$ cells were increased both in CXCR5$^+$ PD1$^+$/CD4$^+$ group and in CXCR5$^-$ PD1$^-$/CD4$^+$ group when treated with dexamethasone, but apoptotic cells were much higher in CXCR5$^+$ PD1$^+$/CD4$^+$ groups (Figure 4E). Based on these findings, it is plausible that IL-21 helps induce Th cell differentiation to Tfh subtypes, while corticosteroid promotes Tfh cell apoptosis. Combined effects of these two factors may counteract each other, resulting in unchanged Tfh cell percentages. In addition, corticosteroid may directly regulate Tfh related cytokines including IL-21 and IL-6 via serum glucocorticoid-regulated kinase 1 (SGK1), an important gene in steroids-related pathway [32,33].

Taken together, here we showed the dynamics of circulating Tfh cells in Chinese SLE populations for the first time. Our results indicated that Tfh cells might interact with B cells and facilitated autoantibodies production in SLE. The proportion of circulating Tfh cells was down-regulated by corticosteroids in a dose-dependent manner, thus providing us a new target in the treatment of SLE patients.

Author Contributions

Conceived and designed the experiments: XF BT. Performed the experiments: DW JC LL. Analyzed the data: XF DW BH. Contributed reagents/materials/analysis tools: XL. Wrote the paper: XF BT. Final approval of the article: LS.

References

1. Deenick EK, Ma CS (2011) The regulation and role of T follicular helper cells in immunity. Immunology 134: 361–367.
2. Good-Jacobson KL, Szumilas CG, Chen L, Sharpe AH, Tomayko MM, et al. (2010) PD-1 regulates germinal center B cell survival and the formation and affinity of long-lived plasma cells. Nat Immunol 11: 535–542.
3. Linterman MA, Beaton L, Yu D, Ramiscal RR, Srivastava M, et al. (2010) IL-21 acts directly on B cells to regulate Bcl-6 expression and germinal center responses. J Exp Med 207: 353–363.
4. Kerfoot SM, Yaari G, Patel JR, Johnson KL, Gonzalez DG, et al. (2011) Germinal center B cell and T follicular helper cell development initiates in the interfollicular zone. Immunity 34: 947–960.
5. Simpson N, Gatenby PA, Wilson A, Malik S, Fulcher DA, et al. (2010) Expansion of circulating T cells resembling follicular helper T cells is a fixed phenotype that identifies a subset of severe systemic lupus erythematosus. Arthritis Rheum 62: 234–244.
6. Zeller GC, Hirahashi J, Schwarting A, Sharpe AH, Kelley VR (2006) Inducible co-stimulator null MRL-Faslpr mice: uncoupling of autoantibodies and T cell responses in lupus. J Am Soc Nephrol 17: 122–130.
7. Zhang W, Wu J, Qiao B, Xu W, Xiong S (2011) Amelioration of lupus nephritis by serum amyloid P component gene therapy with distinct mechanisms varied from different stage of the disease. PLoS One 6: e22659.
8. Lucas JA, Menke J, Rabacal WA, Schoen FJ, Sharpe AH, et al. (2008) Programmed death ligand 1 regulates a critical checkpoint for autoimmune myocarditis and pneumonitis in MRL mice. J Immunol 181: 2513–2521.
9. Herber D, Brown TP, Liang S, Young DA, Collins M, et al. (2007) IL-21 has a pathogenic role in a lupus-prone mouse model and its blockade with IL-21R.Fc reduces disease progression. J Immunol 178: 3822–3830.
10. Nurieva RI, Chung Y, Hwang D, Yang XO, Kang HS, et al. (2008) Generation of T follicular helper cells is mediated by interleukin-21 but independent of T helper 1, 2, or 17 cell lineages. Immunity 29: 138–149.
11. Feng X, Li R, Huang J, Zhang H, Zhu L, et al. (2010) Olfl/EBF associated zinc finger protein interfered with antinuclear antibody production in patients with systemic lupus erythematosus. Arthritis Res Ther 12: R59.
12. Hochberg MC (1997) Updating the American College of Rheumatology revised criteria for the classification of systemic lupus erythematosus. Arthritis Rheum 40: 1725.
13. Bombardier C, Gladman DD, Urowitz MB, Caron D, Chang CH (1992) Derivation of the SLEDAI. A disease activity index for lupus patients. The Committee on Prognosis Studies in SLE. Arthritis Rheum 35: 630–640.
14. Feng J, Lu L, Hua C, Qin L, Zhao P, et al. (2011) High frequency of CD4+ CXCR5+ TFH cells in patients with immune-active chronic hepatitis B. PLoS One 6: e21698.
15. Harrison OJ, Foley J, Bolognese BJ, Long E III, Podolin PL, et al. (2008) Airway infiltration of CD4+ CCR6+ Th17 type cells associated with chronic cigarette smoke induced airspace enlargement. Immunol Lett 121: 13–21.
16. Recher M, Burns SO, de la Fuente MA, Volpi S, Dahlberg C, et al. (2012) B cell-intrinsic deficiency of the Wiskott-Aldrich syndrome protein (WASp) causes severe abnormalities of the peripheral B-cell compartment in mice. Blood 119: 2819–2828.
17. Cepika AM, Bendelja K, Vergles JM, Malenica B, Kapitanovic S, et al. (2010) Monocyte response to LPS after exposure to corticosteroids and chloroquine with implications for systemic lupus erythematosus. Scand J Immunol 72: 434–443.

18. Dolff S, Abdulahad WH, Westra J, Doornbos-van der Meer B, Limburg PC, et al. (2011) Increase in IL-21 producing T-cells in patients with systemic lupus erythematosus. Arthritis Res Ther 13: R157.
19. Nguyen V, Luzina I, Rus H, Tegla C, Chen C, et al. (2012) IL-21 Promotes Lupus-like Disease in Chronic Graft-versus-Host Disease through Both CD4 T Cell- and B Cell-Intrinsic Mechanisms. J Immunol 189: 1081–1093.
20. Alunno A, Bartoloni E, Bistoni O, Nocentini G, Ronchetti S, et al. (2012) Balance between Regulatory T and Th17 Cells in Systemic Lupus Erythematosus: The Old and the New. Clin Dev Immunol 2012: 823085.
21. Shah K, Lee WW, Lee SH, Kim SH, Kang SW, et al. (2010) Dysregulated balance of Th17 and Th1 cells in systemic lupus erythematosus. Arthritis Res Ther 12: R53.
22. Appel H, Maier R, Wu P, Scheer R, Hempfing A, et al. (2011) Analysis of IL-17(+) cells in facet joints of patients with spondyloarthritis suggests that the innate immune pathway might be of greater relevance than the Th17-mediated adaptive immune response. Arthritis Res Ther 13: R95.
23. Prado C, de PB, Gomez J, Lopez P, Rodriguez-Carrio J, et al. (2011) Glucocorticoids enhance Th17/Th1 imbalance and signal transducer and activator of transcription 3 expression in systemic lupus erythematosus patients. Rheumatology (Oxford) 50: 1794–1801.
24. Terrier B, Costedoat-Chalumeau N, Garrido M, Geri G, Rosenzwajg M, et al. (2012) Interleukin 21 Correlates with T Cell and B Cell Subset Alterations in Systemic Lupus Erythematosus. J Rheumatol 39: 1819–1828.
25. Vogelzang A, McGuire HM, Yu D, Sprent J, Mackay CR, et al. (2008) A fundamental role for interleukin-21 in the generation of T follicular helper cells. Immunity 29: 127–137.
26. Ma CS, Deenick EK, Batten M, Tangye SG (2012) The origins, function, and regulation of T follicular helper cells. J Exp Med 209: 1241–1253.
27. Vinuesa CG, Cook MC, Angelucci C, Athanasopoulos V, Rui L, et al. (2005) A RING-type ubiquitin ligase family member required to repress follicular helper T cells and autoimmunity. Nature 435: 452–458.
28. Breitfeld D, Ohl L, Kremmer E, Ellwart J, Sallusto F, et al. (2000) Follicular B helper T cells express CXC chemokine receptor 5, localize to B cell follicles, and support immunoglobulin production. J Exp Med 192: 1545–1552.
29. Patakas A, Platt AM, Butcher JP, Maffia P, McInnes IB, et al. (2011) Putative existence of reciprocal dialogue between Tfh and B cells and its impact on infectious and autoimmune disease. Immunol Lett 138: 38–46.
30. Rhen T, Cidlowski JA (2005) Antiinflammatory action of glucocorticoids–new mechanisms for old drugs. N Engl J Med 353: 1711–1723.
31. King JK, Hahn BH (2007) Systemic lupus erythematosus: modern strategies for management: a moving target. Best Pract Res Clin Rheumatol 21: 971–987.
32. Fagerli UM, Ullrich K, Stuhmer T, Holien T, Kochert K, et al. (2011) Serum/glucocorticoid-regulated kinase 1 (SGK1) is a prominent target gene of the transcriptional response to cytokines in multiple myeloma and supports the growth of myeloma cells. Oncogene 30: 3198–3206.
33. Maranville JC, Luca F, Richards AL, Wen X, Witonsky DB, et al. (2011) Interactions between glucocorticoid treatment and cis-regulatory polymorphisms contribute to cellular response phenotypes. PLoS Genet 7: e1002162.

Bone Disease in Newly Diagnosed Lupus Nephritis Patients

Aline Lázara Resende*, Luciene Machado dos Reis, Cristiane Bitencourt Dias, Melani Ribeiro Custódio, Vanda Jorgetti, Viktoria Woronik

Nephrology Division, Sao Paulo University Medical School, Sao Paulo, Brazil

Abstract

Introduction: Bone loss in Lupus Nephritis (LN) patients is common and multifactorial. The aim of this study was to evaluate the bone status of newly diagnosed LN patients and their correlation with inflammatory factors involved in LN physiopathology.

Methods: We studied 15 pre-menopausal patients with ≤2 months of diagnosed SLE and LN. Patients with prior kidney or bone disease were excluded. In addition to biochemical evaluation (including 25-hydroxyvitamin D_3 [25(OH)D] and Monocyte Chemotactic Protein (MCP1) dosage), we performed bone biopsies followed by osteoblast culture, histomorphometric and immunohistochemistry analysis.

Results: LN patients presented a mean age of 29.5±10 years, a proteinuria of 4.7±2.9 g/day and an estimated glomerular filtration rate (GFR) of 37(31–87) ml/min/1,73 m^2. They were on glucocorticoid therapy for 34±12 days. All patients presented vitamin D insufficiency (9.9±4.4 ng/ml, range 4–20). Urinary MCP1 correlated negatively with 25(OH)D ($r = -0.53$, $p = 0.003$) and positively with serum deoxypyridinoline ($r = 0.53$, $p = 0.004$). Osteoblasts isolated from LN bone biopsies presented a significantly higher expression of MCP-1 when compared to controls (32.0.±9.1 vs. 22.9±5.3 mean fluorescence intensities, $p = 0.01$). LN patients presented a significantly reduced osteoid volume, osteoid thickness, osteoid surface, mineralization surface and bone formation rate, associated with an increased eroded surface and osteoclast surface. Patient's bone specimens demonstrated a reduced immunostaining for osteoprotegerin (0.61±0.82 vs. 1.08±0.50%, $p = 0.003$), and an increased expression of Receptor Activator of NF-κB ligand (RANKL) (1.76±0.92 vs. 0.41±0.28%, $p < 0.001$) when compared to controls.

Discussion: Newly diagnosed LN patients presented a significant disturbance in bone metabolism, characterized by an impaired bone formation and mineralization, associated with an increase in resorption parameters. Glucocorticoid use, vitamin D insufficiency and inflammation might be involved in the physiopathology of bone metabolism disturbance.

Editor: Niels Olsen Saraiva Câmara, Universidade de Sao Paulo, Brazil

Funding: Financial support was provided by the Fundação de Amparo a Pesquisa do Estado de São Paulo (FAPESP, Foundation for the Support of Research in the state of São Paulo) (Grant number 2010/15409-3). The funder had no role in study design, data collection and analysis, decision to publish, or preparation of the manuscript.

Competing Interests: The authors have declared that no competing interests exist.

* Email: alinelr@usp.br

Introduction

Systemic Lupus Erythematosus (SLE) is a chronic autoimmune disease that may compromise multiple organs. Although several mechanisms may influence the loss of self-tolerance, cytokines are thought to initiate and amplify inflammation and organ damage [1]. Because disease survival has improved over the last decades, scientific community has placed a growing emphasis on prevention and treatment of SLE-related comorbidities. Bone loss is not only a common (with osteopenia and osteoporosis been reported in 25–74% and 1.4–68% of patients, respectively), but also a potentially preventable condition associated with SLE [2,3].

The etiology of bone loss in SLE is probably multifactorial, involving both traditional and disease-related risk factors [3]. Glucocorticoid use has been extensively associated with reduced bone mineral density (BMD) in SLE patients [4–7]. Indeed, Glucocorticoid-induced bone disease (GIO) is considered the most common cause of secondary osteoporosis. The loss of BMD in GIO is biphasic: it occurs rapidly (6–12% loss) within the first year and more slowly (3% loss yearly) thereafter [8]. However, the risk of fractures seems to increase 75% within the first 3 months of therapy, before a substantial decline in BMD [9], and possibly due to the loss of bone strength [10]. It is not clear the minimum dose and duration of glucocorticoid therapy that could increase the risk of fracture. Guidelines from the American College of Rheumatology, the National Osteoporosis Foundation and the Royal College of Physicians agree that pharmacologic therapy should be used in patients exposed to glucocorticoid for at least 3 months [11–14]. Nevertheless, the contribution of corticosteroid therapy to bone loss in SLE remains unclear as several studies found no association between reduced BMD and corticosteroid therapy [15–20]. Furthermore, some investigators have reported a relationship between SLE and lower BMD in patients never receiving corticosteroids [19,21,22], suggesting that SLE activity *per se* may be a risk factor for bone loss.

Based on animal and *in vitro* observations [23–27], recent studies have raised the attention on the interplay between inflammatory factors and bone remodeling and metabolism not only in SLE [2,16,28,29], but also in other clinical conditions, such as Rheumatoid Arthritis, Inflammatory Bowel Disease, Idiopathic Hypercalciuria and Estrogen withdrawal [24,26,30–34]. There are many evidences that the immune and skeletal systems not only share a number a regulatory molecules (such as cytokines, receptors, signaling and transcription factors), but also interact in the bone marrow [35].

Lupus nephritis (LN), a major clinical manifestation of SLE, is notably characterized by an intense inflammatory activity. An important mediator of renal injury is a leukocyte chemotactic factor called Monocyte chemoattractant protein-1 (MCP-1). Noteworthy, the urinary levels of MCP-1 are widely recognized as a sensitive and specific biomarker of LN activity [36–41]. Besides inflammation, LN patients may confront an increased risk for bone disturbances due to proteinuria and/or kidney dysfunction, usually aggravating the vitamin D insufficiency [2,16,42,43].

Finally, literature data on SLE-related bone disease are focused in bone mineral density loss (BMD) measured by the most widely used technique known as DEXA (Dual Energy Xray Absorptiometry) [7,19,20,22,44–46]. Although clinically relevant, the decreased BMD might not reflect the bone strength and especially does not help to understand the physiopathology of the bone disorder [10,47]. The aim of this study was evaluate the bone status of newly diagnosed lupus nephritis patients and their correlation with inflammatory factors thought to be involved in LN physiopathology. In addition to biochemical evaluation, we performed bone biopsies followed by osteoblast culture, histomorphometric and immunohistochemistry analysis.

Methods

Subjects

We studied pre-menopausal patients with ≤2 months of diagnosed SLE and LN (according to the American College of Rheumatology classification criteria [48] attended in Sao Paulo University Medical School from December 2010 to December 2012. Patients with prior kidney disease, pregnancy, thyroid dysfunction, currently use of calcium supplements, anticonvulsants, oral anticoagulants, or other drugs affecting bone metabolism were excluded. The local ethics committee of the Sao Paulo University Medical School approved the study protocol, and patients provided written informed consent.

Clinical activity was estimated according to the Systemic Lupus Erythematosus Disease Activity Index (SLEDAI) [49]. Kidney biopsies were performed and LN was classified according to the current International Society of Nephrology (ISN)/Renal Pathology Society classification [50] by an independent pathologist. All patients received glucocorticoids since they were diagnosed. Other immunosuppressive medications were decided by the clinical staff. Of note, proliferative LN patients were treated with monthly intravenous cyclophosphamide (n = 11) or with oral mycophenolate (n = 2), while Membranous LN (n = 1) was treated with oral cyclosporine. Class II LN (n = 1) was treated with a short course of corticosteroid only.

Biochemical analysis

Fasting serum and plasma, 24-hour urine, and early-morning spot urine were all collected at hospital admission (on average three weeks before the bone biopsy). Parathyroid hormone (PTH) was measured by immunochemiluminensce [reference values (RV): 16–87 pg/ml] and 25-hydroxyvitamin D_3 [25(OH)D] by chemoimmunoassay (RV: 30–100 ng/ml). Total calcium (RV: 8.6–10.2 mg/dL), phosphorus (RV: 2.7–4.5 mg/dL) and alkaline phosphatase (RV: 35–104 U/L) were determined by automated routine methods. The Glomerular Filtration Rate (GFR) was estimated by the MDRD simplified formula [51].

The levels of Monocyte Chemotactic Protein (MCP-1) were measured in serum and urine by ELISA assay according to the manufacturer's directions (Human MCP1 ELISA, R&D Systems). Urinary levels of MCP-1 were standardized to urine creatinine (Cr) measured in the same spot urine and expressed as pg/mg Cr.

We also measured the serum levels of Interleukin (IL) 6 and Tumor Necrosis Factor (TNF) α (Human IL-6 and Human TNFα, both from R&D Systems, Minneapolis, MN, USA), considered biomarkers of SLE activity [52–54]. Bone resorption marker deoxypyridinoline was determined by the enzyme-linked immunoassay (Total Deoxypyridinoline ELISA, Quidel, San Diego, CA, USA).

Controls for biochemical analysis were age-matched healthy women, mostly students and employees from our laboratory. Control's samples were taken at the end of winter (September of 2012), period of the year when lowest vitamin D levels are expected. All patients and controls were permanent residents in metropolitan area of Sao Paulo, a city with subtropical climate located at 23°34′S [55,56].

Bone biopsy

After pre-labeling with tetracycline (20 mg/kg/day during 3 days, administered in two time-spaced doses, separated by an interval of 10 days), LN patients were submitted to local anesthesia and light sedation. Bone samples of approximately 1.5 cm in length were obtained from the anterior iliac bone using an electric trephine (Gaulthier Medical, Rochester, MN, USA). Bone specimens were placed in Dulbecco's Modified Eagle's Medium (DMEM) supplemented with HEPES 25 mM, penicillin 250 UI, streptomycin 250 μg/ml and 3 μg/ml of amphotericin B, and divided in 2 parts, one for in vitro analysis, as described next, and the another one for bone histology evaluation (histomorphometry) and immunohistochemistry.

Osteoblast culture

For *in vitro* analysis cancellous bone obtained from bone biopsy were minced into small fragments (1-mm3) that were washed with phosphate buffered saline to remove hematopoietic marrow cells. The bone fragments were first cultured in 100 mm Petri polystyrene dishes (Nunc, Ilinois, USA) with 10 ml of Dulbecco's Modified Eagle's Medium, supplemented with antibiotics (penicillin 50 UI, streptomycin 50 μg/ml, amphotericin B 2.5 μg/ml) and 20% fetal bovine serum (Cultilab, Campinas, Brazil). Culture plates were incubated at 37°C in a humidified atmosphere of 95% of air, 5% CO_2.

The fragments stayed undisturbed for at least 3 days. The medium was replaced three times per week. Outgrowths of spindle-shaped cells became visible in one week or more. After approximately fourteen days, the small fragments were removed and transferred to another Petri dish to continuing primary explant culture. This procedure was repeated three more times to obtain more cells in the first and second passage. Bone cells were cultured until they reached 90% confluence. Bone cells obtained

Table 1. Clinical, biochemical and histological characteristics of lupus nephritis patients.

		mean±sd, median (25–75 IQR) or n/%	Range (when appropriate)
Age (years)		29.5±10	18–47
SLEDAI		21±6	14–32
Cumulative glucocorticoid dose (mg of prednisone)		1953±765	950–3720
Time of glucocorticoid use (days)		34±12	16–62
Use of angiotensin-converting enzyme (ACE) inhibitors or angiotensin receptor blockers		8/53.3%	-
Hemoglobin (g/dL)		9.6±1.1	7.4–11.9
Class of Lupus Nephritis	**II**	1/6.7	-
	III	3/20	
	IV	10/66.6	
	V	1/6.7	
Positive Anti-DNA		11/73.3	-
Decreased C4 complement		13/86.7	-
24 hour proteinuria (g/day)		4.7±2.9	0.8–9.7
Serum albumin (g/dL)		2.4±0.8	1.0–3.9
Total cholesterol (mg/dL)		306±130	152–679
Triglycerides (mg/dL)		268±111	85–480
Serum creatinine (mg/dl)		1.67 (0.89–1.83)	0.57–4.85
Estimated GFR (ml/min/1.73 m²)		37 (31–87)	12–155
Total calcium (mg/dL)		8.2±0.8	6.6–9.5
Phosphorus (mg/dL)		4.9±1.2	3.2–7.6
Alkaline phosphatase (U/L)		58 (45–85)	42–259
25(OH)D (ng/ml)		9.9±4.4	4–20
PTH (pg/ml)		73 (29–102)	14–196

Legend: SLEDAI (Systemic Lupus Erythematosus Disease Activity Index); GFR (Glomerular Filtration Rate estimated by the MDRD simplified formula); 25(OH)D (25-hydroxyvitamin D_3); PTH (parathyroid hormone).

from outgrowths were harvested with trypsin TrypLE Express (Gibco, USA) and separated into three aliquots for cell proliferation, citometry flow experiments, and cryopreservation storage. As the phenotypic expression of human bone cells has been shown to decrease after multiple passages [57], we studied these cells in the first or second passage. The cell population obtained from the trabecular bone surfaces exhibited an osteoblast phenotype, as evidenced by the expression of an early stage marker alkaline phosphatase and the induction of mineralization [58] (data not shown).

Control bone cells were obtained in parallel with the study period from cadaveric age-matched female donor organs (n = 9).

1. Cell proliferation

Bone cells were cultured in 24-well plates (1.8×10^4cells/well) with complete culture medium until they reached 80–90% of confluence. Then, we used serum free medium with ascorbic acid (100 µg/ml) for 16 hours. After this period, we added 5 µCi/ml of Thymidine [Methyl -^{3}H] (Amersham Pharmacia Biotech Brasil Ltda, São Paulo, Brazil) to each well, and the culture was continued for an additional 2 hours. Subsequently, the thymidine was removed, the cells were washed twice with phosphate-buffered saline, and DNA was precipitated with 5% trichloroacetic acid. 300 µl of 0.2 N NaOH/0.3% n-lauroylsarcosine Na salt solution (Sigma) were added at each well, and aliquots of 60 µl were placed at 3 ml of liquid scintillation. Samples were protected from light for 2 hours and then analyzed by a Beckman beta scintillation counter model LS6200 (Beckman Instruments, Palo Alto, CA, USA). Results were expressed as counts per minute (CPM).

2. Flow cytometry

We analyzed the extracellular expression of Alkaline Phosphatase and the intracellular staining of Osteocalcin and MCP-1. Briefly, after dissociation, bone cells (0.5×10^6) were placed in cytometry tubes, washed, centrifuged and incubated with optimal amounts of monoclonal antibodies to detect anti-human bone, liver and kidney alkaline phosphatase −10 µg/ml (US Biological, MA, USA), Phycoerythrin (PE) -conjugated anti-human osteocalcin −0.25 µg/ml (R&D Systems Inc, MN, USA), and anti-human CCL2/MCP1 −2,5 µg/ml (R&D Systems Inc, MN, USA), for 30–45 minutes at 4°C in darkness. For the intracellular staining, cells were first fixed with paraformaldehyde fixative (4% paraformaldehyde in 10 mM phosphate buffered saline) and permeabilized with SAP buffer (0.1% saponin, 0.05% NaN_3 in Hanks Balanced Salt solution HBSS). When necessary, cells were incubated for 30 minutes at 4°C in darkness with a secondary FITC-conjugated antibody to allow binding to the primary antibody. As negative control, we used for each patient an isotype control in the same conditions as for extracellular or intracellular staining. 10^4 events were normally acquired and bone cells were distinguished using light scatter characteristics [forward-scattered light (FSC) that is proportional to cell-surface area or size and side-scattered light (SSC) that is proportional to cell granularity or internal complexity]. Data were analyzedusing a FACSCalibur

Table 2. Clinical and biochemical features of lupus nephritis patients and controls.

	Lupus Nephritis (n = 15)	Controls (n = 15)	p
Age (years)	29.5±10	31.7±6.4	0.25
Body Mass Index (BMI) (Kg/m²)	24±3	24±4	0.74
Estimated GFR (ml/min/1.73 m²)	37 (31–87)	90 (73–100)	0.009
25(OH)D (ng/ml)	9.9±4.4	24.3±6.2	<0.001
Serum MCP1 (pg/ml)	18.3 (16.3–39.9)	11.1 (10.3–13.4)	<0.001
Urinary MCP1 (pg/mg Cr)	1594 (595–2447)	177 (113–267)	<0.001
Serum IL-6 (pg/ml)	5.8 (1.9–11.3)	1.2 (1.1–1.4)	0.002
Serum TNFα (pg/ml)	9.1 (8.2–19.9)	5.6 (5.2–6.7)	<0.001
Serum deoxypyridinoline (nmol/L)	9.1 (5.4–15.5)	3.8 (3.5–4.9)	<0.001

Legend: Results are expressed as mean ± standard deviation, median (25–75 IQR) or n/%. GFR (Glomerular Filtration Rate estimated by the MDRD simplified formula); 25(OH)D (25-hydroxyvitamin D_3); MCP1 (Monocyte Chemoattractant Protein-1); IL-6 (Interleukin 6); TNFα (Tumor Necrosis Factor α).

flow cytometer (Becton Dickinson, San Diego, USA) and a CellQuest Software (Becton Dickinson, San Diego, USA), and the results were expressed as the percentage of positive cells and as mean fluorescence intensities (MFIs), corrected for background fluorescence.

Histomorphometry and immunohistochemistry analysis

Bone material designated to histomorphometry and immunohistochemistry was fixed in 70% ethanol and processed according to Malluche and Faugere [59]. Using a Polycut S equipped with a tungsten carbide knife (Leica, Heidelberg, Germany), undecalcified bone were cut into sections of 5 µm and 10 µm in thickness. Static histomorphometric data were obtained using a semiautomatic image analyser and the software Osteomeasure (Osteometrics Inc., Atlanta, GA, USA). Unstained 10 µm slices were obtained for analysis of dynamic parameters under a microscope with ultraviolet light.

The parameters analyzed were in accordance with the standards set by the American Society for Bone and Mineral Research [60]. The histomorphometric static parameters analyzed were: bone structure, as defined by measuring trabecular volume (BV/TV) (%), trabecular thickness (Tb.Th) (µm), trabecular separation (Tb.Sp) (mm) and trabecular number (Tb.N) (/mm); bone formation, as defined by osteoid volume (OV/BV) (%), osteoblast surface (Ob.S/BS) (%), osteoid thickness (O.Th) (µm) and osteoid surface (OS/BS) (%); and bone resorption, as defined by eroded surface (ES/BS) (%) and osteoclast surface (Oc.S/BS) (%). Kinetic parameters were: mineralizing surface (MS/BS) (%), mineral apposition rate (MAR) (µm/day), bone formation rate (BFR/BS) ($\mu m^3/\mu m^2$/day) and mineralization lag time (MLT) (days). The biopsy samples presented a tissue area of 9.2–54.0 mm^2. Three samples presented a tissue area <30 mm^2.

We performed an immunohistochemistry method for detection of proteins on bone sections embedded in methyl metacrylate [61]. Briefly, bone sections were deacrylated in a mixture of xylene and chloroform, rehydrated in graded alcohol solutions, submitted to a quick decalcification with 1% acetic acid, and treated with 0.1% Tween 20. Endogenous peroxidase activity was inhibited by a mixture of 3% hydrogen peroxide in methanol. Protein Block (DAKO Corporation, California, USA) was used to block nonspecific bindings. Sections were incubated overnight at 4°C in a humidified chamber using the primary goat monoclonal antihuman antibodies Osteoprotegerin (OPG) (1:80) and Receptor Activator of NF-κB ligand (RANKL) (1:150) (Santa Cruz Biotechnology, Santa Cruz, CA, USA). After incubation with the primary antibody, sections were incubated with the biotinylated secondary antibodies (*Biotinylated Link Universal,* DAKO Corporation, California, USA) and with the *Streptavidin-HRP* (DAKO Corporation, California, USA). Antigen-antibody complexes were visualized using a 3-amino-9-ethylcarbazole as chromogen substrate (AEC). The sections were counterstained with Mayer's hemalum solution (Merck, Darmstadt, Germany). Simultaneous negative controls were carried out by omitting primary antibody in all sections. As positive controls, we used bone sections from patients with Chronic Kidney Disease-Mineral and Bone Disease (CKD-MBD). Each bone sample was entirely evaluated in a light microscopy at a magnification of 200×. Immunopositivity was determined as the percentage of positive osteocytes compared with the total osteocyte number in each biopsy.

Controls for histomorphometric static parameters and immunohistochemistry were 15 female age-matched healthy individuals from a large Brazilian bone database [62]. Most subjects had been victims of gunshot or knife wounds, trauma, or traffic accidents and were not known to have any disease. Dynamic parameters were compared to 29 healthy female subjects from Melsen et al (mean age 29 years) [63].

Statistical Analysis

Results are expressed as mean ± stand deviation, median (25–75 IQR) or n/%. For comparisons between groups, we used chi-square and Mann–Whitney tests, as appropriate. Correlations between variables were determined using the Spearman correlation coefficient. Urinary MCP-1 was log transformed and used as a dependent variable in linear regression models. Analyses were performed using the SPSS v 13.0 software. Tests were all two-sided and p value <0.05 was considered as significant.

Results

The results of the clinical, biochemical and histological classification of LN are described in the table 1. LN patients presented a mean age of 29.5±10 years. The mean proteinuria was 4.7±2.9 g/day and the estimated GFR was 37(31–87) ml/min/1,73 m^2. Proliferative Lupus Nephritis was observed in 86.6% of the patients. The mean cumulative prednisone dose was 1953±765 mg in 34±12 days, reflecting that our patients presented a high activity and received an aggressive treatment. All patients presented vitamin D insufficiency (25-hydroxyvitamin $D_3 = 9.9 \pm 4.4$ ng/ml, range 4–20).

Table 2 describes the clinical and biochemical characteristics of the patients and controls. There were no differences in age and body mass index (BMI). LN patients presented lower levels of estimated GFR and 25(OH)D. They also presented significantly higher levels of IL-6, TNFα and MCP-1, reinforcing that they were on high disease activity. Patients also presented higher levels of serum deoxypyridinoline.

The levels of 25(OH)D correlated negatively with serum MCP-1 ($r = -0.53$, $p = 0.003$), IL-6 ($r = -0.58$, $p < 0.001$), TNFα ($r = -0.53$, $p = 0.003$) and deoxypyridinoline ($r = -0.59$, $p < 0.001$), and urinary MCP-1 ($r = -0.63$, $p < 0.001$) (figure 1). We also observed a positive correlation between urinary MCP-1 and serum deoxypyridinoline ($r = 0.53$, $p = 0.004$).

Table 3 describes the results of the Linear regression analysis. The correlation between urinary MCP-1 and 25(OH)D remained unchanged even after adjusted for age, BMI and estimated GFR (beta coeff. −0.585, 95% CI −0.13 to −0.04, $p = 0.001$). The SLEDAI score, the period of use and the cumulative dose of glucocorticoid were not correlated with any of the studied variables.

Osteoblast culture

We obtained bone cells from biopsy fragments of ten patients. There were no differences between NL patients and age-matched female donor organ's controls in osteoblast proliferation measured by incorporation of thymidine (82.22±48.43 *vs* 56.07±23.73 CPM, respectively, $p = 0.21$).

Table 4 shows results from flow cytometry of cultured bone cells. Osteoblasts isolated from LN patients presented a significantly higher expression of MCP-1 (32.0±9.1 *vs* 22.9±5.3 MFIs, $p = 0.01$), while no differences were observed in the expression of osteocalcin or alkaline phosphatase.

We observed no differences between NL patients and controls concerning the percentage of positive MCP-1 and Alkaline Phosphatase cells. There was an increased percentage of osteocalcin positive cells in LN patients (12.25±7.13 *vs* 4.66±3.69%, $p = 0.007$) (Table 4).

Bone histomorphometry

Results of the bone histomorphometry analysis of the patients and controls are summarized in table 5. We did not observe any difference between both groups concerning to structural parameters. LN patients presented a significantly reduced osteoid volume

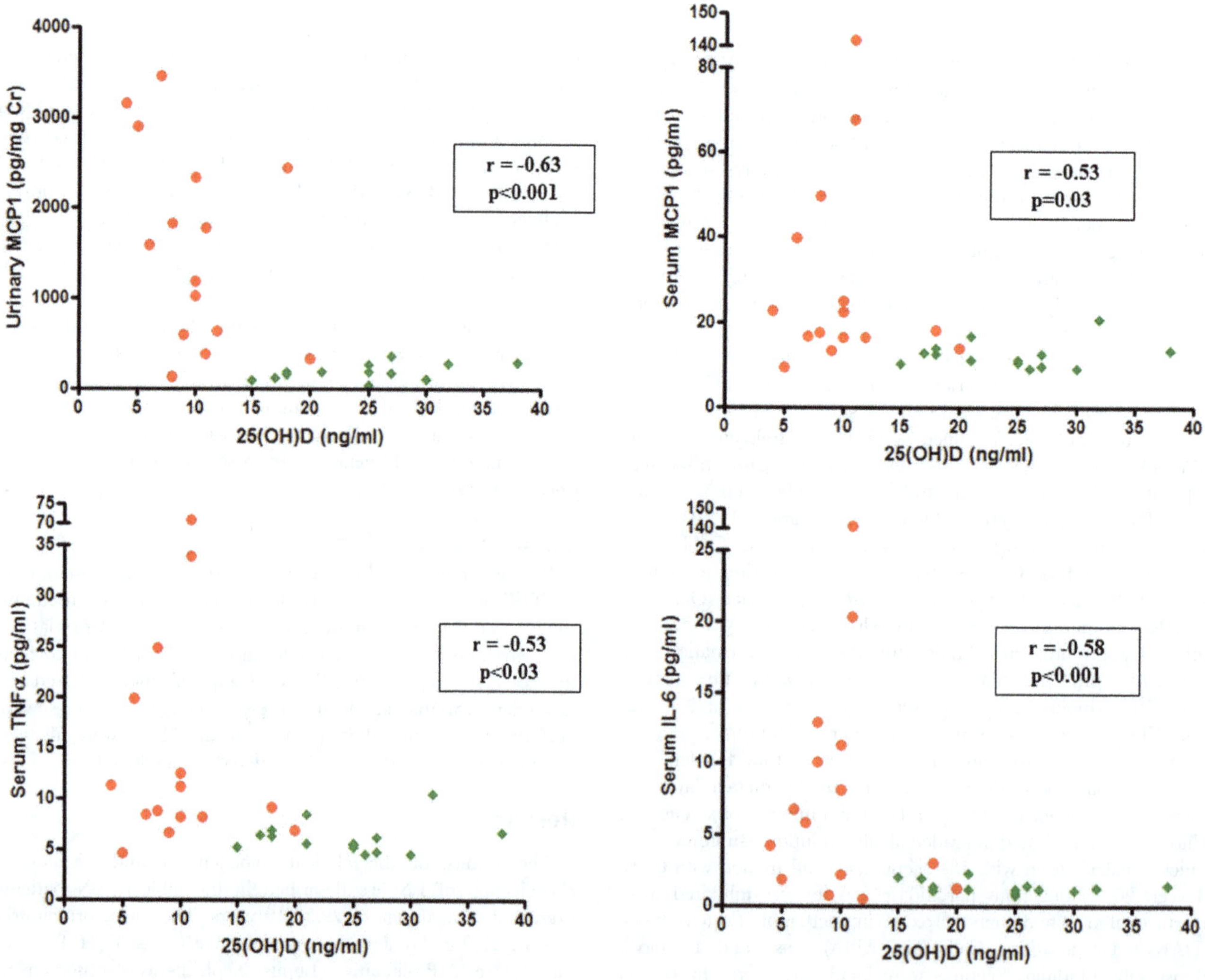

Figure 1. Correlation between 25(OH)D levels and inflammatory markers. Legend: The box contains Spearman's correlation coefficient and *p* value. Green diamonds and red circles represent controls and LN patients, respectively.

Table 3. Linear regression models on Log Urinary MCP1 levels.

	Beta	Se	95% CI	p
25(OH)D (ng/ml)	−0.585	0.02	−0.13– −0.04	0.001
	Beta	**Se**	**95% CI**	**p**
25(OH)D (ng/ml)	−0.387	0.02	−0.11– −0.01	0.03
Age (years)	−0.263	0.02	−0.49–0.01	0.10
Body Mass Index (BMI) (Kg/m²)	0.133	0.06	−0.08–0.19	0.39
Estimated GFR (ml/min/1.73 m²)	−0.360	0.01	−0.02–0.01	0.04

Legend: 25(OH)D (25-hydroxyvitamin D_3); GFR (Glomerular Filtration Rate estimated by the MDRD simplified formula).

(OV/BV), thickness (O.Th) and surface (OS/BS). The mineralization surface (MS/BS) and bone formation rate (BFR/BS) were also reduced in LN patients. The patients also presented higher eroded surface (ES/BS) and osteoclast surface (Oc.S/BS).

Immunohistochemistry

Immunohistochemistry on patient's bone specimens demonstrated a reduced immunostaining for OPG (0.61±0.82 *vs* 1.08±0.50%, p = 0.003), and an increased expression of RANKL (1.76±0.92 *vs* 0.41±0.28%, p<0.001) when compared to controls (figure 2).

Discussion

Our study show that newly diagnosed lupus nephritis patients presented a reduced bone formation and mineralization, associated with an increased bone resorption. Similar findings have already been related to glucocorticoid-induced bone disease. As previously mentioned, it is not clear the minimum dose and duration of glucocorticoid therapy that could significantly impact bone health. Most histomorphometric studies evaluated patients submitted to glucocorticoids for 6 months to 35 years, with current doses of 5 to 12.5 mg of prednisone [64–66]. Despite a limited time of exposure, our patients received high doses of corticosteroids. Thus, it is not possible to exclude the influence of glucocorticoids on our findings.

Vitamin D insufficiency was observed in all of our patients and might also play a role in the bone metabolism disturbance. Reduced calcitriol levels are thought to impair bone mineralization, by limiting the amount of available calcium and phosphorus, and favor bone resorption, by stimulating PTH synthesis and secretion [67,68]. Moreover, recent studies suggest that 25-hydroxivitamin D levels might also influence osteoblast proliferation and functions (through autocrine pathways) [69–72].

Decreased vitamin D levels in SLE patients have been related to several factors. Ruiz-Irastorza et al shown that photosensitivity [odds ratio (OR) 3.5] and photoprotection (OR 5.7) predicted vitamin D insufficiency and deficiency, respectively [73]. It is noteworthy that our patients were all newly diagnosed, and although some required a short hospitalized time, their blood samples were collected at hospital admission and none of them have been previously guided to avoid sun exposure.

Renal involvement is also related to a higher risk for vitamin D deficiency in SLE patients [42,43]. Chronic kidney disease (CKD) may lead to reduced 1.25-dihydroxyvitamin D3 levels by limiting the amount of 1α hydroxylase or suppressing its action through increased fibroblast growth factor-23 [74]. In our patients, reduced GFR was clearly the result of glomerular acute inflammation and not a CKD condition. On follow-up, six months after diagnosed, LN patients presented an estimated GFR of 81(49–121) ml/min/1,73 m^2 and only one of them was still in haemodialysis, reinforcing that at baseline our patients presented primarily an acute kidney injury related to SLE activity.

Proteinuria may also lead to reduced levels of 25(OH)D due to urinary losses of vitamin D binding proteins [75,76], with recognized implications on bone metabolism [77,78]. Using a study protocol similar to ours, Dias et al from our laboratory previously demonstrated that primary Glomerulopathies (PG) patients [69] presented a reduced bone formation and an enhanced bone resorption. When we compared our LN patients to those PG female patients (with author's permission), we observed that, despite a similar age, BMI, estimated GFR and

Table 4. Flow cytometry of cultured osteoblast: labeling of MCP-1, Osteocalcin and Alkaline Phosphatase of Lupus Nephritis patients and controls.

	Lupus Nephritis (n = 10)	Controls (n = 9)	p
MCP-1 (%)	95.1±2.3	92.9±4.3	0.24
MCP-1 (MFIs)	32.0±9.1	22.9±5.3	0.01
Osteocalcin (%)	12.25±7.13	4.66±3.69	0.007
Osteocalcin (MFIs)	1.77±0.61	1.63±0.50	0.63
Alkaline Phosphatase (%)	49.8±17.2	40.5±15.1	0.22
Alkaline Phosphatase (MFIs)	20.9±12.7	16.3±10.9	0.33

Legend: Results are expressed as mean ± standard deviation. MFIs (mean fluorescence intensities); % (percentage of positive cells).

Table 5. Histomorphometric parameters of LN patients and controls.

	Lupus Nephritis (n = 15)	Controls (n = 15) [62] (n = 29) [63]	p
STRUCTURAL			
BV/TV (%)	26.0±6.8	26.4±5.0	0.98
Tb.Th (μm)	130.7±23.7	122.8±21.2	0.49
Tb.Sp (μm)	390.4±110.9	346.8±63.2	0.42
Tb.N (/mm)	1.99±0.39	2.15±0.32	0.22
FORMATION			
OV/BV (%)	0.19 (0.08–0.38)	1.63 (1.10–2.96)	**<0.001**
Ob.S/BS (%)	0.68 (0.20–2.65)	0.80 (0.20–2.66)	0.69
O.Th (μm)	2.85±1.04	11.4±2.1	**<0.001**
OS/BS (%)	3.6 (2.1–8.9)	8.9 (7.2–16.5)	**0.03**
MINERALIZATION			
MS/BS (%)	2.2±1.6	12.0±5.0	**<0.001**
MAR (μm/day)	0.44±0.23	0.64±0.10	0.41
BFR/BS ($\mu m^3/\mu m^2$/day)	0.01±0.01	0.07±0.03	**<0.001**
MLT (days)	28.8±12.8	23.7±2.7	0.71
RESORPTION			
ES/BS (%)	9.78 (5.02–11.80)	2.00 (1.30–3.30)	**<0.001**
Oc.S/BS (%)	0.54 (0.19–0.69)	0.02 (0–0.10)	**<0.001**

Legend: Results are expressed as mean ± standard deviation, median (25–75 IQR). Trabecular volume (BV/TV) (%); trabecular thickness (Tb.Th) (μm); trabecular separation (Tb.Sp) (μm); trabecular number (Tb.N) (/mm); osteoid volume (OV/BV) (%); osteoblast surface (Ob.S/BS) (%); osteoid thickness (O.Th) (μm); osteoid surface (OS/BS) (%); mineralizing surface (MS/BS) (%); mineral apposition rate (MAR) (μm/day); bone formation rate (BFR/BS) ($\mu m^3/\mu m^2$/day); mineralization lag time (MLT) (days); eroded surface (ES/BS) (%); osteoclast surface (Oc.S/BS) (%).

proteinuria (data not shown), LN patients presented significantly lower 25(OH)D levels (9.9±4.4 *vs* 18.4±11.1 ng/ml, p = 0.04), probably contributing to an increase in PTH levels [73 (29–102) *vs* 19 (10–26) pg/ml, p = 0.003]. These findings support the hypothesis that several factors, besides proteinuria and renal dysfunction, may influence the vitamin D status in SLE.

Finally, despite moderate correlation coefficients, 25(OH)D levels were statistically correlated to all inflammatory mediators studied (IL-6, TNFα, and MCP1). The negative correlation between vitamin D and disease activity has already been demonstrated not only in SLE patients, using SLEDAI and Physicians' Global Assessment indexs [28,79,80], but also in rheumatoid arthritis [81], supporting the potential immune modulatory effects of vitamin D.

Cells obtained from the trabecular bone surfaces of LN patients and controls largely expressed alkaline phosphatase, but presented a low expression of osteocalcin, pointing to characteristics of pre-osteoblast phenotype. Patient's osteoblasts presented a significantly higher expression of MCP-1. Recent studies reiterate a cross-talk between bone cell lineages and resident tissue macrophages, as well as Treg cells [82]. Since urine levels and renal tissue expression of MCP-1 has been extensively related to lupus nephritis activity, we can speculate that resident MCP1 primed bone macrophages could stimulate a MCP1 osteoblast phenotype. This speculation needs experimental confirmation.

Interestingly, it has already been shown that this chemokine is produced by osteoblasts and, in response to RANKL, might be expressed by osteoclast precursors, acting as a recruiter of monocytes and other osteoclast precursors [83–86]. MCP-1 expression has already been detected at sites of tooth eruption, bone metastasis and Rheumatoid Arthritis, being regulated by inflammatory cytokines such as TNF-α and Interleukin (IL)-1b and hormones, such as PTH [84,85,87–90]. Therefore, augmented MCP-1 related to LN activity may help to explain the increase in osteoclast activity and bone resorption detected in our patients.

LN patients presented a reduced immunostaining for OPG and an increased expression of RANKL, suggesting that OPG/RANKL system may be involved in the increased bone resorption observed in these patients. As previously mentioned, the OPG/RANKL system, composed by TNF superfamily members, is a final signaling pathway involved in bone resorption modulation. RANKL is a transmembrane protein produced by osteoblastic lineage cells and activated T cells. Besides immunomodulatory effects, binding of RANKL to its specific receptor RANK stimulates osteoclast formation, fusion, differentiation, activation and survival, leading to enhanced bone resorption and loss. Noteworthy, RANKL expression by the osteoblasts might be up-regulated by several cytokines, as previously mentioned [35,91–93].

On the other hand, OPG acts as a solube inhibitor that prevents RANKL binding with RANK, preventing osteoclast differentiation and activation, and promoting osteoclast apoptosis. The production of OPG by a variety of tissues (such as cardiovascular system, bone and immune cells) is also modulated by various cytokines, hormones and drugs. To notice, glucocorticoids, PTH and basic fibroblast growth factor might suppress OPG expression [92,93].

Our study presents several limitations. First, we studied acute and severely ill patients. In this scenario it is very difficult to isolate the possible influence of each factor involved in the pathogenesis of bone disease. Second, the limited time of disease might have prevented us to observe a significant modification on structural parameters of the bone biopsies. Third, osteoblast proliferation was studied in vitro. This method, although standardized and

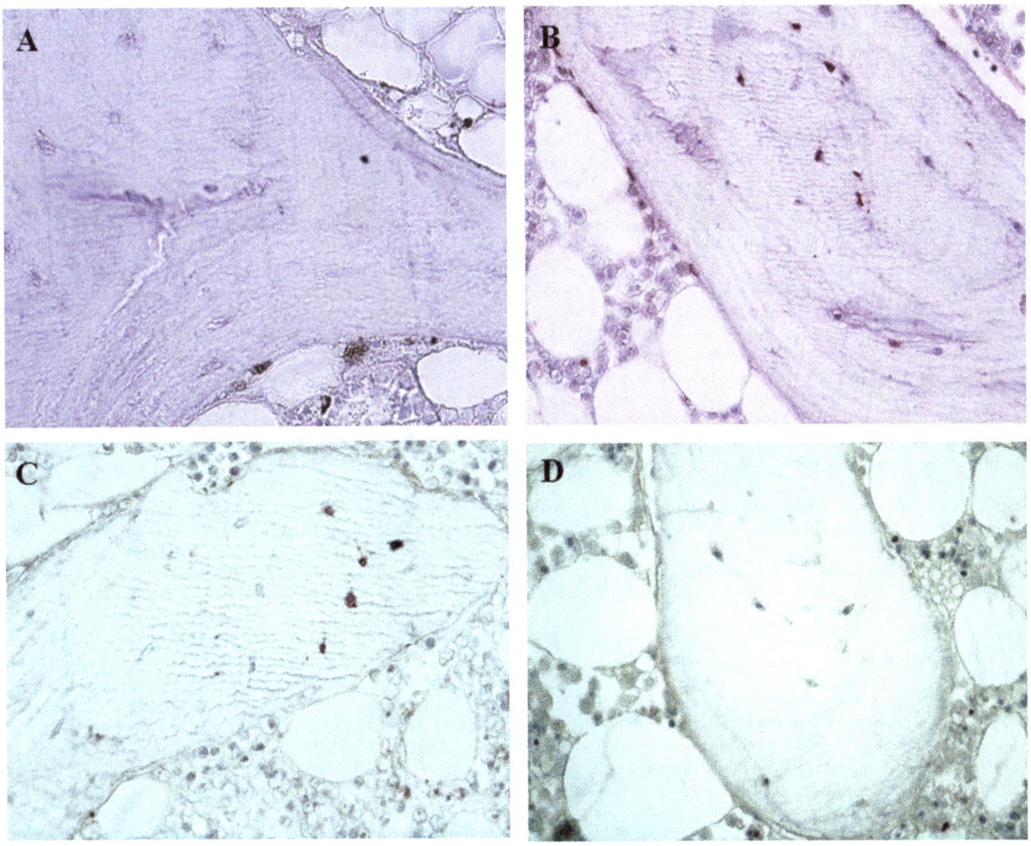

Figure 2. Immunohistochemistry for OPG and RANKL in bone biopsies. Legend: Positive staining appears as brown color (X200). LN patients presented a significantly lower immunostaining for OPG (A) when compared to controls (B). A stronger labeling for RANKL in osteocytes was observed in LN patients (C) when compared to healthy subjects (D).

broadly reproducible, does not reflect local and systemic factors that may influence cell proliferation in vivo.

In conclusion, newly diagnosed lupus nephritis patients present a significant disturbance in bone remodeling, characterized by an impaired bone formation and mineralization, associated with an increase in bone resorption. We believe that glucocorticoid use and vitamin D insufficiency, observed in all of our patients, might have influenced the bone disturbance. Bone tissue showed a reduced immunostaining for OPG and an increased expression of RANKL, suggesting that OPG/RANKL system may be involved in the increased bone resorption. The positive correlation between urinary MCP-1 and serum deoxypyridinoline levels, as well as the increased expression of MCP-1 by cultured bone explants cells suggests that inflammatory background may contribute to bone resorption in LN patients.

Acknowledgments

We thank Wagner Domingues, Fabiana Giorgetti Graciolli and Rita de Cássia Tedeschi Martin for their expert technical assistance.

Author Contributions

Conceived and designed the experiments: ALR LMR VJ VW. Performed the experiments: ALR LMR MRC VJ. Analyzed the data: ALR LMR CBD VW. Contributed reagents/materials/analysis tools: ALR LMR VJ. Wrote the paper: ALR LMR VJ VW.

References

1. Tsokos GC (2011) Systemic lupus erythematosus. N Engl J Med 365: 2110–2121.
2. Bultink IE (2012) Osteoporosis and fractures in systemic lupus erythematosus. Arthritis Care Res (Hoboken) 64: 2–8.
3. Lee C, Ramsey-Goldman R (2005) Osteoporosis in systemic lupus erythematosus mechanisms. Rheum Dis Clin North Am 31: 363–385, viii.
4. Kipen Y, Buchbinder R, Forbes A, Strauss B, Littlejohn G, et al. (1997) Prevalence of reduced bone mineral density in systemic lupus erythematosus and the role of steroids. J Rheumatol 24: 1922–1929.
5. Hansen M, Halberg P, Kollerup G, Pedersen-Zbinden B, Horslev-Petersen K, et al. (1998) Bone metabolism in patients with systemic lupus erythematosus. Effect of disease activity and glucocorticoid treatment. Scand J Rheumatol 27: 197–206.
6. Jardinet D, Lefebvre C, Depresseux G, Lambert M, Devogelaer JP, et al. (2000) Longitudinal analysis of bone mineral density in pre-menopausal female systemic lupus erythematosus patients: deleterious role of glucocorticoid therapy at the lumbar spine. Rheumatology (Oxford) 39: 389–392.
7. Lakshminarayanan S, Walsh S, Mohanraj M, Rothfield N (2001) Factors associated with low bone mineral density in female patients with systemic lupus erythematosus. J Rheumatol 28: 102–108.
8. LoCascio V, Bonucci E, Imbimbo B, Ballanti P, Adami S, et al. (1990) Bone loss in response to long-term glucocorticoid therapy. Bone Miner 8: 39–51.
9. Van Staa TP, Laan RF, Barton IP, Cohen S, Reid DM, et al. (2003) Bone density threshold and other predictors of vertebral fracture in patients receiving oral glucocorticoid therapy. Arthritis Rheum 48: 3224–3229.
10. Seeman E, Delmas PD (2006) Bone quality–the material and structural basis of bone strength and fragility. N Engl J Med 354: 2250–2261.
11. Grossman JM, Gordon R, Ranganath VK, Deal C, Caplan L, et al. (2010) American College of Rheumatology 2010 recommendations for the prevention and treatment of glucocorticoid-induced osteoporosis. Arthritis Care Res (Hoboken) 62: 1515–1526.

12. Foundation NO (2009) National osteoporosis foundation's clinican's guide to the prevention and treatment of osteoporosis.
13. Physicians RCo (2003) Guidelines on the prevention and treatment of glucocorticoid-induced osteoporosis.
14. Weinstein RS (2011) Clinical practice. Glucocorticoid-induced bone disease. N Engl J Med 365: 62–70.
15. Lee C, Almagor O, Dunlop DD, Manzi S, Spies S, et al. (2006) Disease damage and low bone mineral density: an analysis of women with systemic lupus erythematosus ever and never receiving corticosteroids. Rheumatology (Oxford) 45: 53–60.
16. Almehed K, Forsblad d'Elia H, Kvist G, Ohlsson C, Carlsten H (2007) Prevalence and risk factors of osteoporosis in female SLE patients-extended report. Rheumatology (Oxford) 46: 1185–1190.
17. Bultink IE, Lems WF, Kostense PJ, Dijkmans BA, Voskuyl AE (2005) Prevalence of and risk factors for low bone mineral density and vertebral fractures in patients with systemic lupus erythematosus. Arthritis Rheum 52: 2044–2050.
18. Dhillon VB, Davies MC, Hall ML, Round JM, Ell PJ, et al. (1990) Assessment of the effect of oral corticosteroids on bone mineral density in systemic lupus erythematosus: a preliminary study with dual energy x ray absorptiometry. Ann Rheum Dis 49: 624–626.
19. Kalla AA, Fataar AB, Jessop SJ, Bewerunge L (1993) Loss of trabecular bone mineral density in systemic lupus erythematosus. Arthritis Rheum 36: 1726–1734.
20. Formiga F, Moga I, Nolla JM, Pac M, Mitjavila F, et al. (1995) Loss of bone mineral density in premenopausal women with systemic lupus erythematosus. Ann Rheum Dis 54: 274–276.
21. Sels F, Dequeker J, Verwilghen J, Mbuyi-Muamba JM (1996) SLE and osteoporosis: dependence and/or independence on glucocorticoids. Lupus 5: 89–92.
22. Houssiau FA, Lefebvre C, Depresseux G, Lambert M, Devogelaer JP, et al. (1996) Trabecular and cortical bone loss in systemic lupus erythematosus. Br J Rheumatol 35: 244–247.
23. Pacifici R, Rifas L, Teitelbaum S, Slatopolsky E, McCracken R, et al. (1987) Spontaneous release of interleukin 1 from human blood monocytes reflects bone formation in idiopathic osteoporosis. Proc Natl Acad Sci U S A 84: 4616–4620.
24. Mundy GR (2007) Osteoporosis and inflammation. Nutr Rev 65: S147–151.
25. Horton JE, Raisz LG, Simmons HA, Oppenheim JJ, Mergenhagen SE (1972) Bone resorbing activity in supernatant fluid from cultured human peripheral blood leukocytes. Science 177: 793–795.
26. McLean RR (2009) Proinflammatory cytokines and osteoporosis. Curr Osteoporos Rep 7: 134–139.
27. Clowes JA, Riggs BL, Khosla S (2005) The role of the immune system in the pathophysiology of osteoporosis. Immunol Rev 208: 207–227.
28. Borba VZ, Vieira JG, Kasamatsu T, Radominski SC, Sato EI, et al. (2009) Vitamin D deficiency in patients with active systemic lupus erythematosus. Osteoporos Int 20: 427–433.
29. Alele JD, Kamen DL (2010) The importance of inflammation and vitamin D status in SLE-associated osteoporosis. Autoimmun Rev 9: 137–139.
30. Okamoto K, Takayanagi H (2011) Regulation of bone by the adaptive immune system in arthritis. Arthritis Res Ther 13: 219.
31. Ding C, Parameswaran V, Udayan R, Burgess J, Jones G (2008) Circulating levels of inflammatory markers predict change in bone mineral density and resorption in older adults: a longitudinal study. J Clin Endocrinol Metab 93: 1952–1958.
32. Weisinger JR, Alonzo E, Bellorin-Font E, Blasini AM, Rodriguez MA, et al. (1996) Possible role of cytokines on the bone mineral loss in idiopathic hypercalciuria. Kidney Int 49: 244–250.
33. Edwards CJ, Williams E (2010) The role of interleukin-6 in rheumatoid arthritis-associated osteoporosis. Osteoporos Int 21: 1287–1293.
34. Orlic ZC, Turk T, Sincic BM, Stimac D, Cvijanovic O, et al. (2010) How activity of inflammatory bowel disease influences bone loss. J Clin Densitom 13: 36–42.
35. Takayanagi H (2007) Osteoimmunology: shared mechanisms and crosstalk between the immune and bone systems. Nat Rev Immunol 7: 292–304.
36. Rovin BH (2008) The chemokine network in systemic lupus erythematous nephritis. Front Biosci 13: 904–922.
37. Rovin BH, Song H, Birmingham DJ, Hebert LA, Yu CY, et al. (2005) Urine chemokines as biomarkers of human systemic lupus erythematosus activity. J Am Soc Nephrol 16: 467–473.
38. Rovin BH, Zhang X (2009) Biomarkers for lupus nephritis: the quest continues. Clin J Am Soc Nephrol 4: 1858–1865.
39. Kiani AN, Johnson K, Chen C, Diehl E, Hu H, et al. (2009) Urine osteoprotegerin and monocyte chemoattractant protein-1 in lupus nephritis. J Rheumatol 36: 2224–2230.
40. Li Y, Tucci M, Narain S, Barnes EV, Sobel ES, et al. (2006) Urinary biomarkers in lupus nephritis. Autoimmun Rev 5: 383–388.
41. Rosa RF, Takei K, Araujo NC, Loduca SM, Szajubok JC, et al. (2012) Monocyte chemoattractant-1 as a urinary biomarker for the diagnosis of activity of lupus nephritis in Brazilian patients. J Rheumatol 39: 1948–1954.
42. Sumethkul K, Boonyaratavej S, Kitumnuaypong T, Angthararuk S, Cheewasat P, et al. (2013) The predictive factors of low serum 25-hydroxyvitamin D and vitamin D deficiency in patients with systemic lupus erythematosus. Rheumatol Int 33: 1461–1467.
43. Bogaczewicz J, Sysa-Jedrzejowska A, Arkuszewska C, Zabek J, Kontny E, et al. (2012) Vitamin D status in systemic lupus erythematosus patients and its association with selected clinical and laboratory parameters. Lupus 21: 477–484.
44. Sinigaglia L, Varenna M, Binelli L, Zucchi F, Ghiringhella D, et al. (1999) Determinants of bone mass in systemic lupus erythematosus: a cross sectional study on premenopausal women. J Rheumatol 26: 1280–1284.
45. Gilboe IM, Kvien TK, Haugeberg G, Husby G (2000) Bone mineral density in systemic lupus erythematosus: comparison with rheumatoid arthritis and healthy controls. Ann Rheum Dis 59: 110–115.
46. Redlich K, Ziegler S, Kiener HP, Spitzauer S, Stohlawetz P, et al. (2000) Bone mineral density and biochemical parameters of bone metabolism in female patients with systemic lupus erythematosus. Ann Rheum Dis 59: 308–310.
47. Weinstein RS, Wan C, Liu Q, Wang Y, Almeida M, et al. (2010) Endogenous glucocorticoids decrease skeletal angiogenesis, vascularity, hydration, and strength in aged mice. Aging Cell 9: 147–161.
48. Tan EM, Cohen AS, Fries JF, Masi AT, McShane DJ, et al. (1982) The 1982 revised criteria for the classification of systemic lupus erythematosus. Arthritis Rheum 25: 1271–1277.
49. Bombardier C, Gladman DD, Urowitz MB, Caron D, Chang CH (1992) Derivation of the SLEDAI. A disease activity index for lupus patients. The Committee on Prognosis Studies in SLE. Arthritis Rheum 35: 630–640.
50. Weening JJ, D'Agati VD, Schwartz MM, Seshan SV, Alpers CE, et al. (2004) The classification of glomerulonephritis in systemic lupus erythematosus revisited. J Am Soc Nephrol 15: 241–250.
51. Levey AS, Bosch JP, Lewis JB, Greene T, Rogers N, et al. (1999) A more accurate method to estimate glomerular filtration rate from serum creatinine: a new prediction equation. Modification of Diet in Renal Disease Study Group. Ann Intern Med 130: 461–470.
52. Davas EM, Tsirogianni A, Kappou I, Karamitsos D, Economidou I, et al. (1999) Serum IL-6, TNFalpha, p55 srTNFalpha, p75srTNFalpha, srIL-2alpha levels and disease activity in systemic lupus erythematosus. Clin Rheumatol 18: 17–22.
53. Sabry A, Sheashaa H, El-Husseini A, Mahmoud K, Eldahshan KF, et al. (2006) Proinflammatory cytokines (TNF-alpha and IL-6) in Egyptian patients with SLE: its correlation with disease activity. Cytokine 35: 148–153.
54. Chun HY, Chung JW, Kim HA, Yun JM, Jeon JY, et al. (2007) Cytokine IL-6 and IL-10 as biomarkers in systemic lupus erythematosus. J Clin Immunol 27: 461–466.
55. Saraiva GL, Cendoroglo MS, Ramos LR, Araujo LM, Vieira JG, et al. (2005) Influence of ultraviolet radiation on the production of 25 hydroxyvitamin D in the elderly population in the city of Sao Paulo (23 degrees 34'S), Brazil. Osteoporos Int 16: 1649–1654.
56. Unger MD, Cuppari L, Titan SM, Magalhaes MC, Sassaki AL, et al. (2010) Vitamin D status in a sunny country: where has the sun gone? Clin Nutr 29: 784–788.
57. Wergedal JE, Baylink DJ (1984) Characterization of cells isolated and cultured from human bone. Proc Soc Exp Biol Med 176: 60–69.
58. Robey PG, Termine JD (1985) Human bone cells in vitro. Calcif Tissue Int 37: 453–460.
59. Malluche HFM (1986) Methodology of mineralized bone histology. ATLAS of mineralized bone histology. Switzerland: Karger. 17–24.
60. Dempster DW, Compston JE, Drezner MK, Glorieux FH, Kanis JA, et al. (2013) Standardized nomenclature, symbols, and units for bone histomorphometry: a 2012 update of the report of the ASBMR Histomorphometry Nomenclature Committee. J Bone Miner Res 28: 2–17.
61. Gomes SA, dos Reis LM, de Oliveira IB, Noronha IL, Jorgetti V, et al. (2008) Usefulness of a quick decalcification of bone sections embedded in methyl methacrylate[corrected]: an improved method for immunohistochemistry. J Bone Miner Metab 26: 110–113.
62. Dos Reis LM, Batalha JR, Munoz DR, Borelli A, Correa PH, et al. (2007) Brazilian normal static bone histomorphometry: effects of age, sex, and race. J Bone Miner Metab 25: 400–406.
63. Melsen F, Mosekilde L (1978) Tetracycline double-labeling of iliac trabecular bone in 41 normal adults. Calcif Tissue Res 26: 99–102.
64. Dalle Carbonare L, Bertoldo F, Valenti MT, Zenari S, Zanatta M, et al. (2005) Histomorphometric analysis of glucocorticoid-induced osteoporosis. Micron 36: 645–652.
65. Dempster DW (1989) Bone histomorphometry in glucocorticoid-induced osteoporosis. J Bone Miner Res 4: 137–141.
66. Weinstein RS (2012) Glucocorticoid-induced osteoporosis and osteonecrosis. Endocrinol Metab Clin North Am 41: 595–611.
67. Holick MF (2007) Vitamin D deficiency. N Engl J Med 357: 266–281.
68. Holick MFG, Michele (2006) Vitamin D: Photobiology, Metabolism, Mechanism of Action, and Clinical Applications. 2006 American Society for Bone and Mineral Research. 106–114.
69. Dias CB, Dos Reis LM, Caparbo VF, Graciolli FG, Moyses RM, et al. (2007) Decreased in vitro osteoblast proliferation and low turnover bone disease in nonuremic proteinuric patients. Kidney Int 71: 562–568.
70. Atkins GJ, Anderson PH, Findlay DM, Welldon KJ, Vincent C, et al. (2007) Metabolism of vitamin D3 in human osteoblasts: evidence for autocrine and paracrine activities of 1 alpha,25-dihydroxyvitamin D3. Bone 40: 1517–1528.
71. Ormsby RT, Findlay DM, Kogawa M, Anderson PH, Morris HA, et al. (2013) Analysis of vitamin D metabolism gene expression in human bone: Evidence for autocrine control of bone remodelling. J Steroid Biochem Mol Biol.

72. Zhou S, Leboff MS, Waikar SS, Glowacki J (2013) Vitamin D metabolism and action in human marrow stromal cells: effects of chronic kidney disease. J Steroid Biochem Mol Biol 136: 342–344.
73. Ruiz-Irastorza G, Egurbide MV, Olivares N, Martinez-Berriotxoa A, Aguirre C (2008) Vitamin D deficiency in systemic lupus erythematosus: prevalence, predictors and clinical consequences. Rheumatology (Oxford) 47: 920–923.
74. Al-Badr W, Martin KJ (2008) Vitamin D and kidney disease. Clin J Am Soc Nephrol 3: 1555–1560.
75. Khamiseh G, Vaziri ND, Oveisi F, Ahmadnia MR, Ahmadnia L (1991) Vitamin D absorption, plasma concentration and urinary excretion of 25-hydroxyvitamin D in nephrotic syndrome. Proc Soc Exp Biol Med 196: 210–213.
76. Schmidt-Gayk H, Grawunder C, Tschope W, Schmitt W, Ritz E, et al. (1977) 25-hydroxy-vitamin-D in nephrotic syndrome. Lancet 2: 105–108.
77. Malluche HH, Goldstein DA, Massry SG (1979) Osteomalacia and hyperparathyroid bone disease in patients with nephrotic syndrome. J Clin Invest 63: 494–500.
78. Mittal SK, Dash SC, Tiwari SC, Agarwal SK, Saxena S, et al. (1999) Bone histology in patients with nephrotic syndrome and normal renal function. Kidney Int 55: 1912–1919.
79. Abou-Raya A, Abou-Raya S, Helmii M (2013) The effect of vitamin D supplementation on inflammatory and hemostatic markers and disease activity in patients with systemic lupus erythematosus: a randomized placebo-controlled trial. J Rheumatol 40: 265–272.
80. Mok CC, Birmingham DJ, Leung HW, Hebert LA, Song H, et al. (2012) Vitamin D levels in Chinese patients with systemic lupus erythematosus: relationship with disease activity, vascular risk factors and atherosclerosis. Rheumatology (Oxford) 51: 644–652.
81. Cutolo M, Otsa K, Uprus M, Paolino S, Seriolo B (2007) Vitamin D in rheumatoid arthritis. Autoimmun Rev 7: 59–64.
82. Sims NA, Walsh NC (2012) Intercellular cross-talk among bone cells: new factors and pathways. Curr Osteoporos Rep 10: 109–117.
83. Matsuo K, Irie N (2008) Osteoclast-osteoblast communication. Arch Biochem Biophys 473: 201–209.
84. Li X, Qin L, Bergenstock M, Bevelock LM, Novack DV, et al. (2007) Parathyroid hormone stimulates osteoblastic expression of MCP-1 to recruit and increase the fusion of pre/osteoclasts. J Biol Chem 282: 33098–33106.
85. Graves DT, Jiang Y, Valente AJ (1999) The expression of monocyte chemoattractant protein-1 and other chemokines by osteoblasts. Front Biosci 4: D571–580.
86. Kim MS, Magno CL, Day CJ, Morrison NA (2006) Induction of chemokines and chemokine receptors CCR2b and CCR4 in authentic human osteoclasts differentiated with RANKL and osteoclast like cells differentiated by MCP-1 and RANTES. J Cell Biochem 97: 512–518.
87. Koch AE, Kunkel SL, Harlow LA, Johnson B, Evanoff HL, et al. (1992) Enhanced production of monocyte chemoattractant protein-1 in rheumatoid arthritis. J Clin Invest 90: 772–779.
88. Wise GE, Frazier-Bowers S, D'Souza RN (2002) Cellular, molecular, and genetic determinants of tooth eruption. Crit Rev Oral Biol Med 13: 323–334.
89. Lu Y, Cai Z, Xiao G, Keller ET, Mizokami A, et al. (2007) Monocyte chemotactic protein-1 mediates prostate cancer-induced bone resorption. Cancer Res 67: 3646–3653.
90. Aggarwal R, Ghobrial IM, Roodman GD (2006) Chemokines in multiple myeloma. Exp Hematol 34: 1289–1295.
91. Walsh MC, Kim N, Kadono Y, Rho J, Lee SY, et al. (2006) Osteoimmunology: interplay between the immune system and bone metabolism. Annu Rev Immunol 24: 33–63.
92. Caetano-Lopes J, Canhao H, Fonseca JE (2009) Osteoimmunology–the hidden immune regulation of bone. Autoimmun Rev 8: 250–255.
93. Schoppet M, Preissner KT, Hofbauer LC (2002) RANK ligand and osteoprotegerin: paracrine regulators of bone metabolism and vascular function. Arterioscler Thromb Vasc Biol 22: 549–553.

13

Human Parvovirus B19 NS1 Protein Aggravates Liver Injury in NZB/W F1 Mice

Chun-Chou Tsai[1], Chun-Ching Chiu[1,2], Jeng-Dong Hsu[3,4], Huai-Sheng Hsu[1], Bor-Show Tzang[5,6,7]*, Tsai-Ching Hsu[1,7]*

1 Institute of Microbiology and Immunology, Chung Shan Medical University, Taichung, Taiwan, **2** Department of Neurology and Department of Medical Intensive Care Unit, Chunghua Christian Hospital, Chunghua, Taiwan, **3** Department of Pathology, School of Medicine, Chung Shan Medical University, Taichung, Taiwan, **4** Department of Pathology, Chung Shan Medical University Hospital, Taichung, Taiwan, **5** Department of Biochemistry, School of Medicine, Chung Shan Medical University, Taichung, Taiwan, **6** Institute of Biochemistry and Biotechnology, Chung Shan Medical University, Taichung, Taiwan, **7** Clinical Laboratory, Chung Shan Medical University Hospital, Taichung, Taiwan

Abstract

Human parvovirus B19 (B19) has been associated with a variety of diseases. However, the influence of B19 viral proteins on hepatic injury in SLE is still obscure. To elucidate the effects of B19 viral proteins on livers in SLE, recombinant B19 NS1, VP1u or VP2 proteins were injected subcutaneously into NZB/W F1 mice, respectively. Significant expressions of inducible nitric oxide synthase (iNOS) and cyclooxygenase-2 (COX-2) were detected in NZB/W F1 mice receiving B19 NS1 as compared to those mice receiving PBS. Markedly hepatocyte disarray and lymphocyte infiltration were observed in livers from NZB/WF 1 mice receiving B19 NS1 as compared to those mice receiving PBS. Additionally, significant increases of Tumor Necrosis Factor −α (TNF-α), TNF-α receptor, IκB kinase −α (IKK-α), nuclear factor of kappa light polypeptide gene enhancer in B-cells inhibitor (IκB) and nuclear factor-kappa B (NF-κB) were detected in livers from NZB/W F1 mice receiving B19 NS1 as compared to those mice receiving PBS. Accordingly, significant increases of matrix metalloproteinase-9 (MMP9) and U-plasminogen activator (uPA) were also detected in livers from NZB/W F1 mice receiving B19 NS1 as compared to those mice receiving PBS. Contrarily, no significant variation on livers from NZB/W F1 mice receiving B19 VP1u or VP2 was observed as compared to those mice receiving PBS. These findings firstly demonstrated the aggravated effects of B19 NS1 but not VP1u or VP2 protein on hepatic injury and provide a clue in understanding the role of B19 NS1 on hepatic injury in SLE.

Editor: John A. Chiorini, National Institute of Dental and Craniofacial Research, United States of America

Funding: This study was supported by NSC 97-2314-B040-009, NSC 98–2314-B-040-008-MY3, and NSC 101-2314-B-040-008 from the National Science Council, Taiwan, Republic of China. Upright optical microscope, chemiluminescence imaging analyzer and gel digital imaging analyzer from the Instrument center of Chung Shan Medical University were utilized in this study, which is partly supported by National Science Council, Ministry of Education and Chung Shan Medical University. The funders had no role in study design, data collection and analysis, decision to publish, or preparation of the manuscript.

Competing Interests: The authors have declared that no competing interests exist.

* E-mail: bstzang@csmu.edu.tw (BST); htc@csmu.edu.tw (TCH)

Introduction

Systematic lupus erythematosus (SLE) is known as a systemic autoimmune disorder that affects various organs including liver [1]. Various reports have indicated that growing population with liver disease was found in patients with SLE [2–4]. Although the occurrence of liver disease is not routinely screened, the incidence of hepatic abnormality in patients with SLE was reported as varying from 12% to 55% [4].

Human parvovirus B19 (B19) is known as an important human pathogen, which consists a nonstructural protein (NS1) and two capsid proteins, VP1 and VP2 [5]. Notably, B19 infection has been associated with a wide range of different pathologies and clinical manifestations including erythema infectiosum, arthropathy, thrombocytopenia, neurologic disorders, hepatitis, cardiovasculitis and autoimmune disorders [5–8]. Indeed, various studies have postulated a connection between B19 infection and liver injury. A clinical study reported the existence of B19 DNA in a liver biopsy specimen from a patient with acute hepatitis [9]. Another studies also suggested an important role of B19 infection in acute icteric hepatitis liver injury [10] and acute fulminant hepatitis with bone marrow failure [11]. In addition, B19 infection has been recognized to trigger the acute liver failure in a patient with Wilson disease [12].

Although there is no direct evidence of B19 virus in inducing autoimmune diseases, the association between B19 virus and pathogenesis of autoimmunity has been strongly suggested. Recently, human parvovirus B19 has been associated with SLE [6,13–16]. However, little is known about the influence of B19 viral proteins on liver injury in SLE. In the present study, various recombinant B19 viral proteins were prepared and injected subcutaneously into NZB/W F1 mice to elucidate the effects of B19 viral proteins on livers in SLE.

Materials and Methods

Ethics

Animal experiments were approved by the Institutional Animal Care and Use Committee at Chung Shan Medical University.

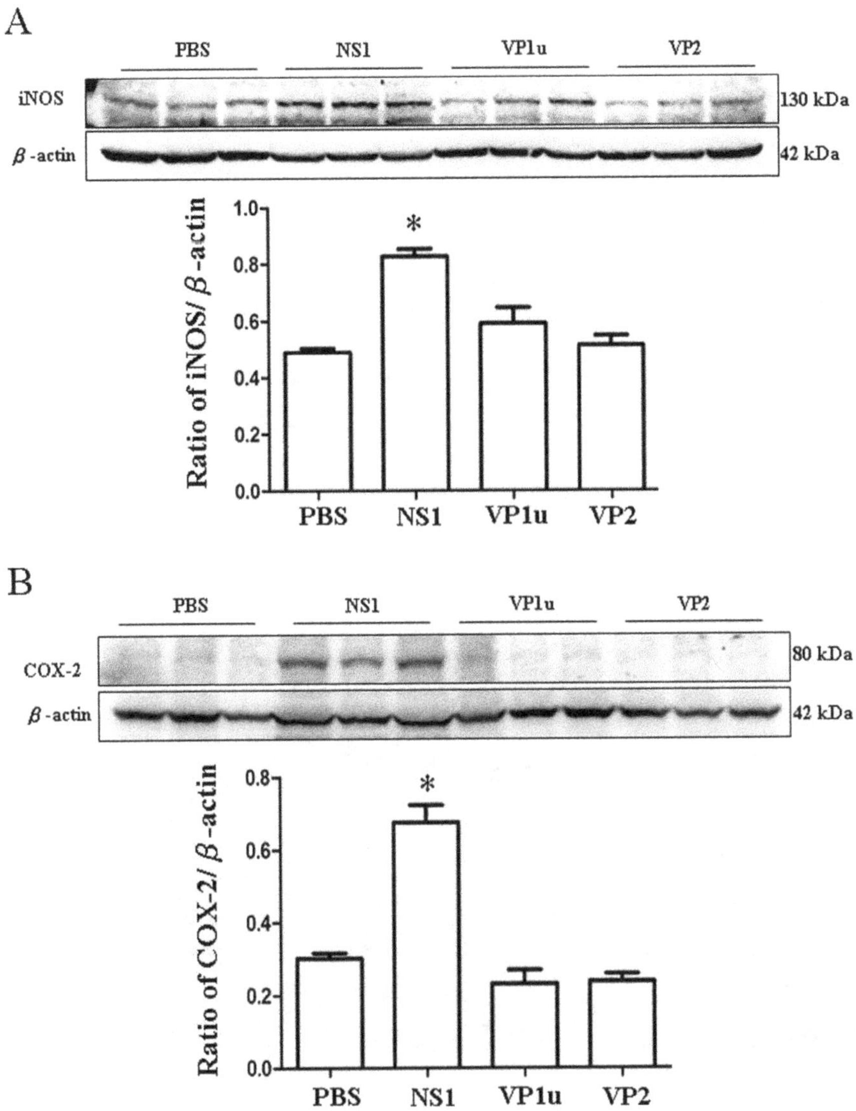

Figure 1. Expression of iNOS and COX-2. Liver lysates obtained from the NZB/W F1 mice receiving PBS, NS1, VP1u or VP2 were probed with antibodies against (A) iNOS and (B) COX-2. Bars represent the relative protein quantification of (A) iNOS and (B) COX-2 on the basis of β-actin. Similar results were observed in three independent experiments, and * indicates the significant difference, $P<0.05$.

Preparation of Recombinant B19 Viral Proteins

The recombinant human parvovirus B19 proteins were prepared as descried elsewhere [17–19]. Briefly, the plasmid pQE40-NS1 containing nonstructural (NS1) gene of human parvovirus B19 was kindly provided by Professor Susanne Modrow, Institute for Medical Microbiology, Universität Regensburg, Regensburg, Germany. The NS1 protein was purified using Profinia denaturing IMAC purification kits and the Profinia protein purification system (Bio-Rad Laboratories, Inc. USA) according to the manufacturer's instructions [17]. The cDNA of B19 VP1u were constructed onto pET-32a plasmid and transformed into E. coli (BL21-DE3). The recombinant B19 VP1u protein were then purified by Ni-NTA spin column (Qiagen, Chatsworth, CA) and spun through P50 and P30 Amicon (Millipore Billerica, MA) to avoid contaminative and degraded proteins [18]. The purified recombinant B19 NS1 and VP1u proteins were also analyzed by HPLC and the purities the three purified recombinant proteins were over 98%. The VP2 open reading frame (ORF) was obtained from the B19 genome (plasmid pYT104-C) by polymerase chain reaction using primers 5′-CGGAATTCCATGACTTCAGTTAATTCTGCA-GAAGCC-3′ and 5′-GCGCGG CCGCTTACAATGGGTGCA-CACGGC-3′ containing *EcoR I* and *Not I* recognition sequences for subsequent cloning to pVL1393 baculoviral transfer vectors (Invitrogen). The constructed transfer vector and the BaculoGold DNA were used to co-transfect *Spodoptera frugiperda* (Sf9) cells by the calcium phosphate coprecipitation method according to the protocol provided by the manufacturer (PharMingen, San Diego, CA). Sf9 cells (Novagen, Merck, Germany) were maintained in Sf-900 II SFM (Invitogen) in 100% room air at 28°C. Sf9 cells were infected with baculovirus stocks at a multiplicity of infection (MOI) of 5 and were harvested 72 h after infection. Recombinant VP2 proteins were purified by using 20% sucrose cushion and CsCl density gradient as described else where [19]. The yields of purified recombinant B19-NS1, -VP1u and VP2 proteins are 6.1, 15.6 and 17.7 mg/l, and the purities are nearly 96.8%, 98.1% and

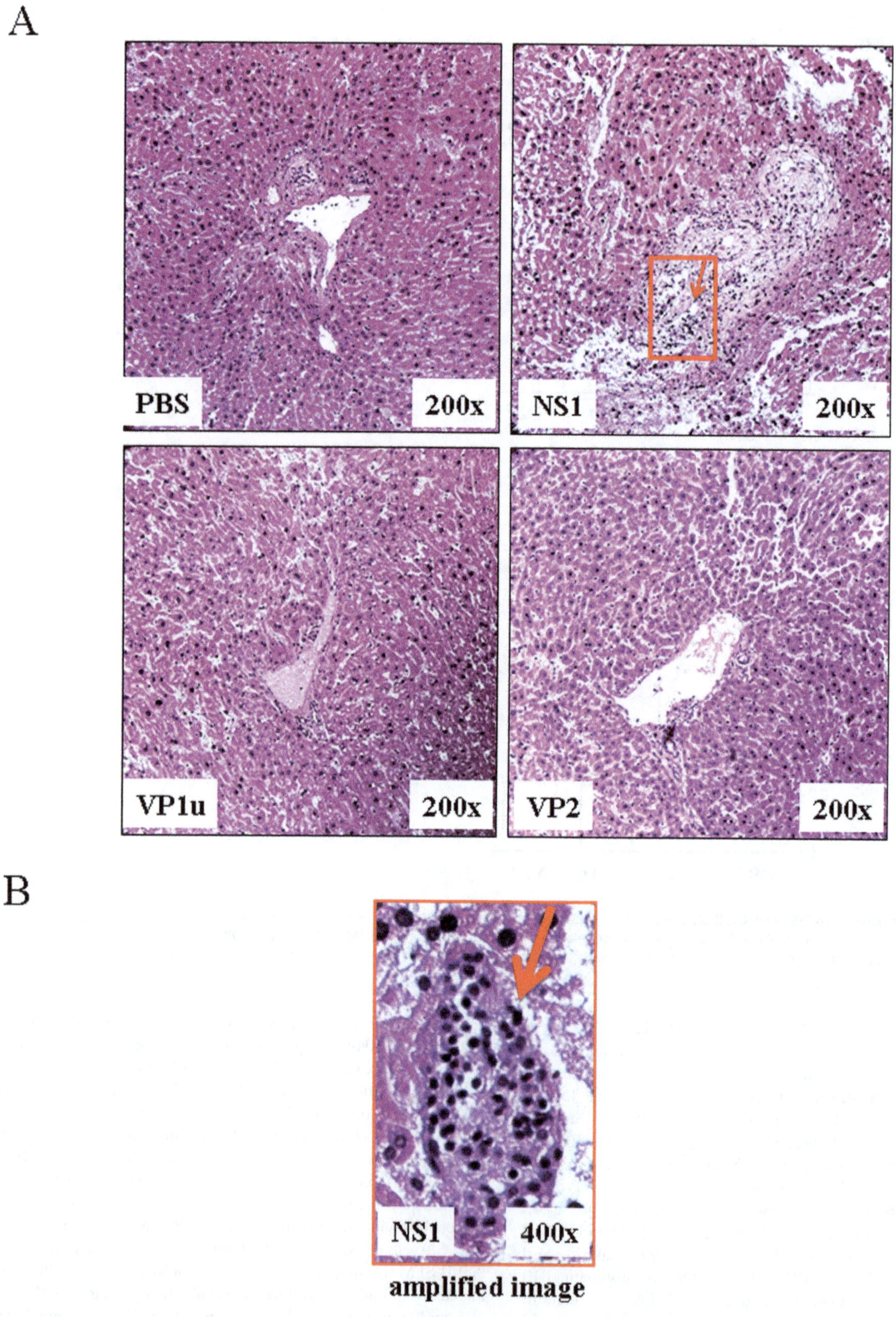

Figure 2. Hepatic histopathological changes in NZB/W F1 mice. (A) Histopathological analysis of hepatic tissue sections with hematoxylin and eosin staining from NZB/W F1 mice receiving PBS, NS1, VP1u or VP2, respectively. These images of hepatic architecture were magnified by 200 times. (B) Amplified image of hepatic tissue sections with hematoxylin and eosin staining from NZB/W F1 mice receiving B19-NS1. The lymphocyte infiltration was indicated by an arrow.

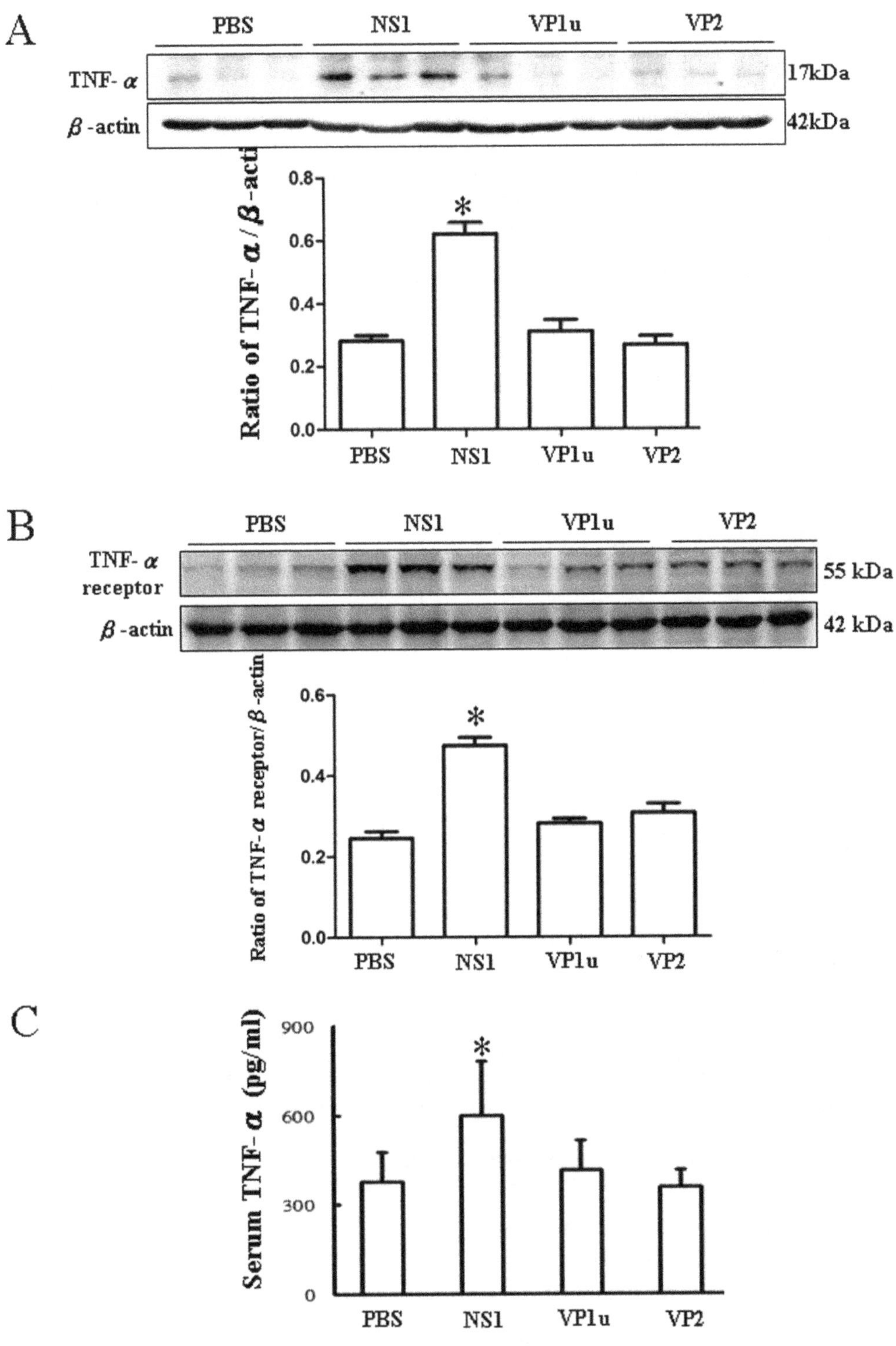

Figure 3. Expression of TNF-α and TNF-α receptor. Liver lysates obtained from the NZB/W F1 mice receiving PBS, NS1, VP1u or VP2 were probed with antibodies against (A) TNF-α and (B) TNF-α receptor. Bars represent the relative protein quantification of (A) TNF-α and (B) TNF-α receptor on the basis of β-actin. (C) Serum TNF-αwas determined with ELISA kit as described in materials and methods (S1). Similar results were observed in three independent experiments, and * indicates the significant difference, $P<0.05$.

97.8%, respectively. Eluted fractions were analyzed by immunoblotting (Figure S1). The endotoxin levels were measured and found to be below the detection limit (0.25 endotoxin unit (EU)/ml) for purified recombinant proteins at the concentration used in the activation assays (Table S1).

Animal and Treatments

Twenty-four female NZB/W F1 mice at week 6 were purchased from Jackson Laboratories (Bar Harbor, ME, USA) and housed under supervision of the Institutional Animal Care and Use Committee at Chung Shan Medical University, Taichung,

Taiwan. The animals were kept under a 12-h light-dark cycle and ambient temperature was maintained at 25°C. Animals were free access to water and standard laboratory chow (Lab Diet 5001; PMI Nutrition International Inc., Brentwood, MO, USA). Animal welfare and experimental procedures were performed according to the NIH Guide for the Care and Use of Laboratory Animals. All the animals at the age of 8 weeks were randomly divided into 4 equal groups (6 mice each group) and injected subcutaneously with 20 ug purified B19-NS1, B19-VP1u, B19-VP2 recombinant proteins or phosphate-buffered saline (PBS) mixed 1:1 (v/v) with Freund's complete adjuvant (Sigma-Aldrich, UK), respectively. The mice were boosted with the same dose mixed 1:1 (v/v) with Freund's incomplete adjuvant (Sigma-Aldrich, UK) twice a week for 3 times and then sacrificed at the age of 16 weeks by CO_2 asphyxiation. The heart blood and liver tissues were collected and stored at −80°C until use. The reactivity of anti-sera to dsDNA and B19 viral proteins was examined (Table S2).

ELISA

Direct antigen-specific ELISA kits were used to detect mouse anti-dsDNA total Ig antibodies (Alpha Diagnostic Intl. Inc., TX, USA) according to the manufacture's description. All serum samples were assayed at a dilution of 1/100. After incubation at room temperature for 60 minutes, liquid of each sample well was removed and washed for four times, and subsequently incubated with anti-mouse Ig-horseradish peroxidase conjugated with HRP at a dilution of 1/100. After incubation at room temperature for 30 min, liquid of each sample well was removed, washed and subsequently incubated with the color reaction TMB Chromogen in the dark for 15 min at room temperature. The 100 μl of stop solution was then added to each well and the absorbance (OD) was

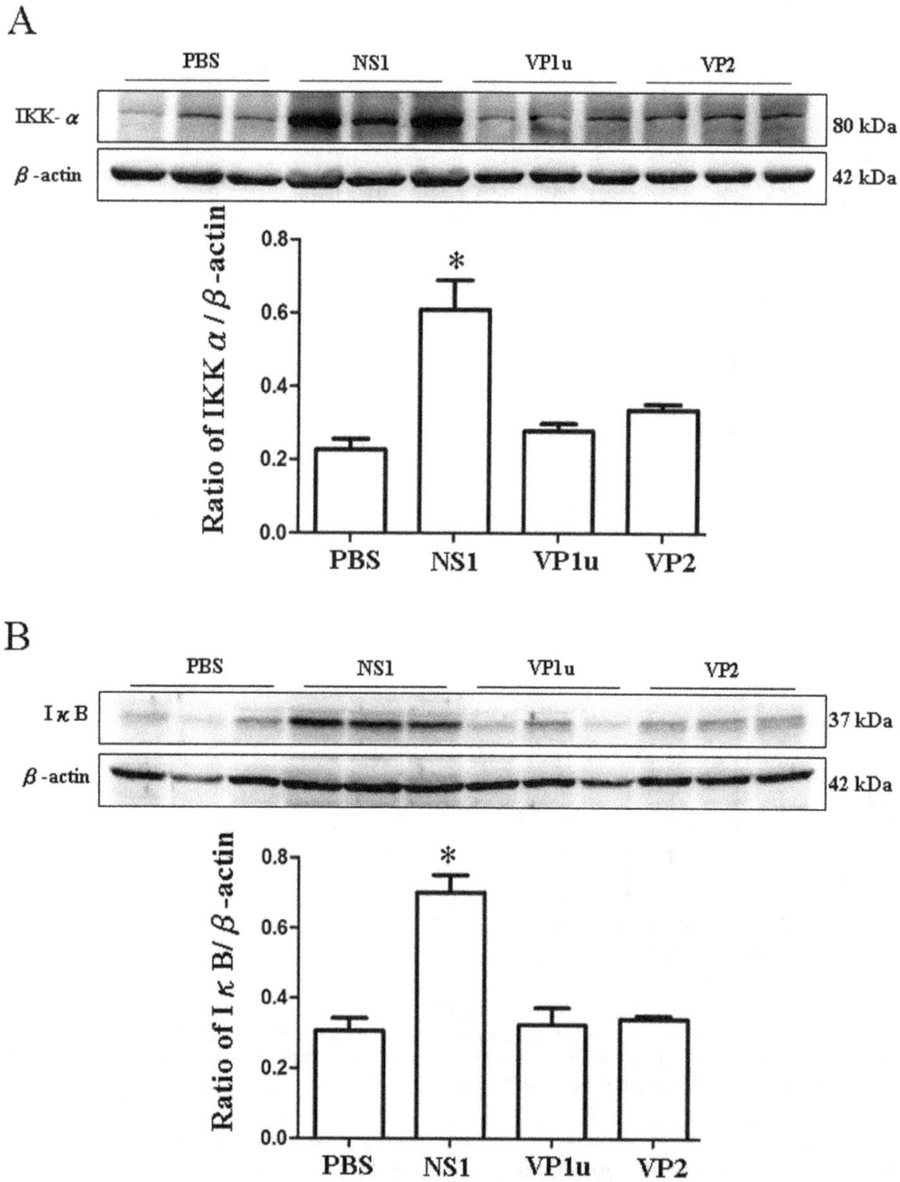

Figure 4. Expression of IKK-α and IκB. Liver lysates obtained from the NZB/W F1 mice receiving PBS, NS1, VP1u or VP2 were probed with antibodies against (A) IKK-α and (B) IκB. Bars represent the relative protein quantification of (A) IKK-α and (B) IκB on the basis of β-actin. Similar results were observed in three independent experiments, and * indicates the significant difference, $P<0.05$.

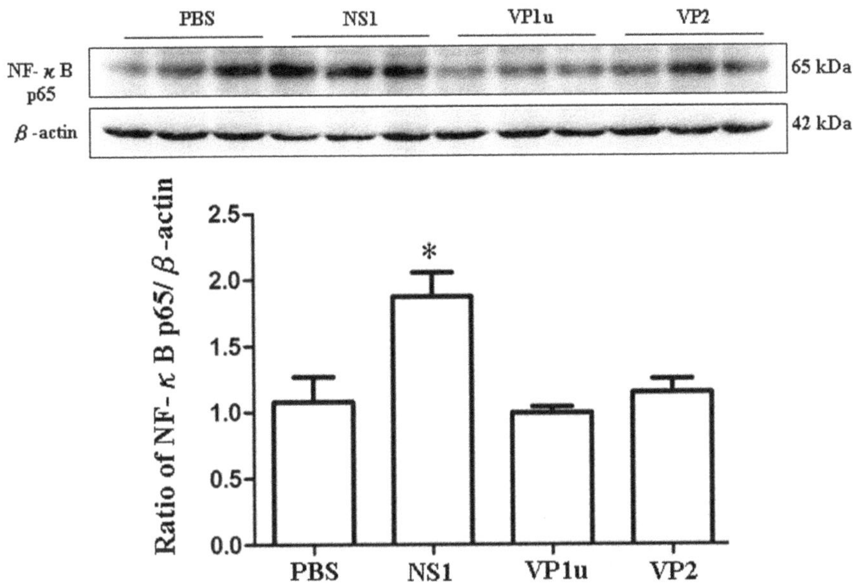

Figure 5. Expression of NF-κB p65. Liver lysates obtained from the NZB/W F1 mice receiving PBS, NS1, VP1u or VP2 were probed with antibodies against NF-κB p65 Bars represent the relative protein quantification of NF-κB p65 on the basis of β-actin. Similar results were observed in three independent experiments, and * indicates the significant difference, $P<0.05$.

read at 450 nm within 1 h. For detecting the reactivity of various anti-sera against B19-NS1, VP1u and VP2, 10 mmol/l of recombinant proteins were immobilized on the surface of each sample well of 96-well plates. All anti-sera were assayed at a dilution of 1/1000. The peroxidase conjugated goat anti-mouse IgG (Sigma, Saint Louis Mo, USA) was assayed at a dilution of 1/1000. The color reaction was done with 1 mg/ml substrate ABTs [2, 2'azino-di-(3- ethylbenzthiazolin-6-sulphonic acid)] (Sigma) in the presence of 0.005% H_2O_2 at room temperature for 15 min.

Hematoxylin-eosin Staining

The liver samples of animals were excised and soaked in formalin and covered with wax. Slides were prepared by deparaffinization and dehydration. They were passed through a series of graded alcohols (100%, 95% and 75%), 15 min of each. The slides were then dyed with hematoxylin. After gently rinsing with water, each slide was then soaked with 85% alcohol, 100% alcohol I and II for 15 min each. At the end, they were soaked with Xylene I and Xylene II. Photomicrographs were obtained using Zeiss Axiophot microscopes.

Preparation of Tissue Extract and Determination of Protein

All procedures were performed at 4°C in a cold room. The tissue samples obtained from NZB/W F1 mice were homogenized in 600 µl PRO-PREP™ solution (iNtRON Biotech, Korea) by 30 strokes using a Dounce Homogenizer (Knotes Glass, Vineland, NJ). The homogenates were centrifuged at 13,000 rpm for 10 min at 4°C and the supernatant was then stored at −80°C until use. Protein concentration of tissue extracts was determined according to the method described elsewhere [20] using bovine serum albumin as standards.

Immunoblotting

Protein samples were separated in 10% or 12.5% SDS-PAGE and electrophoretically transferred to nitrocellulose membrane (Amersham Biosciences, Piscataway, NJ, USA) described elsewhere [21]. After blocking with 5% non-fat dry milk in (PBS), antibodies against TNF-α receptor, TNF-α, iNOS, COX-2, MMP-9, uPA, IKK-α, IκB, NF-κB (p65) (Santa Cruz Biotechnology, CA, USA) and β-actin (Upstates, Charlottesville, VA, USA) were diluted in PBS with 2.5% BSA and incubated for 1.5 h with gentle agitation at room temperature. The membranes were washed twice with PBS-Tween for 1 h and secondary antibody conjugated with horseradish peroxidase (HRP) (Santa Cruz Biotechnology, Santa Cruz, CA, USA) was added. Pierce's Supersignal West Dura HRP Detection Kit (Pierce Biotechnology Inc., Rockford, IL) was used to detect antigen–antibody complexes. Quantified results were performed by densitometry (Appraise, Beckman-Coulter, Brea, CA, USA).

Statistical Analysis

All of the statistical analyses were performed using SPSS 10.0 software (SPSS Inc., Chicago, IL). Three independent experiments were repeated. Statistical analyses were performed using the analysis of variance plus posterior multiple comparison test to test the difference. $P<0.05$ was considered statistically significant. The significant differences were stressed with symbols as shown in figures.

Results

Increased Expression of iNOS and COX-2 Proteins in NZB/W F1 Mice Receiving B19-NS1 Protein

Human parvovirus B19 has been strongly associated with the pathogenesis of SLE. To investigate the influences of B19 viral proteins on livers in SLE, various inflammatory associated proteins including iNOS and COX-2 were examined. Significantly increased iNOS protein level was detected in livers from NZB/W F1 mice receiving B19-NS1 as compared to those mice receiving PBS (Fig. 1A). In contrast, no significant variation on iNOS expression in livers from NZB/W F1 receiving B19-VP1u or VP2 was observed as compared to those mice receiving PBS (Fig. 1A). Additionally, significant increase of COX-2 protein was

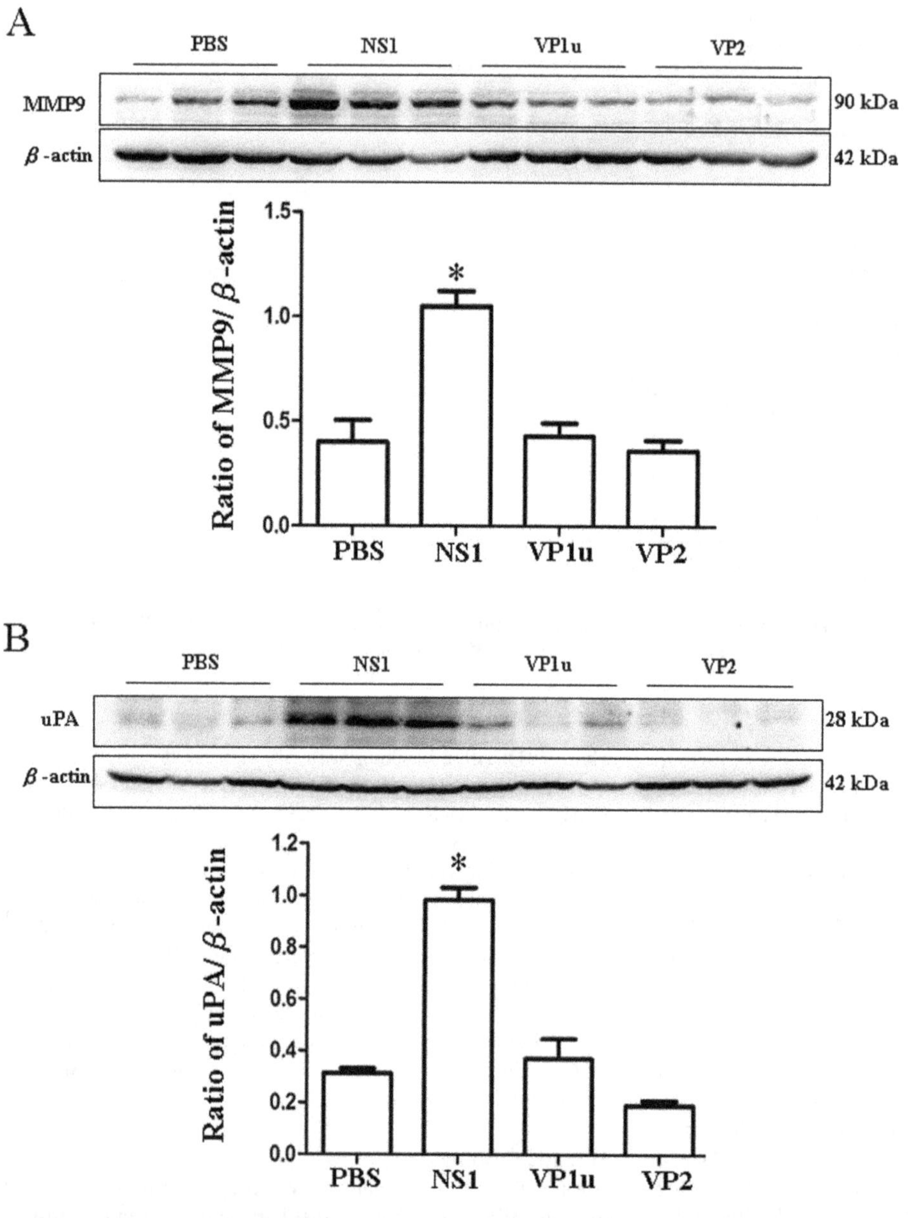

Figure 6. Expression of MMP9 and uPA. Liver lysates obtained from the NZB/W F1 mice receiving PBS, NS1, VP1u or VP2 were probed with antibodies against (A) MMP9 and (B) uPA. Bars represent the relative protein quantification of (A) MMP9 and (B) uPA on the basis of β-actin. Similar results were observed in three independent experiments, and * indicates the significant difference, $P<0.05$.

also detected in livers from NZB/W F1 mice receiving B19-NS1 whereas no significant variation on COX-2 expression in livers from NZB/W F1 receiving B19-VP1u or VP2 was observed as compared to those mice receiving PBS (Fig. 1B). Quantified results were shown in the lower panel of figure 1A and 1B.

Hepatic Architecture Changes in NZB/W F1 Mice Receiving B19-NS1 Protein

To observe the effects of B19-NS1 protein on hepatic architectures in NZB/W F1 mice, we performed a histopathological analysis on liver tissue stained with hematoxylin and eosin (Fig. 2). More abnormal hepatic architecture and increased interstitial space were observed in livers from NZB/W F1 mice receiving B19-NS1 as compared to those mice receiving PBS, B19-VP1u or VP2, respectively (Fig. 2A). Additionally, markedly lymphocyte infiltration was observed in livers from NZB/W F1 mice receiving B19-NS1 protein as compared to those mice from other groups (Fig. 2B).

Increased Expression of TNF-α and TNF-α Receptor in NZB/W F1 Mice Receiving B19-NS1 Protein

To clarify the possible signaling involved in the B19-NS1 aggravated liver injury in NZB/W F1 mice, the expressions of TNF-α and TNF-α receptor were examined. Significant increase of TNF-α was detected in livers from NZB/W F1 mice receiving B19-NS1 as compared to those mice receiving PBS (Fig. 3A). Consequently, significant increase of TNF-α receptor was also detected in livers from NZB/W F1 mice receiving B19-NS1 as compared to those mice receiving PBS (Fig. 3B). In contrast, no significant variation on both TNF-α and TNF-α receptor

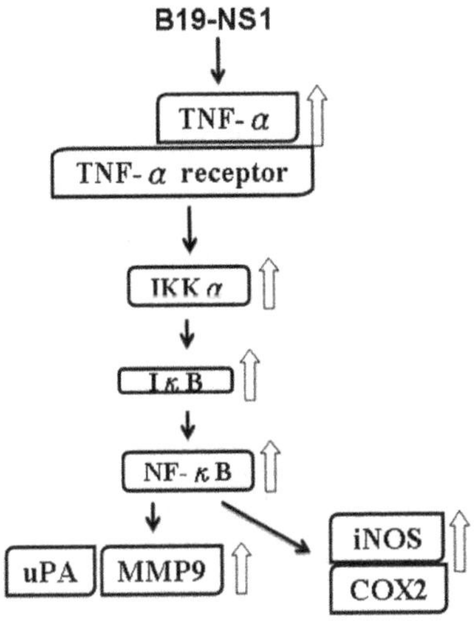

Figure 7. Schematic illustration of the molecular mechanisms involved in the B19 NS1-induced hepatic inflammation in NZB/W F1 mice. B19-NS1 increases the expression of TNF-α and its receptor, which elicit late activation of IKK-αand IκB. Consequently, NF-κB is also activated to induce the expressions of inflammatory associated molecules, uPA and MMP9. The other downstream inflammatory-realted molecules of TNF-α, including iNOS and COX, are also markedly indued.

expression were observed in livers from NZB/W F1 mice receiving B19-VP1u or VP2 as compared to those mice receiving PBS (Fig. 3A and 3B). Meanwhile, significantly increased serum TNF-α level was also detected in NZB/W F1 mice receiving B19-NS1 as compared to those mice receiving PBS (Fig. 3C). Quantified results were shown in the lower panels of figure 3A and 3B.

Increased Expression of IKK-α, IκB and NF-κB (p65) in NZB/W F1 Mice Receiving B19-NS1 Protein

To further investigate the signaling molecules involved in the B19-NS1 enhanced TNF-α expression, the downstream molecules of TNF-α including IKK-α, IκB, NF-κB (p65) were examined. Significant increases of IKK-αand IκB were detected in livers from NZB/W F1 mice receiving B19-NS1 as compared to those mice receiving PBS (Fig. 4A and 4B). In contrast, no significant variation on IKK-αand IκB expression were observed in livers from NZB/W F1 mice receiving B19-VP1u or VP2 as compared to those mice receiving PBS (Fig. 4A and 4B). Quantified results were shown in the lower panels of figure 4A and 4B. Moreover, significant increase of NF-κB (p65) was also detected in livers from NZB/W F1 mice receiving B19-NS1 as compared to those mice receiving PBS whereas no significant variation on NF-κB (p65) level was observed in NZB/W F1 mice receiving B19-VP1 u or VP2 as compared to those mice receiving PBS (Fig. 5). Quantified results were shown in the lower panel of figure 5.

Increased MMP-9 and uPA Expression in NZB/W F1 Mice Receiving B19-NS1 Protein

MMP-9, a consequent molecules in TNF-α signaling, is known as an indicator playing important roles in hepatic disorders. To further examine the effect of B19-NS1 protein on MMP-9 expression, Immunoblots were preformed to examine the expression of MMP-9. Significant increase of MMP-9 was detected in livers from NZB/W F1 mice receiving B19-NS1 as compared to those mice receiving PBS (Fig. 6A). Additionally, the expression of uPA protein, an upstream activator of MMP-9, was also examined. As shown in figure 6B, significant increase of uPA protein was observed in liver from NZB/W F1 mice receiving B19-NS1 as compared to those mice receiving PBS (Fig. 6B). In contrast, no significant variation on both MMP9 and uPA expression were observed in livers from NZB/W F1 mice receiving B19-VP1u or VP2 as compared to those mice receiving PBS (Fig. 6A and 6B). Quantified results were shown in the lower panels of figure 6A and 6B.

Discussion

Although B19 infection has been implicated in pathogenesis of liver diseases and development of SLE, the effects of B19 and its viral proteins including NS1, VP1u and VP2 on hepatic injury in SLE is still obscure [6,9–16]. In the present study, we revealed the aggravated effects of B19 NS1 protein on hepatic injury in NZB/W F1 mice by significantly enhancing the expressions of iNOS and COX-2 proteins and lymphocyte infiltration. Additionally, significant increase of MMP-9 through TNF-α/NF-κB (p65) signaling was also detected.

Elevated inducible nitric oxide synthase (iNOS) has been reported in patients with SLE [22]. According to a recent clinical research of 72 SLE patients, significant higher oxidative stress including iNOS level has been associated with the SLE Disease Activity Index (SLEDAI) and recognized to the pathogenesis of SLE [23]. Similar result was also observed in lupus-prone mice [24]. Accordingly, cyclooxygenase type 2 (COX-2) is also known to play pivotal roles in development of inflammatory diseases and associated with the pathogenesis of SLE [25–26]. A previous study has demonstrated that some COX-2 inhibitors are able to suppress the production of pathogenic autoantibodies to DNA by causing autoimmune T-cell apoptosis [27]. Similar result was also demonstrated in a lupus-prone murine model [28]. These studies did stress the roles of iNOS and COX-2 in development of SLE.

In the current study, significant increases of iNOS and COX-2 expression were detected in livers from NZB/W F1 mice receiving B19-NS1 but not VP1u or VP2 as compared to those mice receiving PBS. By the way, markedly lymphocyte infiltration was observed in NZB/W F1 mice receiving B19-NS1. These findings suggested the effect of B19-NS1 but not VP1u or VP2 on aggravating the hepatic injury in SLE by enhancing the expression of iNOS and COX-2.

Matrix metalloproteinase-9 (MMP-9) has been postulated with the pathogenesis of autoimmune diseases including SLE [29]. Various studies have reported that elevated MMP-9 activity plays crucial role in development of SLE in both human and lupus-prone mice [30–31]. Indeed, the cleavage of myelin basic protein or type II gelatins by MMP-9 will generate remnant epitopes and contribute to develop autoimmunity [32]. Additionally, TNF-α is known to be involved in the signal pathway of MMP-9 induction, which degrades extracellular matrix in the inflammatory responses [33]. Accordingly, IKK and IKB, the downstream molecules for TNF-α induced MMP-9 expression, are known to be activated prior to the transcription of MMP-9 promoter through NF-κB sites [34–35]. Consistently, our experimental results revealed that B19-NS1 aggravatedly induces the expression of MMP-9 in livers of NZB/W F1 mice via TNF-α signaling, which also elicits the activation of IKK-α, IκB and NF-κB (Fig. 7).

B19 NS1 is known as a cytotoxic protein with multi-function. Besides the ATPase and DNA helicase activity [36], B19 NS1 protein has been described as a transactivator of the viral p6- as well as a variety of cellular promoters. These include the promoter region controlling the expression of TNF-α and IL-6 genes [37–

38]. Elevated levels of TNF-α have been shown to be present in patients during the acute and convalescent phases of B19 infection [39]. The prolonged or continuous presence of these proinflammatory cytokines during acute-convalescent and persistent B19 infection, respectively, may result in the induction of long lasting clinical symptoms and autoimmune reactions [6]. Although causality is often difficult to conclude, these studies did imply that B19 NS1 is possibly involved in the induction of autoimmunity and can't be negated [6,39]. Briefly, NZB/W F1 is a well known spontaneously lupus mice model [40], which has been used for investigating SLE for several decades.

Therefore, we simply intend to clarify the influences of B19 NS1 proteins in NZB/W F1 mice and firstly report the aggravated effects of B19 NS1 on liver injury in NZB/W F1 mice. Since B19-infection is commonly detected in patients with SLE [41], these findings may provide a possible explanation on the effects of B19 NS1 in SLE patients with B19-infection.

Supporting Information

Figure S1 SDS-PAGE (A) and Immunoblottings (B) of purified recombinant B19-NS1 (77 kDa), -VP1u (47 kDa) and -VP2 (58 kDa) proteins probed with rabbit anti-B19-NS1 IgG, rabbit anti-B19 VP1u IgG and mouse anti-B19-VP2 IgG, respectively.

Table S1 Endotoxin assay for different preparations of B19 viral proteins.

Table S1 Reactivity of anti-sera to dsDNA and B19 viral proteins.

Acknowledgments

Upright optical microscope, chemiluminescence imaging analyzer and gel digital imaging analyzer from the Instrument center of Chung Shan Medical University were utilized in this study, which is partly supported by National Science Council, Ministry of Education and Chung Shan Medical University.

Author Contributions

Conceived and designed the experiments: BST TCH. Performed the experiments: CCT CCC HSH TCH. Analyzed the data: CCT CCC JDH HSH BST TCH. Contributed reagents/materials/analysis tools: BST TCH JDH. Wrote the paper: BST TCH.

References

1. Hahn BH (1993) An overview of the pathogenesis of systemic lupus erythematosus. In: Wallace DJ, Hahn BH, editors. Dubois' lupus erythematosus. Philadelphia: Williams and Wilkins. 69–76.
2. Mackay IK, Taft LI, Cowling DC (1959) Lupoid hepatitis and the hepatic lesions of SLE. Lancet 5: 65–69.
3. Runyon, LaBrecque DR, Anuras S (1980) The spectrumof liver disease in systemic lupus erythematosus. Report of 33 histologically-proved cases and review of the literature. Am J Med 69: 187–194.
4. Abraham S, Begum S, Isenberg D (2004) Hepatic manifestations of autoimmune rheumatic diseases. Ann Rheum Dis 63: 123–129.
5. Young NS, Brown KE (2004) Parvovirus B19. N Engl J Med 350: 586–597.
6. Lehmann HW, Modrow S (2003) Parvovirus B19 infection and autoimmune disease. Autoimmun Rev 2: 218–223.
7. Bock CT, Klingel K, Aberle S, Duechting A, Lupescu A, et al. (2005) Human parvovirus B19. A new emerging pathogen of inflammatory cardiomyopathy. J. Vet. Med. B: Infect. Dis. Vet. Public Health 52: 340–343.
8. Servant-Delmas A, Lefrère JJ, Morinet F, Pillet S (2010) Advances in human B19 erythrovirus biology. J Virol 84: 9658–9665.
9. Hatakka A, Klein J, He R, Piper J, Tam E, et al. (2011) Acute hepatitis as a manifestation of parvovirus B19 infection. J Clin Microbiol 49: 3422–3424.
10. Sun L, Zhang JC, Jia ZS (2011). Association of parvovirus B19 infection with acute icteric hepatitis in adults. Scand J Infect Dis 43: 547–549.
11. Sun L, Zhang JC (2012) Acute fulminant hepatitis with bone marrow failure in an adult due to parvovirus B19 infection. Hepatology 55: 329–330.
12. Shiraishi A, Hoshina T, Ihara K, Doi T, Ohga S, et al. (2012) Acute liver failure as the initial manifestation of Wilson disease triggered by human parvovirus b19 infection. Pediatr Infect Dis J. 31: 103–104.
13. Von Landenberg P, Lehmann HW, Knöll A, Dorsch S, Modrow S (2003) Antiphospholipid antibodies in pediatric and adult patients with rheumatic disease are associated with parvovirus B19 infection. Arthritis Rheum 48: 1939–1947.
14. Sève P, Ferry T, Koenig M, Cathebras P, Rousset H, et al. (2005) Lupus-like presentation of parvovirus B19 infection. Semin Arthritis Rheum 34: 642–648.
15. Tzang BS, Chen DY, Tsai CC, Chiang SY, Lin TM, et al. (2010) Human parvovirus B19 nonstructural protein NS1 enhanced the expression of cleavage of 70 kDa U1-snRNP autoantigen. J Biomed Sci. 17: 40.
16. Chen DY, Tzang BS, Chen YM, Lan JL, Tsai CC, et al. (2010) The association of anti-parvovirus B19-VP1 unique region antibodies with antiphospholipid antibodies in patients with antiphospholipid syndrome. Clin Chim Acta 411: 1084–1089.
17. Tzang BS, Tsay GJ, Lee YJ, Li C, Sun YS, et al. (2007) The association of VP1 unique region protein in acute parvovirus B19 infection and anti-phospholipid antibody production. Clin Chim Acta 378: 59–65.
18. Tzang BS, Tsai CC, Tsay GJ, Wang M, Sun YS, et al. (2009) Anti-human parvovirus B19 nonstructural protein antibodies in patients with rheumatoid arthritis. Clin Chim Acta 405: 76–82.
19. Kajigaya S, Fujii H, Field AM, Rosenfeld S, Anderson LJ, et al. (1991) Self-assembled B19 parvovirus capsids, produced in a baculovirus system, are antigenically and immunogenically similar to native virions. Proc Natl Acad Sci USA 88: 4646–4650.
20. Bradford MM (1976) A rapid and sensitive method for the quantitation of microgram quantities of protein utilizing the principle of protein-dye binding. Anal Biochem 72: 248–254.
21. Towbin H, Staehelin T, Gordon J (1979) Electrophoretic transfer of proteins from polyacrylamide gels to nitrocellulose sheet: procedure and some applications. Proc. Natl Acad Sci USA 76: 4350–4354.
22. Belmont HM, Levartovsky D, Goel A, Amin A, Giorno R, et al (1997) Rediske J, Skovron ML, Abramson SB. Increased nitric oxide production accompanied by the up-regulation of inducible nitric oxide synthase in vascular endothelium from patients with systemic lupus erythematosus. Arthritis Rheum 40: 1810–1816.
23. Wang G, Pierangeli SS, Papalardo E, Ansari GA, Khan MF (2010) Markers of oxidative and nitrosative stress in systemic lupus erythematosus: correlation with disease activity. Arthritis Rheum. 62: 2064–2072.
24. Wang HP, Hsu TC, Hsu GJ, Li SL, Tzang BS (2009) Cystamine attenuates the expressions of NOS- and TLR-associated molecules in the brain of NZB/W F1 mice. Eur J Pharmacol 607: 102–6.
25. Fung HB, Kirschenbaum HL (1999) Selective cyclooxygenase-2 inhibitors for the treatment of arthritis. Clin. Ther 21: 1131–1157.
26. Weinberg JB (2000) Nitric oxide synthase 2 and cyclooxygenase 2 interactions in inflammation. Immunol Res 22: 319–341.
27. Xu L, Zhang L, Yi Y, Kang HK, Datta SK (2004) Human lupus T cells resist inactivation and escape death by upregulating COX-2. Nat Med 10: 411–415.
28. Zhang L, Bertucci AM, Smith KA, Xu L, Datta SK (2007) Hyperexpression of cyclooxygenase 2 in the lupus immune system and effect of cyclooxygenase 2 inhibitor diet therapy in a murine model of systemic lupus erythematosus. Arthritis Rheum. 56: 4132–4141.
29. Goetzl EJ, Banda MJ, Leppert D (1995). Matrix metalloproteinases and immunity. J Immunol 156: 1–4.
30. Faber-Elmann A, Sthoeger Z, Tcherniack A, Dayan M, Mozes E (2002) Activity of matrix metalloproteinase-9 is elevated in sera of patients with systemic lupus erythematosus. Clin Exp Immunol 127: 393–398.
31. Ainiala H, Hietaharju A, Dastidar P, Loukkola J, Lehtimäki T, et al. (2004) Increased serum matrix metalloproteinase 9 levels in systemic lupus erythematosus patients with neuropsychiatric manifestations and brain magnetic resonance imaging abnormalities. Arthritis Rheum 50: 858–865.
32. Ram M, Sherer Y, Shoenfeld Y (2006) Matrix metalloproteinase-9 and autoimmune diseases. J Clin Immunol 26: 299–307.
33. Prince HE (2005) Biomarkers for diagnosing and monitoring autoimmune diseases. Biomarkers Suppl 1: S44–S49.
34. Sato H, Kita M, Seiki M (1993) v-Src activates the expression of 92-kDa type IV collagenase gene through the AP-1 site and the GT box homologous to retinoblastoma control elements. A mechanism regulating gene expression independent of that by inflammatory cytokines. J Biol Chem 268: 23460–23468.
35. Li W, Li H, Bocking AD, Challis JR (2010) Tumor necrosis factor stimulates matrix metalloproteinase 9 secretion from cultured human chorionic trophoblast cells through TNF receptor 1 signaling to IKBKB-NFKB and MAPK1/3 pathway. Biol Reprod 83: 481–487.
36. Doerig C, Hirt B, Antonietti JP, Beard P (1990) Nonstructural protein of parvoviruses B19 and minute virus of mice controls transcription. J Virol 64: 387–396.

37. Moffatt S, Tanaka N, Tada K, Nose M, Nakamura M, et al. (1996) A cytotoxic nonstructural protein, NS1, of human parvovirus B19 induces activation of interleukin-6 gene expression. J Virol 70: 8485–8491.
38. Sol N, Le Junter J, Vassias I, Freyssinier JM, Thomas A, et al. (1999) Possible interactions between the NS-1 protein and tumor necrosis factor alpha pathways in erythroid cell apoptosis induced by human parvovirus B19. J Virol 73: 8762–8770.
39. Kerr JR, Barah F, Mattey DL, Laing I, Hopkins SJ, et al. (2001) Circulating tumour necrosis factor-alpha and interferon-gamma are detectable during acute and convalescent parvovirus B19 infection and are associated with prolonged and chronic fatigue. J Gen Virol 82: 3011–3019.
40. Burnet FM, Holmes MC (1965) The natural history of the NZB/NZW F1 hybrid mouse: a laboratory model of systemic lupus erythematosus. Australas Ann Med 14: 185–91.
41. Pugliese A, Beltramo T, Torre D, Roccatello D (2007) Parvovirus B19 and immune disorders. Cell Biochem Funct 25: 639–641.

14

Characterization of the Phosphoproteome in SLE Patients

Xinzhou Zhang[1]*, Hualin Ma[1]*, Jianrong Huang[1], Yong Dai[2]*

1 Department of Nephrology, Shenzhen People's Hospital, Second Clinical Medical College, Jinan University, Shenzhen, China, 2 Clinical Medical Research Center, Shenzhen People's Hospital, Second Clinical Medical College, Jinan University, Shenzhen, China

Abstract

Protein phosphorylation is a complex regulatory event that is involved in the signaling networks that affect virtually every cellular process. The protein phosphorylation may be a novel source for discovering biomarkers and drug targets. However, a systematic analysis of the phosphoproteome in patients with SLE has not been performed. To clarify the pathogenesis of systemic lupus erythematosus (SLE), we compared phosphoprotein expression in PBMCs from SLE patients and normal subjects using proteomics analyses. Phosphopeptides were enriched using TiO_2 from PBMCs isolated from 15 SLE patients and 15 healthy subjects and then analyzed by automated LC-MS/MS analysis. Phosphorylation sites were identified and quantitated by MASCOT and MaxQuant. A total of 1035 phosphorylation sites corresponding to 618 NCBI-annotated genes were identified in SLE patients compared with normal subjects. Differentially expressed proteins, peptides and phosphorylation sites were then subjected to bioinformatics analyses. Gene ontology(GO) and pathway analyses showed that nucleic acid metabolism, cellular component organization, transport and multicellular organismal development pathways made up the largest proportions of the differentially expressed genes. Pathway analyses showed that the mitogen-activated protein kinase (MAPK) signaling pathway and actin cytoskeleton regulators made up the largest proportions of the metabolic pathways. Network analysis showed that rous sarcoma oncogene (SRC), v-rel reticuloendotheliosis viral oncogene homolog A (RELA), histone deacetylase (HDA1C) and protein kinase C, delta (PRKCD) play important roles in the stability of the network. These data suggest that aberrant protein phosphorylation may contribute to SLE pathogenesis.

Editor: Leighton R James, University of Florida, United States of America

Funding: This study was financially supported by National Nature Science Foundation of China (grant number 30972741\C080701). The funders had no role in study design, data collection and analysis, decision to publish, or preparation of the manuscript.

Competing Interests: The authors have declared that no competing interests exist.

* E-mail: daiyong22@yahoo.com.cn

These authors contributed equally to this work.

Introduction

Protein phosphorylation is a widespread post-translational modification (PTM). Reversible protein phosphorylation, in which phosphate groups are enzymatically added by protein kinases and removed from proteins by phosphatases, often serves as a molecular switch in signaling pathways. Disruptions in phosphorylation-mediated cell signaling events are connected with numerous diseases [1,2,3,4,5]. Furthermore, the abnormal expression of protein kinases is an important cause or component of many pathologies. Therefore, the characterization of the phosphorylation sites of proteins within various signaling pathways can enhance the understanding of specific disease pathologies [6]. Phosphoproteomics is defined as the study of the components of the proteome that undergo phosphorylation. Systemic lupus erythematosus (SLE) is a classical autoimmune disease. The disease incidence is nine times greater in women than in men [7], and its estimated prevalence in China is 37.7/100,000 persons [8]. However, the details of SLE etiology remain poorly understood. In this study, we thoroughly explored the phosphopeptide proteome of human Peripheral blood mononuclear cells (PBMCs) using a highly sensitive Liquid chromatography-mass spectrometry (LC-MS/MS) system, improved software for phosphopeptide identification and subsequent analysis with an elaborate bioinformatics strategy, including gene ontology (GO) analysis, pathway analysis and protein network analysis. The rich data from the proteomic analysis also provides insight into the pathogenesis of SLE.

Materials and Methods

Patient Assessments and Classifications

This study protocols and consent forms were approved by the Second Clinical Medical College (Shenzhen People's Hospital) of Jinan University and adhere to the Helsinki Declaration guidelines on ethical principles for medical research involving human subjects. Written informed consent was obtained from all participants. A group of 15 SLE patients who had never been treated with disease-modifying antirheumatic drugs (DMARDs) or other immunosuppressive drugs was recruited for this study. Patients treated with nonsteroidal anti-inflammatory drugs or other symptomatic treatments were excluded. All patients satisfied the American College of Rheumatology classification criteria for SLE. In addition, we choose 15 healthy subjects as controls.

Table 1. Demographic and disease manifestation in SLE patients and healthy controls.

characteristic	SLE patients	healthy controls
NO.Female/male	15/0	15/0
Age mean (range) years	33.8(19–54)	33.1(21–55)
SLEDI score	12.2	N/A
Disease manifestation		
Skin rash	3	0
Mucosal ulcers	2	0
Proteinuria	5	0
Hematuria	1	0
Arthritis	4	0
Vasculitis	1	0
Low complement	7	0
Increased dsDNA	8	0
Pericarditis	1	0
Leukopenia	2	0
N/A: not applicable		

PBMCs Isolation and Protein Extraction

Peripheral blood mononuclear cells (PBMCs) were separated by a Ficoll-Paque (Sigma, St. Louis, MO, USA) density gradient centrifugation according to the manufacturer's instructions. In brief, 2 ml blood (with EDTA as an anticoagulant) was layered on 3 ml Ficoll-Hypaque (Sigma) and centrifuged for 25 min at 1300 rpm at room temperature. Mononuclear cells at the interface were aspirated with a Pasteur pipette, washed twice in PBS with centrifugation for 10 min at 900 rpm at room temperature and resuspended in 500 μl SDT lysate (Invitrogen, Carlsbad, USA). The samples were then stored at −80°C until further use.

Phosphopeptide Enrichment

Phosphopeptides from digested peptides were enriched using the Phosphopeptide Enrichment TiO_2 kit (Calbiochem, San Diego, CA) according to the manufacturer's instructions. Briefly, the tryptic digest was dried, dissolved in 200 μL TiO_2 Phosphobind buffer containing 50 g/L 2,5-dihydroxybenzoic acid (DHB) and then mixed with 50 μL TiO_2 Phosphobind Resin. After a 40 minute incubation, the supernatant was discarded, and the TiO_2 resin was washed twice with the washing buffer. Then, elution buffer was added to elute the phosphopeptides in two batches. The eluted supernatant was pooled and dried by evaporation for LC-MS/MS analysis.

LC-MS/MS Analysis

The dried phosphopeptides were subjected to LC-MS/MS analysis with a Finnigan Surveyor High Performance Liquid Chromatography(HPLC) system coupled with a LTQ-Orbitrap XL mass spectrometer (Thermo Electron, San Jose, CA). Briefly, the peptide mixtures were loaded onto a C18 column (100 μm i.d., 10 cm long, 5 μm, resin from Michrom Bioresources, Auburn, CA) using an autosampler. Peptides were eluted in a 5–35% gradient of buffer solution over 180 min and then detected in the LTQ-Orbitrap XL mass spectrometer as described previously [9,10].

Raw MS Data Analysis

Raw Orbitrap full-scan MS and ion trap MSA spectra were processed using the MaxQuant algorithms [11,12]. Peptides and proteins were identified by Mascot through automated database matching of all tandem mass spectra against an in-house curated concatenated target database. Scoring was performed in MaxQuant as described previously. We required strict trypsin enzyme specificity and allowed up to two missed cleavage sites. Cysteine carbamidomethylation (Cys, +57.021464 Da) was searched as a fixed modification, whereas N-acetylation of proteins (N-terminal, +42.010565 Da), oxidized methionine (Met,+15.994915 Da), and serine, threonine, and tyrosine phosphorylations (Ser/Thr/Tyr, +79.966331 Da) were searched as variable modifications.

Peptide filtering and Phosphorylation Site Identification

The Mascot result files were imported into the MaxQuant software suite for further processing. In MaxQuant, we defined the estimated false discovery rate (FDR) of all peptide and protein identifications at 1% by automatically filtering based on peptide length, mass error precision estimates, and the Mascot scores of all forward and reversed peptide identifications. The final estimate of

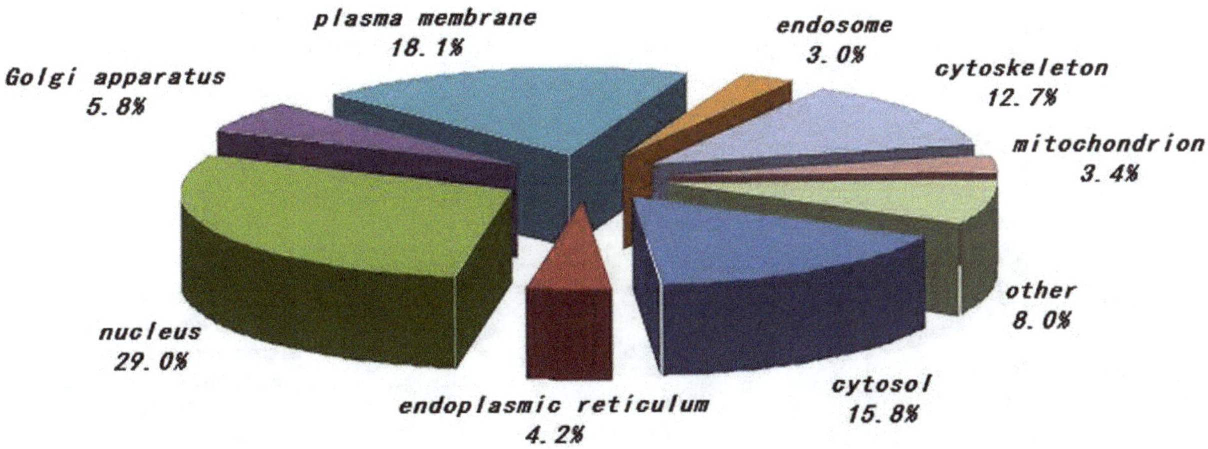

Figure 1. Summary of the cellular components of the PBMCs phosphoproteins characterized by in-gel IEF LC-MS/MS. The most enriched cellular components were nuclear proteins and proteins associated with the plasma membrane, cytosol or cytoskeleton. The information was compiled from Gene Ontology annotations.

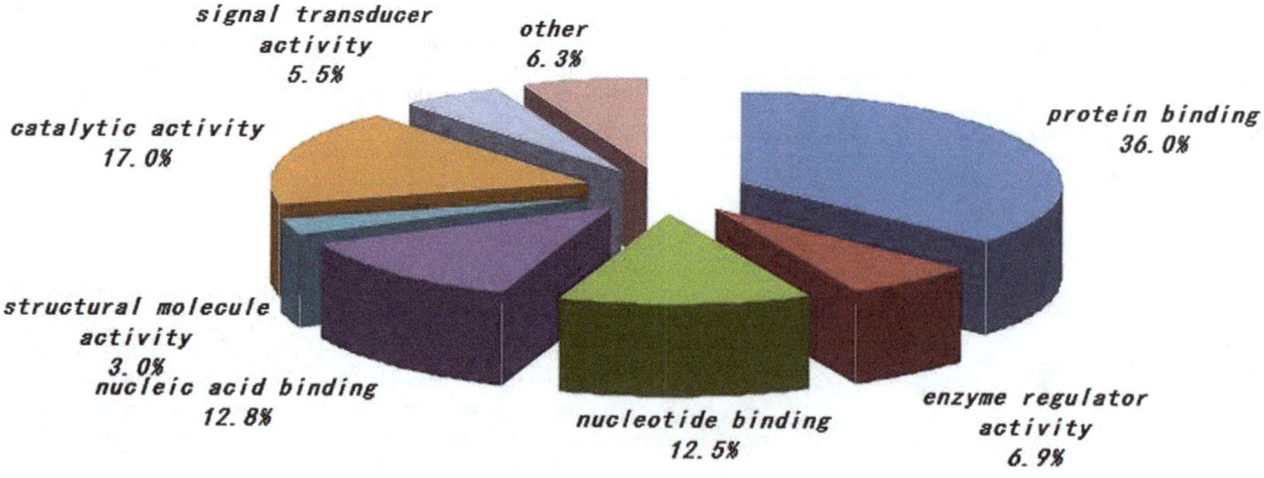

Figure 2. Summary of the molecular functions of the PBMCs phosphoproteins characterized by in-gel IEF LC-MS/MS. The largest group is constituted by protein binding followed by catalytic activity and nucleic acid binding. The information was compiled from Gene Ontology annotations.

true phosphorylated amino acids remaining within all identified phosphopeptide sequences was calculated in MaxQuant based on the localization probabilities of all assumed threonine, serine and tyrosine phosphorylation sites using the PTM score algorithm, as described previously [13].For protein identification, we used IPI database. A protein group was removed if all identified peptides assigned to this protein group were also assigned to another protein group. Tosort out a single protein member from a protein group, we chose the protein from the Swiss-Prot database and with the highest sequence coverage. When using label-free approach to identify differently expressed protein and calculating the coefficient of variance, the number of spectra of each protein was logarithmtransformed.

Different Gene Screening and Statistical Analyses

For screening of phosphorylation sites between the two groups, we used the following method. 1, caculate the fold change between the two groups. 2. set threshold value is 1, that is the average fold change between SLE patients group and healthy controls group was more than or equal to 2 folds; and the p value of single sample t-test was less than or equal to 0.05. T-test was conducted using MATLAB 7.5. 3. labeling the gene name corresponding protein according to the NCBI annotation information.

Bioinformatics Analysis

The expression values calculated for the differential proteins and peptides were used for distance and average to determine linkage for gene ontology (GO) analysis. In pathway analysis, interactions between genes in the range of genomes were analyzed by downloading the pathway data in Kyoto Encyclopedia of Genes and Genomes(KEGG). Finally, the results of the above data were merged into a comprehensive gene inter-relationship network. The established gene network was able to directly reflect the inter-relationships between genes at a whole-cell level, as well as the stability of the gene regulatory network.

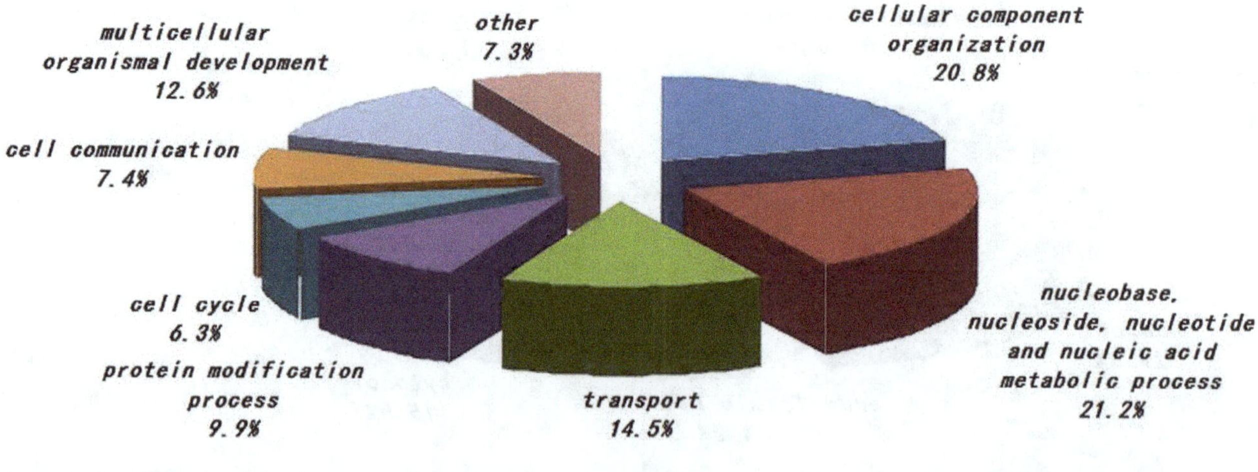

Figure 3. Classification of the characterized PBMCs phosphoproteins based on their involvement in biological processes. The largest group contains proteins related to nucleobase, nucleoside, nucleotide and nucleic acid metabolism. Two other large groups are the proteins involved in cellular component organization and transport. The information was gathered based on Gene Ontology annotations.

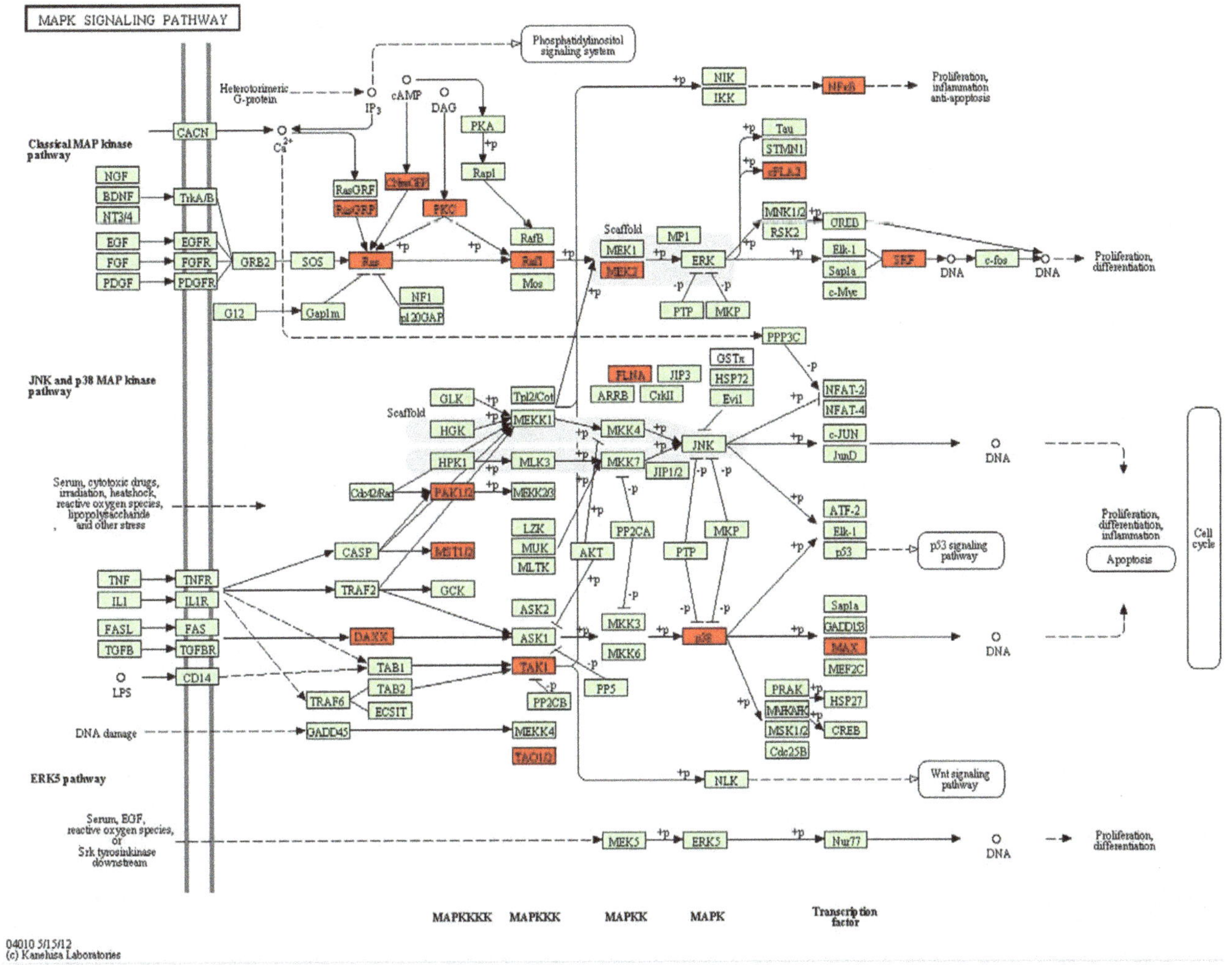

Figure 4. The MAPK signaling pathway showing differentially-expressed gene in SLE patients PBMCs versus healthy controls. Red marks indicate the genes with differential phosphorylation profiles.

Results

The Clinical Characteristics of the Study Population

A total of 30 subjects were in the study group, which included 15 SLE patients and 15 healthy controls. In Table 1, the clinical characteristics of the study population are summarized.

Pretreatment of the Raw Data and Screening of Different Genes

A phosphorylated peptide reagent kit was used to enrich the sample for phosphorylated proteins, thus combining protein separation enrichment technology and mass spectrometry technology. The detailed information on the identified phosphoproteins/phosphopeptides according to the mass spectrometric results (Table S1). A total of 1035 phosphorylation sites, corresponding to 618 NCBI-annotated genes, were identified as differentially modified in SLE patients compared with normal subjects.

GO Annotation and Analysis of the Differences in Phosphoproteins

The phosphoproteins characterized in the study were evaluated based on their molecular function, biological process and cellular component annotations. As shown in Figure 1, proteins from various cellular components (e.g., the nucleus, plasma membrane, cytosol, cytoskeleton, and Golgi apparatus) were included. The most enriched cellular components were nuclear proteins and proteins associated with the plasma membrane, cytosol or cytoskeleton. Functionally, the phosphoproteins characterized in the study are diverse. We grouped the identified phosphoproteins into several categories based on their molecular functions as annotated in the Swiss-Prot database. The distribution of the phosphoproteins among the various functional categories is shown in Figure 2. The largest group is comprised of proteins with roles in protein binding. The other three largest groups are proteins involved in catalytic activity, nucleic acid binding and nucleotide binding. The distribution of phosphoproteins by biological process is shown in Figure 3. The largest group contains proteins related to nucleobase, nucleoside, nucleotide and nucleic acid metabolism. Two other large groups are the proteins involved in cellular component organization and transport.

Signaling Pathway Analyses

We next wanted to determine whether specific pathways are enriched in the set of proteins present in our phosphotyrosine database. Similar to the strategy used for the GO analysis, we

Table 2. KEEG showing differentially-expressed pathways in SLE patients PBMCs versus healty controls.

Pathway	Gene count	P value
Focal adhesion	16	0.001579
Protein processing in endoplasmic reticulum	11	0.024745
Herpes simplex infection	15	0.001521
Long-term potentiation	7	0.004945
Regulation of actin cytoskeleton	20	5.21E-05
Insulin signaling pathway	10	0.016194
Leukocyte transendothelial migration	9	0.012933
Endocrine and other factor-regulated calcium reabsorption	4	0.038077
Glioma	5	0.037015
Fc gamma R-mediated phagocytosis	15	5.43E-07
Fc epsilon RI signaling pathway	12	9.96E-06
Epithelial cell signaling in *Helicobacter pylori* infection	6	0.014573
Salmonella infection	8	0.005302
B cell receptor signaling pathway	7	0.008772
Gap junction	8	0.00664
Spliceosome	14	8.93E-05
ErbB signaling pathway	8	0.005723
Glycolysis/Gluconeogenesis	6	0.011522
Phosphatidylinositol signaling system	9	0.000864
Thyroid cancer	3	0.023349
Pentose phosphate pathway	3	0.020733
Melanogenesis	7	0.038778
Gastric acid secretion	7	0.006928
Starch and sucrose metabolism	5	0.017764
T cell receptor signaling pathway	12	0.000218
Endocytosis	12	0.045153
Pathogenic *Escherichia coli* infection	5	0.017764
Vasopressin-regulated water reabsorption	4	0.025257
Dilated cardiomyopathy	7	0.023862
Natural killer cell mediated cytotoxicity	11	0.00668
Pancreatic secretion	9	0.005007
Ribosome	8	0.007666
MAPK signaling pathway	19	0.00302
Chemokine signaling pathway	17	0.000297
Prostate cancer	8	0.00664
VEGF signaling pathway	7	0.008121
GnRH signaling pathway	12	0.00011
NOD-like receptor signaling pathway	6	0.006232
Long-term depression	8	0.001273
Non-small cell lung cancer	5	0.016332
Shigellosis	6	0.00821
Hypertrophic cardiomyopathy (HCM)	6	0.038708
SNARE interactions in vesicular transport	5	0.002178
RNA transport	13	0.002599
Inositol phosphate metabolism	5	0.024354
Vascular smooth muscle contraction	14	3.07E-05
Adherens junction	6	0.020876
African trypanosomiasis	5	0.002518
Leishmaniasis	6	0.022333
Tight junction	12	0.001512

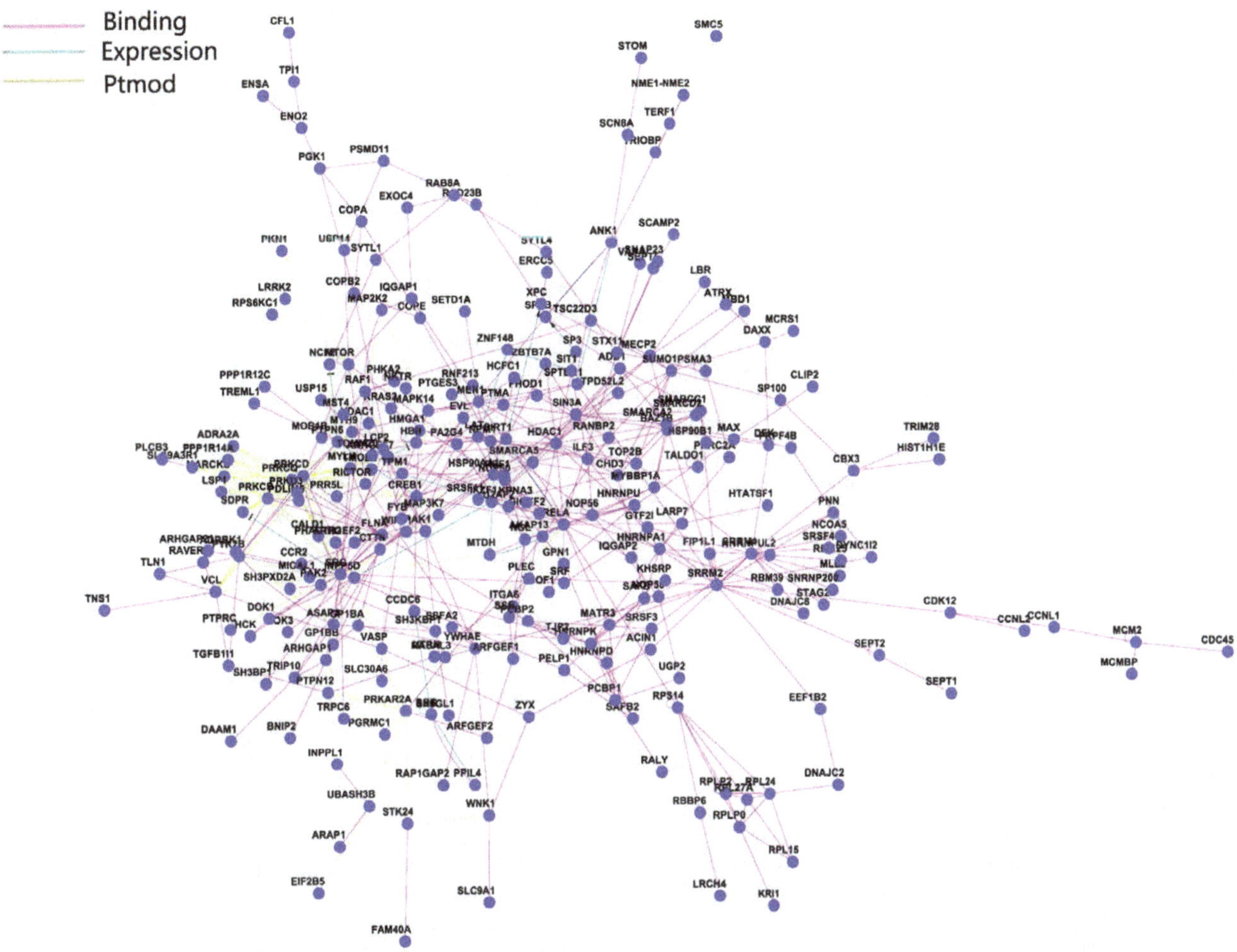

Figure 5. Network analysis of SLE-related genes which were indentified in this analysis. The network can reflect the relationship between genes from the situation as a whole. Blue means expression, gray means binding and purple means ptmod (post-transcription modification).

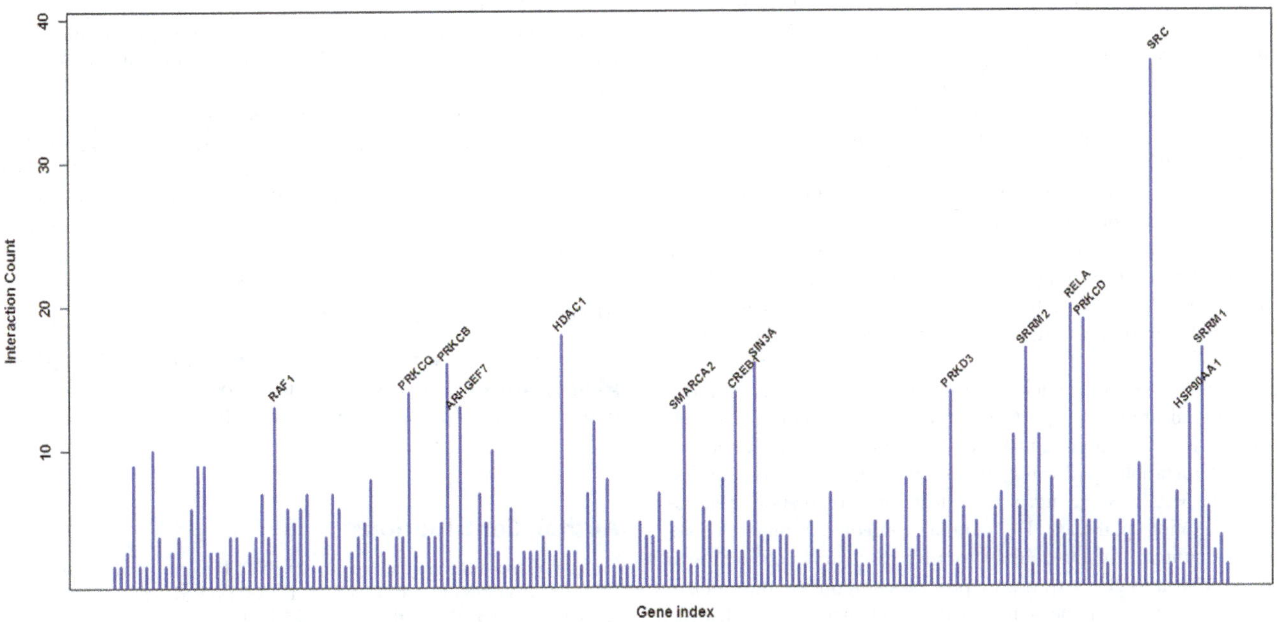

Figure 6. Connectivity analysis of the SLE-related genes. The connectivity of SRC is the highest one in all related-genes.

mapped differentially modified genes to the KEGG pathway database using GenMAPP v2.1 and then performed a statistical test to identify enriched metabolic pathways, using $P<0.05$ as the standard. We selected 50 metabolic pathways (Table 2). The top KEGG pathway was the MAPK signaling pathway (Figure 4).

Gene Network Analysis

We integrated the following three different interaction relationships: 1) the gene regulation and protein modification relationships of genes in the KEGG database and other relationships; 2) interaction data from high-flux experiments, such as protein-protein interactions confirmed by yeast two-hybrid; 3) gene-gene interactions described in the literature. Specifically, we downloaded the pathway data from KEGG database and analyzed genome-wide genetic interactions in R (http://www.r-project.org/) and downloaded the KEGGSOAP package (http://www.bioconductor.org/packages/2.4/bioc/html/KEGGSOAP.html). Finally, we integrated the relationships in a gene network (Figure 5). Genes with large numbers of connections were referred to as "hub" genes. Hub genes often play important roles in network stability. We identified SRC, RELA, HDA1C and PRKCD as hub genes in our network (Figure 6).

Discussion

Protein phosphorylation is the most common posttranslational modification (PTM) in the biosphere [14,15]. Approximately 30% of proteins can be phosphorylated [16] at threonine, tyrosine and serine residues [17]. Protein phosphorylation becomes disordered when protein kinase or phosphatase activity is overexpressed or inhibited, resulting in abnormal cellular activities and producing cell damage or even cancer [18,19]. Phosphoproteomics requires powerful analytical technologies and bioinformatics tools. Several recent reviews have summarized the development of various phosphoproteomic methodologies. These methods typically combine different separation strategies with mass spectrometry [20,21,22]. The successful application of proteomic technologies to biomedical and clinical research has enabled the discovery of disease-specific biomarkers for diagnosis and treatment monitoring, thus offering insight into the underlying pathologies of diseases and identification of new therapeutic targets.

In this study, we used a phosphorylated peptide reagents kit to enrich the samples for phosphorylated proteins and then combined this technique with mass spectrometry technology. A total of 1035 phosphorylation sites corresponding to 618 annotated genes were identified as differentially modified in SLE compared with normal subjects.

GO analyses showed that the most highly differentially expressed genes were related to nucleic acid metabolism, cellular component organization, transportation, protein modification, cell cycle, cell communication, multicellular organismal development, carbohydrate metabolic process, lipid metabolism and protein translation processes. Nucleic acid metabolism, cellular component organization, transport and multicellular organismal development were the dominant processes. Pathway analysis showed that 50 metabolic pathways are modified in SLE pathogenesis. Notably, MAPK signaling, actin cytoskeleton regulation, chemokine signaling pathway, Fc gamma R-mediated phagocytosis, Herpes simplex infection, spliceosome, vascular smooth muscle contraction and RNA transport process components made up a larger proportion of the genes in these 50 metabolic pathways. The MAPK signaling pathway was highlighted as the most important pathway.

SLE is a chronic autoimmune disorder that is characterized by lymphocyte abnormalities and autoantibody production [23]. Hoffmant showed that immune tolerance defects in the peripheral blood T-lymphocytes of SLE patients related to the abnormal regulation of the MAPK signaling pathway, which directly results in abnormal TCR-mediated intracellular signaling and T lymphocyte function [24,25]. The MAPK signaling pathway has important functions in many types of mammalian cells. Mitogen-activated protein kinases (MAPKs) are serine and threonine protein kinases that can be activated by phosphorylation in response to extracellular stimuli, such as mitogens, growth factors, cytokines, and osmotic stress [26,27]. The activation of MAPK pathways has been shown to be a potential pro-inflammatory mechanism in rheumatoid arthritis [28,29,30]. During inflammation, MAPK is activated in various immune cells, and its activation is closely related to stress responses and apoptosis [31]. Our results demonstrated that the MAPK signal pathway is abnormally activated in PBMCs from SLE patients, which provided an experimental basis for researching SLE pathogenesis and exploring new therapies. We believe that interventions in or regulation of this signaling pathway may be useful therapies for treating SLE and related diseases.

SRC was the first protein found to have tyrosine protein kinase activity, and its activity is itself regulated by phosphorylation and dephosphorylation. MAPK signaling pathways control multiple physiological processes and are involved in a variety of diseases. Ras, the activating protein upstream of the MAPK pathway, is directly regulated by SRC activity. The activation of the MAPK pathway downstream of Src phosphorylation leads to transcriptional activation. Meanwhile, the inhibition of MAPK pathway activation can partially reverse the effects of SRC protein activity [32]. In particular, as suggested by protein network analysis, genes with many connections within the network were identified as the hub genes. Hub genes often play an important role in the stability of the network. We found that SRC, RELA, HDA1C and PRKCD were the hub genes in our network. These results demonstrated that SRC plays a central role in the stability of the network, suggesting it is important in the pathogenesis of SLE, which provides an experimental basis for researching the pathogenesis of lupus and exploring new treatment methods for SLE.

This experiment thoroughly characterized the phosphorylated protein expression profile in PBMCs of SLE patients. These data will serve as a reference and supplement to help us better understand the pathogenesis of SLE. Furthermore, interventions that modulate the activities of the involved genes and pathways may be able to block or slow the onset and development of SLE.

Supporting Information

Table S1 The information of phosphoproteins/phosphopeptides. The detailed information on the identified phosphoproteins/phosphopeptides according to the mass spectrometric results.

Author Contributions

Conceived and designed the experiments: YD. Performed the experiments: HM XZ. Analyzed the data: XZ HM. Contributed reagents/materials/analysis tools: JH. Wrote the paper: XZ HM.

References

1. Zahid S, Oellerich M, Asif AR, Ahmed N (2012) Phosphoproteome profiling of substantia nigra and cortex regions of Alzheimer's disease patients. J Neurochem 121: 954–963.
2. Di Domenico F, Sultana R, Barone E, Perluigi M, Cini C, et al. (2011) Quantitative proteomics analysis of phosphorylated proteins in the hippocampus of Alzheimer's disease subjects. J Proteomics 74: 1091–1103.
3. Chien KY, Liu HC, Goshe MB (2011) Development and application of a phosphoproteomic method using electrostatic repulsion-hydrophilic interaction chromatography (ERLIC), IMAC, and LC-MS/MS analysis to study Marek's Disease Virus infection. J Proteome Res 10: 4041–4053.
4. Wu HY, Tseng VS, Chen LC, Chang HY, Chuang IC, et al. (2010) Identification of tyrosine-phosphorylated proteins associated with lung cancer metastasis using label-free quantitative analyses. J Proteome Res 9: 4102–4112.
5. Popova TG, Turell MJ, Espina V, Kehn-Hall K, Kidd J, et al. (2010) Reverse-phase phosphoproteome analysis of signaling pathways induced by Rift valley fever virus in human small airway epithelial cells. PLoS One 5: e13805.
6. Giorgianni F, Zhao Y, Desiderio DM, Beranova-Giorgianni S (2007) Toward a global characterization of the phosphoproteome in prostate cancer cells: identification of phosphoproteins in the LNCaP cell line. Electrophoresis 28: 2027–2034.
7. Rahman A, Isenberg DA (2008) Systemic lupus erythematosus. N Engl J Med 358: 929–939.
8. Xiang YJ, Dai SM (2009) Prevalence of rheumatic diseases and disability in China. Rheumatol Int 29: 481–490.
9. Li X, Zhang Y, Zeng X, Yang L, Deng Y (2011) Chemical profiling of bioactive constituents in Sarcandra glabra and its preparations using ultra-high-pressure liquid chromatography coupled with LTQ Orbitrap mass spectrometry. Rapid Commun Mass Spectrom 25: 2439–2447.
10. Fernbach NV, Planyavsky M, Muller A, Breitwieser FP, Colinge J, et al. (2009) Acid elution and one-dimensional shotgun analysis on an Orbitrap mass spectrometer: an application to drug affinity chromatography. J Proteome Res 8: 4753–4765.
11. Cox J, Matic I, Hilger M, Nagaraj N, Selbach M, et al. (2009) A practical guide to the MaxQuant computational platform· for SILAC-based quantitative proteomics. Nat Protoc 4: 698–705.
12. Cox J, Mann M (2008) MaxQuant enables high peptide identification rates, individualized p.p.b.-range mass accuracies and proteome-wide protein quantification. Nat Biotechnol 26: 1367–1372.
13. Olsen JV, Blagoev B, Gnad F, Macek B, Kumar C, et al. (2006) Global, in vivo, and site-specific phosphorylation dynamics in signaling networks. Cell 127: 635–648.
14. Melo-Braga MN, Braga TV, Leon IR, Antonacci D, Nogueira FC, et al. (2012) Modulation of protein phosphorylation, glycosylation and acetylation in grape (Vitis vinifera) mesocarp and exocarp due to Lobesia botrana infection. Mol Cell Proteomics 11: 945–956.
15. Lin SY, Li TY, Liu Q, Zhang C, Li X, et al. (2012) Protein phosphorylation-acetylation cascade connects growth factor deprivation to autophagy. Autophagy 8: 1385–1386.
16. Raggiaschi R, Gotta S, Terstappen GC (2005) Phosphoproteome analysis. Biosci Rep 25: 33–44.
17. Wu HY, Tseng VS, Liao PC (2007) Mining phosphopeptide signals in liquid chromatography-mass spectrometry data for protein phosphorylation analysis. J Proteome Res 6: 1812–1821.
18. Yang F, Stenoien DL, Strittmatter EF, Wang J, Ding L, et al. (2006) Phosphoproteome profiling of human skin fibroblast cells in response to low- and high-dose irradiation. J Proteome Res 5: 1252–1260.
19. Ge F, Xiao CL, Bi LJ, Tao SC, Xiong S, et al. (2010) Quantitative phosphoproteomics of proteasome inhibition in multiple myeloma cells. PLoS One 5: e13095.
20. Hoffert JD, Knepper MA (2008) Taking aim at shotgun phosphoproteomics. Anal Biochem 375: 1–10.
21. Collins MO, Yu L, Choudhary JS (2007) Analysis of protein phosphorylation on a proteome-scale. Proteomics 7: 2751–2768.
22. Gafken PR, Lampe PD (2006) Methodologies for characterizing phosphoproteins by mass spectrometry. Cell Commun Adhes 13: 249–262.
23. La Cava A (2009) Lupus and T cells. Lupus 18: 196–201.
24. Kyttaris VC, Tsokos GC (2004) T lymphocytes in systemic lupus erythematosus: an update. Curr Opin Rheumatol 16: 548–552.
25. Hoffman RW (2004) T cells in the pathogenesis of systemic lupus erythematosus. Clin Immunol 113: 4–13.
26. De Luca A, Maiello MR, D'Alessio A, Pergameno M, Normanno N (2012) The RAS/RAF/MEK/ERK and the PI3K/AKT signalling pathways: role in cancer pathogenesis and implications for therapeutic approaches. Expert Opin Ther Targets 16 Suppl 2: S17–27.
27. Chang L, Karin M (2001) Mammalian MAP kinase signalling cascades. Nature 410: 37–40.
28. Lopez-Santalla M, Salvador-Bernaldez M, Gonzalez-Alvaro I, Castaneda S, Ortiz AM, et al. (2011) Tyr(3)(2)(3)-dependent p38 activation is associated with rheumatoid arthritis and correlates with disease activity. Arthritis Rheum 63: 1833–1842.
29. Kanbe K, Chen Q, Nakamura A, Hobo K (2011) Inhibition of MAP kinase in synovium by treatment with tocilizumab in rheumatoid arthritis. Clin Rheumatol 30: 1407–1413.
30. Thiel MJ, Schaefer CJ, Lesch ME, Mobley JL, Dudley DT, et al. (2007) Central role of the MEK/ERK MAP kinase pathway in a mouse model of rheumatoid arthritis: potential proinflammatory mechanisms. Arthritis Rheum 56: 3347–3357.
31. Niu X, Fan T, Li W, Xing W, Huang H (2012) The anti-inflammatory effects of sanguinarine and its modulation of inflammatory mediators from peritoneal macrophages. Eur J Pharmacol 689: 262–269.
32. Kline CL, Olson TL, Irby RB (2009) Src activity alters alpha3 integrin expression in colon tumor cells. Clin Exp Metastasis 26: 77–87.

Autoreactive IgE is Prevalent in Systemic Lupus Erythematosus and is Associated with Increased Disease Activity and Nephritis

Barbara Dema[1], Christophe Pellefigues[2], Sarfaraz Hasni[3], Nathalie Gault[6], Chao Jiang[1], Tiffany K. Ricks[1], Michael M. Bonelli[8], Jörg Scheffel[1], Karim Sacré[2,4], Mathieu Jablonski[5], Delphine Gobert[4], Thomas Papo[2,4], Eric Daugas[2,5], Gabor Illei[7], Nicolas Charles[2*⁹], Juan Rivera[1*⁹]

1 Laboratory of Molecular Immunogenetics, National Institute of Arthritis and Musculoskeletal and Skin Diseases, National Institutes of Health, Bethesda, Maryland, United States of America, **2** Institut National de la Santé et de la Recherche Médicale U699, Université Paris Diderot, Paris, France, **3** Office of the Clinical Director, National Institute of Arthritis and Musculoskeletal and Skin Diseases, National Institutes of Health, Bethesda, Maryland, United States of America, **4** Department of Internal Medicine, Hôpital Bichat, Assistance Publique-Hôpitaux de Paris, Université Paris Diderot, Faculté de Médecine site Bichat, Paris, France, **5** Department of Nephrology, Hôpital Bichat, Assistance Publique-Hôpitaux de Paris, Université Paris Diderot, Faculté de Médecine site Bichat, Paris, France, **6** Clinical Research Unit, Hôpital Bichat, Assistance Publique-Hôpitaux de Paris, Université Paris Diderot, Faculté de Médecine site Bichat, Paris, France, **7** Sjogren's Syndrome Clinic, National Institute of Dental and Craniofacial Research, National Institutes of Health, Bethesda, Maryland, United States of America, **8** Lymphocyte Biology Section, National Institute of Arthritis and Musculoskeletal and Skin Diseases, National Institutes of Health, Bethesda, Maryland, United States of America

Abstract

The presence of autoantibodies in systemic lupus erythematosus, particularly those of the IgG subclass, have long been associated with disease onset and activity. Here we explored the prevalence of autoreactive IgE in SLE and its relevance to disease in French (n = 79) and United States (US) (n = 117) cohorts with a mean age of 41.5±12.7 and 43.6±15.3 years and disease duration of 13.5±8.5 and 16.6±11.9 years, respectively. Our findings show that approximately 65% of all SLE subjects studied produced IgE antibodies to the seven autoantigens tested. This positivity was increased to almost 83% when only those subjects with active disease were considered. SLE subjects who were positive for anti-dsDNA, -Sm, and -SSB/La -specific IgE showed a highly significant association in the levels of these antibodies with disease activity similar to that of the corresponding IgG's. A strong association of IgE autoantibodies with active nephritis was also found in the combined cohort analysis. A test of the predictive value of autoreactive IgE's and IgGs for disease activity (SLE Disease Activity Index (SLEDAI) ≥4) revealed that the best predictors were dsDNA-specific IgE and IgG, and that the age of an SLE subject influenced this predictive model. The finding argue that the overall levels of IgE autoantibodies, independently or in combination with IgG autoantibodies, may serve as indicators of active disease.

Editor: Pierre Bobé, INSERM-Université Paris-Sud, France

Funding: This work was supported by the Intramural Program of the National Institute of Arthritis and Musculoskeletal and Skin Diseases (NIAMS) of the National Institutes of Health (NIH), by the French Institut National de la Santé Et de la Recherche Médicale (INSERM), by the Assistance Publique – Hôpitaux de Paris (AP-HP) and by grants from the Mairie de Paris (Emergences 2010), ANR JCJC SVSE1 2011 BASILE and the French Kidney Foundation (Fondation du Rein) to NC. NC is under a translational research contract with the AP-HP (CHRT). The authors wish to acknowledge the invaluable support of the Office of the Clinical Director, NIAMS. The funders had no role in study design, data collection and analysis, decision to publish, or preparation of the manuscript.

Competing Interests: The authors have declared that no competing interests exist.

* E-mail: juan_rivera@nih.gov (JR); nicolas.charles@inserm.fr (NC)

⁹ These authors contributed equally to this work.

Introduction

Systemic Lupus Erythematosus (SLE) is a chronic systemic autoimmune disease characterized by the loss of immune tolerance to self-antigens, dysregulated autoantibody production, and multiple clinical manifestations [1]. A hallmark of the disease is the overproduction of antibodies to nuclear antigens (ANA), dsDNA, Sm, RNP, Ro (SSA), La (SSB), and some phospholipids [2]. The detection of ANA, anti-Ro, anti-La and anti-phospholipid antibodies can occur years in advance of the clinical manifestation and diagnosis of SLE, and these antibodies accumulate with time. In contrast, the presence of anti-dsDNA and anti-Sm antibodies usually precedes by a few months the clinical manifestations of SLE and thus its diagnosis [3]. While the appearance of the different autoantibodies has been associated with diverse clinical manifestations [4], the pathogenesis of disease is most closely linked to the presence of dsDNA-specific IgG antibodies [5] and kidney biopsies reveal that a large proportion of SLE patients, that develop glomerular nephritis, have kidney deposits of dsDNA IgG antibodies [6]. However, not all patients produce dsDNA IgG antibodies and not all of these autoantibodies are pathogenic even though their presence is one criterion for SLE diagnosis [7], thus what other isotypes of autoantibodies might be linked to disease activity and kidney pathology is still a topic of considerable interest.

IgE is the rarest of immunoglobulins in the blood with serum levels in a healthy human at approximately 150 ng/ml whereas

Table 1. Characteristics and demographics of SLE patients and healthy controls in US and French cohorts.

Characteristic	US		France	
	SLE	Controls	SLE	Controls
	(n=117)	(n=79)	(n=79)	(n=32)
Age (years) (Mean, SD)	43.6±15.3	47.3±12.7	41.5±12.7	33.1±8.8
Gender, Females n (%)	99 (84.6)	30 (38.0)	70 (88.6)	15 (46.8)
Ethnicity, n (%)				
European descent	40 (34.2)	45 (56.9)	52 (65.8)	28 (87.5)
African-American/African	35 (29.9)	28 (35.4)	20 (25.3)	1 (3.1)
Hispanic	23 (19.6)	5 (6.3)	3 (3.8)	1 (3.1)
Asian	14 (11.9)	1 (1.3)	4 (5.1)	0
Arabs	1 (0.8)	0	0	0
Unknown	4 (3.4)	0	0	- (6.2)
Disease duration (years), (mean, SD)	16.6±11.9	-	13.5±8.5	-
SLEDAI, IQR (25%, 75%)	4 (0,4)	-	9 (0, 9)	-
Current Prednisone dose (mg/day)				
IQR (25%, 75%)	9.5 (0.5,10)	-	12.25 (1.25, 13.5)	-
Missing values	-		2	
Immunosuppressive therapy, n (%)				
Hydroxychloroquine	89 (76.1)	-	71 (91.0)	-
Mycophenolate mofetil	10 (8.5)	-	25 (33.8)	-
Cyclophosphamide	4 (3.4)	-	45 (60.8)	-
Azathioprine	22 (18.8)	-	11 (14.5)	-
Cyclosporine	2 (1.7)	-	0	-

IQR, Interquartile range.

that of IgG is 10 mg/ml. Normally, IgE functions to protect against various parasitic infections [8], but it is best known to mediate type I hypersensitivity since it binds the high affinity receptor for IgE (FcεRI) on mast cells and basophils (key cells in allergy) and upon allergen recognition causes the activation of these cells and the release of allergic mediators [9]. The presence of IgE autoantibodies has been described in some autoimmune diseases more than three decades ago [10], albeit there has been little advance towards understanding the role of IgE in autoimmunity. Generally, measurement of autoreactive IgE in diseases like SLE has been performed on small patient cohorts using methodologies with poor sensitivity for IgE detection, potentially providing a false perception of the prevalence of these autoantibodies. While some studies suggest that autoreactive IgE's may contribute to autoimmune diseases like SLE and to the underlying pathologies [11,12], the general importance of IgE autoantibodies in SLE has also been questioned [13] based on studies where a small proportion of SLE subjects showed detectable levels of autoreactive IgE's [11]. Nonetheless, the prevalence of autoreactive IgE in SLE and its importance to disease activity and pathologies is underappreciated.

Recently, we reported that the presence of autoreactive (dsDNA) IgE is linked to activation of basophils, which function to amplify autoantibody production in SLE through support of plasma cell survival [12]. In a mouse model of spontaneous lupus-like disease (Lyn-deficient mice), we found that the presence of IgE in circulating immune complexes caused the activation of circulating blood basophils which, upon activation, home to the secondary lymphoid organs by expressing CD62L in their cell surface. In the lymph nodes and the spleen, basophils secreted cytokines (IL-4 and IL-6) and expressed MHC-II and BAFF, enhancing plasma cell survival and autoantibody production [12,14]. Crossing of Lyn-deficient mice to IL-4-deficient or IgE-deficient mice resulted in a marked reduction in Ig autoantibody production and a failure of these double-deficient mice to develop the lupus-like phenotype. Thus, the findings argue for a functional role of autoreactive IgE in amplifying loss of self-tolerance through basophil-mediated support of plasma cell autoantibody production. Analysis of human disease also demonstrated the presence of dsDNA-specific IgE antibodies and activated basophils in a small cohort of SLE subjects [12]. dsDNA-specific IgE autoantibodies were associated with active disease and with lupus nephritis, suggesting that the observed role for autoreactive IgE and basophils in amplifying autoantibody production, in mouse models, might be a plausible immunological mechanism in the progression of human disease.

To further advance the understanding of IgE in SLE we measured the levels of IgE's with specificity to the most common SLE antigens, dsDNA, Sm, SSA (Ro), and SSB (La) in a sample of 196 SLE subjects in France or the US with a mean age of 41.5±12.7 and 43.6±15.3 years and disease duration of 13.5±8.5 and 16.6±11.9 years, respectively (Table 1). The healthy controls used in this study had a mean age 33.1±8.8 and 47.3±12.7 in France and the US, respectively (Table 1). The findings show that autoreactive IgE's are highly prevalent in SLE and that the presence of high levels of dsDNA-specific IgE are tightly linked to disease activity and to parameters of abnormal kidney function similar to dsDNA-specific IgG. We also uncovered autoreactive

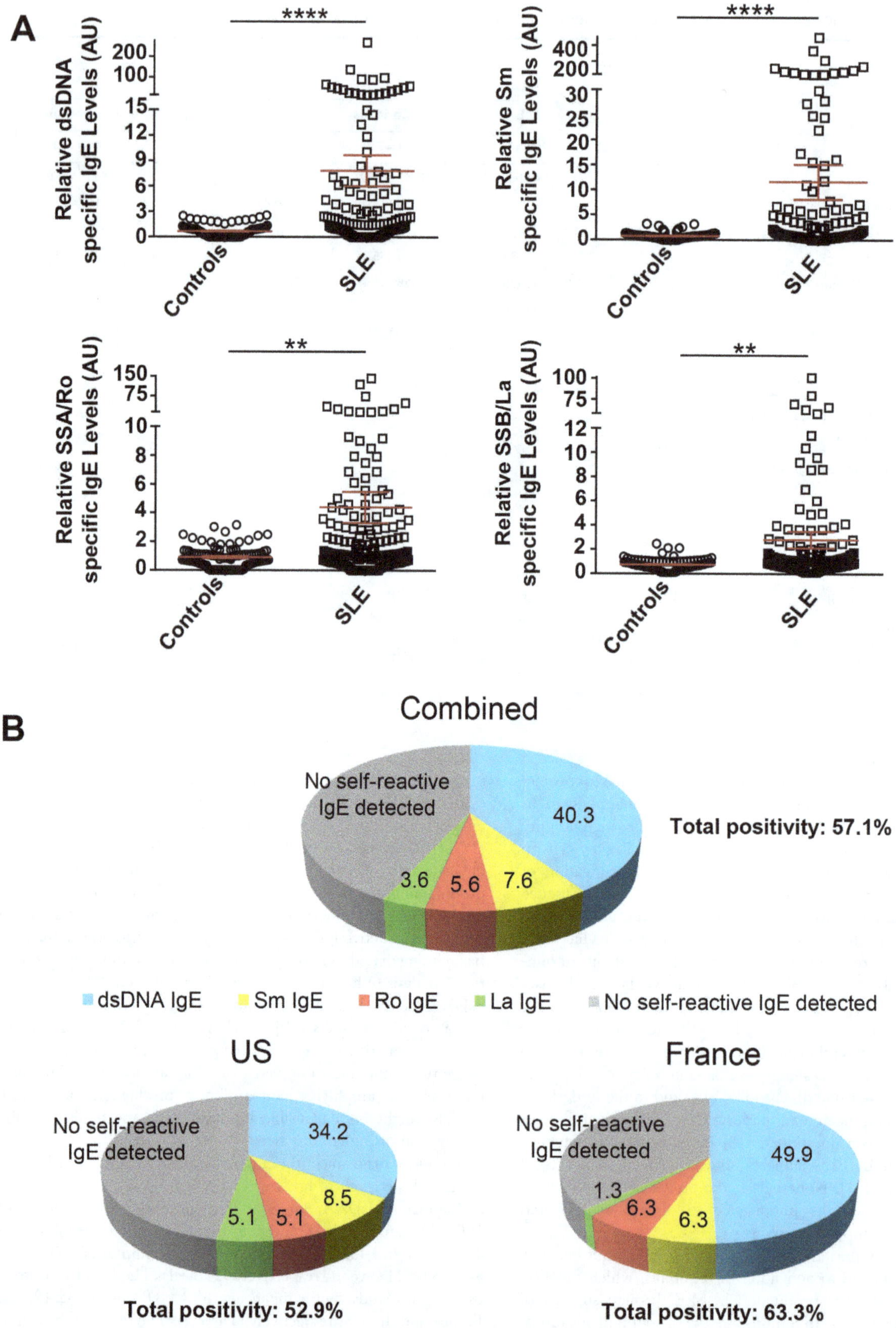

Figure 1. Elevated levels of dsDNA-, Sm-, SSA/Ro- and SSB/La-specific IgE antibodies in SLE subjects versus healthy controls. A. Relative levels from a combined analysis of the US and French SLE cohorts for IgE antibody levels to the four aforementioned antigens. Mann Whitney test was used to compare the different groups. Mean ± SEM is shown. AU, Arbitrary Units. $^{**}p<0.01$; $^{****}p<0.0001$. **B.** Prevalence of IgE

autoantibodies to the aforementioned four common SLE autoantigens. Percentage of patients positive for IgE autoantibodies (2SD over the mean of healthy controls) to at least one of the four autoantigens tested. dsDNA-specific IgE (as the most prevalent autoreactive IgE) was used as the reference. The percent of anti-Sm IgE positive individuals are those without dsDNA-IgE, percent of anti-SSA/Ro positive individuals are without dsDNA- and Sm-IgE's, and anti-SSB/La positive individuals are those without dsDNA, Sm and SSA/Ro reactivties. Therefore, patients in the group of those positive for anti-dsDNA IgE were also positive for the rest of IgE autoantibodies tested, but none of the subjects in the anti-SSB/La IgE positive group had detectable IgE autoantibodies for dsDNA, Sm, or SSA/Ro.

IgE's, but not IgG's, to novel self-antigens that are linked with hypocomplementemia, a serological marker of disease activity. The findings demonstrate that autoreactive IgE is prevalent in SLE and suggest that its detection together with anti-dsDNA IgG, may serve to better predict increased disease activity and/or poor kidney function.

Materials and Methods

Studied Cohorts

This collaborative study was approved by the Institutional Review Board of NIAMS (NIH, Bethesda, USA) and by the Comité Régional de Protection des Personnes (CRPP, Paris, France). A written consent was obtained from all healthy donors and SLE patients. In the US, samples were obtained from SLE patients enrolled in a long-term natural history study of SLE. In France SLE samples were obtained from in- and out- patients enrolled in a long term prospective study of SLE, and clinical data were used after approval by the Comission Nationale de l'Informatique et des Libertés (CNIL). All patients fulfilled the American College of Rheumatology classification criteria for SLE [7,15]. Samples from "healthy" volunteers were obtained from the blood bank at the NIH Clinical Center and from the Université Paris Diderot, Faculté de Médecine site Bichat. The demographics and characteristics of all SLE patients and healthy controls are summarized in Table 1. The data included herein is from one sample provided by each individual SLE subject.

Sample Collection

Whole blood from SLE and healthy donors was collected in 4 ml SST (serum-separating tube) tube for serum. Serum samples were aliquoted and kept at −80°C.

Enzyme-linked Immunosorbent Assays (ELISAs)

The level of antibodies against the four common nuclear antigens (dsDNA, Sm, Ro/SSA, La/SSB) was measured by an ELISA. Horseradish peroxidase-conjugated antibodies to human IgE (Mouse monoclonal anti-human IgE, Immunology Consultants Laboratory) or IgG (Donkey anti-human IgG, Fc fragment specific, Jackson Immunoresearch Laboratory) were used for colorimetric detection was with tetramethylbenzidine substrate (TMB, Invitrogen) and optical density (OD) was measured at 450 nm. Positive values were considered as greater than two standard deviations over the mean absorption units obtained from samples of healthy individuals. dsDNA-specific IgG levels were quantified using standard laboratory procedures by the NIH Clinical Center and by the INSERM U699 Total levels of IgE were determined by ELISA (Calbiotech, for US; Bethyl Laboratories for France) following the manufacturers' instructions.

To determine the level of IgG and IgE autoantibodies to CLIP4, MPG and APEX nuclease 1, we used purified recombinant human proteins, CLIP4 (RSNL2 protein, Abnova), MPG (DNA-3 methyladenine glycosylase, Mybiosource), and APEX nuclease 1 (DNA apurinic or apyrimidinic site lyase, Mybiosource) in ELISA. Detection of reactive autoantibodies was as described above.

Protein Microarray

A Protoarray Human Protein Microarray v5.0 (Invitrogen Life Technologies) with over 9000 purified human proteins was used for novel antigen discovery. The purified recombinant proteins spotted on nitrocellulose-coated glass slides were reacted with the serum of SLE subjects or healthy controls and subsequently incubated with biotinylated goat anti-human IgE antibody (5 µg/ml) (Vector Laboratories) to detect IgE antibody binding. Then either an AlexaFluor 647-conjugated streptavidin (Invitrogen, 1 µg/ml) or an AlexaFluor 647-conjugated anti-V5 antibody (Invitrogen, 0.1 µg/ml) was added for detection and normalization, respectively. Arrays were scanned using fluorescent microarray GenePix 4000B Scanner and GenePix 6.0 software was used for data acquisition. Data analysis was done using Invitrogens proprietary Protoarray Prospector software. For each protein spotted in every array, Z-Score, Z-factor, CI-P value (Chebyshevs Inequality p-Value) was measured. M-Statistic is used to identify those proteins which show a significant differential signal between two populations. The "cutoff" value used corresponded to the value of 200 RFU above the M-Statistic signal threshold established for a specific protein.

Statistics

Student *t* test or a non-parametric Mann-Whitney U-test (when necessary) was used to compare SLE and control samples. A Chi2 assessment of the non-parametric Fisher exact test was used to determine the association of autoreactive IgE with active nephritis as well as the association of autoreactive IgE with active disease. One-way ANOVA with Bonferroni correction test or Kruskal-Wallis with Dunns correction test was applied when more than two groups were compared. Mean and SEM is shown in the scatter plot graphs. The analysis was performed using Graphpad Prism 5.0. Grubbs' outlier test was used to assess the outliers. In some instances some outliers detected in the healthy control group were excluded from the analysis because of the identification of allergic disease or a urine infection and no clinical indications of these conditions in the studied SLE subjects. For forest plot analysis, a fixed effects model was applied and Hedges g statistics was used to calculate the standardized mean difference (SMD).

Stepwise Logistic Regression offered by IBM SPSS Statistics 20 software was used to determine a predictive model of disease activity (Not active, SLEDAI$<$4 vs Active, SLEDAI$\geq$4). Probability to enter a predictor in the model $p<0.1$ and to remove it $p>0.05$. Model 1 included as predictors: positive levels of dsDNA IgE, Sm IgE, SSA/Ro IgE, SSB/La IgE, dsDNA IgG, Sm IgG, SSA/Ro IgG and SSB/La IgG; as confounders age, gender and ethnicity (African American/African, European descendent, Hispanic and others). Model 2 included as predictors: positive levels of autoreactive IgEs, autoreactive IgGs (positive for at least one of the autoantibodies against the four common antigens); as confounders age, gender and ethnicity. Factors not affecting the models were eliminated from consideration. ROC Curve with AUC (area under the curve) analysis and Youden's J Index was calculated by IBM SPSS in order to determine the optimal predictive model selection.

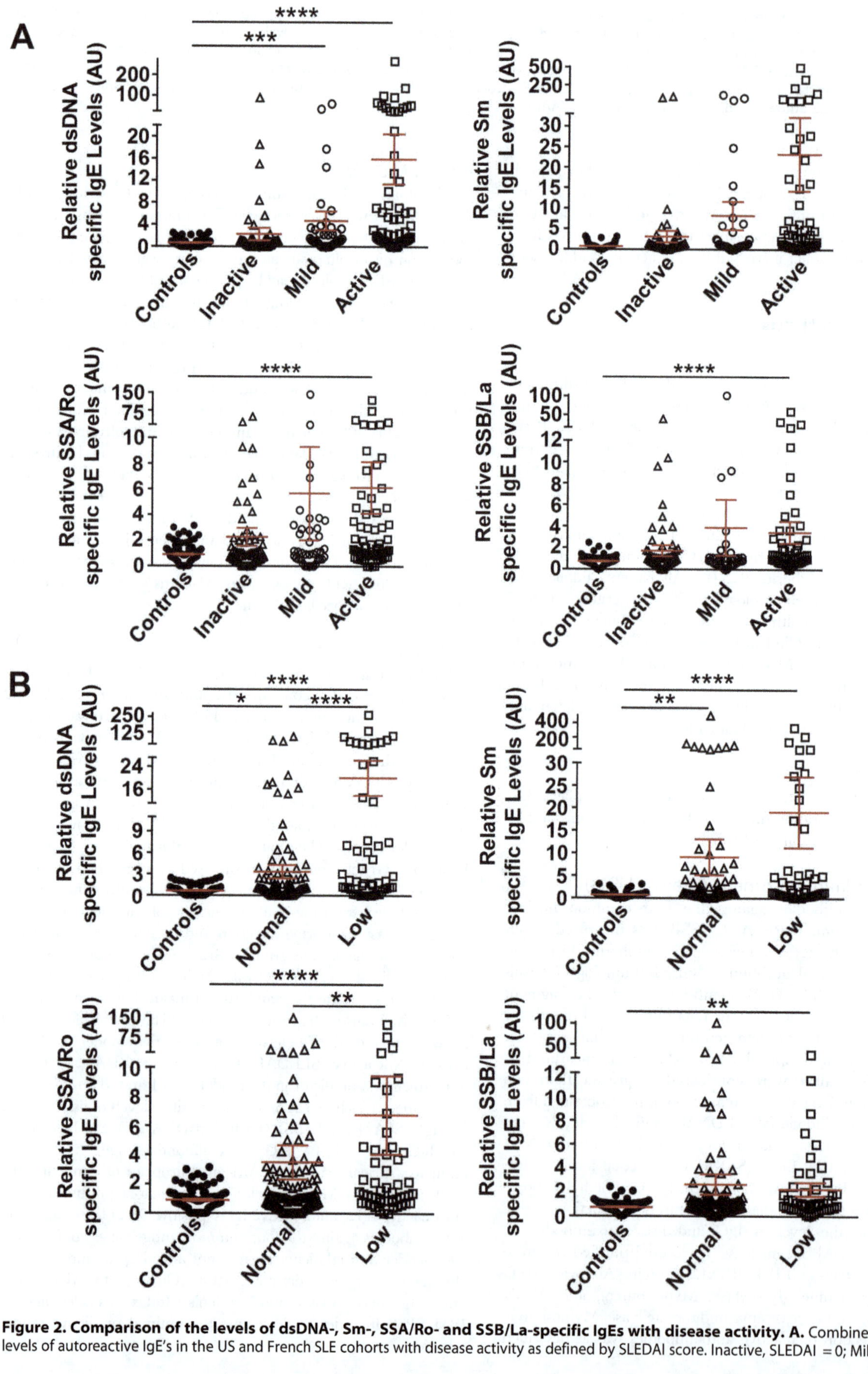

Figure 2. Comparison of the levels of dsDNA-, Sm-, SSA/Ro- and SSB/La-specific IgEs with disease activity. A. Combined analysis of the levels of autoreactive IgE's in the US and French SLE cohorts with disease activity as defined by SLEDAI score. Inactive, SLEDAI = 0; Mild, SLEDAI >0 to

<4; Active, SLEDAI ≥4. **B.** Combined US and French SLE cohort analysis of IgE autoantibodies with complement levels in serum. Low levels of complement were considered as C3<80 mg/dl or C4<15 mg/dl. Kruskal-Wallis with Dunn's multiple comparisons test was used to compare the different groups. Mean ± SEM is shown. AU, Arbitrary Units. *p<0.05; **p<0.01; ***p<0.001; ****p<0.0001.

Results

IgE Auto-antibodies to Common SLE Antigens are Prevalent

The characteristics and demographics of both French and US SLE subjects studied herein are described in Table 1. French SLE subjects were recruited through a long term prospective study of SLE from a primary care center whereas US SLE subjects were part of a long term natural history study of SLE in a secondary care center. Thus, while the mean age of each cohort was similar, the mean years of disease duration was somewhat less in the French subjects (13.5±8.5) versus US subjects (16.6±11.9) and French subjects had a higher SLEDAI score (>9) than US subjects (>4). As might be expected, given that the US subjects were recruited from a secondary care center, only 13 of the 117 US subjects (~11%) had active nephritis whereas 30 of the 79 French subjects (~38%) were active. Treatment regimens were similar in the two cohorts with the exception that a greater number of French subjects (45) were on cyclophosphamide than US subjects (4). The two cohorts also differed in their ethnic composition with fewer Hispanics and Asians present among the French subjects.

It was not known if IgE autoantibodies are generated to all of the antigens most frequently detected in the serologic profile of SLE. Thus, we assayed for the presence of dsDNA, Sm, SSA/Ro and SSB/La in both US and French SLE cohorts. IgE autoantibodies to all four self-antigens were present with anti-dsDNA and anti-Sm IgE antibodies having the most significant association with SLE relative to healthy controls (Figure 1A). Analysis of the overall frequency of all SLE patients with autoreactive IgE positivity (a minimum of one auto-antigen specific IgE) demonstrated a frequency of over 57% (Figure 1B) with the US SLE cohort approaching 53% and the French cohort at 63%. Thus, 47% of the US cohort and 37% of the French cohort did not show IgE reactivity to one of the four auto-antigens tested. Of the four autoantigen specificities, dsDNA specific-IgE was the most frequent with 34.2% and 49.4% of the US and French cohorts, respectively, having this autoantibody (Figure 1B). To test whether the two cohorts had similar characteristics with regards to autoreactive IgE's we performed a forest plot (Figure S1 in File S1) and found no heterogeneity ($I^2 = 0\%$) in the levels of IgE autoantibodies among the cohorts and no significant difference was observed in the effect of the autoreactive IgE on the two cohorts relative to healthy controls as shown by the overall standardized mean difference (SMD) for each individual autoreactive IgE. This argues that the two cohorts showed similar differences in levels of autoreactive IgE relative to healthy controls and that the distribution of the detected autoreactive IgE is similar in these two cohorts. No meaningful differences in the levels of IgE autoantibodies were detected when either gender or ethnicity were considered and no correlation was found between the total levels

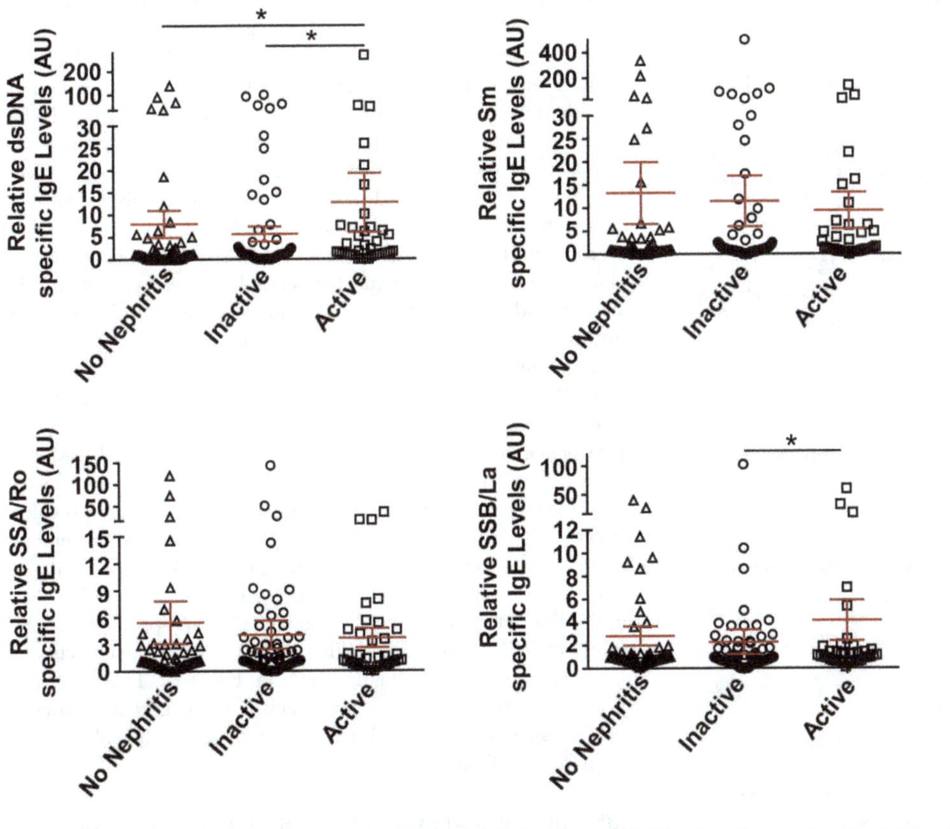

Figure 3. Association of autoreactive IgE's with lupus nephritis. Relative levels of dsDNA-, Sm-, SSA/Ro- and SSB/La-specific IgE autoantibodies in the combined US and French SLE cohort with no nephritis, inactive or active nephritis. Kruskal-Wallis with Dunn's multiple comparisons test was used to compare the different groups. Mean ± SEM is shown. AU, Arbitrary Units. *p<0.05.

Table 2. Correlation of positive levels of autoreactive IgEs and IgGs with disease activity (Active SLEDAI≥4, No Active SLEDAI<4). Analysis of the combined US and French cohorts.

		Anti-dsDNA IgE		Anti-Sm IgE		Anti-Ro/SSA IgE		Anti-La/SSB IgE		Autoreactive IgEs	
		Neg	Pos	Neg	Pos	Neg	Pos	Neg	Pos	Neg	Pos
Active Disease	**No**	90	33	93	28	92	29	99	22	51	32
		(73.2%)	(26.8%)	(76.8%)	(23.1%)	(76.1%)	(23.9%)	(81.8%)	(18.2%)	(61.4%)	(38.5%)
	Yes	27	46	38	33	42	29	45	26	19	54
		(36.9%)	(63.1%)	(53.5%)	(46.5%)	(59.2%)	(40.8%)	(63.4%)	(36.6%)	(26.0%)	(73.9%)
	p value	p<0.0001		p = 0.0008		p = 0.014		p = 0.0044		p<0.0001	
	OR (95% CI)	4.64 (2.49–8.64)		2.84 (1.54–5.41)		2.19 (1.16–4.12)		2.6 (1.33–5.07)		4.53 (2.28–8.98)	
		Anti-dsDNA IgG		**Anti-Sm IgG**		**Anti-Ro/SSA IgG**		**Anti-La/SSB IgG**		**Autoreactive IgGs**	
		Neg	Pos	Neg	Pos	Neg	Pos	Neg	Pos	Neg	Pos
Active Disease	**No**	85	38	75	46	72	49	95	26	38	45
		(69.1%)	(31.2%)	(61.9%)	(38.0%)	(59.5%)	(40.5%)	(78.5%)	(21.5%)	(45.8%)	(54.2%)
	Yes	25	48	31	40	29	42	48	23	10	63
		(34.2%)	(65.7%)	(43.7%)	(56.3%)	(40.8%)	(59.1%)	(67.6%)	(32.3%)	(13.7%)	(86.3%)
	p value	p<0.0001		p = 0.013		p = 0.012		p = 0.09		p<0.0001	
	OR (95% CI)	4.29 (2.32–7.95)		2.10 (1.16–3.82)		2.13 (1.17–3.86)		1.75 (0.90–3.38)		5.32 (2.40–11.78)	

OR, Odds Ratio.
CI, Confidence Interval.

of IgE and the levels of IgE autoantibodies in these cohorts (data not shown).

IgE Autoantibodies are Associated with Increased Disease Activity

The relationship between disease activity and the presence of any one of the four auto-antigen specific IgE's was explored. Disease activity was based on a SLEDAI score of ≥4 as active disease, >0 to <4 for mild disease, and 0 for inactive. As shown in Figure 2A, SLE subjects with autoreactive IgE's were most frequently found in the active disease group. SLE subjects with mild disease also had significantly elevated levels of IgE autoantibodies to dsDNA (Figure 2A).

Table 3. Adjusted results of Multivariate analysis by Stepwise Logistic Regression.

		p value	OR	95% CI	AUC	Youdens J
Model 1	dsDNA IgE	p = 0.004	2.77	1.38–5.55		
	dsDNA IgG	p<0.001	3.43	1.72–6.85	0.769	0.37
	Age	p = 0.008	0.97	0.94–0.99		
Model 2	IgEs Pos	p = 0.011	2.39	1.22–4.67		
	IgGs Pos	p = 0.022	2.58	1.14–5.81	0.735	0.32
	Age	p = 0.003	0.97	0.94–0.99		

ROC curve and Youden's J Index analysis of both models.
OR, Odds Ratio.
CI, Confidence Interval.
AUC, Area under the curve.

To further verify the association of autoreactive IgE's with disease activity, we analyzed its relationship to hypocomplementemia, a commonly used serological marker of increased disease activity or disease relapses [16,17]. The levels of IgE autoantibodies to the tested autoantigens (dsDNA, Sm, SSA/Ro, SSB/La) were significantly elevated in SLE subjects with hypocomplementemia (C3<80 mg/dl, C4<15 mg/dl) (Figure 2B). However, dsDNA and Sm-specific IgE's were also significantly elevated in SLE subjects with normal complement levels. When the cohorts were analyzed individually, only ds-DNA-specific IgE showed a significant association with hypocomplementemia in both the French and US cohorts (data not shown), demonstrating that this autoreactive IgE is most significantly associated with hypocomplementemia.

While more than 50% of SLE subjects had autoreactive IgE to one or more of the four common SLE auto-antigens, the prevalence of these IgE's in active SLE subjects (SLEDAI ≥4) was 73.7% and 74.1% for the French and US subjects, respectively, with dsDNA specific-IgE being the most prevalent (US = 62.8%, French = 63.2%) (Figure S2A in File S1). When we analyzed the prevalence of these autoreactive IgE's in SLE subjects with hypocomplementemia, it was higher in the French cohort (90%) than in the US cohort (72%) with dsDNA-specific IgE being found in 60% of the US and 80% of the French SLE subjects with hypocomplementemia (Figure S2B in File S1). These findings argue that the presence of autoreactive IgE's (and in particular dsDNA-specific IgE) in SLE may be a reasonable clinical indicator of increased disease activity.

IgE Autoantibodies are Associated with Active Nephritis and Other Clinical Parameters of Disease Activity

Forty three of the 196 SLE subjects under study were determined to have active nephritis based on a protein/creatinine

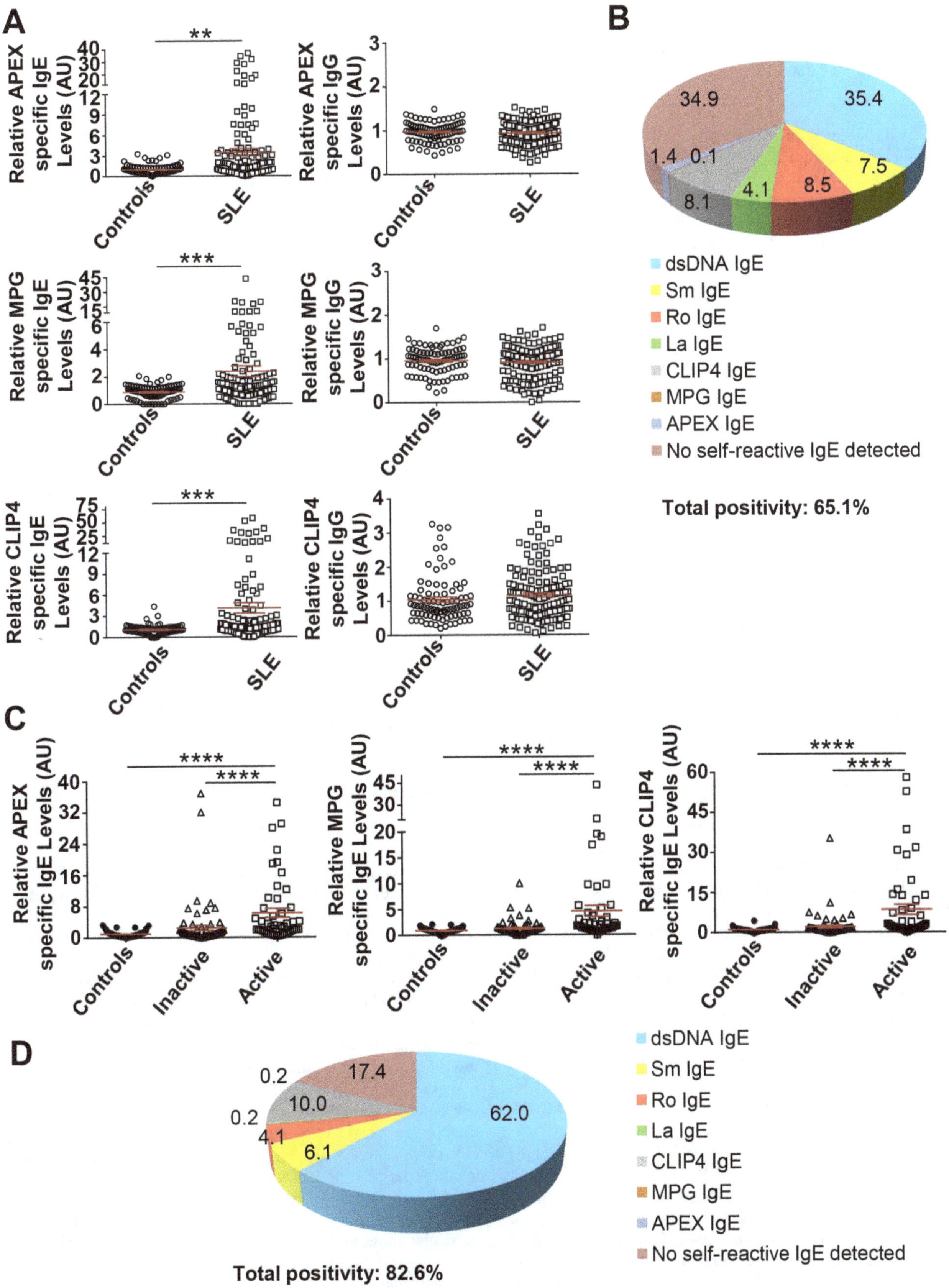

Figure 4. Identification of novel IgE autoantigens in SLE, overall prevalence, and association of all tested autoreactive IgE's with SLE disease activity. A. Relative levels of APEX, MPG and CLIP4 specific IgEs and IgGs in US and French SLE cohorts. **B.** Overall prevalence of IgE autoantibodies in SLE for seven tested autoantigens tested (dsDNA, Sm, SSA/Ro and SSB/La, APEX, MPG and CLIP4). **C.** Comparison of the levels of all

tested autoreactive IgE antibodies (as in B) in US and French cohorts with disease activity as measured by SLEDAI score. Inactive, SLEDAI =0; Mild, SLEDAI >0 to <4; Active, SLEDAI ≥4. **D.** Prevalence of all tested autoreactive IgE's in US and French SLE subjects with active disease. Mann Whitney test or Kruskal-Wallis with Dunn's multiple comparisons test (more than two groups) was used to compare the different groups. Mean ± SEM is shown. **p<0.01; ***p<0.001, ****p<0.0001.

ratio of ≥0.5, positivity for dsDNA IgG, and hypocomplementemia. As shown in Figure 3, a significant association of active nephritis with increased levels of dsDNA–specific IgE's (no nephritis vs active nephritis, p = 0.02) was observed. If the analysis is limited to those individuals in the combined cohort who were positive for increased levels of autoreactive IgE's (Table S1 in File S1), the association with dsDNA-IgE was highly significant. Univariate analysis of the individual cohorts (Table S1 in File S1) revealed no significant association in the US SLE subjects, even for dsDNA-specific IgE (p = 0.20). In contrast, in French cohort where 30 of 79 SLE subjects (~38%) had active nephritis, both dsDNA and Sm- specific IgE's showed a significant association (p = 0.017 and 0.021, respectively) with this clinical diagnosis (Table S1 in File S1).

Since the titer of circulating IgG autoantibodies (in particular dsDNA-specific IgG) is known to be associated with SLE disease activity, we set out to compare the relationship of autoreactive IgG and IgE with disease activity. Analysis of SLE subjects, with active disease, having positivity for autoreactive IgE or IgG to the four common SLE autoantigens showed a similar significance (p< 0.0001) in the association of anti-dsDNA IgE or IgG with active disease (Table 2). However, anti-Sm IgE showed a more significant association with active disease than anti-Sm IgG (p = 0.0008 vs. p = 0.013) and anti-SSB/La IgE also showed a significant (p = 0.0044) association whereas the association of its IgG counterpart did not achieve significance (Table 2).

Analysis of the predictive value of autoreactive IgE's or IgG's for active disease in SLE subjects demonstrated that anti-dsDNA IgE and anti-dsDNA IgG were significant in predicting SLE subjects with active disease (Table 3, AUC = 0.769, Youden's J = 0.37), compared to the individual analysis of each of the predictors (dsDNA-IgE: AUC = 0.72, Youden's J = 0.36; dsDNA-IgG: AUC = 0.737, Youden's J = 0.347). However, anti-dsDNA IgG was a modestly stronger predictor (OR adjusted = 3.43 versus OR 2.77 for anti-dsDNA IgE) perhaps due to inclusion of dsDNA-IgG's as a determinant of SLEDAI. Inclusion of autoreactive IgG's and IgE's with other specificities (Sm, SSA/Ro, SSB/La) reduced the overall sensitivity of the model indicating that these were not strong indicators of disease activity (data not shown). Introduction of ethnicity, gender, and age as confounding factors revealed that only age influenced the predictive model (Table 3). Thus, the findings show that, like anti-dsDNA IgG, anti-dsDNA IgE is useful in predicting disease activity and the use of both of these autoantibodies increases the predictive ability (Table 3).

Discovery of Novel Auto-antigens for IgE in SLE and their Relationship with Disease Activity

Roughly, 40–50% of SLE subjects tested did not have IgE autoantibodies to the four common SLE autoantigens (Figure 1B). To explore whether IgE antibodies to other autoantigens might be present in these subjects, we used Invitrogen's ProtoArray to screen the sera of subjects from both the US and French cohort. As shown in Figure 4A, high levels of IgE autoantibodies to APEX nuclease 1 (APEX), N-methylpurine-DNA glycosylase (MPG), and CAP-GLY domain containing linker protein family member 4 (CLIP4) were found in some SLE subjects but were minimally detected in healthy controls. The difference in the relative amounts of these IgE autoantibodies between healthy controls and SLE subjects was significant. Minimal levels of IgG antibodies to these autoantigens were detected and no changes in their levels were observed in SLE subjects (Figure 4A). Inclusion of SLE subjects with these novel IgE reactivities with those having at least one of the four common SLE autoantibodies increased the prevalence of autoreactive IgE's from approximately 57% (Figure 1B) to 65% (Figure 4B). Analysis of the association between these new IgE autoantibodies with disease activity revealed a highly significant association of APEX-, MPG-, and CLIP4–specific IgE's with active disease (Figure 4C). Approximately 74% of SLE subjects who had active disease also had IgE's that reacted to the four common SLE autoantigens (Figure S2A in File S1). The inclusion of IgE reactivity to at least one or more of the three novel autoantigens increased the proportion of active SLE subjects with these autoantibodies to almost 83% (Figure 4D). Thus, a large majority of SLE subjects with active disease have the presence of a circulating autoreactive IgE. Autoreactive IgE's to APEX, MPG, and CLIP4 also showed a highly significant association with hypocomplementemia (Figure S3A in File S1) and with active nephritis (Figure S3B in File S1).

Of the 146 SLE subjects analyzed from the US and French cohort who were positive for autoreactive IgE's to all seven autoantigens tested, 94 were positive for increased levels of autoreactive IgE whereas 107 were found to have increased levels of autoreactive IgG's. Of this latter group, 76 subjects (71.1%) were positive for both (Figure S4A in File S1). Of the autoantigens tested, dsDNA-specific IgG and IgE and Sm-specific IgG and IgE showed a significant (p = 0.046) or highly significant (p<0.0001) correlation, respectively (Figure S4B in File S1).

Discussion

It is well known that the presence of circulating autoantibodies of the IgA, IgM, and IgG isotypes are found in SLE. Moreover, the presence of circulating IgE autoantibodies has also been reported [10]. The presence of this diverse immunoglobulin response is not surprising given that SLE is characterized by abnormalities that involve hyperactive B and T cells (as well as other cell types like monocytes) resulting in polyclonal B-cell activation, increased numbers of plasma cells and autoantibody production. The mechanistic role of the different immunoglobulin isotypes in the onset and progression of SLE is, for the most part, still unclear. However, clues are emerging from studies in both mouse models and human disease. For example, IgA autoantibodies to phospholipids (anti-cardiolipin) have been shown to be a risk factor for thrombosis in SLE [18,19] and in some SLE patients dsDNA-specific IgA is linked to active disease [20,21,22]. However, there are also reports that incidence of IgA-deficiency (characterized by the lack of IgA-producing B cells) is also higher in SLE and in such cases there appears to be no association to clinical parameters of disease [23,24]. IgM autoantibodies (and in particular those to dsDNA) are also frequent in lupus. However, unlike their IgG counterpart, anti-dsDNA IgM appears to be inversely linked to the development of nephritis [25] and in mouse models there is evidence that such autoantibodies may have a protective role [26]. It has been proposed that the ratio of IgG/IgM anti-dsDNA antibodies might be a useful prognostic marker for lupus nephritis [27], although rigorous studies to test this hypothesis are yet to be conducted. The levels of IgG autoantibodies to dsDNA in serum are known to fluctuate with disease activity in SLE and they often increase prior to the flaring of disease activity. Because of their prevalence and specificity in SLE and their association with disease activity as well as with lupus nephritis, elevated levels of anti-dsDNA IgG is one accepted criterion in the diagnosis of SLE. In fact, anti-dsDNA of the IgG subclass is also frequently found in the kidney of SLE subjects with nephritis [28,29] and some of these autoantibodies have been shown in various animal models to have pathogenicity [30,31].

An understanding of the role of IgE autoantibodies in this disease and their link to clinical parameters of disease has been lacking. In the present work, we set out to rigorously explore the prevalence and the relevance of autoreactive IgE in SLE. Here, we find that autoreactive IgE to four common and three newly identified SLE autoantigens is present in 65% of SLE subjects as determined in both the US and French cohorts. This frequency is increased to almost 83% when one limits the cohort analysis to only SLE subjects with active disease, demonstrating that the prevalence of autoreactive IgE's in SLE is not only common but that it is most often found in individuals with active disease. The findings clearly establish a link between autoreactive IgE and active nephritis, consistent with our previous preliminary results [12,32], but also extend the previous findings by demonstrating that autoreactive IgE may be a reasonable predictor of SLE disease activity. Perhaps, the most unexpected finding of this study is that anti-dsDNA IgE can serve as a predictor of active disease and in combination with anti-dsDNA IgG enhances the predictive value. These findings suggest that measurement of the serum levels of autoreactive IgE's (in combination with autoreactive IgG's) may perhaps be a useful and more sensitive criterion in the diagnosis of SLE but further studies are clearly required.

An important question that remains to be addressed is the role of IgE in human SLE disease pathology. Although, some studies have demonstrated the presence of IgE in the kidney of SLE subjects [33] these reports are limited and the occurrence appears to be infrequent. This is consistent with mouse models of spontaneous lupus (such as the *lyn*$^{-/-}$ mice) where detection of IgE in the kidney has been difficult. One must also consider that the concentration of IgE in both the circulation and tissues is extremely low and that this immunoglobulin does not fix complement (a major participant in tissue damage in the lupus kidney), thus the pathological consequence of any IgE deposition in the kidney is unclear and the contribution of IgE to tissue damage would most likely occur through induction of proinflammatory responses. While the relationship between autoreactive IgE and autoantibody production in human disease is difficult to unravel, our current analysis on the combined cohorts tested for the common SLE autoantigens uncovered evidence of a significant correlation between increased levels of autoreactive IgE and increased levels of autoreactive IgG (Figure S4 in File S1). Since the absolute levels of autoreactive IgG's or other immunoglobulins produced by a given SLE subject is highly variable (and influenced by the genetic makeup of the individual), evidence of a significant correlation in the levels of these two immunoglobulins was rather unexpected. This demonstrates that even in the presence of the multiple variables that can influence immunoglobulin responses in SLE, high levels of IgE are significantly correlated with the presence of high levels of IgG and vice versa, suggesting intimate co-regulation and perhaps supporting and/or complementary roles in disease progression.

Conclusions

Increased IgE production has been documented in various autoimmune, inflammatory, and genetic diseases [34,35], but beyond the role of IgE in allergic inflammation there is a lack of knowledge on the role of IgE in such diseases. The analysis conducted herein advances the relevance of IgE beyond allergies. It demonstrates that the incidence of autoreactive IgE in cohorts of both US and French SLE subjects is common and that IgE antibodies are generated to the common SLE autoantigens, as well as to autoantigens that appear to selectively elicit IgE and not IgG responses. The current analysis also demonstrates a significant relationship between the presence of high levels of autoreactive IgE, active disease and lupus nephritis. It suggests that autoreactive IgE (perhaps in combination with autoreactive IgG) may serve as a potential predictor of SLE. Replication of these findings in larger cohorts is essential. Moreover, longitudinal studies to assess the relationship of autoreactive IgE's with disease onset or flares is necessary to ascertain its true relevance to disease activity and as potential predictors of disease onset. Additional studies are also required to determine the importance of autoreactive IgE's, if any, in the development of lupus nephritis. Nonetheless, the findings clearly extend the relevance of IgE beyond allergies and demonstrate that autoantibody production of the IgE subclass is not rare in lupus, and perhaps is present in other autoimmunities.

Supporting Information

File S1 This file contains Figure S1–S4 and Table S1. Figure S1, Combined analysis of US and French cohorts demonstrates similarities in the distribution of autoreactive IgE's in the two cohorts. The forest plot represented, used a fixed-effect model of the mean relative levels of dsDNA, Sm, SSA/Ro and SSB/La IgE autoantibodies for the two distinct cohorts. SMD, standardized mean difference. Figure S2, High prevalence of IgE autoantibodies in SLE subjects with active disease. The prevalence of IgE autoantibodies to dsDNA, Sm, SSA/Ro and SSB/La in SLE subjects with active disease (SLEDAI $\geq$4) (A) or in SLE subjects with hypocomplementenemia (B, C3<80 mg/dl or C4<15 mg/dl) is shown. The percent of SLE subjects with positive dsDNA IgE levels was the reference point. Percent of subjects with Sm IgE had no dsDNA IgE, percent of subjects with SSA/Ro IgE had no dsDNA or Sm IgE, and the percent of subjects with SSB/La IgE had no detectable levels of dsDNA, Sm or SSA/Ro IgE. Figure S3, Association of novel autoreactive IgE levels (APEX, MPG and CLIP4) with nephritis (A) and complement levels (B). Low levels of complement were defined as C3<80 mg/dl or C4<15 mg/dl. Kruskal-Wallis with Dunn's multiple comparisons test was used to compare the different groups. AU, Arbitrary Units. Mean ± SEM is shown. *p<0.05; **p<0.01; ***p<0.001; ****p<0.0001. Figure S4, Increased levels of dsDNA and Sm –specific IgE's are associated with increased levels of their respective IgG counterparts. A. Analysis of the relationship between IgE and IgG in SLE subjects positive for all seven autoantigens (dsDNA, Sm, SSA/Ro, SSB/La, APEX, MPG, and CLIP4) tested in this study. Stacked bar (left panel) and analysis (table, right panel) of the combined number of French and US SLE subjects. Positivity was considered as a value over the mean +2SD of healthy controls for at least one of the aforementioned autoantigens. B. Spearman correlation between autoreactive IgE and IgG levels for dsDNA and Sm in the group of subjects with double positivity shown on a logarithmic scale. Table S1, Correlation of positive levels of autoreactive IgE with active nephritis. Analysis of the combined and individual US and French cohorts.

Acknowledgments

The authors wish to acknowledge the invaluable support of the Office of the Clinical Director, National Institute of Arthritis and Musculoskeletal and Skin Diseases, National Institutes of Health.

Author Contributions

Conceived and designed the experiments: BD NC SH ED GI JR. Performed the experiments: BD CP MMB JS CJ TKR. Analyzed the data: BD NG MMB SH GI NC JR. Contributed reagents/materials/analysis tools: SH KS MJ DG TP ED. Wrote the paper: BD SH NG MJ DG ED GI NC JR.

References

1. Frieri M (2013) Mechanisms of disease for the clinician: systemic lupus erythematosus. Ann Allergy Asthma Immunol 110: 228–232.
2. Sawalha AH, Harley JB (2004) Antinuclear autoantibodies in systemic lupus erythematosus. Curr Opin Rheumatol 16: 534–540.
3. Arbuckle MR, McClain MT, Rubertone MV, Scofield RH, Dennis GJ, et al. (2003) Development of autoantibodies before the clinical onset of systemic lupus erythematosus. N Engl J Med 349: 1526–1533.
4. Rahman A, Isenberg DA (2008) Systemic lupus erythematosus. N Engl J Med 358: 929–939.
5. Schroeder K, Herrmann M, Winkler TH (2012) The role of somatic hypermutation in the generation of pathogenic antibodies in SLE. Autoimmunity 46: 121–127.
6. Kalaaji M, Fenton KA, Mortensen ES, Olsen R, Sturfelt G, et al. (2007) Glomerular apoptotic nucleosomes are central target structures for nephritogenic antibodies in human SLE nephritis. Kidney Int 71: 664–672.
7. Hochberg MC (1997) Updating the American College of Rheumatology revised criteria for the classification of systemic lupus erythematosus. Arthritis Rheum 40: 1725.
8. Capron A, Dessaint JP (1977) IgE and cells in protective immunity. Pathol Biol (Paris) 25: 287–290.
9. Blank U, Rivera J (2004) The ins and outs of IgE-dependent mast-cell exocytosis. Trends Immunol 25: 266–273.
10. Permin H, Wiik A (1978) The prevalence of IgE antinuclear antibodies in rheumatoid arthritis and systemic lupus erythematosus. Acta Pathol Microbiol Scand C 86C: 245–249.
11. Atta AM, Santiago MB, Guerra FG, Pereira MM, Sousa Atta ML (2010) Autoimmune response of IgE antibodies to cellular self-antigens in systemic Lupus Erythematosus. Int Arch Allergy Immunol 152: 401–406.
12. Charles N, Hardwick D, Daugas E, Illei GG, Rivera J (2010) Basophils and the T helper 2 environment can promote the development of lupus nephritis. Nat Med 16: 701–707.
13. Bosch X, Lozano F, Cervera R, Ramos-Casals M, Min B (2011) Basophils, IgE, and autoantibody-mediated kidney disease. J Immunol 186: 6083–6090.
14. Rodriguez Gomez M, Talke Y, Goebel N, Hermann F, Reich B, et al. (2010) Basophils support the survival of plasma cells in mice. J Immunol 185: 7180–7185.
15. Tan EM, Cohen AS, Fries JF, Masi AT, McShane DJ, et al. (1982) The 1982 revised criteria for the classification of systemic lupus erythematosus. Arthritis Rheum 25: 1271–1277.
16. Kallenberg CG, Stegeman CA, Bootsma H, Bijl M, Limburg PC (2006) Quantitation of autoantibodies in systemic autoimmune diseases: clinically useful? Lupus 15: 397–402.
17. Livingston B, Bonner A, Pope J (2012) Differences in autoantibody profiles and disease activity and damage scores between childhood- and adult-onset systemic lupus erythematosus: a meta-analysis. Semin Arthritis Rheum 42: 271–280.
18. Sweiss NJ, Bo R, Kapadia R, Manst D, Mahmood F, et al. (2010) IgA anti-beta2-glycoprotein I autoantibodies are associated with an increased risk of thromboembolic events in patients with systemic lupus erythematosus. PLoS One 5: e12280.
19. Mehrani T, Petri M (2011) Association of IgA Anti-beta2 glycoprotein I with clinical and laboratory manifestations of systemic lupus erythematosus. J Rheumatol 38: 64–68.
20. Miltenburg AM, Roos A, Slegtenhorst L, Daha MR, Breedveld FC (1993) IgA anti-dsDNA antibodies in systemic lupus erythematosus: occurrence, incidence and association with clinical and laboratory variables of disease activity. J Rheumatol 20: 53–58.
21. Witte T, Hartung K, Matthias T, Sachse C, Fricke M, et al. (1998) Association of IgA anti-dsDNA antibodies with vasculitis and disease activity in systemic lupus erythematosus. SLE Study Group. Rheumatol Int 18: 63–69.
22. Villalta D, Bizzaro N, Bassi N, Zen M, Gatto M, et al. (2013) Anti-dsDNA antibody isotypes in systemic lupus erythematosus: IgA in addition to IgG anti-dsDNA help to identify glomerulonephritis and active disease. PLoS One 8: e71458.
23. Latiff AH, Kerr MA (2007) The clinical significance of immunoglobulin A deficiency. Ann Clin Biochem 44: 131–139.
24. Mantovani AP, Monclaro MP, Skare TL (2010) Prevalence of IgA deficiency in adult systemic lupus erythematosus and the study of the association with its clinical and autoantibody profiles. Rev Bras Rheumatol 50: 273–282.
25. Witte T, Hartung K, Sachse C, Matthias T, Fricke M, et al. (1998) IgM anti-dsDNA antibodies in systemic lupus erythematosus: negative association with nephritis. SLE Study Group. Rheumatol Int 18: 85–91.
26. Werwitzke S, Trick D, Kamino K, Matthias T, Kniesch K, et al. (2005) Inhibition of lupus disease by anti-double-stranded DNA antibodies of the IgM isotype in the (NZB x NZW)F1 mouse. Arthritis Rheum 52: 3629–3638.
27. Forger F, Matthias T, Oppermann M, Becker H, Helmke K (2004) Clinical significance of anti-dsDNA antibody isotypes: IgG/IgM ratio of anti-dsDNA antibodies as a prognostic marker for lupus nephritis. Lupus 13: 36–44.
28. Kenderov A, Minkova V, Mihailova D, Giltiay N, Kyurkchiev S, et al. (2002) Lupus-specific kidney deposits of HSP90 are associated with altered IgG idiotypic interactions of anti-HSP90 autoantibodies. Clin Exp Immunol 129: 169–176.
29. Bijl M, Dijstelbloem HM, Oost WW, Bootsma H, Derksen RH, et al. (2002) IgG subclass distribution of autoantibodies differs between renal and extra-renal relapses in patients with systemic lupus erythematosus. Rheumatology (Oxford) 41: 62–67.
30. Madaio MP, Carlson J, Cataldo J, Ucci A, Migliorini P, et al. (1987) Murine monoclonal anti-DNA antibodies bind directly to glomerular antigens and form immune deposits. J Immunol 138: 2883–2889.
31. Pankewycz OG, Migliorini P, Madaio MP (1987) Polyreactive autoantibodies are nephritogenic in murine lupus nephritis. J Immunol 139: 3287–3294.
32. Charles N, Rivera J (2011) Basophils and autoreactive IgE in the pathogenesis of systemic lupus erythematosus. Current allergy and asthma reports 11: 378–387.
33. Tuma SN, Llach F, Sostrin S, Dubois EL, Massry SG (1981) Glomerular IgE deposits in patients with lupus nephritis. Am J Nephrol 1: 31–36.
34. Altin J, Shen C, Liston A (2010) Understanding the genetic regulation of IgE production. Blood Rev 24: 163–169.
35. Pate MB, Smith JK, Chi DS, Krishnaswamy G (2010) Regulation and dysregulation of immunoglobulin E: a molecular and clinical perspective. Clin Mol Allergy 8: 3.

16

RNA-Seq for Enrichment and Analysis of *IRF5* Transcript Expression in SLE

Rivka C. Stone[1,2], Peicheng Du[3], Di Feng[1,2], Kopal Dhawan[4], Lars Rönnblom[5], Maija-Leena Eloranta[5], Robert Donnelly[4], Betsy J. Barnes[1,2]*

1 Department of Biochemistry & Molecular Biology, New Jersey Medical School, UMDNJ, Newark, New Jersey, United States of America, **2** New Jersey Medical School-University Hospital Cancer Center, UMDNJ, Newark, New Jersey, United States of America, **3** High Performance and Research Computing, Department of Information Systems and Technology, UMDNJ, Newark, New Jersey, United States of America, **4** Molecular Resource Facility, New Jersey Medical School, UMDNJ, Newark, New Jersey, United States of America, **5** Department of Medical Sciences, Section of Rheumatology, Uppsala University, Uppsala, Sweden

Abstract

Polymorphisms in the interferon regulatory factor 5 (*IRF5*) gene have been consistently replicated and shown to confer risk for or protection from the development of systemic lupus erythematosus (SLE). IRF5 expression is significantly upregulated in SLE patients and upregulation associates with *IRF5*-SLE risk haplotypes. *IRF5* alternative splicing has also been shown to be elevated in SLE patients. Given that human *IRF5* exists as multiple alternatively spliced transcripts with distinct function(s), it is important to determine whether the *IRF5* transcript profile expressed in healthy donor immune cells is different from that expressed in SLE patients. Moreover, it is not currently known whether an *IRF5*-SLE risk haplotype defines the profile of *IRF5* transcripts expressed. Using standard molecular cloning techniques, we identified and isolated 14 new differentially spliced *IRF5* transcript variants from purified monocytes of healthy donors and SLE patients to generate an *IRF5* variant transcriptome. Next-generation sequencing was then used to perform in-depth and quantitative analysis of full-length *IRF5* transcript expression in primary immune cells of SLE patients and healthy donors by next-generation sequencing. Evidence for additional alternatively spliced transcripts was obtained from *de novo* junction discovery. Data from these studies support the overall complexity of *IRF5* alternative splicing in SLE. Results from next-generation sequencing correlated with cloning and gave similar abundance rankings in SLE patients thus supporting the use of this new technology for in-depth single gene transcript profiling. Results from this study provide the first proof that 1) SLE patients express an *IRF5* transcript signature that is distinct from healthy donors, 2) an *IRF5*-SLE risk haplotype defines the top four most abundant *IRF5* transcripts expressed in SLE patients, and 3) an *IRF5* transcript signature enables clustering of SLE patients with the H2 risk haplotype.

Editor: George C. Tsokos, Beth Israel Deaconess Medical Center, United States of America

Funding: This work was supported by grants from the National Institute of Health (NIH)/National Institute of Arthritis and Musculoskeletal and Skin Diseases (NIAMS; 5R03AR054070), the Arthritis Foundation and the Alliance for Lupus Research (to BJB), the Swedish Research Council, the Swedish Rheumatism Association, the Torsten and Ragnar Söderberg Foundation, the King Gustaf V 80-year Foundation and Combine, the Alliance for Lupus Research (to LR), and the King Gustaf V 80-year Foundation (to MLE). The funders had no role in study design, data collection and analysis, decision to publish, or preparation of the manuscript.

Competing Interests: The authors have declared that no competing interests exist.

* E-mail: barnesbe@umdnj.edu

Introduction

Systemic lupus erythematosus (SLE) is a complex systemic autoimmune disease characterized by elevated type I interferon (IFN) production, a break of immune tolerance to self-antigens, persistent production of pathogenic autoantibodies, complement activation, and immune complex (IC) deposition resulting in inflammation and end organ damage [1]. While the underlying etiology of SLE remains obscure, several lines of evidence document the importance of genetic factors [2–3]. One such factor, the interferon regulatory factor 5 (*IRF5*) gene, was identified in the susceptibility to develop SLE [4]. This initial finding, and the subsequent replication in numerous patient cohorts [4–10], marked an important break-through in our understanding of SLE pathogenesis given the critical role of IRF5 in regulating type I IFN expression and mediating Toll-like receptor (TLR) signaling [11–14]. Polymorphisms in the *IRF5* gene have been robustly associated with susceptibility to SLE in multiple populations with varying ethnic ancestries [4–10]. In each population, a distinct group of *IRF5* single nucleotide polymorphisms (SNPs) and genetic variants form haplotypes that confer risk for, or protection from, the development of SLE. It has recently been demonstrated that IRF5 expression and alternative splicing are significantly elevated in primary purified peripheral blood mononuclear cells (PBMC) from SLE patients; enhanced transcript and protein levels were associated with the *IRF5*-SLE H2 homozygous full risk haplotype in purified monocytes (Mo) [15]. The *IRF5*-SLE H2 haplotype consists of two copies of the 4xCGGGG promoter indel, the T-allele of SNP rs2004640, A-allele of SNP rs10954213, and C-allele of SNP rs10488631 [16]. Further studies have shown that *IRF5*-SLE risk haplotypes are associated with serum IFNα activity in SLE patients [17–18].

IRF5 is a member of the IRF family of transcription factors [11] and exists as multiple alternatively spliced 1.6-kb transcripts each encoding proteins with distinct cell type-specific expression, regulation and function [19]. IRF5 is a DNA binding protein primarily studied for its role in controlling inflammatory and immune responses, as well as mediating DNA damage- and death receptor-induced apoptosis [11–14,19–29]. Given its important role(s) in host immunity, it is not surprising to find that it is constitutively expressed in cells of the immune system, particularly plasmacytoid dendritic cells (PDC), Mo, Mo-derived dendritic cells, and activated B cells [11,19,30].

Recent data in mice support a critical role for IRF5 in SLE pathogenesis. Consistent observations in murine models of lupus indicate that loss of *Irf5* protects mice from lupus-like disease [31–33]. In the pristane-induced model, *Irf5*$^{-/-}$ mice lack pathogenic autoantibodies and glomerular deposits as seen in their wild-type counterparts [32]. IRF5 is absolutely required for disease development in *FcγRIIB*$^{-/-}$*Yaa* and *FcγRIIB*$^{-/-}$ mice [31] and Mrl/lpr *Irf5*$^{-/-}$ mice survived longer and had lower levels of autoantibodies as well as inflammatory cytokines and IFNα in their serum [33]. Additionally, autoimmune disease-prone NZB/W mice that spontaneously develop lupus-like disease were shown to display elevated constitutive levels of *Irf5* [34]. However, unlike human *IRF5* that exists as multiple alternatively spliced variants [19], murine *IRF5* appears to exist as a single major variant [28], suggesting inherent complexities between studies of IRF5 in human SLE and murine lupus-like disease; nevertheless, current data support a critical role for IRF5 in both human and murine SLE pathogenesis.

Results from genetic association studies have begun to shed light on the genetic risk conferred by an *IRF5* risk haplotype; however, to date, these studies have only been associative/correlative with other clinical manifestations of SLE, *e.g.* serum IFNα activity, autoantibody production and gene expression [18,35]. One might speculate that if the IRF5 protein(s) encoded by the genetic variation is a mediator of such effects, then we should theoretically be able to detect this in the profile of *IRF5* transcripts expressed. Indeed, it has been hypothesized that an *IRF5*-SLE risk haplotype will confer changes in *IRF5* transcription, protein/isoform expression, and biological function [4,7–8,10,36]; however, recent data from traditional cloning and sequencing suggests that haplotype does not alter the profile of transcripts expressed [8]. The aim of this study was to use a combination of molecular cloning and next-generation sequencing technologies to obtain sufficient coverage depth in primary immune cells of SLE patients and healthy donors to clearly determine 1) whether SLE patients express an *IRF5* transcript signature that is distinct from healthy donors, and 2) whether an *IRF5*-SLE risk haplotype determines the *IRF5* transcript signature, thus controlling and/or contributing to the global pathologic function(s) of IRF5 in SLE.

Results

Profiling IRF5 Transcript Expression by Traditional Molecular Cloning

Significant differences in *IRF5* expression levels have been detected in purified PBMC of healthy donors and SLE patients [7–8,15]; yet, in general, this heterogeneous population of cells expresses low levels of total *IRF5* [19]. IRF5 expression has been shown to differ between immune cell subpopulations with Mo expressing the highest levels [19,30,37]. We have demonstrated a significant association between elevated IRF5 expression in primary Mo of SLE patients with the *IRF5*-SLE H2 risk haplotype [15]; in addition, we recently showed that IRF5 is constitutively activated in Mo, and not T or natural killer (NK) cells, from SLE patients compared to healthy donors [37]. Based on these data, we focused our expression profiling experiments on purified Mo from healthy donors and SLE patients. Given that new alternatively spliced *IRF5* transcript variants continue to be identified [7–8,19], we initiated our study with the molecular cloning of full-length transcripts from this cell population. One-step RT-PCR was performed using primers that amplify all transcripts originating from the non-coding exon 1a (Ex1a) of *IRF5* [15,19]. At least four non-coding alternative first exons (Ex1a, 1b, 1c and 1d) in the 5'-untranslated region (5'-UTR) of the *IRF5* gene have been identified [19]. We focused this study on transcripts that utilize Ex1a only since it has previously been shown that Ex1a transcripts are expressed at higher levels than other Ex1 transcripts [8,19] and expression of known transcripts (V1, V4, V5 and V6) appears to be equivalent independent of Ex1 alternative utilization [8]. Indeed, cloning from Ex1a or Ex1c gave nearly identical expression of known *IRF5* variants V1, V2/V6, V3/V4 and V5 (data not shown). Results in Fig. 1A summarize the data illustrating the complete absence of V1 transcripts and significantly elevated V6 transcripts in SLE patients (n = 6) as compared to healthy donors (n = 3). Mo from both healthy donors and SLE patients shared predominant expression of known variants V4, V5 and V6, as well as the novel variant NV1. A total of five new *IRF5* variants were identified in Mo of healthy donors (Fig. 1A; NV1, NV2, NV3, NV7, NV8), four of which were exclusive to these healthy donors; nine new *IRF5* transcript variants were identified in the SLE patients examined.

A unique combination of insertions and deletions in coding exons 2–9 define the 14 new transcripts (NV1-NV14) isolated from purified Mo (Fig. 1B). Some of the new transcripts share deletions previously observed; the 30-nucleotide deletion seen in V1 and V4 is also seen in transcripts NV7, NV13 and NV14. Transcripts NV2, NV5, NV7 and NV13 share a common 28-nucleotide deletion at the end of exon 3 that has been described previously [7]. New deletions were observed as well; exon 5 is completely deleted in transcripts NV1, NV2, NV3, NV6, NV7 and NV11, and large internal deletions spanning more than 2 exons are seen in transcripts NV3 and NV6. Transcripts NV3 and NV8 share a common 19-nucleotide deletion in exon 8, and NV12 is identical to NV1 except it contains a duplication of 12 nucleotides in exon 8. Transcripts NV4, NV6, NV9 and NV14 have internal deletions in exon 7. Transcripts were also identified that contain combinations of insertions and deletions in exon 6, as diagrammed in Fig. 1C; exon 6A and 6C deletions were previously reported in known transcripts V1, V4, and V6 [19] while a novel 47-bp intronic insertion was identified in transcript NV10. Sequences of newly cloned transcripts are listed in Dataset S1.

PCR Enrichment and Next-generation Sequencing

The power of standard molecular cloning to accurately profile *IRF5* expression in SLE patients and healthy donors is limited by the number of *IRF5*-positive clones analyzed; a large number of clones would be required to attain a statistically rigorous profile, requiring great resources and financial expenditure. Additionally, it has been observed that certain cDNAs cannot be obtained by molecular cloning techniques [38]; thus, a transcript profile obtained by cloning alone may be inaccurate. To overcome some of these issues, we utilized the power of next-generation sequencing to gain an unbiased view of *IRF5* transcript profiles in primary healthy donor and SLE patient samples. For these studies, we focused on Mo from genotyped healthy donors and SLE patients given our recent findings of elevated IRF5 expression and constitutive activation in these cells [15,37]. Similar to the molecular cloning described above, a portion of PCR-amplified full-length *IRF5* cDNA from Mo was subjected to deep sequencing

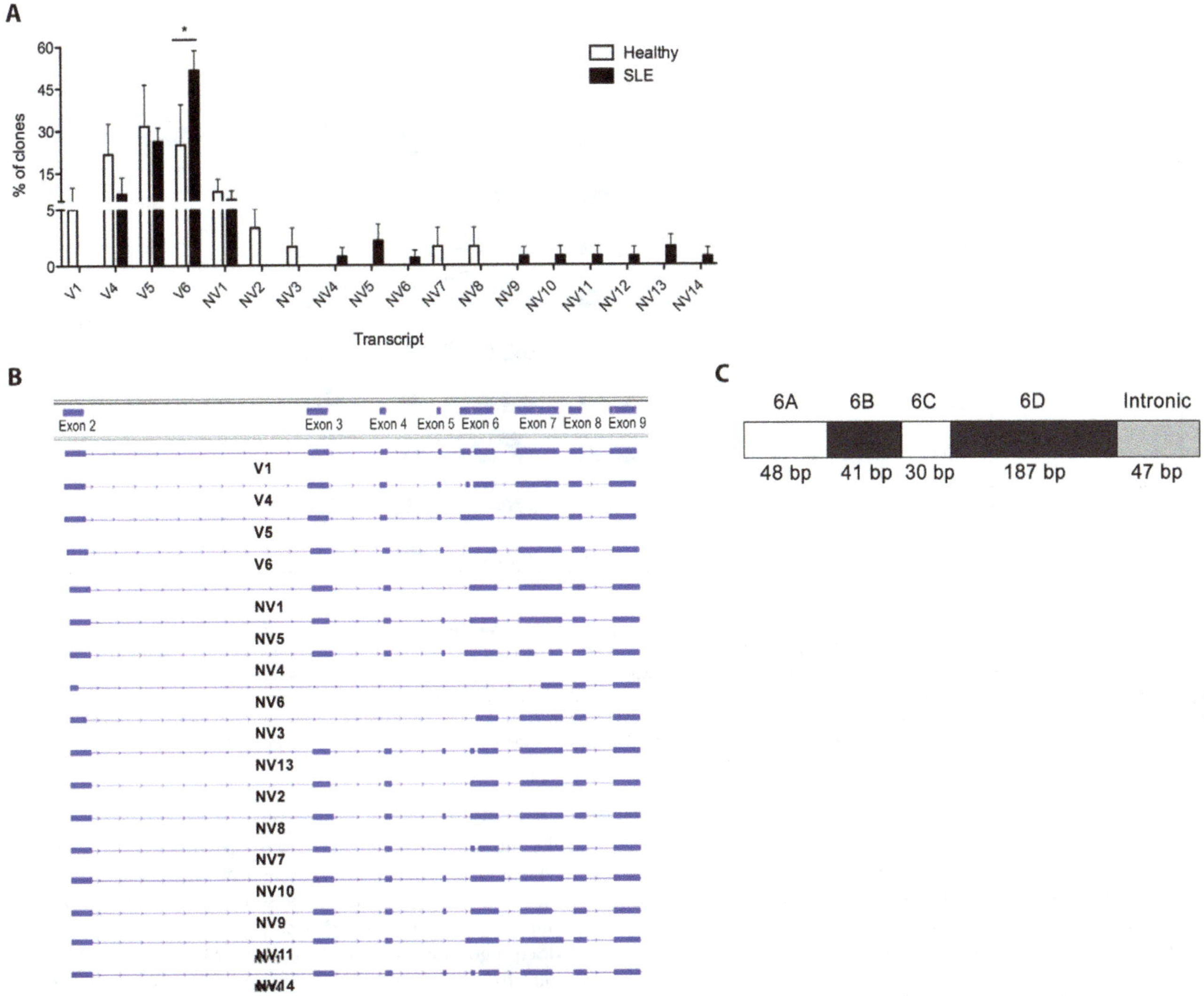

Figure 1. Identification of *IRF5* transcript variants expressed in immune cells of SLE patients and healthy donors. *A*, A profile of *IRF5* transcripts expressed in purified Mo of healthy donors (n = 3) and SLE patients (n = 6) was generated by molecular cloning and sequencing. PCR amplification was from non-coding Ex1a through Exon 9. At least 20 clones from each donor were obtained. Data are represented as a pooled % of total clones after calculating % of clones per variant per donor. Statistical analysis was performed using the two-way Anova with Bonferroni post-test. Known transcript variants V1, V4, V5 and V6 are depicted with novel variants (NV1-NV14). *B*, Scheme illustrating all *IRF5* transcripts cloned from purified Mo of healthy donors and SLE patients in a display generated using IGV software. Transcripts are comprised of exons (blue rectangles) spliced from the full *IRF5* genomic sequence (horizontal lines with arrowheads). Transcript NV12 is not shown since IGV software displays each transcript using the *IRF5* genomic sequence as a reference and is thus unable to represent duplications; NV12 contains a 12-bp internal duplication of a portion of exon 8 but is otherwise identical to transcript NV1. *C*, Diagram of exon 6 divided into portions 6A-6D as found in alternatively spliced *IRF5* transcripts. Ex6a and/or Ex6c (white rectangles) are deleted in several of the transcripts. The intronic insertion of transcript NV10 is shown as well.

analysis. cDNA libraries were generated and sequenced on the ABI SOLiD 3 Plus system. At least 2 million 50-bp reads were obtained from each sample, providing an unprecedented coverage depth of *IRF5*>3,000-fold. To achieve this depth of coverage with traditional molecular cloning, we would have to sequence 27,000 clones per donor. The number of reads obtained per sample are given in Table S1.

A visual perspective of the pile-up view of sequencing reads from individual samples mapped to the full-length *IRF5* genomic sequence reveals strong coverage across the entire exons span (Fig. 2A). In order to determine whether the observed structural features, i.e. "hills" and "valleys", reflect alternative splicing events or just position/sequence-bias, we examined reads mapping to the common valley seen in exon 7. We found multiple individual 50 bp reads that contain the exon 7 deletion supporting the existence of extensive alternative splicing in this region (Fig. 2B). In some samples, we also observed the utilization of unannotated exons, shown by the arrows. These data provide further evidence of widespread *IRF5* alternative splicing [15,19].

In order to obtain a more accurate and in-depth estimate of the differences between *IRF5* transcript expression in healthy donors and SLE patients, we developed a comprehensive workflow for the analysis of the 50-bp reads obtained from next-generation sequencing (Fig. 3). Estimates of transcript expression were generated in two ways. First, we created an "*IRF5* variant transcriptome" consisting of the 18 transcripts identified from cloning (4 known - V1, V4, V5, V6 and 14 new - NV1-NV14; Fig. 1B). Reads were mapped to this full-length transcriptome and

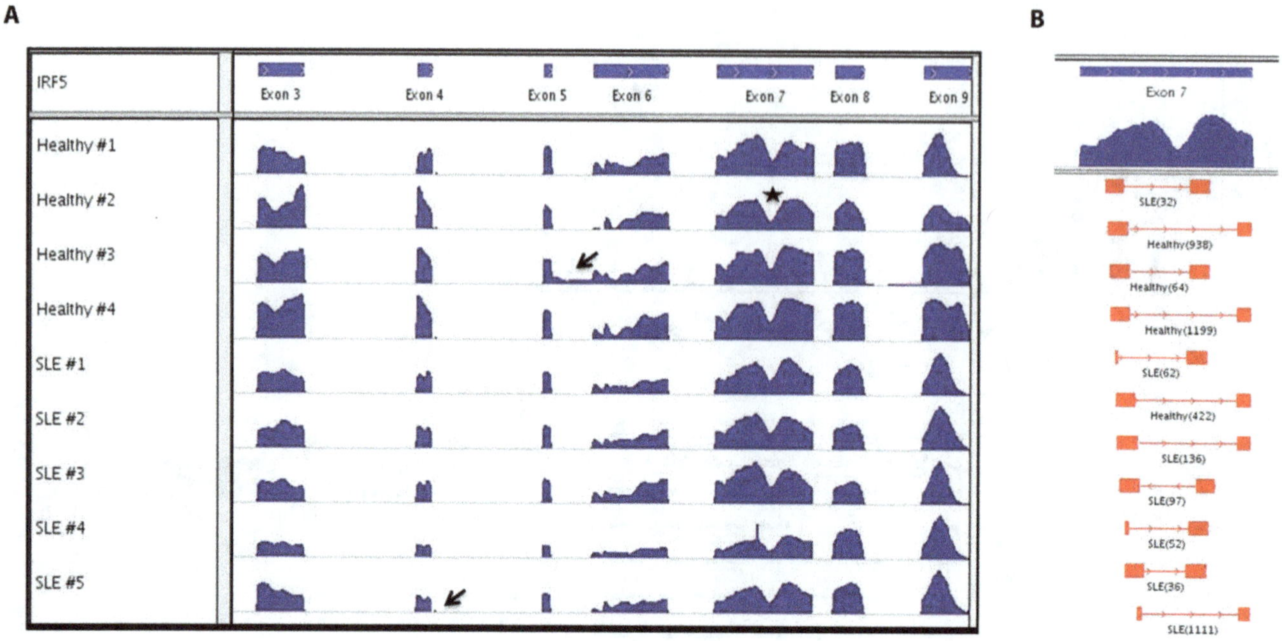

Figure 2. Pile-up view of reads from deep sequencing of PCR-amplified *IRF5* fragments. *A*, Pile-up view of *IRF5* sequencing reads mapped to the *IRF5* genomic sequence was generated with IGV. Peak heights represent the relative frequency of mappings to the indicated regions - hills reflect a high mapping frequency of reads to a particular region and valleys indicate low mapping frequency or deletions (example shown with star); arrows point to areas of reads aligning to previously unannotated exons. Results shown are from 4 independent healthy donors and 5 independent SLE patients. *B*, Reads from healthy donors and SLE patients that mapped to exon 7, shown by the star in *A* above, and reflect true internal deletions of exon 7 are shown. Junction reads are aligned by position and labeled as to whether it was detected in a healthy or SLE sample; the exact number of reads per sample that contained the junction is shown in parentheses.

expression profiles between healthy donors and SLE patients were determined. Second, we mapped reads to a list of junctions contained in the *IRF5* variant transcriptome and used junction counts to approximate transcript expression. Results obtained from these two methods are compared.

Profiling IRF5 Expression by Mapping to the Full-length "IRF5 Variant Transcriptome"

Similar to molecular cloning, next-generation sequencing has its own limitations when it comes to single gene profiling; since each read is only 50 bp in length, it is impossible to obtain complete full-length (~1600 bp) *IRF5* transcripts from raw sequencing data. As such, in the first approach, we mapped the 50 bp reads from each healthy donor (n = 4) or SLE patient (n = 5) Mo sample to the *IRF5* variant transcriptome and examined their assembly into full-length transcripts in order to obtain expression measures for each transcript. Mapping details are given in the Materials and Methods, as well as Table S1. To estimate the relative abundance of each transcript within a given sample, we used the recently published MMSeq algorithm that accounts for reads that map to multiple transcripts for obtaining expression estimates [39]. Transcript expression between healthy donors and SLE patients was then compared by converting MMSeq estimates (Gibbs values) to count equivalents and normalizing to total mapped reads; this conversion is necessary to compare expression estimates between samples. As a group, SLE patients had significantly higher normalized read counts for some of the alternatively spliced transcripts, providing support for the existence of an *IRF5*-SLE transcript profile that is distinct from that seen in representative healthy donors (Fig. 4A). A comparison of total transcript expression between pooled healthy donors (n = 4) and pooled SLE patients (n = 5) gave a $p = 0\ (10^{-10})$ by the χ^2-test supporting a significant difference in *IRF5* transcript profiles between SLE patients and healthy donors. To confirm the validity of this new method for analyzing *IRF5* transcript expression in primary immune cells, we performed a series of simulations to test the MMSeq algorithm, as described in the Materials and Methods. Results from a representative simulation is shown in Fig. 4B supporting the use of MMSeq for estimating the expression of highly similar transcripts. The overall correlation between MMSeq-derived expression estimates and true assigned expression levels of the 18 transcript variants is highly significant with $p<0.001$.

We next compared data obtained from next-generation sequencing to that from molecular cloning to determine whether this new method could be used instead of traditional cloning. By plotting MMSeq model transcript estimates from next-generation sequencing with clone count obtained from molecular cloning, we found that a greater clone count generally correlated with a higher estimated abundance ranking; R^2 correlation coefficients from scatter plots were all significant ($p<0.01$) at alpha = 0.05 further supporting the validity of this new method (Fig. 5). Data in Fig. 5 from MMSeq analysis are presented as Gibbs expression measures with calculated Monte Carlo standard errors for each transcript. This representation allows us to directly compare, within a single sample, the differential expression between transcripts. A statistical comparison can be made between individual transcripts within a single sample, revealing statistically significant differences between every transcript detected ($p<0.001$). However, the Monte Carlo standard errors are highly simplified in our experimental setup given the depth in our coverage and the redundancy in our transcripts (communicated by Dr. Ernest Turro, author of the MMSeq algorithm [39]); thus, data in Fig. 4A is a "truer"

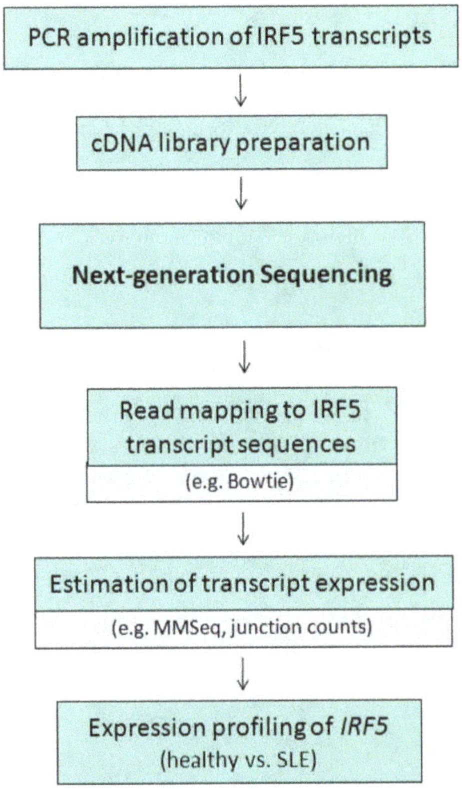

Figure 3. Workflow for enrichment and analysis of single gene profiling by RNA-Seq. Following PCR amplification of RNA of a single gene, cDNA is sequenced by next-generation sequencing and reads are mapped to sequences of alternatively spliced transcripts to obtain expression estimates and to compare transcript expression profiles across samples.

representation of transcript expression allowing for the direct statistical comparison of individual transcripts across samples.

By ranking transcript abundances and stratifying SLE patients by genotype, we found, quite strikingly, that patients with the *IRF5* H2 homozygous full risk haplotype [15] had identical rankings of the top four most abundant transcripts (Fig. 6A). Ranking of these four transcripts in H2 patients was different than in a patient with the H3 homozygous full protective haplotype or healthy donors. Haplotypes of the four healthy donors are shown at the bottom of Fig. 6. Permutation analysis revealed that the probability of observing a shared ranking of the top four transcripts among any four samples by chance is $p = 2.52 \times 10^{-15}$, indicating the significance of this abundance profile as being unique to the *IRF5*-SLE H2 risk haplotype. All four H2 samples were estimated to express V6 in the greatest proportion, followed by V5, then V1, then V4. In order to obtain a visual perspective of *IRF5* transcript expression profiles between healthy donors and SLE patients, hierarchial clustering was performed on the nine samples using expression profiles of the 18 *IRF5* transcript variants. Results from this unrestricted analysis provide additional support that the *IRF5* transcript signature found in SLE patients carrying the H2 risk haplotype is highly related to genotype as these four patients (SLE 1–4) clustered very tightly together (Fig. 6B).

Profiling IRF5 Expression by Junction Counts

Another method for comparing *IRF5* transcript expression between healthy donors and SLE patients is by aligning sequencing reads to junctions contained in the *IRF5* variant transcriptome and using counts to approximate transcript expressions. A list of 19 junctions was compiled, each ~94 bp in length, spanning the joined exons (~47 bp each of the proximal and distal portions). Junctions are described in Table S2 and sequences listed in Dataset S2. Most of these junctions are shared by multiple variants (Table S3) and thus cannot be used on their own to predict full-length *IRF5* transcript expression. However, we have found that six junctions in the *IRF5* transcriptome are exclusive to single transcript variants (junctions B, C, G, M, Q, and R); thus counts obtained for these 6 junctions might be expected to independently approximate expression of those transcripts. We therefore compared counts for these junctions in pooled healthy donor (n = 4) and SLE patients (n = 5) as a measure of differential expression of these transcript variants between the two groups. Data in Fig. 7A depict that proportionally more transcripts containing junction B (Ex2-6), C (Ex2-7), G (Ex4-6A), M (Ex6insert-7), and Q (Ex7deletion) were found in SLE patients, corresponding to new transcript variants NV3, NV6, NV11, NV10, and NV4, respectively. In healthy donors, we found only transcripts containing junction R (NV12) were elevated. Indeed, we found that these pooled data are in agreement with data from MMSeq analysis of full-length transcript expression (Fig. 4A).

Expression of IRF5 Transcript Variants Containing the Exon 6 Insertion/deletion

It has recently been demonstrated that a structural insertion/deletion (in/del) variation in exon 6 of the *IRF5* gene is associated with an *IRF5*-SLE haplotype [8,10]; the presence of the 30-nt insertion (Fig. 1C; exon 6c) is correlated with a risk haplotype for SLE development. This 30-bp in-frame in/del is considered/expected to be a functional genetic variant since it is located in the PEST (proline-, glutamic acid-, serine-, and threonine-rich) domain of IRF5 and protein isoforms that contain alterations in this region, *i.e.* V1, V3/V4, V5 and V2/V6, have differential ability to regulate type I *IFN* promoter reporters [19] and IL6 expression in mouse embryonic fibroblasts (MEFs) [40]. Using the MMSeq model of transcript expression estimates, we were able to demonstrate that as a group, transcripts containing the Ex6c 30-bp deletion (V1, V4, NV7, NV13, NV14) were expressed in significantly lower proportion in SLE patients with the H2 risk haplotype (Table 1). Furthermore, counts for Junction K, which represents the Ex6c deletion, were proportionately lower in these patients as well. As a result, by analyzing our next-generation sequencing data in this way, we were able to detect and support the differential expression of the Ex6C in/del genetic variant in SLE patients carrying the H2 risk haplotype. These data provide independent confirmation of Graham et al's findings [10] and significant support for the screening of the exon 6 in/del in SLE patients as a single pathogenic region conferring risk in SLE.

De Novo Junction Discovery Provides Evidence for Additional IRF5 Transcript Variants

The primary limitation of transcriptome-based expression analysis is that it requires *a priori* knowledge of all the alternatively spliced transcripts, and the use of molecular cloning to generate the transcript sequences may be defined in part by the abundance of a given transcript, *i.e.* we only sequenced ~20–25 clones per sample and likely missed low-abundant transcripts. Thus, although we observed congruity between expression estimates obtained by quantifying the 18 full-length transcripts in our *IRF5* transcriptome by MMSeq (Figs. 4A) and by

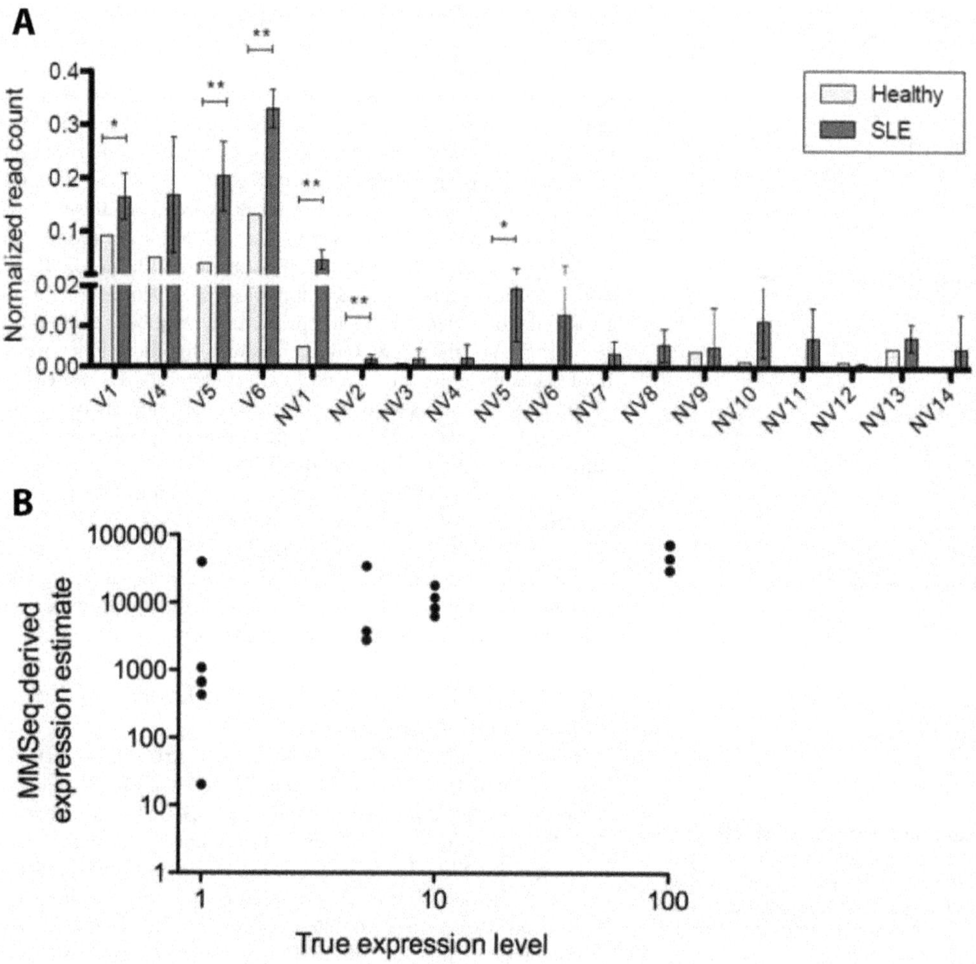

Figure 4. Expression estimates of *IRF5* alternatively spliced transcripts in healthy donors and SLE patients. *A,* Gibbs expression estimates were obtained with MMSeq and converted to raw read counts, then normalized to total read counts. Normalized read counts for each transcript in 5 SLE patients and a representative healthy donor (#1) are plotted; read counts were compared between the two sets using a student's *t*-test. *$p<0.05$; **$p<0.01$. *B,* Scatter plot showing the correlation between MMSeq-derived expression estimates and true (assigned) expression levels of the 18 transcript variants. $R^2 = 0.6532$ at alpha = 0.05 and $p<0.0001$ indicating a highly significant correlation.

quantifying the six junctions that were "unique" to individual transcripts (Fig. 7A), we sought to examine the possibility that additional transcripts exist that are not currently annotated in our transcriptome. Indeed, the raw pile-up view of aligned sample reads (Fig. 2) supports the existence of coding regions within the *IRF5* gene that are not represented in the variants currently contained in our transcriptome. Given these considerations, we hypothesized that additional *IRF5* transcript variants, not yet identified, may be expressed in purified Mo of SLE patients and/or healthy donors. Since next-generation sequencing is unbiased, evidence for the existence of these transcripts should be found in our data; *de novo* junction discovery should help us determine whether additional transcripts exist. We therefore used TopHat software, which compiles exon coverage data, constructs a list of potential splice junctions, and systematically maps the sequencing data to this list to yield a complete set of predicted junctions [41]. We identified a number of new splice junctions that were not found in any of our 18 cloned transcripts, several of which are depicted and described in Fig. 7B and Table 2. In new junctions 1–3, we observed splicing and alignments to areas of *IRF5* which were previously believed to be noncoding, indicating the presence of newly discovered coding exons in *IRF5* full-length transcripts (Fig. 7B). New junctions 4–9 contain deletions of varying sizes, ranging from a novel 218-nucleotide internal deletion in exon 7 (junction 5) to a full deletion of exons 5 and 6 (junction 6).

We also analyzed the newly identified junction splice sites to classify as canonical or non-canonical (Table 2) and found that most of the junctions featured the canonical dinucleotides GT and AG, indicating that they reflect a predicted alternative splicing event in *IRF5* and further support that they are not false discoveries generated by random by-products of a large sequencing depth. Further characterization of splice sites identified in our samples by TopHat support that random splicing events are unlikely to contribute significantly to the profile of *IRF5* transcripts detected by the next-generation sequencing analyses in our healthy and SLE patient samples (Figure S1 and Methods S1). Moreover, TopHat also identified the majority of known (canonical and non-canonical) junctions found in our *IRF5* variant transcriptome, thus further supporting the validity of this approach (Table S4).

As a final validation of TopHat and the overall next-generation sequencing approach [42], we used quantitative real-time PCR (qPCR) to examine whether the new junctions

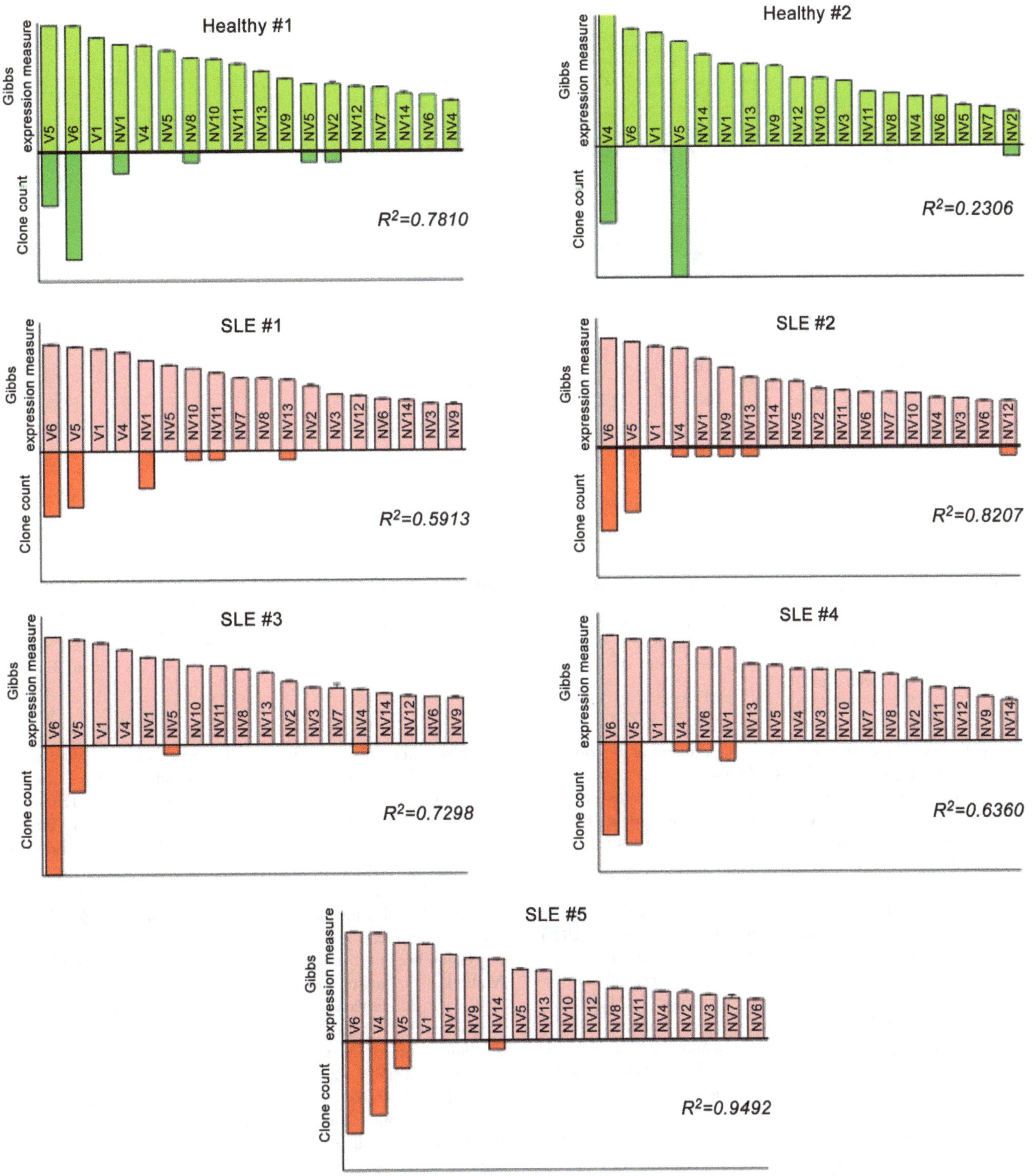

Figure 5. Correlation between Gibbs expression estimates and clone count. Gibbs expression estimates and Monte Carlo standard errors were generated by MMSeq. Bar graphs show Gibbs expression measures from next-generation sequencing versus clone counts from traditional cloning and sequencing. Data from n = 2 healthy donors and n = 5 SLE patients is shown; at least 20 *IRF5*-positive clones from each donor were used for this analysis.

reported by TopHat for each healthy donor and patient sample could be detected in the original Mo RNA. Data in Fig. 7C depict the successful confirmation of expression of individual TopHat-discovered junctions within the corresponding samples (Fig. 7C).

Functional Consequence of an IRF5-SLE H2 Risk Haplotype

Our data thus far supports the existence of an *IRF5* transcript signature in SLE patients that is distinct from that expressed in

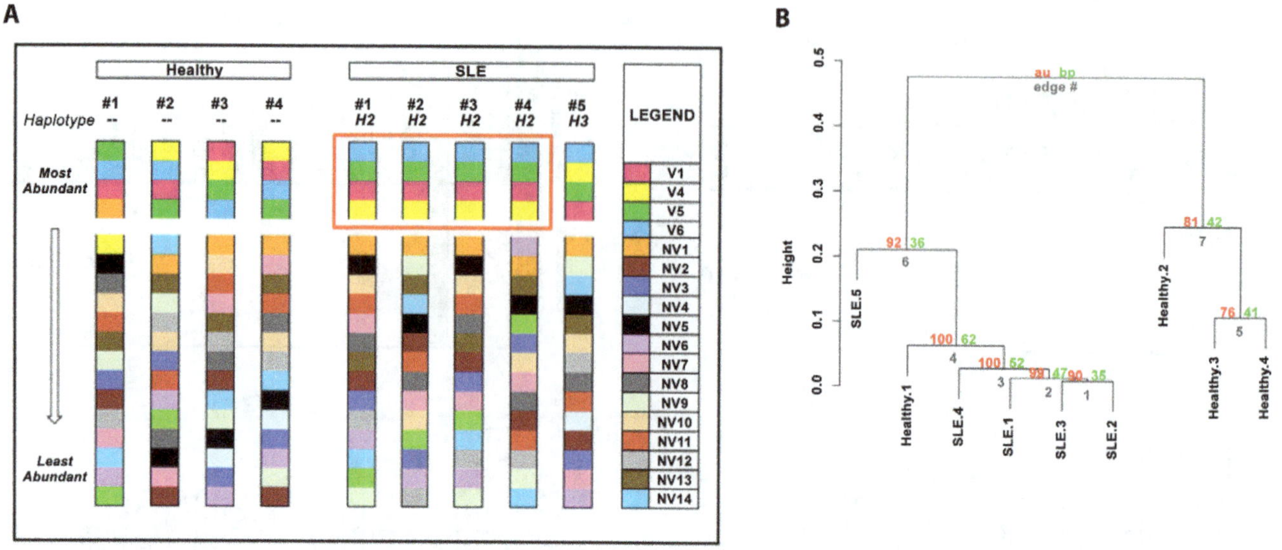

Healthy	GC-indel	rs2004640	rs10954213	rs10488631
#1	0	GG	AG	TT
#2	1	GT	AG	CT
#3	1	GT	AA	CT
#4	1	GT	AG	TT

Figure 6. Top four most abundant transcripts are shared by SLE patients with the H2 full risk haplotype. *A,* Relative abundance ranking of transcripts from 4 healthy donors, 1 SLE patient with the H3 full protective haplotype, and 4 SLE patients with the H2 full risk haplotype is shown. Transcripts were ranked from most to least abundant using MMSeq-generated Gibbs expression estimates; individual transcripts are represented by distinct colors. *B,* Hierarchial clustering was performed on the nine samples using expression profiles of the 18 *IRF5* transcript variants. Height represents the difference between samples. Red values are AU *p*-values and green values are BP values. Clusters with AU larger than 95% are statistically significant with a $p<0.05$.

healthy donors. The dramatic findings that ranking of the top four most abundant transcripts (V1, V4, V5 and V6) and clustering of total transcript signatures are shared by the SLE patients carrying the H2 risk haplotype (Fig. 6) prompted us to investigate further the function(s) of these top four variants that might contribute to SLE risk. Previous studies in human fibroblasts showed that the identical polypeptide encoded by *IRF5* V3/V4 is the most potent inducer of virus-mediated type I IFN [19]. More recent studies indicate that deletions in exon 6 determine the ability of IRF5 isoforms to mediate LPS-induced production of IL6 in MEFs [40]. Given that recent data in *irf5*$^{-/-}$ mice reveal a critical role for IRF5 in regulating TLR-mediated proinflammatory cytokines IL6, TNFα, and IL12 [13], which have been shown, along with IFNα, to be pathologically elevated in the circulation of SLE patients [43–45], we performed a comparative analysis of human promoter transactivation by the top four most abundant isoforms. Transient transfection to Hek293T cells resulted in equal expression of individual isoforms, as determined by immunoblot (data not shown), yet differential transactivation of each promoter was observed, except for the *IL6* promoter in which all isoforms gave similar transactivation (Fig. 8A). The patterns of transactivation were fairly well-conserved with isoform V2/V6 showing the greatest constitutive transactivation, followed by V1, then V3/V4 and V5. Interestingly, a significantly different pattern of transactivation was observed with the artificially constructed reporter containing 5 copies of the ISRE consensus sequence.

Another manner by which we compared functional differences between these isoforms was by measuring protein stability. For years, others and we have hypothesized [8,19,40] that alterations in exon 6 might affect protein stability since this region localizes to the PEST domain [46–47]. These top four most abundant isoforms differ only in their exon 6 deletion pattern; V5 has no deletions, V1 has the single 30 bp Ex6c deletion, V2/V6 has the single 48 bp Ex6a deletion, and V3/V4 contains both Ex6a and 6c deletions [19]. Using a modified cycloheximide chase technique [48], we determined the relative stability of GFP-tagged isoforms (Fig. 8B). GFP was used as a positive control with a known 26 hr half-life [49] and V8 as a control isoform lacking the PEST domain [19]. Results from analysis of covariance (ANCOVA) reveal that there is statistical difference between the slopes of the regression lines of these top four most abundant isoforms (Fig. 8B). Multiple comparison/post-hoc testing identified a statistically significant difference between V3/V4 and V5, V3/V4 and V2/V6, V1 and V2/V6, V5 and V2/V6, with *p* values <0.05. The absolute slopes of the regression lines for each isoform indicated that the most stable was V3/V4≅V1<V5<V2/V6<V8, with V8 being the least stable. As expected, GFP gave the greatest relative stability, with only a small decrease in mean fluorescence intensity (MFI) over time (data not shown). Surprisingly, based on the PEST domain alone, we would have predicted a different pattern of stability, with V8 being the most stable and V5 being the least. These data indicate that the PEST domain of IRF5 is not the determining factor for relative stability.

Discussion

High-throughput mRNA sequencing (RNA-Seq) of mammalian transcriptomes can provide a wealth of information on transcript assembly and abundance estimates [50]. Major challenges arise, however, when attempting to measure the differential expression of multiple alternatively spliced transcripts from a single gene [51–53]. Given that many of these transcripts will be expressed at low

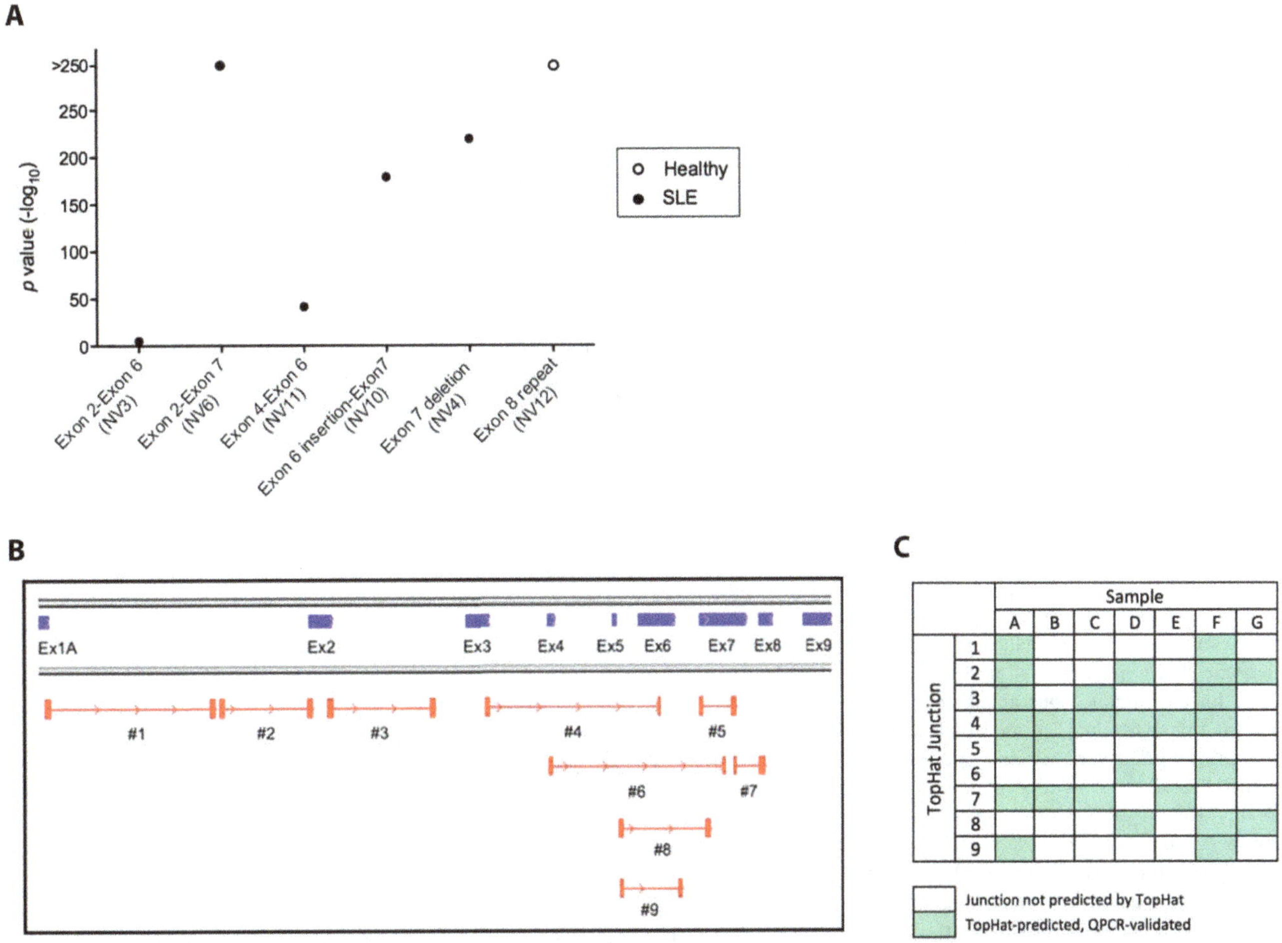

Figure 7. Profiling *IRF5* alternative splicing using junction counts and *de novo* junction discovery. *A,* Counts were obtained for the 6 junctions unique to single cloned transcripts by aligning reads from healthy donor (n = 4) and SLE patient samples (n = 5) to 94-bp junction sequences. Proportionally more transcripts containing each junction were found in either healthy donors (open circles) or SLE patients (closed circles); plotted are the *p* values obtained by the Pearson's χ^2-test. *B, De novo* junction discovery was performed using TopHat to identify novel alternative splicing events. Representative junctions are displayed using IGV with the *IRF5* genomic sequence as a reference. Each pair of red blocks represents one junction, and lines joining two blocks denote spliced-out portions of *IRF5*. Junctions 1-3 show evidence of splicing to unannotated intronic regions of *IRF5*; junctions 4–9 have novel inter- and intra-exonic deletions. *C,* Schematic illustration of junctions in *B* confirmed by qPCR.

levels [54], we chose to enrich for our gene of interest first, before sequencing, in order to alleviate some of these later challenges in analysis. While enrichment of *IRF5* by PCR amplification may introduce artifactual changes in transcript quantity due to structural variation in the material being sequenced; for example, certain nucleotide strings may be less efficiently amplified than others or they may form higher-order structures that cannot be amplified, we would expect this to be minimized in the current

Table 1. Analysis of *IRF5* transcripts containing the Ex6 in/del.

Full-length transcripts	**Healthy** (Σ **read counts**)	**SLE** (Σ **read counts**)
Containing the Ex6c deletion *(V1, V4, NV7, NV13, NV14)*	7865656[a]	3920591[a]
Missing the Ex6c deletion *(All other variants)*	1054066[a]	2333273[a]
Junction	**Healthy** (Σ junction counts)	**SLE** (Σ junction counts)
Exon 6c deletion *(Junction K)*	142709[b]	30640[b]
Other junctions	2606821[b]	574378[b]

Using estimated transcript read counts obtained from MMSeq, expression of transcripts containing vs. those missing the Ex6c deletion was compared in healthy donors (n = 4) and SLE patients carrying the H2 risk haplotype (n = 4). Shown are the total number of reads aligned per group of patients. $^{a}\chi^2 = 1377726$ with $p < 2.2 \times 10^{-16}$; *p* values were obtained by the Pearson's χ^2-test with Yates continuity correction. Totaled reads mapping to the Ex6C deletion were similarly compared across grouped healthy vs. SLE (risk) patients; $^{b}\chi^2 = 16.0379$ with $p < 6.209 \times 10^{-15}$. Σ = sum.

Table 2. Representative novel splice junctions identified by *de novo* junction discovery.

Junction	Predicted spliced regions	Canonical (Yes/No)
1	Ex1a – new exon	Yes
2	New exon – Ex2	Yes
3	Ex2- new exon	Yes
4	Ex3- Ex6	No
5	Ex7- Ex7	No
6	Ex4- Ex7	No
7	Ex7- Ex8	Yes
8	Ex5- Ex7	Yes
9	Ex5- Ex6	Yes

Individual junctions identified by TopHat and illustrated in Fig. 7B are listed and defined as canonical or non-canonical; Ex = exon.

study given the high similarity and redundancy in *IRF5* transcript variants. *IRF5* alternatively spliced transcripts are a family of very similar molecules, thus the efficiency of PCR amplification should theoretically be similar for all transcripts.

To further enhance our ability to analyze results from next-generation sequencing, we used data from molecular cloning to generate an *IRF5* variant transcriptome. We developed a newly defined workflow of next-generation sequencing whereby differentially spliced transcripts of a single gene could be rapidly enriched and quantified in donor RNA samples. Results obtained from these various steps of the pipeline confirmed what was found by molecular cloning but at a much greater depth. Some examples of this include, but are not limited to, the finding that 1) MMSeq estimates were comparable to cloning estimates (Fig. 5), and 2) TopHat *de novo* discovery detected essentially all of the junctions found in our newly cloned transcripts (Table S4). Using these methods, we were also able to confirm previous findings that support a role for the Ex6c in/del in SLE (Table 1) [8,10]. Altogether, findings presented herein support the use of this newly defined workflow of next-generation sequencing to 1) confirm the contribution of genotype to the profile of *IRF5* transcripts expressed, and 2) address the question of what *cis* polymorphisms in the *IRF5*-SLE haplotype regulate *IRF5* alternative splicing? Both of these studies will require sequencing on larger cohorts of genotyped healthy donor and SLE patient samples; however, the first critical support and proof-of-principle for additional studies, such as these, is now provided. Data in the current study support a significant role for genotype in defining the top four most abundant transcripts expressed, yet little is still known of the mechanisms regulating *IRF5* alternative splicing. *Cis*-acting variants have been identified in the *IRF5* gene that associate with elevated expression, but the data on *cis* regulation of *IRF5* alternative splicing is unclear [7–8,55]. Indeed, recent findings by Alonso-Perez et al. indicate that *cis*-regulation of *IRF5* expression is not enough to fully account for *IRF5* association with SLE susceptibility, suggesting that other mechanisms exist that regulate functional changes in *IRF5* [56]. These data are confirmatory of earlier work in the lab revealing that genotype alone was not enough to account for elevated IRF5 expression in primary immune cells of SLE patients and enhanced *IRF5* alternative splicing was, at least in part, due to elevated levels of spliceosome components in SLE patients as overexpression of many of these factors led to increased *IRF5* alternative splicing [15].

There are currently numerous software programs available for the assembly and analysis of the short reads obtained by RNA-Seq. Due to the high level of redundancy in our transcriptome (Fig 1B), after testing a number of these programs (MMSeq, Cufflinks, RSEM), we chose to primarily use MMSeq to quantify *IRF5* transcript expression since its algorithm was specially designed to account for reads that map to multiple transcripts [39]. We found that many of the other expression estimate algorithms discard these reads, thus underestimating expression [39]. Indeed, simulation experiments testing the validity of this approach, whereby arbitrary expression values were assigned to each of the 18 transcripts and reads simulated using WGSIM [57], gave significant correlation between the assigned true expression level and MMSeq-derived expression estimates (Fig. 4B). We found in the simulations that MMSeq is most accurate with the more abundant transcripts thus providing additional confidence in the statistical findings of Fig. 4A since significance was only obtained in the more abundant transcripts. This makes sense since the relative error in MMSeq estimates is larger for less abundant transcripts and relatively small for highly abundant transcripts based on the algorithm used by MMSeq that assigns reads to each iteration probabilistically [39].

Our results also support the use of next-generation sequencing to broaden the *IRF5* transcriptome contained in primary immune cells of SLE patients and healthy donors. The unbiased junction discovery performed by TopHat produced an assortment of new junctions whose expression was confirmed by qPCR in original RNA from healthy donors and SLE patients (Fig. 7B&C). Ultimately, these data suggest that new full-length transcripts could be cloned and sequences input back into the pipeline (Fig. 3) so as to obtain an even closer approximation of the "true" *IRF5* transcript signature in SLE patients. Moreover, the successful *in vitro* detection of these new junctions derived solely from raw next-generation sequencing reads provides additional validation for the use of RNA-Seq in *IRF5* transcript expression profiling.

Results from these studies significantly enhance our current understanding of *IRF5* expression in monocytes of SLE patients and provide critical insight into how genotype might contribute to and/or alter IRF5 function. Further studies will be required to determine if unique transcript profiles will be obtained between purified B cells of SLE patients, where IRF5 has recently been proposed to function [32,58], and Mo, and whether a distinct difference in transcript expression will be necessary to predict altered function(s) for IRF5 in these two immune cell populations. Data in Table 1, from analyzing the exon 6 in/del, supports that this region alone may be sufficient to define SLE risk and thus could be used as a potential marker of IRF5 pathogenic function. Future studies will be important to confirm this finding in additional healthy donor and SLE patient samples, along with determining the functional consequence of the in/del as many variations in exon 6 have been observed (Fig. 1B).

Conversely, it may be that all immune cells share the same *IRF5* pathogenic signature in SLE. Nevertheless, data from all three methods of analyses (molecular cloning, MMSeq, and junction counts) support the presence of an *IRF5*-SLE transcript signature in purified Mo of SLE patients that is significantly different from that expressed in healthy donor Mo. To this end, we provide intriguing data to be built upon in the near future that suggests genotype may define, not only the top four most abundant transcripts expressed in Mo of SLE patients with the H2 risk haplotype, but the *IRF5* transcript signature itself, as patients carrying the H2 risk haplotype clustered tightly together (Fig. 6B). It is important to point out the relevance of the different abundance rankings as slight changes in the order of the top four

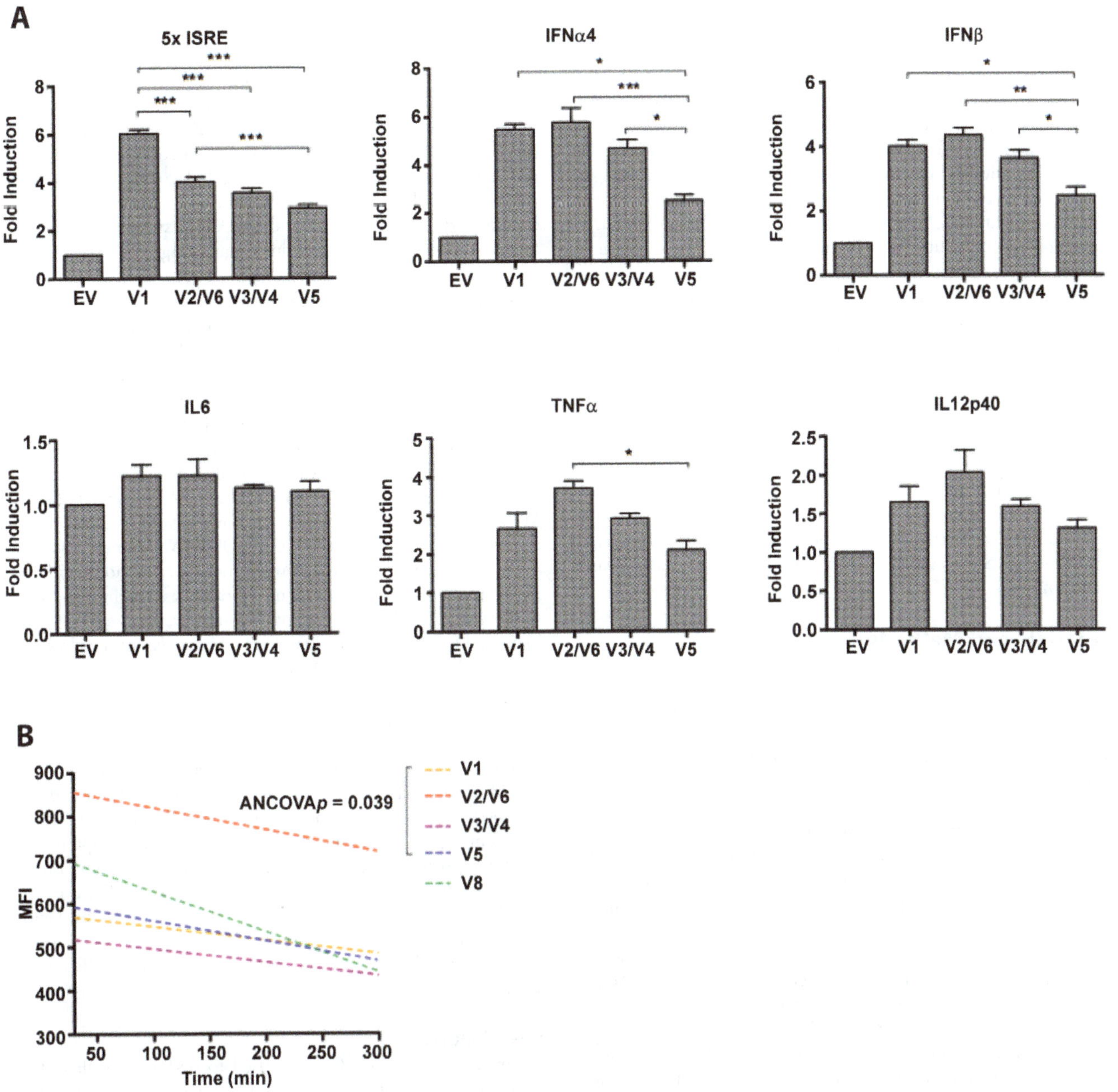

Figure 8. Distinct transactivation potential and stability for IRF5 isoforms associated with the *IRF5*-SLE H2 risk haplotype. *A*, Flag-tagged *IRF5* V1, V2/V6, V3/V4, V5, and empty vector (EV) were co-transfected with the indicated luciferase reporters - 5x*ISRE*, *IFNα4*, *IFNβ*, *IL6*, *TNFα*, or *IL12p40*, and promoter transactivation determined by dual luciferase assay. Independent experiments were repeated in duplicate wells at least three times; mean ± S.D. are plotted. Statistical analysis was performed by one-way ANOVA with Bonferroni post-test; *$p<0.05$, **$p<0.01$, ***$p<0.001$. Promoter induction by each IRF5 isoform was significantly greater than empty vector (EV) controls in all experiments (astericks not shown). *B*, Relative half-lives of IRF5 isoforms V1, V2/V6, V3/V4, and V5 were determined by cycloheximide chase experiments (see Materials & Methods). Similar to *A*, GFP-tagged *IRF5* variants were transfected to Hek293T cells; V8 was included as a comparative control lacking the PEST-rich exons 5–7. Representative data from 2–3 independent experiments is shown as mean fluorescence intensity (MFI) of GFP-IRF5 over the indicated time period. Analysis of covariance (ANCOVA) was used to determine if regression lines between isoforms differed significantly.

most abundant transcripts are likely to result in significant differences in expression. This is best shown in Fig. 4A through the statistical comparison of normalized expression levels between healthy donor #1, that has the abundance ranking of **V5**> **V6**> V1> NV1, and patients with the H2 haplotype (**V6**> **V5**> V1> V4). We found a significant difference in the levels of V5 and V6 between the healthy donor and SLE patients even though these top two ranked variants only changed order position. Whether all of these data together define the exact *IRF5*-SLE pathogenic signature that delineates its global function in SLE is still unclear. Future studies will be necessary that focus on identifying new transcripts, determining their abundance, and characterizing their function(s) in the immune system.

To this extent, we present data that supports the premise that IRF5 isoforms have differential abilities to regulate proinflammatory cytokines associated with SLE pathogenesis (Fig. 8) [19,40]. In this study, we focused on characterizing further the function of the top four expressed transcripts (V6>V5>V1>V4) identified in SLE patients with the H2 risk haplotype. We found that V6 had the greatest transactivation function yet the lowest stability of the four isoforms (V4>V1>V5>V6). These data are intriguing and support a complex scenario in SLE where a particular IRF5 isoform might have enhanced transactivation potential, yet decreased relative stability that may instead diminish its pathologic contribution. An important question to be addressed in future studies is - what is the functional consequence of an altered *IRF5* expression profile? Current preliminary data on some of the new variants has yet to point toward distinct functions (data not shown) [19]; although, one might argue the relevance of analyzing the function of individual encoded isoforms since it is clear in SLE that isoforms are not expressed in a singular fashion and instead are expressed all together. IRF5, like other IRF family members, forms homodimers and/or heterodimers with other proteins resulting in function [26,59–60]. The complexity of this system is thus obvious and future studies on isoform function will have to take into account the aspects of differential protein stability, DNA binding potential and interaction with other IRF5 isoforms and proteins. Additional work in this area will be essential to our understanding of exactly how elevated and altered *IRF5* transcript expression in SLE patients contributes functionally to disease pathogenesis.

Materials and Methods

Ethics Statement

All study subjects provided written informed consent to participate in the study, and the study was approved by institutional and regional ethical boards at both the University of Medicine and Dentistry of New Jersey and Uppsala University.

Study Participants and Genotyping

Purified monocyte (Mo) samples from 6 Swedish patients with SLE were obtained from the rheumatology clinic at Uppsala University Hospital (UUH) in Sweden; Mo (n = 4) from healthy controls were obtained from Uppsala University Hospital. Each of the patients fulfilled at least four of the classification criteria for SLE as defined by the American College of Rheumatology (ACR) with a median ACR index of 6 (range 5–8). Clinical disease activity at the time of blood sampling was assessed with the modified SLE disease activity index (mSLEDAI-2K) where complement and anti-DNA antibodies were omitted. The median mSLEDAI-2K value was 1 (range 0–26) showing that most patients had low or no clinical disease activity at the time of blood collection.

Genotyping

Subjects were genotyped at the rs2004640, rs10954213, and rs10488631 SNPs in 250 ng of DNA extracted from blood samples of study subjects using the Illumina Golden Gate assay (Illumina, San Diego, CA, USA), as described [4,16]. The 5 bp CGGGG indel of *IRF5* was genotyped by PCR amplification followed by size separation using 4% agarose gels, or using an ABI 3770 capillary sequencer (Applied Biosystems, Foster City, CA, USA).

RNA Extraction and PCR Amplification

Mo were purified immediately following phlebotomy from peripheral blood of healthy donors and SLE patients by positive selection with CD14 magnetic beads (Miltenyi Biotech). RNA was extracted using the RNEasy Mini kit (Qiagen) and genomic DNA was removed by DNase treatment (Promega). One-step RT-PCR Kit (Qiagen) was used to amplify full-length *IRF5* transcripts from non-coding Ex1A through 9. PCR conditions were as follows: 1 cycle of 50°C for 30 minutes and 95°C for 15 minutes, followed by 30–40 cycles of 94°C for 30 seconds, 62°C for 30 seconds, and 68°C for 2 min 30 seconds, then 1 cycle of 72°C for 10 minutes. In some cases, a second round of nested PCR was performed with an exon 2 primer spanning the ATG start codon sequence. PCR products were separated by agarose gel electrophoresis on a 1% gel. The amplified band corresponding to MW 1600 bp was excised and purified with the QiaQuick gel extraction kit (Qiagen) and used for downstream cloning/sequencing.

Molecular Cloning of Transcripts

Gel-purified PCR products were ligated into the pCR®2.1-TOPO vector (Invitrogen) or pDrive UA cloning vector (Qiagen) and heat-transformed as per manufacturer's instructions. Following blue/white selection, plasmids were extracted from individually grown colonies with the Plasmid Miniprep kit (Qiagen) and checked for correctly sized inserts by EcoR1/BamH1 digestion. Plasmids were sequenced with the ABI 3130xl Genetic Analyzer (Applied Biosystems, Inc., Foster City, CA) using M13R and M13F sequencing primers. Forward and reverse sequences were assembled and analyzed using CLC DNA Workbench 5 software (CLC bio, Cambridge, MA). Annotations were made to indicate exons and junctions (known or novel) present in each transcript. A minimum of 20 *IRF5*-positive clones were sequenced and identified from each individual donor. Sequences of novel variants NV1-NV14 are found in Dataset S1.

High-throughput Sequencing

PCR products were sheared into 100–150 base pair (bp) fragments, ligated to sequencing adapters, nick-translated, and amplified to yield a library for each individual. Gel-purified PCR products from each donor were sheared into 100–150 bp fragments and ligated to barcoded sequencing adapters. The resulting products were nick translated and amplified three to five cycles to yield a library for each donor. These libraries were attached to beads by emulsion PCR and sequenced by ligation on the ABI SOLiD 3 plus system (Life Technologies, Carlsbad, CA). Greater than 2×10^6 50-bp reads were obtained from each sample.

Read Mapping

Bowtie software [61–62] was used to perform all alignments, using default mapping/quality parameters unless otherwise specified below. Mapping statistics for each set of alignments are found in Table S1. For MMSeq-based analyses, reads were aligned to an index of the 18 *IRF5* transcript sequences identified by cloning. Parameters were set to report all alignments of equivalent alignment score, thus accounting for reads that could originate from multiple transcripts sharing common exons (Bowtie parameters "–a –best –strata"). SAMTools software [57] was used to convert alignment files to BAM format. Mappings of reads to the transcript set were generated using MMSeq feature "bam2hits" in preparation for running the MMSeq software pipeline [39]. For junction-based quantitation, reads were aligned to an index of 19 junction sequences (94 bp each) obtained from sequences of cloned transcripts (Table S2). Bowtie parameters were set to report the single best alignment for each read ("-k 1–best"). For alignments to the *IRF5* gene, an index was built from the *IRF5* genomic sequence retrieved from NCBI RefSeq# NC_000007.13 (128577994.128590089) on Chromosome 7. Reads were mapped with parameters "-n 2–k 40–m 40."

Determination of Coverage Depth and Cloning Estimates

A minimum of 800,000 50-bp reads per sample aligned to *IRF5* sequences (Table S1). The *IRF5* gene is approximately 12,000 bp; 800,000 reads $\times$50 bp per read/12,000 bp in *IRF5* = a minimum of 3,000-fold coverage of *IRF5*. Each *IRF5* alternatively spliced transcript is approximately 1600 bp, which corresponds to ~30 50-bp sequencing reads. 800,000 reads divided by 30 reads per transcript yields the equivalent of 27,000 *IRF5* transcript-containing clones.

Transcript Expression Estimates and Abundance Rankings with MMSeq

Following mapping of reads to the *IRF5* transcriptome, alignments were input to the MMSeq pipeline [39] to obtain mean log Gibbs expression estimates and Monte Carlo standard errors for each of the 18 transcripts within a given donor sample. Abundance rankings were obtained by listing transcripts in order of magnitude of Gibbs values within each sample. To obtain "counts" for comparing transcript expression across samples, Gibbs expression measures for each transcript were converted to raw read counts by multiplying by the transcript length (in kb) and then by the total number of reads (in millions) in the alignments file from each sample. Raw read counts were then normalized to total read counts in the sample, and values were compared across healthy and SLE samples.

Transcript Expression Estimates by Quantification of Unique Junctions

Counts for each of the junctions unique to one of the 18 alternatively spliced transcripts were used to construct six 2×2 contingency tables. Rows contained pooled counts of each unique junction vs. counts of other junctions (rows) for grouped healthy donors vs. SLE patients (columns). The Pearson's χ^2-test was then performed on each 2×2 contingency table; the two-tailed *p*-value reported represents the probability of observing the data by chance if there is no differential expression between healthy donors and SLE patients.

MMSeq Simulations

Arbitrary expression values of 1, 5, 10, or 100 were randomly assigned to each of the 18 transcript variants. 50 bp reads were simulated separately for each transcript by WGSIM, part of the SAMtools distribution [57], at high coverage (>600x) so as to minimize sampling bias. Read mapping and MMSeq-based analyses was performed as described above.

Analysis of Exon 6C Insertion/deletion

The χ^2-test was used to examine the differential expression of the exon 6C in/del in healthy donors vs. SLE patients. Raw read counts from MMSeq-based estimates were summed to obtain totals for transcripts containing vs. not containing the exon 6C deletion; counts for multiple transcripts in each group of healthy vs. SLE patient samples formed the rows of a contingency table. Alignments to Junction K (representing the Exon 6C deletion) vs. other junctions were similarly totaled for both groups. The Pearson's χ^2-test was performed on each 2×2 contingency table; the two-tailed *p*-value reported represents the probability of observing the data in the contingency table by chance if there is no differential expression between healthy donors and SLE patients.

De Novo Identification and Confirmation of Splice Junctions

Using Bowtie default mapping parameters contained within the TopHat software pipeline [41], reads were aligned to the *IRF5* genomic sequence (NCBI RefSeq# NC_000007.13 (128577994.128590089)), and iterative mappings to predicted splice junctions were performed and quantified by TopHat. To control for false positive junctions found by TopHat, splice sites of reported junctions were classified as canonical or non-canonical; a junction was considered non-canonical if its splice site was none of the following: GT...AG, GC...AG, AT...AC, GG...AG, GT...TG, GT...GG, CT...AG [63–64]. A threshold value of 0.01% of total mapped reads, where the fraction of non-canonical junction sites levels off, was set to exclude junctions reported by chance (described further in Method S1 and Figure S1).

To confirm TopHat findings, junction-specific quantitative PCR (qPCR) was performed on original monocyte RNA using a modified approach described in [42]. Individual primer sets (shown in Table S5) were designed with one primer corresponding to the splice-specific region of each junction (containing portions of the two spanned exons), and the other primer corresponding to neighboring exonic sequences; detection of an amplified product confirmed junction presence. qPCR conditions were: 1 cycle of 45°C for 3 minutes and 95°C for 10 minutes, followed by 40 cycles of 95°C for 15 seconds and 60°C for 1 minute.

Dual Luciferase Assays and Protein Stability

HEK-293T cells were transfected using Lipofectamine 2000 (Invitrogen). For dual luciferase assays, a 1:1 ratio (2 µg each) of luciferase reporter and IRF5 expression plasmid along with 0.1 µg of pRL-CMV as an internal control were used. Cells were harvested 24 h post-transfection and lysed with Passive Lysis Buffer (Promega). Luciferase assays were carried out using the Dual Luciferase Assay kit according to the manufacturer's specifications. Levels of reporter firefly luciferase activity were normalized to a constant level of pRL-CMV activity; values were normalized to the luciferase readings from an empty vector control. Experiments were repeated at least three times in duplicate and data are presented as fold induction; mean ± S.D. are plotted. Statistical analysis was performed by one-way ANOVA with Bonferroni post-test. For the determination of IRF5 stability, cells were transfected with 8 µg GFP-IRF5 plasmids. 48 hr post-transfection, cells were fractionated by fluorescence activated cell sorting (FACS) into subpopulations expressing low, medium, and high levels of GFP, as described [48]. Cells with medium expression of GFP were treated with 100 µg/mL cycloheximide for 5 hr. Cells were collected at 30–60 min intervals and analyzed by flow cytometry for mean GFP fluorescence. Linear regression analysis of mean fluorescence vs. time was performed for each isoform, and analysis of covariance (ANCOVA) with multiple comparison test (by Tukey's HSD test and Bonferroni's post-hoc) was used to determine if regression lines between isoforms differed significantly.

Data Display

The Integrative Genomics Viewer (IGV) [65] was used to display transcripts, read alignments, and junctions as they map to coordinates of the *IRF5* genomic sequence.

Statistical Analysis of IRF5 Expression Profiles in Healthy vs. SLE

The two-way ANOVA with Bonferroni post-test was used to detect differences in *IRF5* transcript profiles obtained by cloning from healthy and SLE Mo. For the testing of differential expression between healthy donors and SLE patients, the mean ± S.D. of normalized raw read counts (MMSeq-based predictions) or normalized expression level for each transcript was calculated and pooled for the SLE subjects, and the student's *t*-test was used to test the null hypothesis that a healthy subject is the same as the SLE group. Pearson correlation coefficient was used to detect differences between MMSeq-derived expression estimates and true expression levels (in the simulation study) and MMSeq-derived Gibbs expression measures and clone count at alpha = 0.05 with a 95% confidence interval. Hierarchial clustering on the samples using expression profiles of the 18 transcripts was performed by multiscale bootstrapping using the pvclust package of R.

Calculating the Probability of Transcript Rankings

Given 7 independent subjects, where each subject has 18 transcripts, we used combinatorics to determine the probability that the top 4 most abundant transcripts in any 4 subjects are the same: $p = (14!/18!)^3((18!\text{-}4!14!)/18!)^3 = 2.522181E^{-15}$.

Supporting Information

Figure S1 Filtering TopHat junctions by relative hits excludes non-canonical junctions likely to represent random splicing. TopHat-reported junctions for two representative samples (1 healthy donor, 1 SLE patients) are grouped by "relative hits", or the percentage of total mapped reads aligning to them, and the fraction of junctions containing a non-canonical splice site is plotted versus the relative hits %. The frequency of non-canonical junctions levels off as the relative hits % approaches 0.01%.

Table S1 Read mapping statistics. For each sequenced healthy donor and SLE patient sample, the number of reads as well as percentages of reads mapped within each Bowtie alignment is shown. For MMSeq-based expression estimates, mapping was performed to transcript variants (column 3); to *IRF5* genomic sequence for pile-up views (column 4); to junction sequences for junction-based expression estimates (column 5); and iteratively to *IRF5* and its predicted junctions by TopHat *de novo* junction detection software (column 6).

Table S2 List of splice junctions identified in the *IRF5* variant transcriptome. Junctions were considered canonical if splice sites consisted of nucleotides GT…AG, GC…AG, AT…AC, GG…AG, GT…TG, GT…GG, or CT…AG [62]. Del = deletion; ins = insertion; N/A - not applicable (*junction R represents an internal duplication).

Table S3 List of junctions contained in each full-length alternatively spliced *IRF5* transcript. Each of the 18 transcripts contains a unique combination of junctions.

Table S4 List of junctions in the *IRF5* variant transcriptome that were detected by TopHat. Junctions were considered canonical if splice sites consisted of nucleotides GT…AG, GC…AG, AT…AC, GG…AG, GT…TG, GT…GG, or CT…AG [62]. Individual junctions present in each sample are shown by the x.

Table S5 List of primers used to confirm TopHat discovered junctions 1–9.

Dataset S1 Sequences of the 14 novel alternatively spliced *IRF5* transcripts. New variants were identified by cloning from purified monocytes of healthy donors and SLE patients.

Dataset S2 Sequences of the 19 junctions derived from the *IRF5* variant transcriptome. Each junction is 94 bp in length and consists of 47-bp blocks of the two spliced exons at the area of intersection.

Method S1 Filtering *de novo* junctions reported by TopHat to exclude random splicing. True splice junctions are more likely to have a canonical or near canonical splice site, while random (non-significant) splicing is more likely to use non-canonical splice sites [62–63]; thus the fraction of non-canonical sites among junctions reported can serve as an indicator of the false positive rate. Data in Table S2 reveal that the majority of junction splice sites found in the *IRF5* variant transcriptome feature the canonical dinucleotides GT and AG as intronic donor and acceptor splice sites, respectively. However, well-known *IRF5* variants V1 and V4 contain the non-canonical junction K that generates one of the Ex6 deletions [19]. Thus, validity of junctions discovered *de novo* might better be determined with a cut-off. When we define "relative hits" as the number of reads mapping to a TopHat-reported junction per fraction of all reads for all reported junctions, we observe that the fraction of non-canonical splice sites for discovered junctions decreases when the number of relative hits to the junctions increase (Figure S1). When the relative hits for a junction reaches 0.01%, the frequency of having a non-canonical splicing site tends to level off to near zero. Based on these findings, we set a threshold of 0.01% and discard reported junctions with relative hits below this value, thus more likely including junctions that represent true, non-random splicing.
(TIF)

Acknowledgments

We thank Dr. Ernest Turro for his comments and critical reading of the manuscript. We thank Ms. Rezvan Kiani for collecting the blood samples and Asiel Benitez for aiding in the cloning optimization. We express extreme gratitude to the Molecular Resource Facility at the New Jersey Medical School for sharing of reagents and time. We thank IST/High Performance and Research Computing for their contributions and resources, and Gedaliah Wolosh for writing scripts to run BOWTIE, TOPHAT and MMSEQ.

Author Contributions

Conceived and designed the experiments: BJB RCS DF RD LR MLE. Performed the experiments: RCS DF KD MLE RD. Analyzed the data: RCS PD DF KD BJB. Contributed reagents/materials/analysis tools: PD KD LR MLE RD BJB. Wrote the paper: BJB RCS PD DF LR MLE RD.

References

1. Rahman A, Isenberg DA (2008) Systemic lupus erythematosus. N Engl J Med 358: 929–939.
2. Flesher DL, Sun X, Behrens TW, Graham RR, Criswell LA (2010) Recent advances in the genetics of systemic lupus erythematosus. Expert Rev Clin Immunol 6: 461–479.

3. Deng Y, Tsao BP (2010) Genetic susceptibility to systemic lupus erythematosus in the genomic era. Nat Rev Rheumatol 6: 683–692.
4. Sigurdsson S, Nordmark G, Harald Goring HH, Lindroos K, Wiman C, et al. (2005) Polymorphisms in the tyrosine kinase 2 and interferon regulatory factor 5 genes are associated with systemic lupus erythematosus. Am J Hum Genet 76: 528–537.
5. Demirci FY, Manzi S, Ramsey-Goldman R, Minster RL, Kenney M, et al. (2006) Association of a common interferon regulatory factor 5 (IRF5) variant with increased risk of systemic lupus erythematosus (SLE). Ann Hum Genet 71: 308–311.
6. Cunninghame Graham DS, Manku H, Wagner S, Reid J, Timms K, et al. (2007) Association of IRF5 in UK SLE families identifies a variant involved in polyadenylation. Hum Mol Genet 16: 579–591.
7. Graham RR, Kozyrev SV, Baechler EC, Reddy MV, Plenge RM, et al. (2006) A common haplotype of interferon regulatory factor 5 (IRF5) regulates splicing and expression and is associated with increased risk of systemic lupus erythematosus. Nat Genet 38: 550–555.
8. Kozyrev SV, Lewen S, Reddy PM, Pons-Estel B, Argentine Collarborative Group, et al. (2007) Structural insertion/deletion variation in IRF5 is associated with a risk haplotype and defines the precise IRF5 isoforms expressed in systemic lupus erythematosus. Arthritis Rheum 56: 1234–1241.
9. Shin HD, Sung YK, Choi CB, Lee SO, Lee HW, et al. (2007) Replication of genetic effects of interferon regulatory factor 5 (IRF5) on systemic lupus erythematosus in a Korean population. Arthritis Res Ther 9, R32.
10. Graham RR, Kyogoku C, Sigurdsson S, Vlasova IA, Davies LR, et al. (2007) Three functional variants of IFN regulatory factor 5 (IRF5) define risk and protective haplotypes for human lupus. Proc Natl Acad Sci USA 104: 6758–6763.
11. Barnes BJ, Moore PA, Pitha PM (2001) Virus-specific activation of a novel interferon regulatory factor, IRF-5, results in the induction of distinct interferon alpha genes J Biol Chem 276: 23382–23390.
12. Schoenemeyer A, Barnes BJ, Mancl ME, Latz E, Goutagny N, et al. (2005) The Interferon Regulatory Factor, IRF-5, Is a Central Mediator of Toll-like Receptor 7 Signaling. J Biol Chem 280: 17005–17012.
13. Takaoka A, Yanai H, Kondo S, Duncan G, Negishi H, et al. (2005) Integral role of IRF-5 in the gene induction programme activated by Toll-Like Receptors. Nature 434: 243–249.
14. Yanai H, Chen HM, Inuzuka T, Kondo S, Mak TW, et al. (2007) Role of IFN regulatory factor 5 transcription factor in antiviral immunity and tumor suppression. Proc Natl Acad Sci USA 104: 3402–3407.
15. Feng D, Stone RC, Eloranta ML, Sangster-Guity N, Nordmark G, et al. (2010) Genetic variants and disease-associated factors contribute to enhanced IRF-5 expression in blood cells of systemic lupus erythematosus patients. Arthritis Rheum 62: 562–573.
16. Sigurdsson S, Goring HHH, Kristjandsdottir G, Milani L, Nordmark G, et al. (2008) Comprehensive evaluation of the genetic variants of interferon regulatory factor 5 reveals a novel 5 bp length polymorphism as strong risk factor for systemic lupus erythematosus. Hum Mol Genet 17: 872–881.
17. Niewold TB, Hua J, Lehman TJ, Harley JB, Crow MK (2007) High serum IFN-alpha activity is a heritable risk factor for systemic lupus erythematosus. Genes Immun 56: 3995–4004.
18. Niewold TB, Kelly JA, Flesch MH, Espinoza LR, Harley JB, et al. (2008) Association of the IRF5 risk haplotype with high serum interferon-α activity in systemic lupus erythematosus patients. Arthritis Rheum 58: 2481–2487.
19. Mancl ME, Hu G, Sangster-Guity N, Olshalsky SL, Hoops K, et al. (2005) Two distinct promoters regulate the alternative-spliced human Interferon regulatory factor-5 variants: Multiple variants with distinct cell-type specific expression, localization, regulation and function. J Biol Chem 280: 21078–90.
20. Barnes BJ, Kellum MJ, Field AE, Pitha PM (2002) Multiple regulatory domains of IRF-5 control activation, cellular localization and induction of chemokines that mediate T-lymphocyte recruitment. Mol Cell Biol 22: 5721–5740.
21. Barnes BJ, Richards J, Mancl M, Hanash S, Beretta L, et al. (2004) Global and distinct targets of IRF-5 and IRF-7 during innate response to viral infection. J Biol Chem 279: 45194–45207.
22. Barnes BJ, Kellum MJ, Pinder KE, Frisancho JA, Pitha PM (2003) Interferon regulatory factor 5, a novel mediator of cell cycle arrest and cell death. Cancer Res 63: 6424–6431.
23. Hu G, Mancl M, Barnes BJ (2005) Signaling through IFN regulatory factor-5 sensitizes p53-deficient tumors to DNA damage-induced apoptosis and cell death. Cancer Res 65: 7403–7412.
24. Couzinet A, Tamura K, Chen HM, Nishimura K, Wang Z, et al. (2008) A cell-type-specific requirement for IFN regulatory factor 5 (IRF5) in Fas-induced apoptosis. Proc Natl Acad Sci U S A 105: 2556–2561.
25. Hu G, Barnes BJ (2009) IRF-5 is a mediator of the death receptor-induced apoptotic signaling pathway. J Biol Chem 284: 2767–2777.
26. Feng D, Sangster-Guity N, Stone R, Korczeniewska J, Mancl ME, et al. (2010) Differential requirement of histone acetylase and deacetylase activities for IRF5-mediated proinflammatory cytokine expression. J Immunol 185: 6003–6012.
27. Yasuda K, Richez C, Maciaszek JW, Agrawal N, Akira S, et al. (2007) Murine dendritic cell type I IFN production induced by human IgG-RNA immune complexes is IFN regulatory factor (IRF)5 and IRF7 dependent and is required for IL-6 production. J Immunol 178: 6876–6885.
28. Paun A, Reinert JT, Jiang Z, Medin C, Balkhi MY, et al. (2008) Functional characterization of murine interferon regulatory factor 5 (IRF-5) and its role in the innate antiviral response. J Biol Chem 283: 14295–14308.
29. Krausgruber T, Blazek K, Smallie T, Alzabin S, Lockstone H, et al. (2011) IRF5 promotes inflammatory macrophage polarization and TH1-TH17 responses. Nat Immunol 12: 231–238.
30. Izaguirre A, Barnes BJ, Amrute S, Yeow WS, Megjugorac N, et al. (2003) Comparative analysis of IRF and IFN-alpha expression in human plasmacytoid and monocyte-derived dendritic cells. J Leukoc Biol 74: 1125–1138.
31. Richez C, Yasuda K, Bonegio RG, Watkins AA, Aprahamian T, et al. (2010) IFN regulatory factor 5 is required for disease development in the FcgammaRIIB−/−Yaa and FcgammaRIIB−/− mouse models of systemic lupus erythematosus. J Immunol 184: 796–806.
32. Savitsky DA, Yanai H, Tamura T, Taniguchi T, Honda K (2010) Contribution of IRF5 in B cells to the development of murine SLE-like disease through its transcriptional control of the IgG2a locus. Proc Natl Acad Sci USA 107: 10154–10159.
33. Tada Y, Kondo S, Aoki S, Koarada S, Inoue H, et al. (2011) Interferon regulatory factor 5 is critical for the development of lupus in MRL/lpr mice. Arthritis Rheum 63: 738–748.
34. Shen H, Panchanathan R, Rajavelu P, Duan X, Gould KA, et al. (2010) Gender-dependent expression of murine Irf5 gene: implications for sex bias in autoimmunity. J Mol Cell Biol 2: 284–290.
35. Rullo OJ, Woo JM, Wu H, Hoftman AD, Maranian P, et al. (2010) Association of IRF5 polymorphisms with activation of the interferon alpha pathway. Ann Rheum Dis 69: 611–617.
36. Kozyrev SV, Alarcon-Riquelme ME (2007) The genetics and biology of Irf5-mediated signaling in lupus. Autoimmunity 40: 591–601.
37. Stone RC, Feng D, Deng J, Singh S, Yang L, et al. (2012) Interferon regulatory factor 5 activation in monocytes of SLE patients is triggered by circulating autoantigens independent of type I IFN. Arthritis Rheum 64: 788–798.
38. Sambrook J, Russell DW (2001) Preparation of cDNA libraries and gene identification. In: Molecular Cloning: a laboratory manual. Cold Spring Harbor Laboratory Press, 11.69–11.70.
39. Turro E, Su SY, Goncalves A, Coin LJ, Richardson S, et al. (2011) Haplotype and isoform specific expression estimation using multi-mapping RNA-seq reads. Genome Biol 12: R13.
40. Wen F, Ellingson SM, Kyogoku C, Peterson EJ, Gaffney PM (2010) Exon 6 variants carried on systemic lupus erythematosus (SLE) risk haplotypes modulate IRF5 function. Autoimmunity 44: 82–89.
41. Trapnell C, Pachter L, Salzberg SL (2009) TopHat: discovering splice junctions with RNA-Seq. Bioinformatics 25: 1105–1111.
42. Griffith M, Griffith OL, Mwenifumbo J, Goya R, Morrissy AS, et al. (2010) Alternative expression analysis by RNA sequencing. Nature Methods 7: 843–847.
43. Lauwerys BR, Van Snick J, Houssiau FA (2002) Serum IL-12 in systemic lupus erythematosus: absence of p70 heterodimers but presence of p40 monomers correlating with disease activity. Lupus 11: 384–387.
44. Linker-Israeli M, Deans RJ, Wallace DJ, Prehn J, Ozeri-Chen T, et al. (1991) Elevated levels of endogenous IL-6 in systemic lupus erythematosus. A putative role in pathogenesis. J Immunol 147: 117–123.
45. Aringer M, Smolen JS (2003) SLE - Complex cytokine effects in a complex autoimmune disease: tumor necrosis factor in systemic lupus erythematosus. Arthritis Res Ther 5: 172–177.
46. Rogers S, Wells R, Rechsteiner M (1986) Amino acid sequences common to rapidly degraded proteins: the PEST hypothesis. Science 234: 364–368.
47. Shumway SD, Maki M, Miyamoto S (1999) The PEST domain of IkappaBalpha is necessary and sufficient for in vitro degradation by mu-calpain. J Biol Chem 274: 30874–30881.
48. Jiang X, Coffino P, Li X (2004) Development of a method for screening short-lived proteins using green fluorescent protein. Genome Biol 5: R81.
49. Corish P, Tyler-Smith C (1999) Attenuation of green fluorescent protein half-life in mammalian cells. Protein Eng 12: 1035–1040.
50. Mortazavi A, Williams BA, McCue K, Schaeffer L, Wold B (2008) Mapping and quantifying mammalian transcriptomes by RNA-Seq. Nat Methods 5: 621–628.
51. Hiller D, Jiang H, Xu W, Wong W (2009) Identifiability of isoform deconvoluation from junction arrays and RNA-Seq. Bioinformatics 25: 3056–3059.
52. Jiang H, Wong WH (2009) Statistical inferences for isoform expression in RNA-Seq. Bioinformatics 25: 1026–1032.
53. Li B, Ruotti V, Stewart RM, Thomson JA, Dewey CN (2010) RNA-Seq gene expression estimation with read mapping uncertainty. Bioinformatics 26: 493–500.
54. Roberts A, Pimentel H, Trapnell C, Pachter L (2011) Identification of novel transcripts in annotated genomes using RNA-Seq. Bioinformatics 27: 2325–2329.
55. Morley M, Molony CM, Weber TM, Devlin JL, Ewens KG, et al. (2004) Genetic analysis of genome-wide variation in human gene expression. Nature 430: 743–747.
56. Alonso-Perez E, Suarez-Gestal M, Calaza M, Kwan T, Majewski J, et al. (2011) *Cis*-regulation of IRF5 expression is unable to fully account for systemic lupuserythematosus association: analysis of multiple experiments with lymphoblastoid cell lines. Arthritis & Therap 13: R80.

57. Li H, Handsaker B, Wysoker A, Fennell T, Ruan J, et al. (2009) The Sequence Alignment/Map format and SAMtools. Bioinformatics 25: 2078–2079.
58. Jarvinen TM, Hellquist A, Zucchelli M, Koskenmies S, Panelius J, et al. (2012) Replication of genome-wide association study identified systemic lupus erythematosus susceptibility genes affirms B-cell receptor pathway signalling and strengthens the role of IRF5 in disease susceptibility in a Northern European population. Rheumatology 51: 87–92.
59. Barnes BJ, Field A, Pitha-Rowe PM (2003) Virus-induced heterodimer formation between IRF-5 and IRF-7 modulates assembly of the IFNA enhanceosome in vivo and transcriptional activity of IFNA genes. J Biol Chem 278: 16630–16641.
60. Cheng TF, Brzostek S, Ando O, Van Scoy S, Kumar KP, et al. (2006) Differential activation of IFN regulatory factor (IRF)-3 and IRF-5 transcription factors during viral infection. J Immunol 176: 7462–7470.
61. Langmead B (2010) Aligning short sequencing reads with Bowtie. Curr Protoc Bioinformatics Chapter 11, Unit 11 7.
62. Langmead B, Trapnell C, Pop M, Salzberg SL (2009) Ultrafast and memory-efficient alignment of short DNA sequences to the human genome. Genome Biol 10: R25.
63. Burset M, Seledtsov IA, Solovyev VV (2000) Analysis of canonical and non-canonical splice sites in mammalian genomes. Nucl Acids Res 28: 4364–4375.
64. Houseley J, Tollervey D (2010) Apparent non-canonical trans-splicing is generated by reverse transcriptase *in vitro*. PLoS ONE 5(8): e12271.
65. Robinson JY, Thorvaldsdóttir H, Winckler W, Guttman M, Lander ES, et al. (2011) Integrative Genomics Viewer. Nature Biotechnology 29: 24–26.

17

Decreased Frequencies of Circulating Follicular Helper T Cell Counterparts and Plasmablasts in Ankylosing Spondylitis Patients Naïve for TNF Blockers

María-Belén Bautista-Caro[1], Irene Arroyo-Villa[1], Concepción Castillo-Gallego[1], Eugenio de Miguel[1], Diana Peiteado[1], Chamaida Plasencia-Rodríguez[1], Alejandro Villalba[1], Paloma Sánchez-Mateos[2], Amaya Puig-Kröger[2], Emilio Martín-Mola[1], María-Eugenia Miranda-Carús[1]*

1 Department of Rheumatology, Hospital Universitario La Paz-IdiPAZ, Madrid, Spain, **2** Laboratorio de Inmuno-Oncología, Hospital General Universitario Gregorio Marañón, Madrid, Spain

Abstract

Follicular helper T cells (Tfh), localized in lymphoid organs, promote B cell differentiation and function. Circulating CD4 T cells expressing CXCR5, ICOS and/or PD-1 are counterparts of Tfh. Three subpopulations of circulating CD4+CXCR5+ cells have been described: CXCR3+CCR6- (Tfh-Th1), CXCR3-CCR6+ (Tfh-Th17), and CXCR3-CCR6- (Tfh-Th2). Only Tfh-Th17 and Tfh-Th2 function as B cell helpers. Our objective was to study the frequencies of circulating Tfh (cTfh), cTfh subsets and plasmablasts (CD19+CD20-CD27+CD38^{high} cells), and the function of cTfh cells, in patients with Ankylosing Spondylitis (AS). To this end, peripheral blood was drawn from healthy controls (HC) (n = 50), AS patients naïve for TNF blockers (AS/nb) (n = 25) and AS patients treated with TNF blockers (AS/b) (n = 25). The frequencies of cTfh and plasmablasts were determined by flow cytometry. Cocultures of magnetically sorted CD4+CXCR5+ T cells with autologous CD19+CD27- naïve B cells were established from 3 AS/nb patients and 3 HC, and concentrations of IgG, A and M were measured in supernatants. We obseved that AS/nb but not AS/b patients, demonstrated decreased frequencies of circulating CD4+CXCR5+ICOS+PD-1+ cells and plasmablasts, together with a decreased (Tfh-Th17+Tfh-Th2)/Tfh-Th1 ratio. The amounts of IgG and IgA produced in cocultures of CD4+CXCR5+ T cells with CD19+CD27- B cells of AS/nb patients were significantly lower than observed in cocultures established from HC. In summary, AS/nb but not AS/b patients, demonstrate a decreased frequency of cTfh and plasmablasts, and an underrepresentation of cTfh subsets bearing a B helper phenotype. In addition, peripheral blood CD4+ CXCR5+ T cells of AS/nb patients showed a decreased capacity to help B cells ex vivo.

Editor: Peter Szodoray, Institute of Immunology, Rikshospitalet, Norway

Funding: This work was supported by Fondo de Investigación Sanitaria grant PI-13/00084 from Ministerio de Economía y Competitividad/Instituto de Salud Carlos III (MINECO/ISCIII) (www.isciii.es), by RETICS Program RD12/0009/0012 (Red de Investigación en Inflamación y enfermedades Reumáticas - RIER) from MINECO/ISCIII (www.isciii.es), and by Comunidad Autónoma de Madrid/Fondo Europeo de Desarrollo Regional RAPHYME (http://www.madrimasd.org). The funders had no role in study design, data collection and analysis, decision to publish, or preparation of the manuscript.

Competing Interests: The authors have declared that no competing interests exist.

* Email: mariaeugenia.miranda@salud.madrid.org

Introduction

Ankylosing spondylitis (AS) is the prototype of Spondyloarthritis (SpA) [1,2], a group of diseases sharing clinical, radiographic and genetic features [1,2]. Despite intensive research, the pathogenesis of SpA is not well understood, and evidence suggesting the implication of either autoinflammatory or autoimmune mechanisms has been reported [3].

The role of B cells and of humoral immunity in SpA is not clear. Several autoantibodies have been observed in patients with SpA [4–7], but their poor sensitivity or specificity have not allowed to establish a clear pathogenic association. More recently, reactivity against CD74 has been proposed as a marker for SpA [8,9]. Also, increased numbers of CD5+ B lymphocytes have been described in SpA [10]. Furthermore, it has been reported that some patients with AS seem to benefit from B cell depleting therapeutic strategies [11].

Follicular helper T cells (Tfh) are a major subset of effector T lymphocytes specialized in the provision of help to B cells [12–17], and characterized by their surface phenotype (CD4+CXCR5+ ICOS+PD-1+), cytokine profile (IL-21, IL-10, IL-17) and transcriptional program (BCL-6) [12–17]. Tfh cells seem to be implicated in autoimmunity [18], and increased numbers are found in murine models of Systemic Lupus Erythematosus (SLE) [18–20] and inflammatory arthritis [21]; furthermore, strategies directed at reducing Tfh cell generation ameliorate disease manifestations in these animal models [20,22].

The initial definition of Tfh cells was based on both their phenotype and their characteristic location in secondary lymphoid organs [12–17]. Several reports have subsequently described circulating populations of CD4 T cells that express CXCR5 and share both phenotypical and functional properties of classical Tfh cells [23–26]. Increased frequencies of circulating Tfh cell counterparts (cTfh), have been associated with autoimmune diseases such as SLE [23], Rheumatoid Arthritis (RA) [27], Sjögren's Syndrome [28], autoimmune thyroiditis [29], chronic active hepatitis [30] and myasthenia gravis [31]. More recently, three subpopulations of cTfh cells have been described, based on their differential expression of the chemokine receptors CXCR3 and CCR6 and on their distinct functional capacities [24]. An altered balance of these cTfh subsets has been associated with autoimmunity in juvenile dermatomyositis and SLE [24,32].

The features of cTfh cells or their subsets in SpA have not been fully characterized, and to our knowledge only two articles with discordant results have been published on this matter [33,34]. Therefore, our objective was to study the frequency and function of cTfh cells, together with the frequency of cTfh subsets and plasmablasts (CD19+CD20-CD27+CD38^{high} B cells), in patients with Ankylosing Spondylitis (AS). We observed that AS patients naïve for TNF blockers (AS/nb) but not those receiving TNF blocking agents (AS/b), demonstrate a decreased frequency of cTfh and plasmablasts, and an underrepresentation of cTfh subsets bearing a B helper phenotype. In addition, peripheral blood CD4+CXCR5+ T cells of AS/nb patients showed a decreased capacity to help B cells ex vivo.

Patients and Methods

Ethics Statement

The study was approved by the Hospital La Paz - IdiPAZ Ethics Committee, and all subjects provided written informed consent according to the Declaration of Helsinki.

Patients

Peripheral blood was obtained from 25 AS patients who had never received TNF blockers (AS/nb), 25 AS patients treated with TNF blockers (AS/b) and from 50 age and gender-matched healthy controls (HC). AS was diagnosed according to the 1984 modified New York criteria [35]. For patients receiving TNF blockers, blood was drawn immediately before the infusion/administration of the drug. All subjects were of Western European descent.

Among AS/nb patients, 16 were taking non-steroidal anti-inflammatory drugs (NSAIDs) and 4 were receiving sulfasalazine (SSZ); 5 of them did not take any medication regularly. Among AS/b patients, 20 were receiving infliximab, 4 etanercept and 1 adalimumab. In addition to TNF blockers, 7 patients were taking NSAIDs, and 8 were taking SSZ. Clinical characteristics of all patients are shown in Tables 1 and 2.

Isolation of CD4+ T cells and B cells from human peripheral blood

Peripheral blood mononuclear cells (PBMCs) were separated immediately after blood sample collection, by Ficoll-Hypaque (GE Healthcare Biosciences AB, Uppsala, Sweden) density gradient centrifugation. CD4+ T or B cells were purifed from freshly isolated PBMCs by exhaustive immunomagnetic negative selection in an Automacs (Miltenyi Biotec, Bergisch Gladbach, Germany), using the "CD4+ T Cell Isolation Kit" or the "B Cell Isolation Kit II" from Miltenyi Biotec. Isolated CD4+ T cells or CD19+ B cells were >98% pure. CXCR5+ and CXCR5- subpopulations were subsequently isolated from total CD4+ T cells using PE-labeled CXCR5 microbeads (Miltenyi Biotec). Naïve (CD19+CD27-) and memory (CD19+CD27+) B cells were selected from total CD19+ B cells using CD27+ microbeads (Miltenyi Biotec). T and B cell subpopulations were >98% pure and used immediately after isolation.

B cell/T cell cocultures

To assess the functional capacity of circulating CD4+CXCR5+ T cells, sorted CXCR5+ cells (2×10^5 cells/well) were cocultured for 13 days with autologous naïve B (CD19+CD27-) cells (1×10^5 cells/well) in U-bottom 96-well plates containing RPMI 1640 medium (Lonza, Alendale, NJ, USA) with 10% FCS, 2 mM L-glutamine, 50 U/ml penicillin, 50 µg/ml streptomycin and 50 µM 2-mercapto-ethanol. Endotoxin-reduced staphylococcal enterotoxin B (SEB) (1 mg/ml) (Sigma-Aldrich) was also added to the cultures, since the production of immunoglobulins in Tfh/B cell cocultures has been shown to depend on cognate T/B cell interactions [24]. For comparison, autologous cocultures of CD4+ CXCR5+ T cells with CD19+CD27+ memory B cells and cocultures of CD4+CXCR5- T cells with naïve or memory B cells were also established. Concentrations of IgG, IgA and IgM were measured in coculture supernatants at different time points by ELISA.

Cell Surface Staining and Flow Cytometry

The frequency and phenotype of Tfh-like cells and of plasmablasts present in the peripheral blood of AS patients and HC was assessed by flow cytometry after staining freshly isolated PBMCs with antibodies directed against surface phenotypical markers. Fluorochrome-conjugated mAbs from BD Pharmingen (San Diego, CA, USA) were used to examine the expression of CD3, CD4, CD8, CXCR5, ICOS, PD-1, CCR6, CXCR3, CD19, CD20, CD27 and CD38 in a FACSCalibur flow cytometer with CellQuest software (BD Biosciences).

ELISAs

Cell-free coculture supernatants were collected and stored at −80°C. The concentrations of immunoglobulins were measured by ELISA. In brief, 96-well plates (MaxiSorp, Thermo Fisher Scientific, Waltham, MA, USA) were coated overnight at 4°C with 10 µg/ml mouse monoclonal anti-human IgG, IgA or IgM (AbD Serotec, Munich, Germany), and subseqently blocked with 2% BSA/PBS. Standard curves of human IgG, IgA or IgM (Sigma-Aldrich) together with culture supernatants diluted in 2% BSA/PBS were incubated for 3 hours at room temperature, washed and developed with HRP-conjugated goat anti-human IgG, IgA or IgM (ABD serotec) followed by TMB substrate solution (BD-Pharmingen). Absorbance was measured at 450 nm in a Synergy H4 Hybrid Multi-Mode Microplate Reader (BioTec Instruments, Inc., Winoosi, VT, USA).

Determination of serum IgG, IgA and IgM concentrations

Sera from all studied subjects were collected on the day when phenotypical studies were done, and stored at −80°C. Concentrations of IgG, IgA and IgM were subsequently examined in sera of AS/nb, AS/b patients and HC by nephelometry in an Immage 800 Immunochemistry System (Beckman Coulter, Brea, CA, U.S.A). For AS/b patients, determinations of Igs were also performed in serum that had been collected just before initiation of treatment with TNF blockers.

Statistical Analysis

Comparison between groups was by Mann-Whitney or Kruskal-Wallis test. When appropriate, Bonferroni correction for multiple comparisons was applied. Correlations were analyzed using Spearman's rank correlation coefficients. All analyses were performed using Prism version 5.0 software (GraphPad Software, San Diego, CA, USA).

Table 1. Clinical characteristics of AS/nb and AS/b patients.

	AS/nb (n = 25)	AS/b (n = 25)
Age (years); median (IQR)	56 (45.5–65.5)	53 (45–61.5)
Male; n° (%)	12 (48)	16 (64)
HLA-B27+; n° (%)	22 (88)	23 (92)
Duration of symptoms (yrs); median (IQR)	25.5 (17.5–35)	24.5 (14–36)
Time since diagnosis (yrs); median (IQR)	11.5 (5.5–20)	15 (9–22.5)
Time on TNF blockers (yrs); median (IQR)	-	7 (5–9)
BASDAI; median (IQR)	3.9 (2.8–4.8)	2.6 (1.3–6.1)
BASFI; median (IQR)	1.8 (0.5–4.9)	3 (0.6–5.8)
ASDAS-ESR; median (IQR)	2.14 (1.89–2.72)	2.22 (1.41–3.15)
ASDAS-CRP; median (IQR)	2.55 (1.9–3.13)	2.34 (1.07–3.02)
CRP; median (IQR)	7.37 (2.51–11.1)	4.52 (1.44–15.4)
Pt. global assessment; median (IQR)	3 (2–6)	3 (2–6.5)

AS/nb: AS patients naïve for TNF blockers; AS/b: AS patients treated with TNF blockers.

Results

Patients with AS naïve for TNF blockers demonstrate decreased numbers of circulating Tfh counterparts

We first sought to examine the expression of Tfh phenotypical surface markers on peripheral blood CD4+ T cells. The frequency of CXCR5+ cells contained in circulating CD4+ T lymphocytes was not different among the three groups of studied subjects: 18.3±5.8 % in HC, 18.6±7.6 % in AS patients naïve for TNF blockers (AS/nb) and 18.1±5.6 % in AS patients treated with TNF blockers (AS/b) (mean ± SD). However, the frequencies of circulating total CD4+CXCR5+ICOS+ and of CD4+CXCR5+ICOS^{high}, together with the frequencies of total CD4+CXCR5+ICOS+ PD-1+ and of CD4+CXCR5+ICOS^{high}PD-1^{high} T cells, that are currently considered as circulating counterparts of classical Tfh cells (cTfh) [23,25,26], were significantly decreased in AS/nb patients (Figure 1, A, B) but were not different from controls in AS/b patients (Figure 1, A, B). In parallel, the absolute numbers of cTfh were also decreased in AS/nb patients (Figure 1 C).

Patients with AS naïve for TNF blockers demonstrate an altered balance of circulating Tfh subsets

We then examined the frequency of cTfh cell subsets as described by Morita et al. [24], based on the combined expression on CD4+ T cells of CXCR5 with CCR6 or CXCR3, that are characteristic chemokine receptors expressed on Th17 or Th1 cells, respectively. AS/nb patients demonstrated an increased frequency of circulating CD4+CXCR5+CXCR3+CCR6- (Tfh-Th1) cells together with a decreased frequency of CD4+CXCR5+CXCR3-CCR6+ (Tfh-Th17) cells, whereas the frequency of CD4+CXCR5+CXCR3-CCR6- (Tfh-Th2) cells was not different from controls (Figure 2A). Furthermore, the sum of %Tfh-Th2 plus %Tfh-Th17 cells and the ratio (%Tfh-Th2+%Tfh-Th17)/%Tfh-Th1, were decreased in AS/nb patients (Figure 2B). That is, AS/nb but not AS/b patients demonstrated a relative deficiency of cTfh cell subsets bearing a phenotype associated with B cell helping capacity [24].

Patients with AS naïve for TNF blockers demonstrate decreased numbers of circulating plasmablasts

The frequency of circulating plasmablasts among CD19+ cells, defined as CD19+CD20-CD27+CD38^{high} B cells, was decreased in AS/nb but not in AS/b patients (Figure 3, A, B). In parallel, the absolute number of circulating plasmablasts was also decreased in AS/nb (Figure 3C).

Interestingly, in AS/nb patients, the frequency of circulating plasmablasts was positively correlated not only with the frequency of cTfh counterparts, but also with the sum %Tfh-Th2+%Tfh-Th17 and with the ratio (%Tfh-Th2+%Tfh-Th17)/%Tfh-Th1 cells (Figure 3D). Conversely, the frequency of circulating plasmablasts was negatively correlated with the frequency of Tfh-Th1 cells in AS/nb (Figure 3D).

In addition, the absolute number of circulating plasmablasts was positively correlated with the absolute numbers of CD4+CXCR5+ICOS+ ($r = 0.40$, $p < 0.05$), CD4+CXCR5+ICOS^{high} ($r = 0.46$, $p < 0.05$) and CD4+CXCR5+ICOS^{high}PD-1^{high} T cells ($r = 0.41$, $p < 0.05$).

Functional capacity of circulating CD4+CXCR5+ T cells

We then went on to examine the functional capacity of circulating total CD4+CXCR5+ T cells, which in AS/nb patients contain decreased proportions of cTfh, together with decreased proportions of cTfh cell subsets bearing a phenotype associated

Table 2. Number of patients according to disease activity state based on ASDAS-CRP values [38].

ASDAS-CRP = =>	< 1.3 (inactive disease)	1.3–2.1 (moderate activity)	2.1–3.5 (high activity)	>3.5 (very high activity)
AS/nb (# of patients)	2	7	13	3
AS/b (# of patients)	7	1	13	4

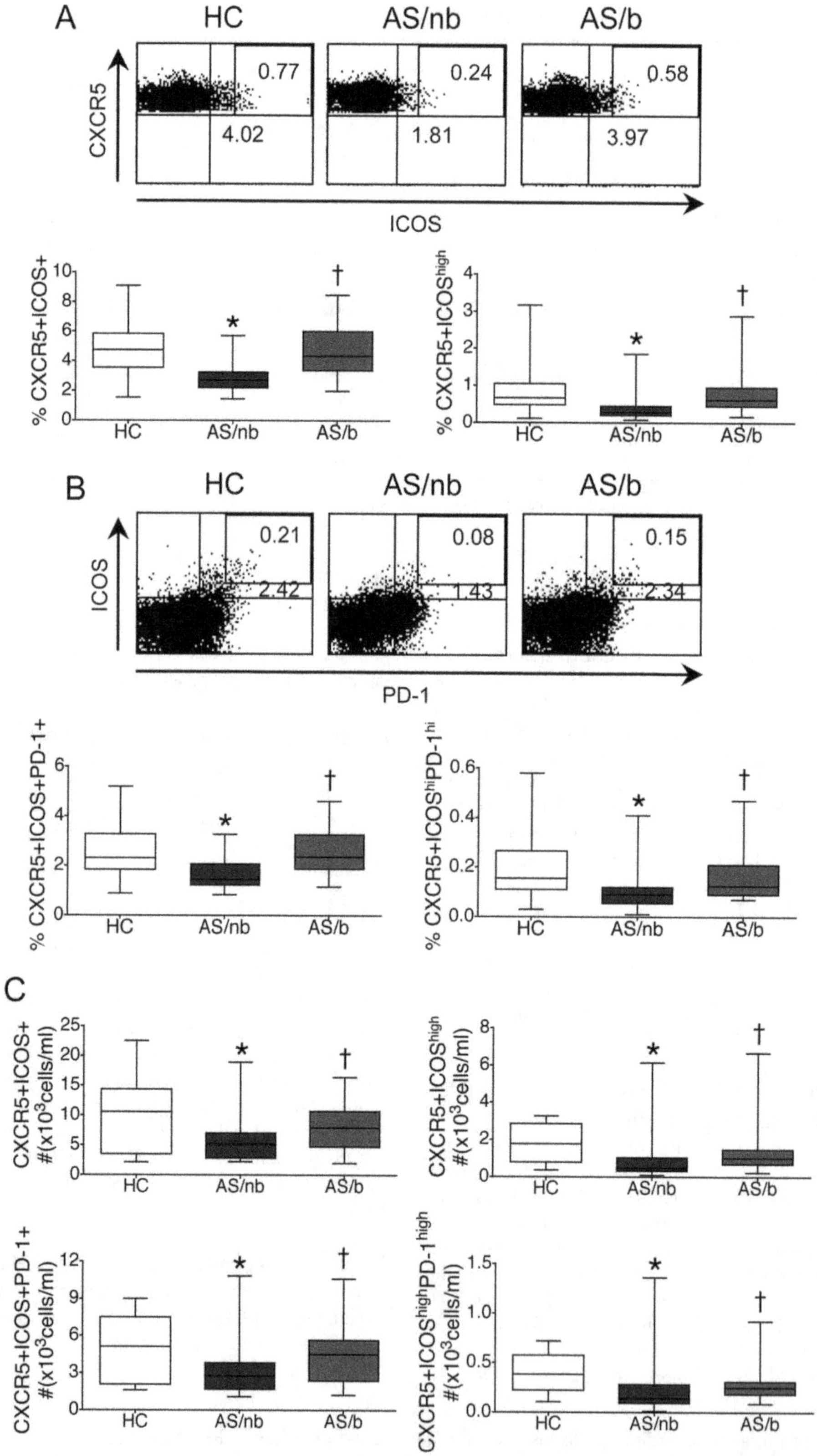

Figure 1. Numbers of circulating Tfh counterparts (cTfh) in patients with AS. AS/nb but not AS/b patients demonstrate decreased frequencies and absolute numbers of cTfh. A, B. Frequency of cTfh in HC, AS/nb and AS/b patients. Representative dot plots demonstrate ICOS and CXCR5 expression (A) or ICOS and PD-1 expression (B) in cells gated for CD3, CD4 and CXCR5. C. Absolute numbers of circulating Tfh counterparts (cTfh) in HC, AS/nb and AS/b patients. Box and whiskers plots represent the median, interquartile range, maximum and minimum values calculated from 25 AS/nb patients, 25 AS/b patients and 50 HC. *p<0.0001 vs HC; † p<0.01 vs AS/nb patients.

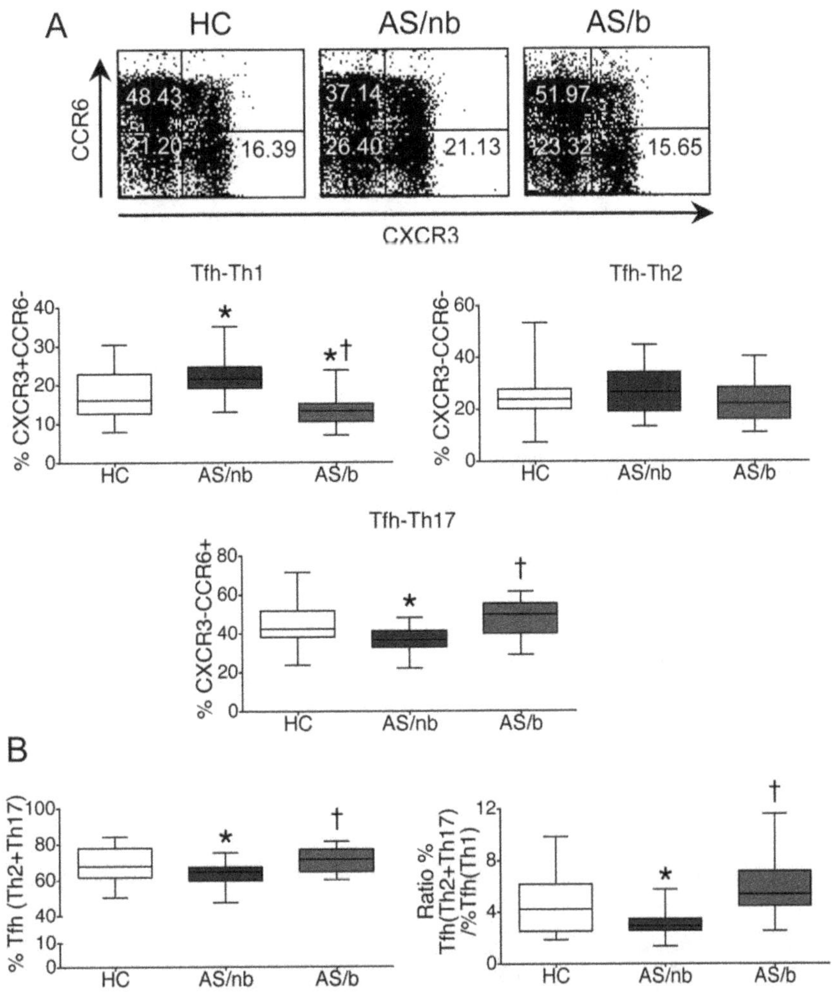

Figure 2. Frequency of circulating Tfh subsets in patients with AS. A. AS/nb, but not AS/b patients, demonstrate an increased frequency of circulating CD4+CXCR5+CXCR3+CCR6- (Tfh-Th1) cells and a decreased frequency of CD4+CXCR5+CXCR3-CCR6+ (Tfh-Th17) cells as compared with HC, whereas the frequency of CD4+CXCR5+CXCR3-CCR6- (Tfh-Th2) cells is not different among the three groups. Representative dot plots demonstrate CXCR3 and CCR6 expression in cells gated for CD3, CD4 and CXCR5. B. Underrepresentation of cTfh subsets with a B cell helper phenotype (Tfh-Th17 plus Tfh-Th2 cells) in AS/nb but not in AS/b patients. Box and whiskers plots represent the median, interquartile range, maximum and minimum values calculated from 25 AS/nb patients, 25 AS/b patients and 50 HC. $^*p<0.05$ vs HC, $^\dagger p<0.005$ vs AS/nb.

with B cell helping capacity. To this end, cocultures of sorted CD4+CXCR5+ T cells from 3 AS/nb patients and 3 age and gender-matched healthy controls were established with autologous naïve CD19+CD27- B cells; secretion of IgG and IgA in supernatants were measured as a readout of B cell maturation. All three patients were male, aged 45, 51 and 57 years and were taking NSAIDs. Two of them were HLA B27+ and one was HLA B27-. Duration of symptoms was 28, 33 and 36 years and time since diagnosis was 25, 27 and 13 years, respectively. Their ASDAS-CRPs were 3.4, 2.75 and 2.05.

In cocultures of naïve B cells with CD4+CXCR5+ T cells, increased proportions of CD19+CD20-CD38^{high} plasmablasts (Figure 4A) were observed; in addition, IgG and IgA were detected in supernatants from the 6th day on, with increasing concentrations up to the 13th day (Figure 4B,C). Interestingly, in cocultures established with T and B cells of AS/nb patients, lower proportions of CD19+CD20-CD38^{high} plasmablasts and lower concentrations of both IgG and IgA were observed as compared with with HC (Figure 4, A-C). In contrast, the amount of secreted IgM was not different in cocultures of naïve B cells with CD4+ CXCR5+ T cells established from HC or AS/nb patients (Figure 4B, C). Of note, the number of recovered viable B cells was not different in cocultures established from HC or AS/nb patients (Figure 4D).

No IgG or IgA could be detected in coculture supernatants of naïve B cells with CD4+ CXCR5- T cells from either AS/nb patients or healthy controls (Figure 4B,C), which only produced low amounts of IgM (Figure 4B, C). This was not attributable to poor T cell survival since the amount of recovered viable T cells was comparable in cocultures of naïve B cells established with either CXCR5+ or CXCR5- CD4+ T cells (Figure 4D).

In addition, isolated CD4+CXCR5+ of HC or AS/nb patients were more efficient than CD4+CXCR5- T cells at helping memory CD19+CD27+ B cells to secrete IgG, IgA and IgM. No differences between HC and AS/nb were observed when measuring the secreted amounts of IgG, IgA or IgM in these CD4+CXCR5+/CD19+CD27+ or CD4+CXCR5-/CD19+CD27+ cocultures (data not shown).

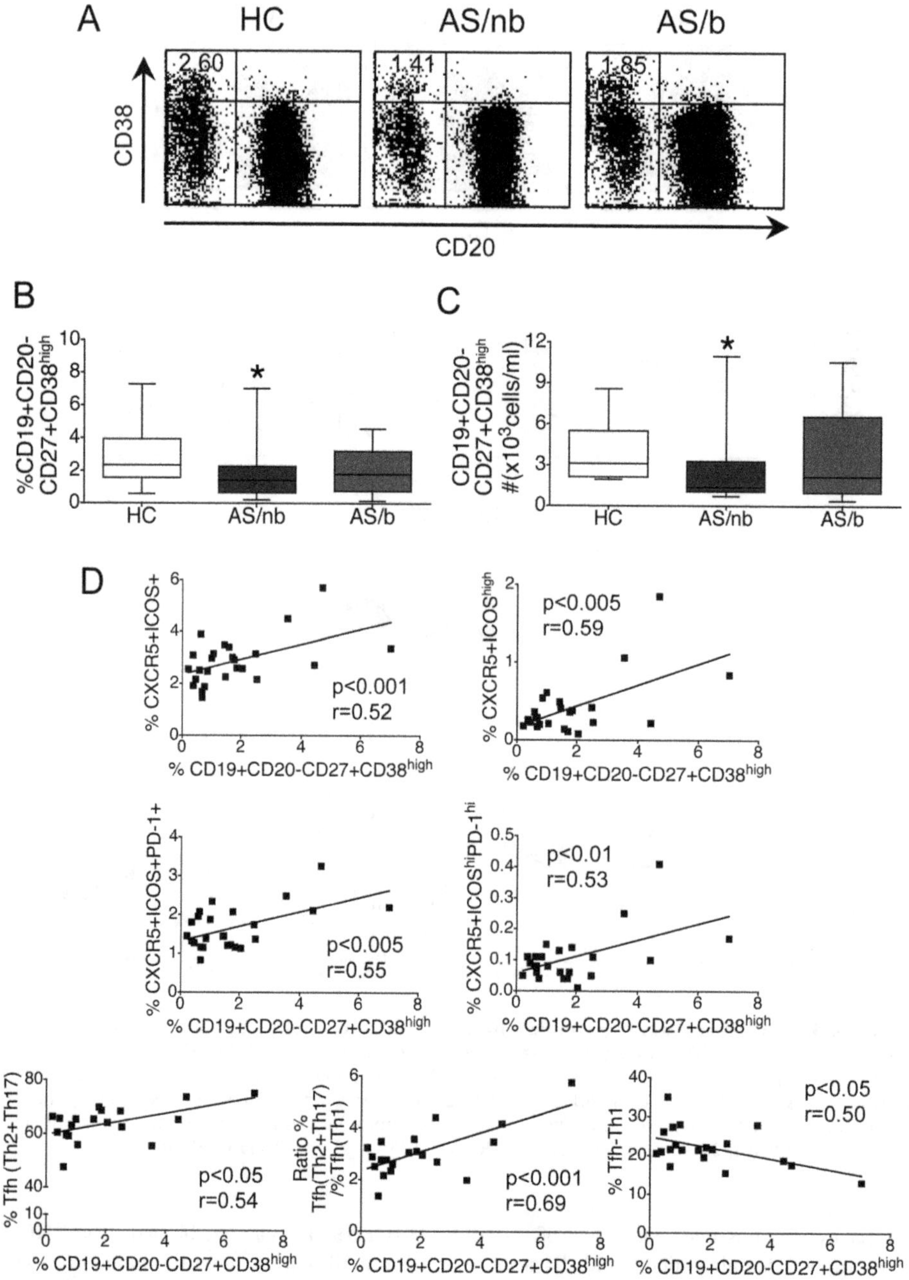

Figure 3. Numbers of circulating plasmablasts in patients with AS. A, B. AS/nb but not AS/b patients demonstrate a decreased frequency of circulating plasmablasts. Shown are representative dot plots of CD20 and CD38 expression on CD19+ cells (A). C. Decreased absolute numbers of circulating plasmablasts in AS/nb patients. B and C represent box and whiskers plots from 25 AS/nb patients, 25 AS/b patients and 50 HC; * $p < 0.005$ vs HC. D. The frequency of circulating plasmablasts in AS/nb patients is positively correlated with the frequency of circulating Tfh counterparts, with the frequency of Tfh(Th2+Th17) and with the ratio [%Tfh(Th2+Th17)]/%Tfh(Th1) cells, and negatively correlated with the frequency of Tfh-Th1 cells.

Serum levels of IgG, IgA and IgM in AS/nb and AS/b patients, and their relation with disease activity and cTfh numbers

As previously described [36,37], serum IgA levels were elevated in AS patients (Figure 5A, B). Interestingly, among our AS/nb patients, serum IgA was ony increased in those who had high or very high activity as determined by an ASDAS-CRP > 2.1 [38] (Figure 5B). In contrast, all of our AS/b patients demonstrated elevated serum IgA, even those with inactive disease or moderate activity, as determined by an ASDAS-CRP < 2.1 [38], although levels were higher in patients with high or very high activity (Figure 5B). In addition, AS/b patients had elevated serum IgG and IgM levels, that were more marked in subjects with high or very high activity (Figure 5B). Importantly, increased serum IgA and IgM levels in this group were already present in sera taken just before initiation of treatment with TNF blockers (Figure 5A). This is consistent with previous observations indicating that AS patients with severe disease can demonstrate increased levels of all three IgG, IgA and IgM [39]. Interestingly, the above described normal or increased Ig levels did not parallel the decreased or normal cTfh and plasmablast numbers observed in AS/nb or AS/b subjects,

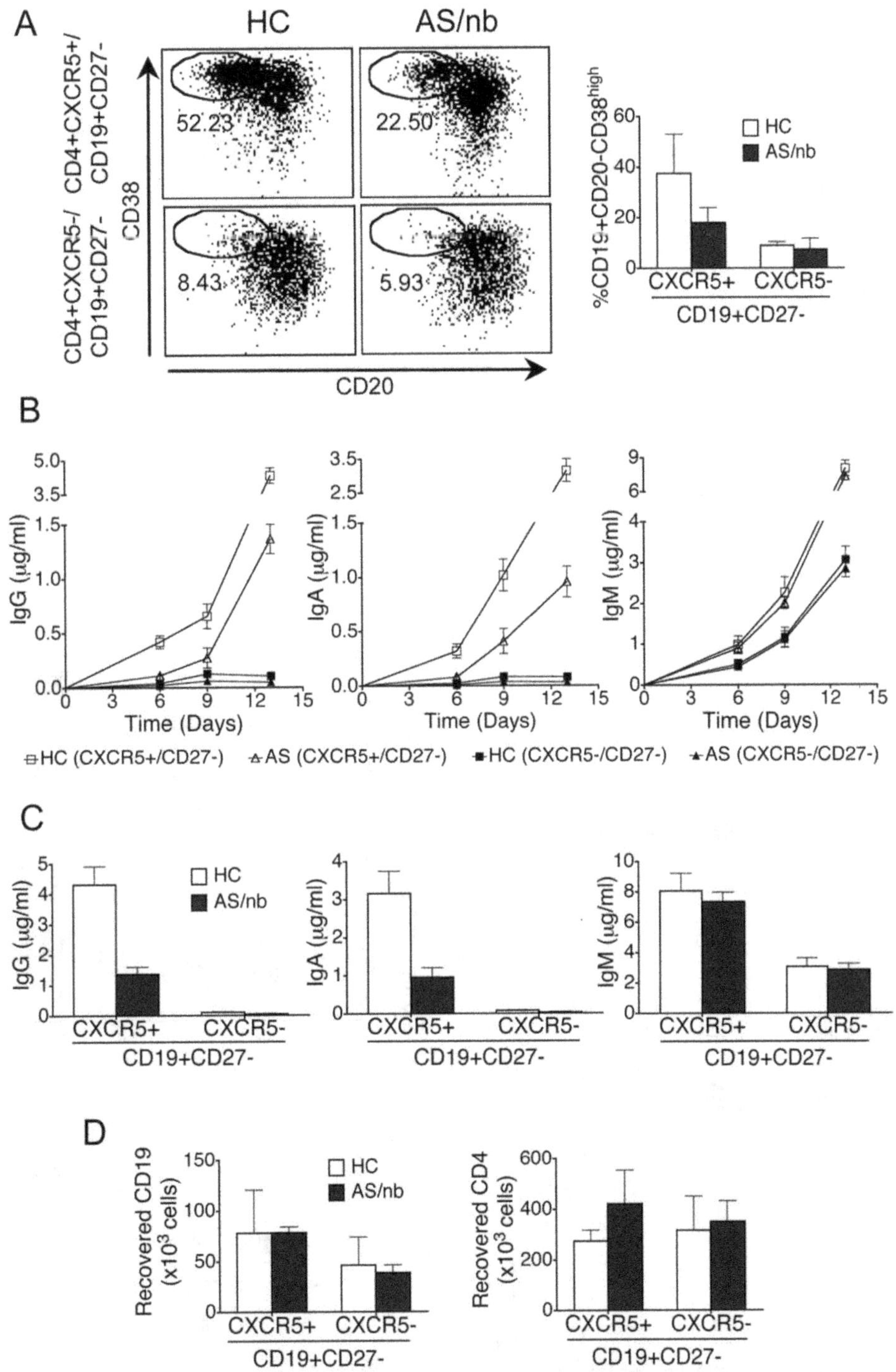

Figure 4. Functional capacity of circulating CD4+CXCR5+ T cells. CD4+CXCR5+ T cells isolated from peripheral blood of HC are more efficient than cells from AS/nb patients at inducing maturation of cocultured autologous naïve B cells. A. CD19+CD20-CD38^{high} plasmablasts in 9-day cocultures of naïve B cells from AS/nb patients or HC with autologous CXCR5+ or CXCR5- CD4+ T cells. B, C. Concentrations of IgG, A and M at different time points (B) or at 13 days (C) in cocultures of naïve B cells from AS/nb patients or HC with autologous CXCR5+ or CXCR5- CD4+ T cells. D. Recovered viable B and T cells in 9-day cocultures of naïve B cells from AS/nb patients or HC with autologous CXCR5+ or CXCR5- CD4+ T cells. Line and bar graphs represent the mean and SD of 3 independent experiments.

respectively (Figure 5B). That is, AS/nb patients showed normal or increased IgA levels in the presence of decreased cTfh and plasmablasts and altered cTfh subset ratio (Figure 5B). In addition, AS/b patients demonstrated increased Ig levels in the presence of cTfh, cTfh subset ratio and plasmablast values that were not different from HC (Figure 5B). Furthermore, whereas serum Ig concentrations paralleled disease activity, cTfh and plasmablast numbers did not (Figure 5B).

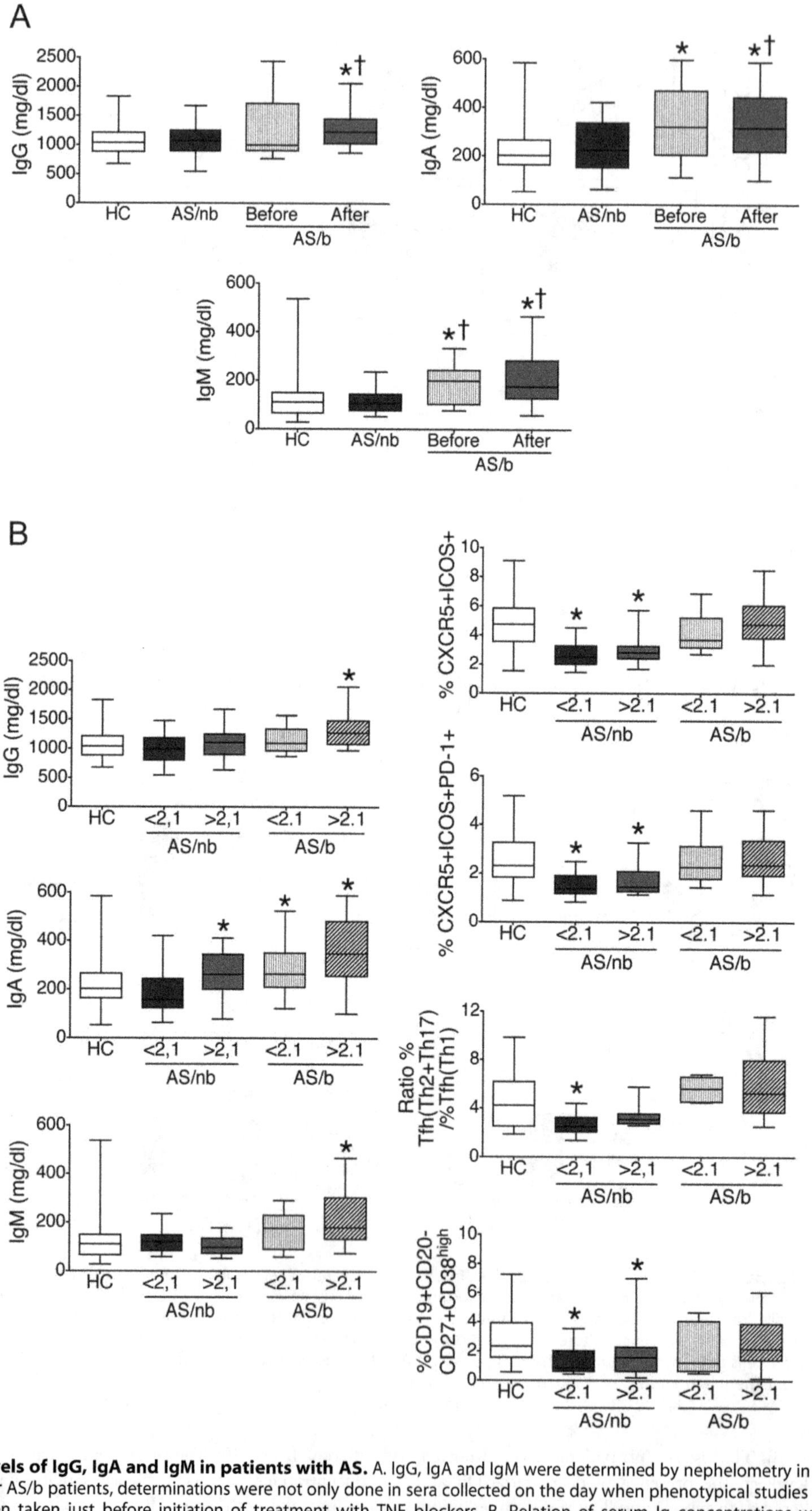

Figure 5. Serum levels of IgG, IgA and IgM in patients with AS. A. IgG, IgA and IgM were determined by nephelometry in the serum of AS/nb and AS/b patients. For AS/b patients, determinations were not only done in sera collected on the day when phenotypical studies were done, but also on sera that had been taken just before initiation of treatment with TNF blockers. B. Relation of serum Ig concentrations with cTfh, circulating plasmablasts and disease activity. Shown are cTfh proportions, cTfh subset ratio and circulating plasmablast proportions together with serum IgG, IgA and IgM concentrations in HC, AS patients with inactive disease or moderate disease activity (ASDAS-CRP < 2.1) [38] and AS patients with high or very high disease activity (ASDAS-CRP > 2.1) [38]. Normal or elevated serum Ig levels are observed despite the presence of decreased or normal cTfh

and plasmablasts, respectively. Note that serum Ig concentrations vary with disease activity whereas cTfh and plasmablast numbers do not. Box and whiskers plots represent the median, interquartile range, maximum and minimum values. *$p<0.05$ vs HC, †$p<0.05$ vs AS/nb.

Discussion

Spondyloarthritis (SpA) and their prototype disease, AS, are typically not associated with circulating autoantibodies [1–3] and therefore, the role of B cells or B-helper T cells (Tfh) in their pathogenesis has not been thoroughly investigated. There is more recent evidence indicating that B cells may indeed be implicated in SpA [8–11], and we deemed it interesting to study the frequency of cTfh cells and plasmablasts in AS.

We have herein described that AS/nb patients demonstrate a decreased frequency of cTfh cells, together with a decreased frequency of circulating plasmablasts. Furthermore, an altered proportion of cTfh subpopulations is observed: AS/nb patients showed a predominance of Tfh-Th1 cells, that lack B cell helping capacity in healthy subjects [24], over Tfh-Th17 and Tfh-Th2 cells, that do have B cell helping capacity as described by Morita et al. [24]. In contrast, AS/b patients do not display these alterations. Discordance with previously published observations [33,34] may be attributable to different treatment, ethnicity, disease duration or activity.

Because AS/nb patients were not receiving methotrexate or other drugs that may interfere with the cell cycle, the observed alterations in cTfh and plasmablasts in this patient group are not attributable to a drug effect. Conversely, the finding of normal frequencies of cTfh and plasmablasts in AS patients receiving TNF blockers suggests that these drugs may restore the initial immune alteration. Because the ASDAS-CRP and ASDAS-ESR indexes were comparable beween AS/nb and AS/b patients, the observed differences in cTfh numbers and cTfh subset balance do not seem related with different disease activity. In addition, there was no correlation of cTfh cell numbers or subsets with disease activity in either group; this parallels the observation that increased numbers of cTfh in SLE do not associate with disease activity [23] but are related to the pathogenesis of the disease [23].

Of note, the ex vivo functional studies herein described demonstrated that isolated peripheral blood CD4+CXCR5+ T cells are indeed able to provide B cell help as previously reported [24–26]: CD4+CXCR5+ but not CD4+CXCR5- T cells, induced IgG and IgA secretion in cocultured CD19+CD27- B cells. In the presence of CD4+CXCR5- T cells, CD19+CD27- B cells only produced low amounts of IgM as expected [24,25]. In addition, CD4+CXCR5+ T cells were more efficient than CD4+CXCR5- T cells at helping memory CD19+CD27+ B cells to produce Igs. Interestingly, we observed that total CD4+CXCR5+ T cells from AS/nb patients, containing decreased proportions of cTfh and an altered balance of cTfh subpopulations, do have a reduced capacity to promote maturation of naïve B cells, as indicated by a lower induced secretion of IgG and IgA from naïve B cells when compared with HC. In contrast, the amount of IgM produced in cocultures of CD4+CXCR5+ T with autologous naïve B cells of AS/nb patients or HC was comparable. To our knowledge, this is the first functional study directed to assessing the B cell helping capacity of cTfh cells in patients with a rheumatic disease.

Our findings in AS/nb patients are in contrast with the elevated frequency of cTfh and plasmablasts described in autoimmune diseases characterized by autoantibody production [23,27–31]. In fact, it has been proposed that increased numbers of cTfh can be a signature of human immune-mediated diseases [26]. Specifically, a causal relation between accumulation of Tfh cells, autoantibody production and lupus nephritis has been demonstrated in mice [20], and augmented numbers of Tfh counterparts in the peripheral blood of patients with SLE have been associated with disease severity [23]. Conversely, patients with deficiency of CD40-ligand or ICOS demonstrate a severely impaired generation of GC together with decreased circulating CD4+CXCR5+ T cells [40], suggesting that the numbers of cTfh are a reflection of the pool of typical Tfh in lymphoid organs.

The lower frequency of cTfh and plasmablasts in AS/nb might be related with a predominant contribution of innate versus acquired immune mechanisms to the pathogenesis of the disease [3] or with a lower capacity of AS/nb patients to produce T-dependent antibodies. However, AS has not been associated with immunodeficiency, and AS/nb patients are able to mount good antibody responses to vaccination with T-dependent antigens [41]. Alternatively, Tfh could be sequestered in the gut-associated lymphoid tissue (GALT) of AS/nb patients. In fact, subclinical gut inflammation has been described in up to 65% of AS patients [42], and is associated with increased numbers of lymphoid follicles in the ileum and colon [43]; furthermore, increased intestinal permeability has been observed not only in AS patients but also in their relatives [44]. In this context, normal numbers of cTfh cells and plasmablasts in our AS/b patients, the majority of which were receiving infliximab or adalimumab, could parallel an improvement of subclinical gut inflammation induced by these drugs. This would be consistent with studies indicating the leading role of TNF-α in intestinal homeostasis, gut barrier integrity, and pathogenesis of inflammatory bowel disease [45]. However, the levels of serum IgG, IgA and IgM in AS/nb or AS/b patients were discordant with the numbers of cTfh, cTfh subset ratio or plasmablasts: AS/nb patients, with decreased cTfh and plasmablasts, demonstrated normal or high serum IgA concentrations whereas AS/b patients, with normal cTfh and plasmablast numbers, demonstrated increased Ig concentrations. In addition, whereas numbers of cTfh or plasmablasts did not parallel disease activity parameters in AS/nb or AS/b patients, serum IgA in AS/nb or serum IgG, IgA and IgM levels in AS/b patients did, which is consistent with previous observations [36,37,39].

Interestingly, patients with AS/b demonstrated increased IgA and IgM concentrations before TNF blockade was started, which did not return to normal levels with treatment, even in patients who achieved a state of inactive or moderate disease activity as determined by ASDAS-CRP values. This suggests that AS/b patients do have a more severe disease as compared with AS/nb subjects, and that increased Ig concentrations in this group are not a side effect of treatment with TNF blockers. In addition, this observation reflects the difficulty in assessing disease activity and severity in AS with the currently available tools [38].

The lack of parallelism of cTfh and plasmablast numbers with serum Ig levels may be explained by two different mechanisms. First, Tfh and plamablasts may be sequestered in the GALT as mentioned above. Also, the altered cTfh subset ratio of AS/nb patients could result from preferential accumulation of Tfh-Th17 over Tfh-Th1 cells in the gut: whereas CCL20, the ligand for CCR6, is normally expressed in the GALT and intestinal epithelium [46,47], its expression level significantly increases in states of gut inflammation, which conditions local accumulation of CCR6 expressing cells [46,47]. Local sequestration would lead to decreased cTfh and circulating plasmablast numbers, together with altered cTfh subset ratio, in AS/nb patients. In turn, AS/b patients, with a more severe disease and a more marked alteration of intestinal permeability, would have an even higher accumulation of Tfh and plasmablasts in the GALT, with a higher rate of local Ig production and an increased number of lymphocytes available for recirculation, resulting not only in elevated serum Ig levels [48] but also in apparently normal numbers of cTfh and plasmablasts.

Of note, and as mentioned above, local Tfh sequestration at the inflammatory sites does not seem to occur in autoimmune diseases such as SLE, where increased numbers of total classical Tfh in lymphoid organs are associated with increased numbers of cTfh and autoantibody production [23]. Therefore, local sequestration of Tfh in the gut would be a mechanism operating differentially in AS. An alternative explanation for our findings would be that the number of cTfh does indeed parallel the number of true Tfh in lymphoid organs of AS patients: that is, decreased cTfh in AS/nb or normal cTfh numbers in AS/b patients would be a reflection of a decreased or "normal" pool of classsical Tfh. In this setting, innate immunity with T cell independent class switch recombination, would have a pivotal contribution to Ig production in both AS/nb and AS/b [49–51]; in turn, normal numbers of cTfh in AS/b patients would reflect activation of the acquired immune system in patients with a more severe disease [51,52]. In fact, it has been proposed that the role of innate immunity is predominant at initial stages of bowel inflammation in SpA [51], and as disease progresses or advances in severity, the contribution of acquired immunity tends to become more prominent [51,52].

Finally, both mechanisms, local Tfh sequestration and increased Ig production by innate mechanisms, may operate simultaneously in AS.

In summary, we have herein described decreased circulating Tfh and plasmablast numbers in AS/nb but not in AS/b patients, in the presence of normal or augmented serum levels of Igs. This observation sheds new light into the pathogenesis of AS and suggests that Tfh cells and plasmablasts may be sequestered in the GALT and/or innate immune mechanisms in the gut have a leading role in the pathogenesis of the disease.

Acknowledgments

We wish to thank Dr. Margarita López Trascasa (Immunology Department, Hospital Universitario La Paz, IdiPAZ, Madrid, Spain) and Dr. Joaquín Navarro Caspistegui (Hospital Universitarion Gregorio Marañón, Madrid, Spain) for their invaluable help in determinining serum Ig concentrations.

Author Contributions

Conceived and designed the experiments: MEMC. Performed the experiments: MBBC IAV. Analyzed the data: MEMC IAV MBBC PSM APK EDM CCG EMM. Contributed reagents/materials/analysis tools: IAV MBBC CCG EDM DP CPR AV EMM PSM APK. Contributed to the writing of the manuscript: MEMC.

References

1. Rudwaleit M, van der Heijde D, Landewé R, Akkoc N, Brandt J, et al. (2011) The Assessment of SpondyloArthritis International Society classification criteria for peripheral spondyloarthritis and for spondyloarthritis in general. Ann Rheum Dis 70: 25–31.
2. Rudwaleit M, van der Heijde D, Landewé R, Listing J, Akkoc N, et al. (2009) The development of Assessment of SpondyloArthritis international Society classification criteria for axial spondyloarthritis (part II): validation and final selection. Ann Rheum Dis 68: 777–783.
3. Ambarus C, Yeremenko N, Tak PP, Baeten D (2012) Pathogenesis of spondyloarthritis: autoimmune or autoinflammatory? Curr Opin Rheumatol 24: 351–358.
4. Chou CL, Wu MJ, Yu CL, Lu MC, Hsieh SC, et al. (2010) Anti-agalactosyl IgG antibody in ankylosing spondylitis and psoriatic arthritis. Clin Rheumatol 29: 875–881.
5. Wang M, Li X, Chen J, Zhou Y, Cao H, et al. (2011) Screening and evaluating the mimic peptides as a useful serum biomarker of ankylosing spondylitis using a phage display technique. Rheumatol Int 31: 1009–1016.
6. Duftner C, Dejaco C, Klauser A, Falkenbach A, Lakomek HJ, et al. (2006) High positive predictive value of specific antibodies cross-reacting with a 28-kDa Drosophila antigen for diagnosis of ankylosing spondylitis. Rheumatology (Oxford) 45: 38–42.
7. Georgopoulos K, Dick WC, Goodacre JA, Pain RH (1985) A reinvestigation of the cross-reactivity between Klebsiella and HLA-B27 in the aetiology of ankylosing spondylitis. Clin Exp Immunol 62: 662–671.
8. Baerlecken NT, Nothdorft S, Stummvoll GH, Sieper J, Rudwaleit M, et al. (2014) Autoantibodies against CD74 in spondyloarthritis. Ann Rheum Dis 73: 1211–1214.
9. Baraliakos X, Baerlecken N, Witte T, Heldmann F, Braun J (2014) High prevalence of anti-CD74 antibodies specific for the HLA class II-associated invariant chain peptide (CLIP) in patients with axial spondyloarthritis. Ann Rheum Dis 73:1079–1082.
10. Cantaert T, Doorenspleet ME, Francosalinas G, Paramarta JE, Klarenbeek PL, et al. (2012) Increased numbers of CD5+ B lymphocytes with a regulatory phenotype in spondylarthritis. Arthritis Rheum 64:1859–1868.
11. Song IH, Heldmann F, Rudwaleit M, Listing J, Appel H, et al. (2010) Different response to rituximab in tumor necrosis factor blocker-naive patients with active ankylosing spondylitis and in patients in whom tumor necrosis factor blockers have failed: a twenty-four-week clinical trial. Arthritis Rheum 62:1290–1297.
12. Craft JE (2012) Follicular helper T cells in immunity and systemic autoimmunity. Nat Rev Rheumatol 8:337–347.
13. Fazilleau N, Mark L, McHeyzer-Williams LJ, McHeyzer-Williams MG (2009) Follicular helper T cells: lineage and location. Immunity 30: 324–335.
14. Breitfeld D, Ohl L, Kremmer E, Ellwart J, Sallusto F, et al. (2000) J Exp Med 192:1545–1552.
15. Schaerli P, Willimann K, Lang AB, Lipp M, Loetscher P, et al. (2000) CXC chemokine receptor 5 expression defines follicular homing T cells with B cell helper function. J Exp Med 192:1553–1562.
16. Kim CH, Rott LS, Clark-Lewis I, Campbell DJ, Wu L, et al. (2001) Subspecialization of CXCR5+ T cells: B helper activity is focused in a germinal center-localized subset of CXCR5+ T cells. J Exp Med 193:1373–1381.
17. Crotty S (2011) Follicular helper CD4 T cells (TFH). Annu Rev Immunol 29: 621–663.
18. Vinuesa CG, Cook MC, Angelucci C, Athanasopoulos V, Rui L, et al. (2005) A RING-type ubiquitin ligase family member required to repress follicular helper T cells and autoimmunity. Nature 435(7041): 452–458.
19. Subramanian S, Tus K, Li QZ, Wang A, Tian XH, et al. (2006) A Tlr7 translocation accelerates systemic autoimmunity in murine lupus. Proc Natl Acad Sci U S A 103: 9970–9975.
20. Linterman MA, Rigby RJ, Wong RK, Yu D, Brink R, et al. (2009) Follicular helper T cells are required for systemic autoimmunity. J Exp Med 206: 561–576.
21. Ji YR, Kim HJ, Yu DH, Bae KB, Park SJ, et al. (2012) Enforced expression of roquin protein in T cells exacerbates the incidence and severity of experimental arthritis. J Biol Chem 287: 42269–42277.
22. Hron JD, Caplan L, Gerth AJ, Schwartzberg PL, Peng SL (2004) SH2D1A regulates T-dependent humoral autoimmunity. J Exp Med 200: 261–266.
23. Simpson N, Gatenby PA, Wilson A, Malik S, Fulcher DA, et al. (2010) Expansion of circulating T cells resembling follicular helper T cells is a fixed phenotype that identifies a subset of severe systemic lupus erythematosus. Arthritis Rheum 62: 234–244.
24. Morita R, Schmitt N, Bentebibel SE, Ranganathan R, Bourdery L, et al. (2011) Human blood CXCR5(+)CD4(+) T cells are counterparts of T follicular cells and contain specific subsets that differentially support antibody secretion. Immunity 34: 108–121.
25. Chevalier N, Jarrossay D, Ho E, Avery DT, Ma CS, et al. (2011) CXCR5 expressing human central memory CD4 T cells and their relevance for humoral immune responses. J Immunol 186: 5556–5568.
26. Vinuesa CG, Cook MC (2011) Blood relatives of follicular helper T cells. Immunity 34: 10–12.
27. Wang J, Shan Y, Jiang Z, Feng J, Li C, et al. (2013) High frequencies of activated B cells and T follicular helper cells are correlated with disease activity in patients with new-onset rheumatoid arthritis. Clin Exp Immunol 174: 212–220.
28. Szabo K, Papp G, Barath S, Gyimesi E, Szanto A, et al. (2013) Follicular helper T cells may play an important role in the severity of primary Sjögren's syndrome. Clin Immunol 147: 95–104.
29. Zhu C, Ma J, Liu Y, Tong J, Tian J, et al. (2012) Increased frequency of follicular helper T cells in patients with autoimmune thyroid disease. J Clin Endocrinol Metab 97: 943–950.
30. Feng J, Lu L, Hua C, Qin L, Zhao P, et al. (2011) High frequency of CD4+ CXCR5+ TFH cells in patients with immune-active chronic hepatitis B. PLoS One 6(7): e21698.

31. Luo C, Li Y, Liu W, Feng H, Wang H, et al. (2013) Expansion of circulating counterparts of follicular helper T cells in patients with myasthenia gravis. J Neuroimmunol 256: 55–61.
32. Le Coz C, Joublin A, Pasquali JL, Korganow AS, Dumortier H, et al. (2013) Circulating TFH subset distribution is strongly affected in lupus patients with an active disease. PLoS One 8(9): e75319.
33. Xiao F, Zhang HY, Liu YJ, Zhao D, Shan YX, et al. (2013) Higher frequency of peripheral blood interleukin 21 positive follicular helper T cells in patients with ankylosing spondylitis. J Rheumatol 40: 2029–2037.
34. Wu S, Yang T, Pan F, Xia G, Hu Y, et al. (2014) Increased frequency of circulating follicular helper T cells in patients with ankylosing spondylitis. Mod Rheumatol [Epub ahead of print] PMID: 24716597.
35. van der Linden S, Valkenburg HA, Cats A (1984) Evaluation of diagnostic criteria for ankylosing spondylitis. A proposal for modification of the New York criteria. Arthritis Rheum 27: 361–368.
36. Trull A, Ebringer A, Panayi G, Ebringer R, James DC (1984) HLA-B27 and the immune response to enterobacterial antigens in ankylosing spondylitis. Clin Exp Immunol 55: 74–80.
37. Franssen MJ, van de Putte LB, Gribnau FW (1985) IgA serum levels and disease activity in ankylosing spondylitis: a prospective study. Ann Rheum Dis 44: 766–771.
38. Machado P, Landewé R, Lie E, Kvien TK, Braun J, et al. (2011) Assessment of SpondyloArthritis international Society. Ankylosing Spondylitis Disease Activity Score (ASDAS): defining cut-off values for disease activity states and improvement scores. Ann Rheum Dis 70: 47–53.
39. Richter MB, Woo P, Panayi GS, Trull A, Unger A, et al. (1983) The effects of intravenous pulse methylprednisolone on immunological and inflammatory processes in ankylosing spondylitis. Clin Exp Immunol 53:51–59.
40. Bossaller L, Burger J, Draeger R, Grimbacher B, Knoth R, et al. (2006) ICOS deficiency is associated with a severe reduction of CXCR5+CD4 germinal center Th cells. J Immunol 177: 4927–4932.
41. Salinas GF, De Rycke L, Barendregt B, Paramarta JE, Hreggvidstdottir H, et al. (2013) Anti-TNF treatment blocks the induction of T cell-dependent humoral responses. Ann Rheum Dis 72:1037–1043.
42. Mielants H, Veys EM, Goemaere S, Goethals K, Cuvelier C, et al. (1991) Gut inflammation in the spondyloarthropathies: clinical, radiologic, biologic and genetic features in relation to the type of histology. A prospective study. J Rheumatol 18:1542–1551.
43. Demetter P, Van Huysse JA, De Keyser F, Van Damme N, Verbruggen G, et al. (2002) Increase in lymphoid follicles and leukocyte adhesion molecules emphasizes a role for the gut in spondyloarthropathy pathogenesis. J Pathol 198: 517–522.
44. Martínez-González O, Cantero-Hinojosa J, Paule-Sastre P, Gómez-Magán JC, Salvatierra-Ríos D (1994) Intestinal permeability in patients with ankylosing spondylitis and their healthy relatives. Br J Rheumatol 33:644–647.
45. Gibson PR (2004) Increased gut permeability in Crohn's disease: is TNF the link? Gut 53:1724–1725.
46. Wang C, Kang SG, Lee J, Sun Z, Kim CH (2009) The roles of CCR6 in migration of Th17 cells and regulation of effector T-cell balance in the gut. Mucosal Immunol 2: 173–183.
47. Izadpanah A, Dwinell MB, Eckmann L, Varki NM, Kagnoff MF (2001) Regulated MIP-3alpha/CCL20 production by human intestinal epithelium: mechanism for modulating mucosal immunity. Am J Physiol Gastrointest Liver Physiol 280: G710–719.
48. Zimmermann K, Haas A, Oxenius A (2012) Systemic antibody responses to gut microbes in health and disease. Gut Microbes 3:42–47.
49. Macpherson AJ, Gatto D, Sainsbury E, Harriman GR, Hengartner H, et al. (2000) A primitive T cell-independent mechanism of intestinal mucosal IgA responses to commensal bacteria. Science 288(5474): 2222–2226.
50. Bergqvist P, Stensson A, Lycke NY, Bemark M (2010) T cell-independent IgA class switch recombination is restricted to the GALT and occurs prior to manifest germinal center formation. J Immunol 184: 3545–3553.
51. Van Praet L, Jacques P, Van den Bosch F, Elewaut D (2012) The transition of acute to chronic bowel inflammation in spondyloarthritis. Nat Rev Rheumatol 8:288–295.
52. Iwasaki A, Medzhitov R (2010) Regulation of adaptive immunity by the innate immune system. Science 327(5963): 291–295.

18

Impaired Clearance of Early Apoptotic Cells Mediated by Inhibitory IgG Antibodies in Patients with Primary Sjögren's Syndrome

Menelaos N. Manoussakis[1,2]*, George E. Fragoulis[1], Aigli G. Vakrakou[1], Haralampos M. Moutsopoulos[1]

1 Department of Pathophysiology, School of Medicine, University of Athens, Athens, Greece, **2** Hellenic Pasteur Institute, Athens, Greece

Abstract

Objectives: Deficient efferocytosis (i.e. phagocytic clearance of apoptotic cells) has been frequently reported in systemic lupus erythematosus (SLE). Todate, patients with primary Sjögren's syndrome (SS) have not been assessed for phagocytosis of apoptotic cells (ApoCell-phagocytosis) and of particulate targets (microbeads, MB-phagocytosis).

Design: ApoCell-phagocytosis and MB-phagocytosis were comparatively assessed by flow cytometry in peripheral blood specimens and monocyte-derived macrophage (MDM) preparations from healthy blood donors (HBD) and consecutive SS, SLE and rheumatoid arthritis (RA) patients. Cross-admixture ApoCell-phagocytosis experiments were also performed using phagocytes from HBD or patients, and apoptotic cells pretreated with whole sera or purified serum IgG derived from patients or HBD.

Results: Compared to HBD, approximately half of SS and SLE patients studied (but not RA) manifested significantly reduced ApoCell-phagocytosis ($p<0.001$) and MB-phagocytosis ($p<0.003$) by blood-borne phagocytes that correlated inversely with disease activity ($p\leq0.004$). In cross-admixture assays, healthy monocytes showed significantly reduced ApoCell-phagocytosis when fed with apoptotic cells that were pretreated with sera or purified serum IgG preparations from SS and SLE patients ($p<0.0001$, compared to those from HBD or RA). Such aberrant effect of the SS and SLE sera and IgG preparations correlated linearly with their content of IgG antibodies against apoptotic cells ($p\leq0.0001$). Phagocytic dysfunction maybe also present in certain SS and SLE patients, as supported by deficient capacity of MDM for ApoCell-phagocytosis and MB-phagocytosis under patients' serum-free conditions.

Conclusion: Similarly to SLE, efferocytosis is frequently impaired in SS and is primarily due to the presence of inhibitory IgG anti-ApoCell antibodies and secondarily to phagocytes' dysfunction.

Editor: Masataka Kuwana, Keio University School of Medicine, Japan

Funding: The study was supported by grants from the Hellenic Rheumatology Society (ERE141/10 to M.N.M), the Propondis Foundation (to A.G.V.) and the Lillian Voudouri Foundation. The funders had no role in study design, data collection and analysis, decision to publish, or preparation of the manuscript.

Competing Interests: The authors have declared that no competing interests exist.

* Email: menman@med.uoa.gr

Introduction

Apoptosis represents a major mechanism of programmed cell death that is essential for the regulation of tissue growth and homeostasis [1]. Normally, cells dying by apoptosis undergo specific changes that target them for rapid clearance by professional phagocytes, such as macrophages. This process leads to the active production of anti-inflammatory mediators by phagocytes and thus facilitates the "immunologically silent" removal of apoptotic cells [2]. The prompt elimination of apoptotic cells (also termed "efferocytosis") [3] is a very crucial biological process, since lingering apoptotic cells eventually proceed to the state of "late apoptosis" or "secondary necrosis" wherein they may contribute to inflammatory reactions via the release of immunogenic intracellular components, including modified autoantigens and "danger signals" [4]. In fact, apoptosis and efferocytosis act in concert to regulate various processes, such as embryogenesis, tissue homeostasis, tolerance the elimination of damaged cells, and the resolution of inflammation [5–7].

The occurrence of defective efferocytosis in certain inflammatory diseases is thought to have pathogenetic significance, based on the pro-inflammatory potential of secondary necrotic cells [8] Among them, systemic lupus erythematosus (SLE) is regarded as the archetypical disease model where the impaired clearance of apoptotic cells by macrophages represents a possible mechanism for the development of chronic autoimmune reactions and organ damage [9–11]. Apart from defective efferocytosis, various in vitro clearance defects of macrophages have been described in SLE, including aberrant Fc-gamma receptor-mediated uptake of IgG ligand-coated erythrocytes [12] and decreased phagocytosis of yeast cells [13] and particulate targets [10]. These aberrations have been attributed to intrinsic defects of patients' phagocytes [9], to the decreased density of circulating macrophages [14], as well as to the effect of serum components [11,15–17].

Primary Sjögren's syndrome (SS), which is characterized by mononuclear cell infiltrates in exocrine glands and parenchymal organs, shares several immunologic manifestations with SLE. These include various features of B-cell hyperactivity, such as the profound hypergammaglobulinemia, multiple autoantibodies, circulating immune complexes and evidence of complement consumption [18]. In this context, we presently sought to comparatively investigate the capacity of peripheral blood monocytes and monocyte-derived macrophages (MDM) of SS and SLE patients for phagocytosis of apoptotic cells and of particulate targets. For this purpose, we established ex-vivo phagocytosis assays and assessed patients with SLE, SS and RA, as well as healthy individuals. Our findings indicate that considerable proportions of SS and SLE patients (but not RA) manifest deficient phagocytosis of apoptotic cells and of particulate targets that correlate with the activity of these diseases, and apparently owes primarily to inhibitory IgG anti-ApoCell antibodies and secondarily to the dysfunction of phagocytes.

Patients and Methods

Patients

Specimens of peripheral blood were obtained after informed consent from 43 consecutive unselected Greek Caucasian patients with primary-SS, 27 with SLE and 14 with RA [19–21] (**Table 1**), as well as from Greek Caucasian healthy blood donors (2 groups; HBD-1 and HBD-2, 17 each, age- and sex-matched to the SS and SLE groups, respectively). In all assays, HBD-1 and HBD-2 groups exhibited similar results, without statistical difference to each other. Thus, they were subsequently considered as a single group (HBD) in the comparative analyses. The study was approved by the Medical council of "Laikon" University Hospital (Research Ethics Committee). Written informed consent was given by all individuals for their participation in the study, as well as for the usage of their clinical records. Patients' medical records were retrospectively analyzed for demographic variables, clinical and laboratory features. At the time of the study, patients studied were assessed for disease activity by calculation of ESSDAI (for SS) [22], SLEDAI (for SLE), DAS28 (for RA) and for disease severity by SSDDI (for SS) [23], SLICC-ACR (for SLE) [24] and by global disease severity index (for RA). None of the SLE or RA patients studied manifested any evidence of secondary or associated Sjögren's syndrome. SS patients were also analyzed for the presence of extraglandular manifestations and of type-I disease, as previously [25]. At the time of investigation, none of the patients or controls studied displayed evidence of infection or had history of infection with hepatitis viruses or HIV. Sera were tested for anti-Ro/SSA, anti-La/SSB by counter-immunoelectrophoresis, for anti-C1q, anti-native histone and anti-chromatin antibodies by ELISA (QuantaLite), for C3 and C4 complement levels by radial immunodiffusion and for C1q levels by nephelometry. Total immunoglobulin IgG was isolated from serum samples of patients and HBD using the Melon Gel purification Kit (Pierce), according to the manufacturer's protocol, aliquoted and stored at −20°C. Protein yields were quantified spectrophotometrically and purification was routinely found to be more than 95% by SDS-PAGE electrophoresis.

Generation of early apoptotic cells

The Jurkat cell line (ATCC) was grown in RPMI-1640 medium (Gibco) supplemented with 10% heat-inactivated human AB-serum and 0.1% gentamicin. Apoptosis was induced in Jurkat cells by exposure to Ultraviolet-B irradiation (800 mJ/cm^2) at room temperature using Stratalinker-1800 (Stratagene), as previously [26]. Subsequently, cells were washed twice with PBS, seeded into Petri dishes 60×15 mm in the above culture medium (0.7×10^7 cells/mL) and incubated for 4-hrs at 37°C. The percentage of apoptotic cells was determined by flow cytometry (Facscalibur, BD) using annexin-V/propidium iodide staining (R&D). As determined in extensive preliminary experiments and verified at each preparation, after the 4-hrs incubation, approximately 60% of Jurkat cells were early apoptotic (annexin-V-positive/propidium iodide-negative, mean ±SEM: 61.2±5.0%, n = 10 experiments), with the remaining of cells being viable (negative for both annexin-V and propidium iodide, 37.5±4.3%). In such preparations, late apoptotic cells (positive for both annexin-V and propidium iodide) were typically <2% of cells (1.9±0.2%).

Assessment of serum IgM and IgG immunoglobulin binding to apoptotic cells

The levels of IgM and IgG antibodies to early apoptotic cells (anti-ApoCell) were assayed in serum specimens (diluted to 20% and 5% v/v, respectively) by flow cytometry as previously [16], using early apoptotic Jurkat cells prepared as above and FITC-labeled rabbit antisera to human IgM or IgG immunoglobulin as secondary antibody (Dako), respectively. In each experiment, the reproducibility and inter-assay variation was evaluated by testing two standard specimens (aliquoted and stored at 20°C) in duplicates consisted of pooled sera from 3 healthy donors (negative control) and 3 SLE patients (positive control), respectively. For the estimation of ApoCell-specific serum IgM or IgG antibody binding, the non-specific binding of the secondary antibody was considered as baseline, the values obtained were normalized to the standard negative control specimen and the results were expressed as binding index (percent gated by mean fluorescence intensity). Coefficient variation for standard specimens was less than 12.5% between different experiments. The occurrence of anti-ApoCell antibodies in purified IgG preparations (50 µg/mL) of patients and controls was also assessed by flow cytometry as above.

Assessment of phagocytosis of apoptotic cells (ApoCell-phagocytosis) by peripheral blood monocytes

For the assessment of ApoCell-phagocytosis by peripheral blood phagocytes, freshly prepared early apoptotic Jurkat cells were labeled with the fluorescent dye carboxylfluorescein diaceteate-succinimidylester (CFSE, Molecular Probes) and were added (1×10^6 cells) in duplicate samples (100 µl) of freshly drawn heparinized peripheral blood. Mixtures were incubated for 90-min at 37°C and subsequently, erythrocytes were destroyed with a lysis buffer (Pharmingen). In preliminary experiments, using fluorescence microscopy, normal peripheral blood monocytes and polymorphonuclear cells were found to ingest appreciable amounts of CFSE-stained apoptotic cells, but not viable cells. ApoCell-phagocytosis by monocytes was quantitatively assessed in peripheral blood samples from HBD and patients by flow cytometry, using the appropriate forward/side scatter pattern gate and confirmation by staining with CD14 monoclonal antibody (Santa Cruz). Monocytes were electronically gated, and the uptake of fluorescent CFSE-stained apoptotic Jurkat cells by these cells was estimated as ApoCell-phagocytosis index (ApoCell-PhI), which was calculated as the product of the percentage of gated fluorescent-positive cells by their mean fluorescence intensity. The localization of apoptotic Jurkat cells in the gate of granulocytes had precluded the assessment of ApoCell-phagocytosis by the latter type of cells.

Table 1. Selected anthropometric, clinical and laboratory features of the patients studied.

Disease Features	SS (n=43)	SLE (n=27)	RA (n=14)
Age, years, median (range)	52.5 (33–67)	37.5 (19–45)	60.0 (38–75)
Sex, female:male	43:0	25:2	7:7
Disease duration, years, median (range)	11 (2–23)	11 (1–20)	10 (1–17)
Sicca man manifestations, no. positive (%)	43 (100)	0 (0.0)	0 (0.0)
Disease activity, median (range) [a]	9 (0–41)	4 (0–16)	5.2 (3.5–7.0)
Disease severity, median (range) [a]	2 (2–11)	2 (0–6)	2.9 (1.3–5.4)
Type-I SS disease, no. positive (%) [a]	25 (58.1)	NA	NA
ANA, titer^{-1}, median (range)	320 (0–2560)	640 (0–2560)	0
Anti-Ro/SSA, no. positive (%)	29 (67.4)	15 (40.5)	0 (0.0)
Anti-La/SSB, no. positive (%)	13 (30.2)	0 (0.0)	0 (0.0)
Anti-dsDNA, no. positive (%)	0 (0.0)	18 (47.4)	0 (0.0)
Anti-chromatin, no. positive (%)	0/27 (0.0)	4/19 (21.1)	0 (0.0)
Anti-histone, no. positive (%)	0/27 (0.0)	5/19 (26.3)	0 (0.0)
Low serum C3 and/or C4, no. positive (%) [b]	18 (41.9)	23 (60.5)	0 (0.0)
Low serum C1q, no. positive (%) [c]	5/17 (29.4)	5/15 (33.3)	ND
Rheumatoid factor, no. positive (%)	20 (46.5)	ND	11 (78.6)

a: disease activity, disease severity and Type-I SS disease were defined as described in Patients and Methods,
b: low serum C3<90 mg/dl and C4<20 mg/dl,
c: low serum C1q<15 mg/dl, NA: not applicable, ND: not done.

ApoCell-phagocytosis by monocyte-derived macrophages (MDM)

For the preparation of MDM, mononuclear cells were isolated from peripheral blood of patients and healthy donors by density-gradient centrifugation (BD-Vacutainer), washed thrice with HBSS (Gibco) and plated onto 24-well plates (Corning, 4×10^6 cells/well) in DMEM (Gibco) supplemented with 10% heat-inactivated FBS. Following 1-hour incubation at 37°C, 5% CO_2, non-adherent cells were removed by washing with HBSS and the adherent monocytes were allowed to mature to macrophages by cultivation for 8-days in X-VIVO-10 medium (Lonza) containing 10% heat-inactivated AB human serum, as previously [26]. Culture medium was changed at day-3, and following an additional 5-day culture, the supernatant was aspirated and fresh preparations of early apoptotic cells were added in each well, in X-VIVO-10 (3×10^6 cells/ml). MDM were washed thrice with cold PBS to remove the non-ingested apoptotic cells, were detached with EDTA-lidocaine solution and ApoCell-phagocytosis was analyzed by flow cytometry, as above. MDM preparations were typically 50-65% CD14-positive.

Cross-admixture experiments for the assessment of the influence of serum factors in ApoCell-phagocytosis

To assess the influence of serum components in ApoCell-phagocytosis, apoptotic cells were pre-treated (for 15-min at 37°C) with DMEM culture medium alone, with whole serum or with purified IgG preparations (50 μg/ml) derived from autoimmune patients or HBD. Apoptotic cells were washed and incubated (1×10^6 cells) with preparations of isolated peripheral blood mononuclear cells (1×10^6 cells) or MDM (1×10^5 cells) derived from a healthy donor, and the samples were analyzed for ApoCell-phagocytosis, as above. In separate experiments, prior the addition to mixtures, serum samples from HBD were heat-inactivated (56°C, 30-min) to destroy complement. The rates of ApoCell-phagocytosis by healthy MDM of apoptotic cells pretreated with purified IgG preparations (50 μg/ml) derived from either autoimmune patients or HBD were also comparatively investigated by two-color flow cytometry analyses of healthy MDM stained with CD14-PE (BD-Pharmingen) and CFSE-labelled IgG-pretreated apoptotic cells, as well as by single-color flow cytometry using apoptotic cells labelled with the pH-sensitive fluorescent dye pHrodo succinimidyl ester (pHrodo-SE, Life Technologies, 20 ng/ml at room temperature for 30-min), which allows the actual detection of ingested apoptotic cells owing to increased light emission in the acidic environment of the phagosomes of phagocytes [27].

Phagocytosis assay of fluorescent microbeads (MB-phagocytosis) by peripheral blood phagocytes and MDM

Fluorescent monodisperse polystyrene microbeads (MB) with 1-μm diameter (Fluoresbrite YG, Polysciences) were used. The experimental conditions were optimized in preliminary experiments, where the ingestion of MB was verified by fluorescent microscopy. In such experiments, the application of uncoated microbeads or microbeads coated with human immunoglobulin or human serum albumin had yielded equivalent results, whereas no discernible uptake was observed upon incubation of blood samples with microbeads at 4°C. In brief, duplicate samples of heparinized peripheral blood (200 μl) were mixed with MB (4×10^7 beads/ml) and were incubated for 30-min at 37°C. Erythrocytes were lysed as above, and following three washings with cold PBS to remove the non-ingested MB, the samples were analyzed by flow cytometry. Typical laser scatter properties were used to determine separate acquisition gates for granulocytes and monocytes. MB-phagocytosis index (MB-PhI) was calculated as the product of the percentage of gated fluorescence-positive cells by their mean fluorescence intensity. MB-phagocytosis by MDM preparations was also assessed as above.

Statistical analyses

Correlations were calculated using the Spearman's rank correlation coefficient. Group comparisons were performed by Mann-Whitney rank sum test. For paired comparisons, Wilcoxon signed-rank test and one-way analysis of variance were used, when appropriate. Analyses were conducted using SPSS 15.0 and Graph Pad 5.0 softwares. The results were expressed as median and range, and correlations with two-tailed p-values less than 0.05 were considered statistically significant.

Results

Serological aberrations in SS and SLE patients studied

Serological analyses had revealed several aberrations, including the presence of various anti-nuclear autoantibodies in the serum samples from the SS and SLE patients studied, but not in those from RA (**Table 1**).

Significantly impaired ApoCell-phagocytosis by peripheral blood monocytes of SS and SLE patients

The study of ApoCell-phagocytosis had yielded similar results between RA patients and HBD, but significantly decreased ApoCell-PhI values in both SS and SLE patient groups, compared to HBD ($p = 0.0002$ and $p < 0.0001$, respectively) and to RA patients ($p = 0.0009$ and $p = 0.0004$, respectively) (**Figure 1A**). Conversely, ApoCell-PhI values were not statistically different between SS and SLE patients. Decreased ApoCell-phagocytosis was observed in approximately half of SS and SLE patients, compared to none of RA patients studied (**Figure 1A**).

Among SS patients, ApoCell-phagocytosis by monocytes (ApoCell-PhI values) was found to correlate inversely with ESSDAI scores ($r = -0.559$, $p = 0.004$, **Figure 1B**) and to be significantly impaired among patients with type-I disease (in type-I disease; median: 168, range: 119–206, in type-II disease; median: 221, range: 130–338, $p = 0.04$) or with anti-Ro/SSA autoantibodies (in anti-Ro/SSA-positive; median: 164, range: 119–227, in anti-Ro/SSA-negative; median: 190, range: 142–338, $p = 0.03$). In SLE patients, ApoCell-phagocytosis by monocytes (ApoCell-PhI values) correlated inversely with SLEDAI scores ($r = -0.627$, $p = 0.0008$, **Figure 1C**) and to be significantly impaired among patients with serum anti-Ro/SSA antibodies (in anti-Ro/SSA-positive; median: 149, range: 47–191, in anti-Ro/SSA-negative; median: 194, range: 136–308, $p = 0.002$), anti-dsDNA antibodies (in anti-dsDNA-positive; median: 154, range: 110–213, in anti-dsDNA-negative; median: 194, range: 47–308, $p = 0.02$) and low C3 complement levels (in those with low C3; median: 162, range: 47–212, in those with normal C3; median: 193, range: 123–308, $p = 0.03$).

Impaired ApoCell-phagocytosis by MDM preparations of SS and SLE patients

The in-vitro differentiation of monocytes to macrophages (MDM) represents a surrogate for tissue macrophages [28] and a convenient means for the study of ApoCell-phagocytosis in the absence of direct influence of serum factors. In this context, ApoCell-phagocytosis was comparatively investigated in preparations of MDM derived from HBD and from SS and SLE patients. All HBD studied manifested substantial ApoCell-phagocytosis by MDM, whereas a significant number of SS and SLE cases showed impaired ApoCell-phagocytosis (ApoCell-PhI values less than two SD below the mean of HBD; in 4/9 of SS and in 7/10 of SLE) (**Figure 1D**). Parallel ApoCell-phagocytosis assays of peripheral blood monocytes from these individuals revealed significant agreement with those of MDM, being normal in all HBD (10/10), but impaired in the majority of patients (in 9/9 of SS and in 8/10 of SLE). In these patients, the occurrence of deficient ApoCell-phagocytosis by MDM always (in 11/11 of cases) correlated with decreased ApoCell-phagocytosis by peripheral blood monocytes. However, in 6 MDM preparations from patients (5 with SS and 1 with SLE), normal ApoCell-phagocytosis was associated with defective uptake by peripheral blood monocytes, a fact which likely suggests the influence of serum factors that operated only in the peripheral blood assays.

ApoCell-phagocytosis by healthy monocytes is inefficiently supported by sera from SS and SLE patients

In preliminary experiments, the addition of serum specimens from healthy individuals was found to promote the ApoCell-phagocytosis by healthy peripheral blood monocytes. In fact, the replacement of healthy serum by DMEM resulted in significantly lower uptake of apoptotic cells ($n = 13$; median reduction: 48.0%, range: 34.2–56.9%, $p = 0.001$). In addition, the heat-treatment of HBD sera ($n = 6$) was also found to result in considerable reduction of ApoCell-phagocytosis by healthy monocytes (median reduction: 22.9%, range: 18.9–45.8%, $p = 0.004$), indicating the physiologic participation of heat-labile serum factors in the ingestion of apoptotic cells by monocytes.

In cross-admixture experiments, the application of apoptotic cells pre-treated with sera from SS and SLE patients (but not RA patients) resulted in significantly reduced ApoCell-phagocytosis by healthy peripheral blood monocytes (both for $p < 0.0001$), compared to pretreatment with sera from HBD (**Figure 1E**). In those experiments, ApoCell-PhI values obtained following the pretreatments with SS and SLE sera showed positive correlations with C3 and C4 complement levels (for SS sera; $r = 0.510$, $p = 0.007$ and $r = 0.447$, $p = 0.02$, respectively, for SLE sera; $r = 0.467$, $p = 0.03$ and $r = 0.546$, $p = 0.008$, respectively). Among SS and SLE sera used, those with reactivity to Ro/SSA and to native histones, respectively, showed significantly decreased ApoCell-phagocytosis (among SS sera: the anti-Ro/SSA-positive; median: 206, range: 118–320, the anti-Ro/SSA-negative; median: 356, range: 289–462, $p = 0.0008$, among SLE sera: the anti-histone-positive; median: 255, range: 209–300, the anti-histone-negative; median: 327, range: 245–450, $p = 0.02$).

Additional cross-admixture ApoCell-phagocytosis assays were also performed using peripheral blood monocytes obtained from selected SS and SLE patients with deficient ApoCell-phagocytosis (6 from SS and 3 from SLE patients) and apoptotic cells pre-treated with either the autologous serum or serum from a HBD. In these experiments, the pre-treatment of apoptotic cells with HBD serum was found to increase significantly ApoCell-phagocytosis values over those obtained with the autologous sera (median increase: 21.8%, range: 18.7–79.9%, $p = 0.02$). In fact, the incubation of apoptotic cells with HBD serum was found to confer normal ApoCell-phagocytosis values to the monocytes of 4/6 SS patients and of 1/3 SLE patients studied, a finding which suggests the key contribution of serum factor(s) in the aberrations observed, in a loss-of-function and/or a gain-of-function mode.

Purified serum IgG from SS and SLE patients display inhibitory activity against ApoCell-phagocytosis that correlates with its binding to apoptotic cells

Sera from autoimmune patients (SS; $n = 20$, SLE; $n = 14$, RA; $n = 5$) and HBD ($n = 12$) were screened by flow cytometry for IgM and IgG immunoglobulin reactivity to early apoptotic cells. Such analyses had revealed that the levels of IgM anti-ApoCell

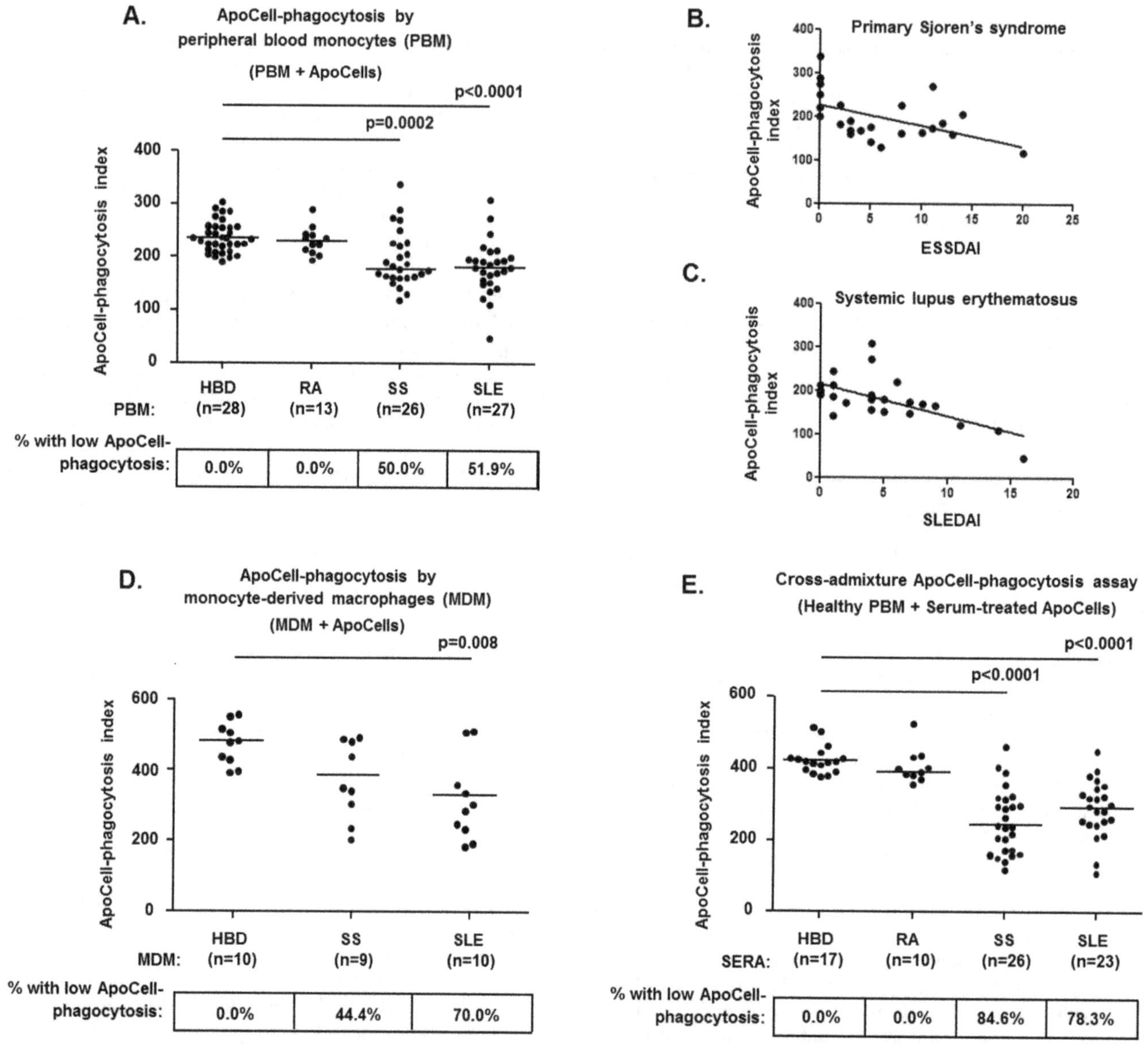

Figure 1. The peripheral blood (PB) monocytes and monocyte-derived macrophages (MDM) of SS and SLE patients manifest significantly impaired ApoCell-phagocytosis. The aberrant uptake of apoptotic cells by blood-borne phagocytes largely resides in the patients' sera. **A.** Significantly decreased ApoCell-phagocytosis by PB monocytes in SS and SLE patients, but not in RA. **B–C.** The ApoCell-phagocytosis index values observed in SS and SLE patients correlated inversely with the disease activity indices of these diseases. **D.** Decreased ApoCell-phagocytosis by MDM in SS and SLE patients. **E.** Cross-admixture experiments illustrating the significantly reduced capacity of sera from SS and SLE patients to support ApoCell-phagocytosis by normal peripheral blood (PB) monocytes, in contrast to sera from HBD and from RA patients. In panels A, C and D the horizontal lines indicate the median levels in each group, whereas the numbers in boxes indicate the percentages of individuals with decreased ApoCell-phagocytosis, as defined by the presence of ApoCell-PhI values that were two standard deviations below the corresponding mean of HBD. Statistically significant comparisons of patient groups to HBD are shown. In panel B, the mean ApoCell-PhI values of SS-derived MDM were marginally different compared to MDM (p = 0.06).

antibodies were significantly decreased in the sera of SS patients (median IgM anti-ApoCell binding index [range]: 1.34 [0.22–5.05]) compared to HBD (3.26 [1.44–5.97], p = 0.0079), but not in those from SLE and RA patients (SLE: 4.91 [0.60–8.50], RA: 2.48 [1.58–3.28], differences not significant). In direct contrast, significantly increased levels of IgG anti-ApoCell antibodies were observed in the sera of SS and SLE patients (median IgG anti-ApoCell binding index [range]; SS: 1.70 [0.33–6.63], SLE: 1.57 [0.41–5.13]), compared to HBD (0.54 [0.38–0.73], for p = 0.035 and p = 0.001, respectively), but not in those from RA patients (0.70 [0.55–1.17], difference not significant). Rheumatoid factor positivity was not found to influence the IgG or IgM anti-ApoCell binding assay results (data not shown).

The rates of ApoCell-phagocytosis that were observed in the cross-admixture experiments presented above (application of healthy peripheral blood monocytes and sera-pretreated apoptotic cells) correlated inversely and highly significantly with the levels of IgG anti-ApoCell antibodies in those sera, (r = −0.631, p = 0.0009), but not those of IgM (r = 0.284, difference not significant). Therefore, to address whether the IgG anti-ApoCell antibodies that were present in the sera of SS and SLE patients may interfere adversely with the ingestion of apoptotic cells, serum

IgG immunoglobulins were purified from the sera of autoimmune patients and controls and subsequently analyzed for anti-ApoCell reactivity, as well as in cross-admixture ApoCell-phagocytosis assays. The levels of anti-ApoCell antibodies were significantly increased in the IgG preparations derived from SS and SLE patients (both for $p<0.0001$, compared to HBD), but in not those from RA (**Figure 2A**). In addition, anti-ApoCell levels were significantly higher among anti-Ro/SSA antibody-positive patients (median: 1.033, range: 0.426-5.500) compared to antibody-negative ones, (median: 1.030, range: 0.445–2.020, $p=0.019$). In cross-admixture ApoCell-phagocytosis assays, the application of healthy MDM and purified IgG-pretreated early apoptotic cells had revealed significantly reduced ApoCell-phagocytosis upon the application of IgG preparations derived from SS and SLE patients (for $p<0.0001$ and $p=0.0002$, respectively, compared to HBD) but not from RA (**Figure 2B & 2C**) suggesting the inhibitory effect of IgG anti-ApoCell antibodies in SS and SLE on ApoCell-phagocytosis. The significantly impaired engulfment of apoptotic cells following their pretreatment with purified IgG from SS and SLE patients compared to that from HBD, was also demonstrated by comparative ApoCell-phagocytosis assays using pHrodo-SE-labelled apoptotic cells (**Figure 2D**). Importantly, highly significant inverse correlation was found between the rate of ApoCell-phagocytosis obtained by the various IgG preparations used and the levels of anti-ApoCell antibodies in those preparations ($r=-0.661$, $p<0.0001$, **Figure 2E**). Similar inverse correlation was observed between the ApoCell-PhI values obtained with the application of whole sera in the cross-admixture experiments described earlier, and the anti-ApoCell levels that were detected in purified IgG preparations from the respective sera used (in 25 sera; 8 from SS, 7 from SLE, 4 from RA patients and 6 from HBD, $r=-0.595$, $p=0.0017$).

Significantly impaired MB-phagocytosis by peripheral blood monocytes of SS and SLE patients

RA patients displayed similar MB-phagocytosis indices to those of HBD. In direct contrast, both SS and SLE groups were found to manifest highly significantly decreased levels of MB-phagocytosis by granulocytes and by monocytes compared to HBD, as well as to RA (**Figure 3A & 3B**). Conversely, there were no differences of MB-phagocytosis indices between SS and SLE patients for either granulocytes or monocytes (**Figure 3A & 3B**). The overall analysis of phagocytosis index values had revealed a highly significant correlation between the levels of MB-phagocytosis and ApoCell-phagocytosis by monocytes in the various groups studied ($r=0.432$, $p=0.001$).

Among the various clinical and serological parameters examined, the degree of MB-phagocytosis by monocytes was found to positively correlate with the C4 serum complement levels in both SS and SLE patients (SS; $r=0.377$, $p=0.03$, SLE; $r=0.520$, $p=0.03$). Furthermore, in SS patients, the occurrence of extraglandular disease correlated with significantly lower levels of MB-phagocytosis by granulocytes (glandular SS; median = 41, range: 5–84, extraglandular SS; median = 14, range: 3–63, $p=0.003$), as well as by monocytes (glandular SS; median = 58, range: 11–132, extraglandular SS; median = 24, range: 1–87, $p=0.002$). Finally, MB-phagocytosis indices in SS patients also inversely correlated with ESSDAI (for granulocytes; $r=-0.432$, $p=0.01$, for monocytes; $r=-0.520$, $p=0.002$) and SSDDI (for granulocytes; $r=-0.355$, $p=0.02$, for monocytes; $r=-0.475$, $p=0.006$).

Impaired MB-phagocytosis by MDM preparations of SS and SLE patients

The study of MB-phagocytosis by MDM had yielded similar results between RA patients and HBD, whereas significantly decreased MB-phagocytosis was observed in both SS and SLE patient groups, compared to HBD ($p=0.01$ and $p=0.004$, respectively), as well as to RA patients (**Figure 3C**). The overall analysis of MB-PhI values had revealed a significant correlation of the levels of MB-phagocytosis by MDM with those obtained by peripheral blood monocytes in the various groups studied ($r=0.552$, $p=0.01$). In SS patients, MB-phagocytosis by MDM was marginally lower among patients with extraglandular disease (median = 184, range: 34–312), compared to those with disease confined in glands (median = 282, range: 252–468, $p=0.07$), as well as among patients with type-I SS (median = 183, range: 34–312), compared to those without (median = 281, range: 252–468, $p=0.06$). Among the SLE patients studied, the occurrence of decreased MB-phagocytosis by MDM was not found to correlate significantly with any of the clinical and serological parameters examined.

Discussion

Several previous studies had documented that the monocytes of SLE patients manifest reduced clearance of various targets [29], including defective efferocytosis [9,11,17,26]. In fact, the accumulation of apoptotic cells in lymph node and skin biopsies of SLE patients is thought to signify the deficient phagocytic clearance of apoptotic cells in vivo [30]. These data had provided a mechanistic explanation for the development of chronic inflammatory and autoimmune reactions in SLE patients, via the progression of uncleared apoptotic cells to the state of secondary necrosis and the release thereof of alarmins and modified self antigens that activate innate and acquired immune system [31]. In fact, experimental mice that are deficient for molecules involved in the phagocytosis of apoptotic cells display defective efferocytosis, as well as features of SLE, such as the development of antinuclear antibodies and glomerulonephritis [32]. In the same context, lupus-prone strains of mice are reported to display decreased phagocytosis of apoptotic cells by macrophages [33].

SLE and SS are immunologically similar disorders in several respects [18], therefore in this study we sought to evaluate directly the capacity of the peripheral blood monocytes of SS and SLE patients for uptake of early apoptotic cells, employing simple and reproducible ex-vivo ApoCell-phagocytosis assays. In addition, several lines of experimental evidence from mice and human studies indicate that apoptosis plays a crucial role in the pathophysiology of SS [34–36], whereas SS-related autoantigens, such as Ro(SSA) and La(SSB), have been shown to be clustered at the surface of apoptotic cells [37].

In good concordance with previous studies [9,26], our findings indicate that compared to healthy individuals, approximately half of the SLE patients tested manifested significantly impaired ApoCell-phagocytosis by monocytes. In addition, this study provides first evidence that, in a manner similar to SLE, deficient uptake of early apoptotic cells by monocytes also characterizes a significant proportion of SS patients, whereas such aberration is not apparently present among RA patients. Interestingly, previous studies of experimental animal models had indicated decreased ApoCell-phagocytosis by macrophages not only in lupus-prone strains of mice [33] but also in mice susceptible to SS-like sialadenitis [38]. In addition, defective efferocytosis has been described to occur in the heart of fetuses of certain SS and SLE patients owing to aberrant opsonization of apoptotic cells by

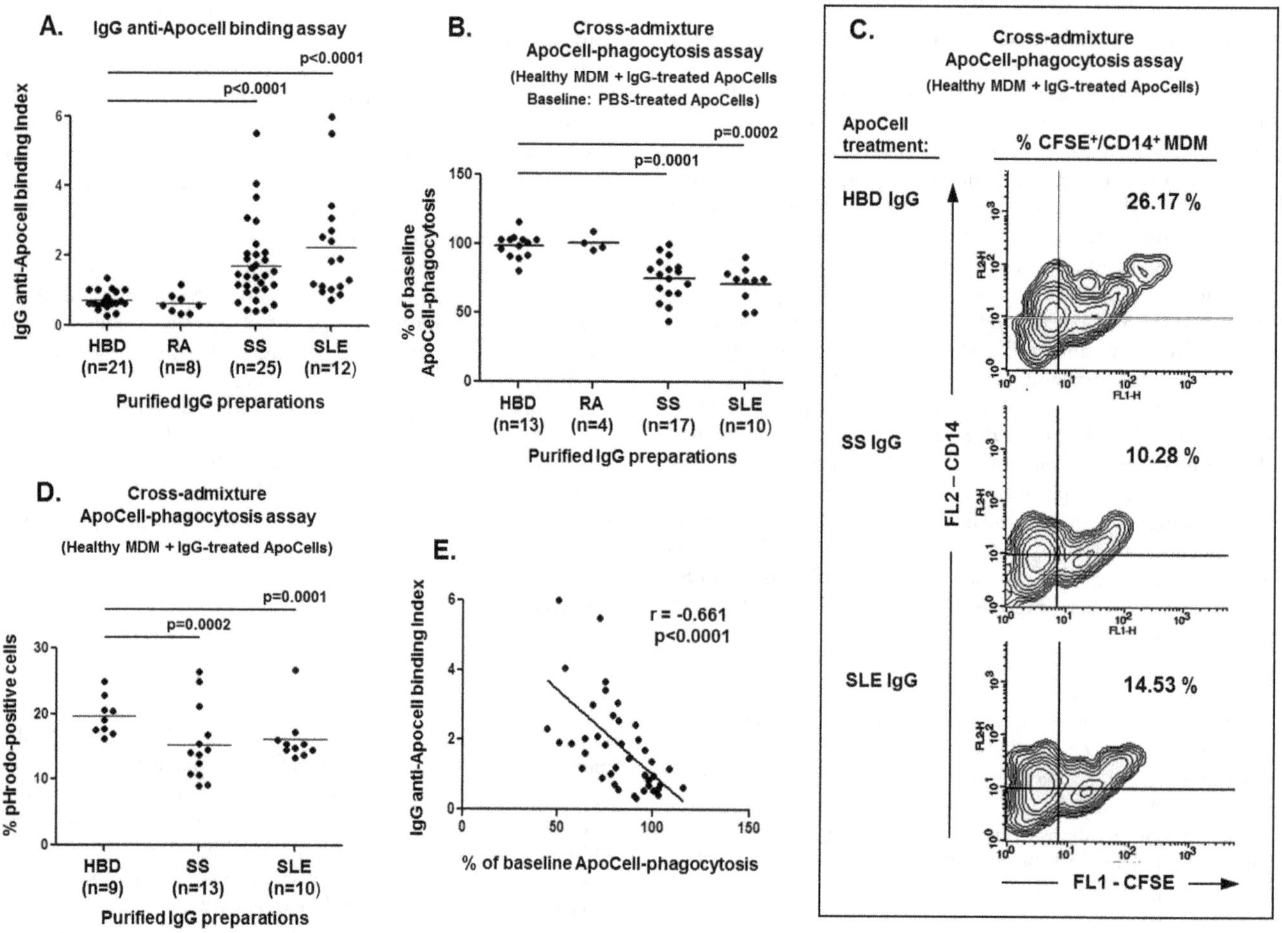

Figure 2. Inhibitory effect of IgG on ApoCell-phagocytosis. Purified serum IgG preparations from SS and SLE patients display inhibitory activity on ApoCell-phagocytosis by healthy MDM that correlates with its binding activity to early apoptotic cells. **A.** Purified serum IgG preparations from SS and SLE patients (but not RA) display significantly increased binding to early apoptotic cells. Binding index was normalized and expressed as fold increase over the binding of a purified IgG preparation from a HBD used in all experiments. **B–D.** Cross-admixture ApoCell-phagocytosis experiments demonstrating that the pretreatment of early apoptotic cells with purified serum IgG preparations derived from SS and SLE (but not from RA) results in decreased ApoCell-phagocytosis by healthy MDM, as compared to treatment with IgG from HBD. In **B**, data are expressed as percent of baseline ApoCell-phagocytosis values (e.g. treatment of apoptotic cells with PBS only, considered as 100%). Similar results were obtained by slightly different experimental setups assaying the ingestion of CFSE-labelled IgG-pretreated apoptotic cells by electronically gated CD14-stained MDM in dual-color flow cytometry (**C**; representative results from 3 independent experiments) or the uptake of pHrodo-SE-labelled apoptotic cells in single-color flow cytometry (**D**). **E.** Highly significant inverse correlation between the rates of ApoCell-phagocytosis obtained by the various purified serum IgG preparations used (shown in A) and the levels of anti-ApoCell antibodies in those preparations (shown in A).

maternal IgG anti-Ro/SSA and anti-La/SSB antibodies [39]. Furthermore, in the present study the rates of ApoCell-phagocytosis in SS and SLE patients correlated inversely and highly significantly with the activity indices of these disorders. Although larger cohort studies with a wide sampling of patients are needed, our findings support aberrant efferocytosis as an important pathogenetic mechanism for both SS and SLE and as a promising field of search for novel biomarkers for these diseases. In fact, the inverse correlation between deficient ApoCell-phagocytosis and disease activity has been also previously observed in SLE patients [11].

The underlying cause of defective efferocytosis in SLE has been attributed to the presence of intrinsic functional defects in patients' phagocytes [9,11,17,26] and/or aberrant serum factors [16,17]. Our findings mainly indicate that serum factors in SS and SLE patients are mostly responsible for the observed impairment of ApoCell-phagocytosis; however, certain lines of evidence may be also supportive to the notion of disordered function of patients' phagocytes per se. First, in line with previous reports in SLE patients [9], [26], our data indicate that ApoCell-phagocytosis is deficient in several MDM preparations that were derived from SS and SLE patients by cultivation in the absence of patients' sera, a fact that may at least partly support a model of intrinsically defective monocyte in these disorders. Alternatively, the impaired capacity of phagocytes of SS and SLE patients for uptake of prey may be viewed as a result of cellular activation taking place in vivo, a notion probably also implied by the significant correlation between the findings in the various phagocytosis assays and the activity indices of these diseases. Finally, the notably low capacity of SS and SLE patients for phagocytosis of particulate targets by blood-borne monocytes and MDM that was observed may reflect an overall dysfunction of phagocytes in the proper engulfment of certain preys in these disorders. Interestingly, deficient phagocytosis of particulate targets is also reported in primary biliary cirrhosis [40], a disease with striking clinicopathologic similarities to SS [41]. On the other hand, it should be noticed that in sharp

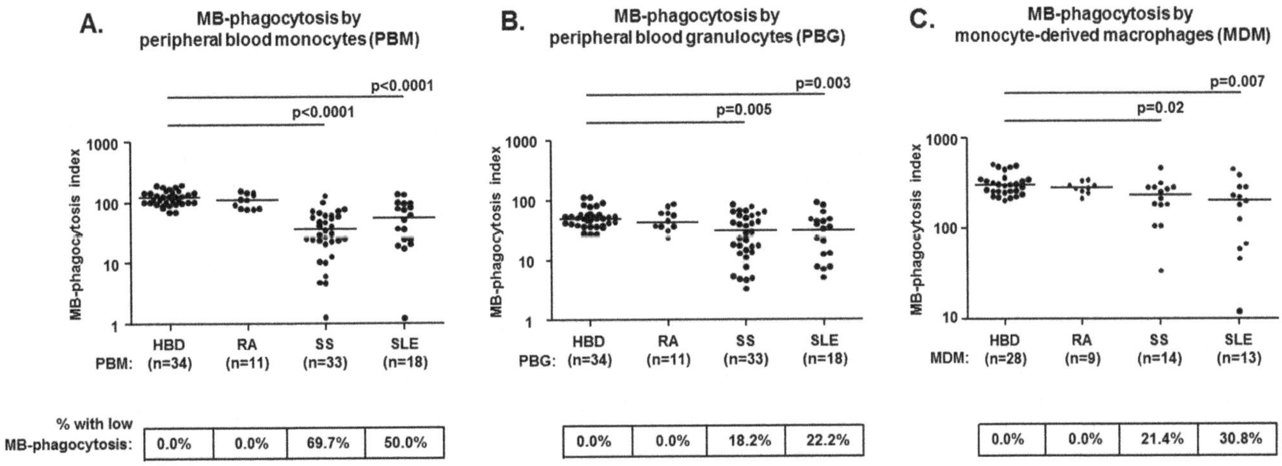

Figure 3. Impaired MB-phagocytosis by peripheral blood (PB) phagocytes (A; monocytes B; granulocytes) and by monocyte-derived macrophages (MDM, C) obtained from SS and SLE patients, but not from RA patients. The horizontal lines indicate the median levels in each group, whereas the numbers in boxes indicate the percentages of individuals with decreased MB-phagocytosis, as defined by the presence of MB-PhI values that were two standard deviations below the corresponding mean of HBD. Statistically significant comparisons of patient groups to HBD are shown.

contrast to the above deficient phagocytic capacities, the blood-borne monocytes of SS and SLE were found remarkably hyperfunctional in the phagocytosis of necrotic cell debris [42].

The addition of healthy serum was found to facilitate significantly the ingestion of apoptotic cells by blood-borne monocytes derived from healthy individuals, as well as from SLE or SS patients. These findings are in good agreement with the previously observed capacity of sera from healthy individuals to restore the phagocytic ability of macrophages from SLE patients [11]. In addition, ApoCell-phagocytosis by healthy monocytes was presently shown to be severely impaired following the substitution of HBD sera by sera derived from SS and SLE patients. Consistent with previous observations [17], the sera from approximately 80% of SLE patients studied were not as efficient as healthy sera in supporting of ApoCell-phagocytosis by normal blood-borne monocytes. In this study, we present first evidence that such incapacity is also manifested by the vast majority of sera from SS patients studied. The precise nature of this aberration in SS and SLE patients is unclear. Normally, several serum proteins (such as complement C1q, IgM, C-reactive protein, serum amyloid protein, milk fat globule-EGF factor 8 protein [MFG-e8] and mannose-binding lectin) attach to apoptotic cells and induce the deposition of C3 and its degradation products C3b and iC3b, thus enhancing efferocytosis by phagocytes via recognition by complement receptors CR3 and CR4 [43]. In this context, mice lacking such bridging molecules, such as MFG-e8, Mer or C1q are reported to develop lupus-like manifestations associated with inefficient removal of apoptotic cells [32]. In line to these observations, several quantitative and functional aberrations of the above opsonins have been described in SLE and SS patients, including hypocomplementemia, which is considered as one of the major immunological markers and of key clinical importance for both disorders [44,45]. In fact, an intact classical complement pathway is essential for the phagocytic removal of apoptotic cells [46], whereas the deficient ApoCell-phagocytosis in SLE patients has been previously attributed to defective opsonization of apoptotic cells by aberrantly low levels of C1q, C3, and C4 complement proteins [17]. Our results from the cross-admixture experiments also implicate the role of aberrant serum complement function in SS and SLE patients in the observed defect of ApoCell-phagocytosis. The capacity of the SS and SLE patients' sera to assist ApoCell-phagocytosis by healthy monocytes was found to inversely correlate with C3 and C4 complement levels in these sera. In line with these observations, the decomplementation of normal sera by heat-inactivation largely diminished their capacity to support ApoCell-phagocytosis by healthy monocytes.

Most remarkably however, our results had indicated that the inhibitory component of SS and SLE sera to ApoCell-phagocytosis largely resides in the IgG immunoglobulin fraction. Serum IgG preparations from SS and SLE patients (but not from controls) were very frequently found to possess significant inhibitory activity on ApoCell-phagocytosis by normal monocytes, as well as enhanced binding capacity for the surface of early apoptotic cells. Moreover, the rate of ApoCell-phagocytosis obtained by the various IgG preparations used in cross-admixture experiments was presently found to correlate significantly in an inverse manner with the levels of anti-ApoCell antibodies in those preparations. In fact, serum antibodies against late, but not against early apoptotic cells, have been previously reported in the serum of SLE patients and to prevent the uptake of opsonized late apoptotic cells by phagocytes [16].

The nature of IgG antibodies to early apoptotic cells that we have detected in the sera of SS and SLE patients is presently unclear. In the recent years, growing evidence indicates that various types of serum autoantibodies may interfere with the clearance of apoptotic cells by phagocytes. Such autoantibody responses may involve reactivities against surface membranous molecules of the apoptotic cells and/or the phagocytes [16,47], as well as against bridging molecules that normally facilitate ApoCell-phagocytosis [48]. Recently, the occurrence of anti-C3 complement autoantibodies in SLE patients has been shown to react to C3 bound on apoptotic cells and thus to interfere with the proper C3-mediated recognition and clearance of apoptotic cells by phagocytes [49]. Anti-nuclear antibodies, which are a hallmark feature of SLE and SS, may also hamper the uptake of apoptotic cells by phagocytes. In fact, autoantibodies from SLE and SS patients are reported to opsonize late apoptotic cells and to inhibit their uptake by macrophages via an Fc-gamma receptor-dependent mechanism [16]. In line with these observations, our results from cross-admixture experiments had also indicated that the occurrence of specific anti-nuclear antibodies in the sera of SLE (anti-histones) and SS patients (anti-Ro/SSA) is associated with failure to support the ApoCell-phagocytosis by healthy monocytes, whereas we have found increased IgG binding activity to early apoptotic cells among anti-Ro/SSA-positive sera. Notably, apoptotic cells are reportedly characterized by surface translocation of various nuclear constituents, including the ribonucleoproteins Ro/SSA and La/SSB [37], which represent the major targets of autoimmune responses in SS. Importantly also, IgG anti-Ro/SSA and anti-La/SSB antibodies have been previously shown to opsonize in-vitro apoptotic cardiocytes and thus to inhibit their clearance by phagocytes [39]. To this end, detailed autoantibody depletion and antigen inhibition experiments are in progress in this laboratory to delineate the characteristics and role of particular antibody specificities in the clearance of apoptotic cells. On the other hand, loss-of-function processes involving the natural IgM immunoglobulins of SS patients may also have a role, as indicated by the occurrence of significantly decreased IgM anti-ApoCell levels that we observed in the SS patients, compared to healthy individuals. In fact, the important role of natural IgM antibodies for the clearance of apoptotic cells, microbes and various small particles is well-described [50].

In conclusion, this study demonstrates that in a manner similar and comparable to SLE, a significant portion of SS patients is characterized by impaired uptake of early apoptotic cells, as well as of particulate targets by blood-borne phagocytes and macrophages that apparently involves both loss-of-function and gain-of-function processes. Importantly, these aberrations were found to correlate with various clinico-serologic disease indices of SS and SLE, and thus may represent promising areas of search for novel biomarkers for these disorders. The defective clearance of apoptotic cells in SS and SLE appears primarily to depend on serologic aberrations, such as the occurrence of inhibitory IgG anti-ApoCell antibodies and hypocomplementemia, and secondarily on the dysfunction of phagocytes. Such failure of efferocytosis may lead to the accumulation of immunogenic and inflammagenic secondary necrotic cells and debris and the perpetuation thereof of a vicious cycle of inflammatory and autoimmune reactions. In fact, we have recently demonstrated that, SS and SLE patients also manifest impaired serum-mediated degradation of necrotic cell debris that leads to increased amounts of circulating nuclear material and their massive uptake by blood-borne phagocytes [42]. Altogether, these aberrations may represent major causes of the inflammatory and autoimmune reactions that characterize SS and SLE, and may thus hold key roles in the pathogenesis of these disorders.

Author Contributions

Conceived and designed the experiments: MNM. Performed the experiments: GEF AGV. Analyzed the data: MNM GEF AGV HMM. Wrote the paper: MNM GEF AGV HMM.

References

1. Majno G, Joris I (1995) Apoptosis, oncosis, and necrosis. An overview of cell death. Am J Pathol 146: 3–15.
2. Voll RE, Herrmann M, Roth EA, Stach C, Kalden JR, et al. (1997) Immunosuppressive effects of apoptotic cells. Nature 390: 350–351.
3. Vandivier RW, Henson PM, Douglas IS (2006) Burying the dead: the impact of failed apoptotic cell removal (efferocytosis) on chronic inflammatory lung disease. Chest 129: 1673–1682.
4. Munoz LE, van Bavel C, Franz S, Berden J, Herrmann M, et al. (2008) Apoptosis in the pathogenesis of systemic lupus erythematosus. Lupus 17: 371–375.
5. Cohen JJ, Duke RC, Fadok VA, Sellins KS (1992) Apoptosis and programmed cell death in immunity. Annu Rev Immunol 10: 267–293.
6. Han H, Iwanaga T, Uchiyama Y, Fujita T (1993) Aggregation of macrophages in the tips of intestinal villi in guinea pigs: their possible role in the phagocytosis of effete epithelial cells. Cell Tissue Res 271: 407–416.
7. Hopkinson-Woolley J, Hughes D, Gordon S, Martin P (1994) Macrophage recruitment during limb development and wound healing in the embryonic and foetal mouse. J Cell Sci 107 (Pt 5): 1159–1167.
8. Munoz LE, Janko C, Grossmayer GE, Frey B, Voll RE, et al. (2009) Remnants of secondarily necrotic cells fuel inflammation in systemic lupus erythematosus. Arthritis Rheum 60: 1733–1742.
9. Herrmann M, Voll RE, Zoller OM, Hagenhofer M, Ponner BB, et al. (1998) Impaired phagocytosis of apoptotic cell material by monocyte-derived macrophages from patients with systemic lupus erythematosus. Arthritis Rheum 41: 1241–1250.
10. Gaipl US, Munoz LE, Grossmayer G, Lauber K, Franz S, et al. (2007) Clearance deficiency and systemic lupus erythematosus (SLE). J Autoimmun 28: 114–121.
11. Ren Y, Tang J, Mok MY, Chan AW, Wu A, et al. (2003) Increased apoptotic neutrophils and macrophages and impaired macrophage phagocytic clearance of apoptotic neutrophils in systemic lupus erythematosus. Arthritis Rheum 48: 2888–2897.
12. Kimberly RP, Salmon JE, Edberg JC, Gibofsky A (1989) The role of Fc gamma receptors in mononuclear phagocyte system function. Clin Exp Rheumatol 7 Suppl 3: S103–108.
13. Svensson BO (1975) Serum factors causing impaired macrophage function in systemic lupus erythematosus. Scand J Immunol 4: 145–150.
14. Shoshan Y, Shapira I, Toubi E, Frolkis I, Yaron M, et al. (2001) Accelerated Fas-mediated apoptosis of monocytes and maturing macrophages from patients with systemic lupus erythematosus: relevance to in vitro impairment of interaction with iC3b-opsonized apoptotic cells. J Immunol 167: 5963–5969.
15. Sarmiento LF, Munoz LE, Chirinos P, Bianco NE, Zabaleta-Lanz ME (2007) Opsonization by anti-dsDNA antibodies of apoptotic cells in systemic lupus erythematosus. Autoimmunity 40: 337–339.
16. Reefman E, Horst G, Nijk MT, Limburg PC, Kallenberg CG, et al. (2007) Opsonization of late apoptotic cells by systemic lupus erythematosus autoantibodies inhibits their uptake via an Fcgamma receptor-dependent mechanism. Arthritis Rheum 56: 3399–3411.
17. Bijl M, Reefman E, Horst G, Limburg PC, Kallenberg CG (2006) Reduced uptake of apoptotic cells by macrophages in systemic lupus erythematosus: correlates with decreased serum levels of complement. Ann Rheum Dis 65: 57–63.
18. Manoussakis MN, Georgopoulou C, Zintzaras E, Spyropoulou M, Stavropoulou A, et al. (2004) Sjogren's syndrome associated with systemic lupus erythematosus: clinical and laboratory profiles and comparison with primary Sjogren's syndrome. Arthritis Rheum 50: 882–891.
19. Vitali C, Bombardieri S, Jonsson R, Moutsopoulos HM, Alexander EL, et al. (2002) Classification criteria for Sjogren's syndrome: a revised version of the European criteria proposed by the American-European Consensus Group. Ann Rheum Dis 61: 554–558.
20. Tan EM, Cohen AS, Fries JF, Masi AT, McShane DJ, et al. (1982) The 1982 revised criteria for the classification of systemic lupus erythematosus. Arthritis Rheum 25: 1271–1277.
21. Aletaha D, Neogi T, Silman AJ, Funovits J, Felson DT, et al. (2010) 2010 Rheumatoid arthritis classification criteria: an American College of Rheumatology/European League Against Rheumatism collaborative initiative. Arthritis Rheum 62: 2569–2581.
22. Seror R, Ravaud P, Bowman SJ, Baron G, Tzioufas A, et al. (2010) EULAR Sjogren's syndrome disease activity index: development of a consensus systemic disease activity index for primary Sjogren's syndrome. Ann Rheum Dis 69: 1103–1109.
23. Vitali C, Palombi G, Baldini C, Benucci M, Bombardieri S, et al. (2007) Sjogren's Syndrome Disease Damage Index and disease activity index: scoring systems for the assessment of disease damage and disease activity in Sjogren's syndrome, derived from an analysis of a cohort of Italian patients. Arthritis Rheum 56: 2223–2231.
24. Gladman D, Ginzler E, Goldsmith C, Fortin P, Liang M, et al. (1996) The development and initial validation of the Systemic Lupus International Collaborating Clinics/American College of Rheumatology damage index for systemic lupus erythematosus. Arthritis Rheum 39: 363–369.
25. Ioannidis JP, Vassiliou VA, Moutsopoulos HM (2002) Long-term risk of mortality and lymphoproliferative disease and predictive classification of primary Sjogren's syndrome. Arthritis Rheum 46: 741–747.
26. Tas SW, Quartier P, Botto M, Fossati-Jimack L (2006) Macrophages from patients with SLE and rheumatoid arthritis have defective adhesion in vitro, while only SLE macrophages have impaired uptake of apoptotic cells. Ann Rheum Dis 65: 216–221.
27. Esmann L, Idel C, Sarkar A, Hellberg L, Behnen M, et al. (2010) Phagocytosis of apoptotic cells by neutrophil granulocytes: diminished proinflammatory neutrophil functions in the presence of apoptotic cells. J Immunol 184: 391–400.
28. Gantner F, Kupferschmidt R, Schudt C, Wendel A, Hatzelmann A (1997) In vitro differentiation of human monocytes to macrophages: change of PDE

profile and its relationship to suppression of tumour necrosis factor-alpha release by PDE inhibitors. Br J Pharmacol 121: 221–231.

29. Katsiari CG, Liossis SN, Sfikakis PP (2010) The pathophysiologic role of monocytes and macrophages in systemic lupus erythematosus: a reappraisal. Semin Arthritis Rheum 39: 491–503.
30. Baumann I, Kolowos W, Voll RE, Manger B, Gaipl U, et al. (2002) Impaired uptake of apoptotic cells into tingible body macrophages in germinal centers of patients with systemic lupus erythematosus. Arthritis Rheum 46: 191–201.
31. Urbonaviciute V, Furnrohr BG, Meister S, Munoz L, Heyder P, et al. (2008) Induction of inflammatory and immune responses by HMGB1-nucleosome complexes: implications for the pathogenesis of SLE. J Exp Med 205: 3007–3018.
32. Viorritto IC, Nikolov NP, Siegel RM (2007) Autoimmunity versus tolerance: can dying cells tip the balance? Clin Immunol 122: 125–134.
33. Licht R, Dieker JW, Jacobs CW, Tax WJ, Berden JH (2004) Decreased phagocytosis of apoptotic cells in diseased SLE mice. J Autoimmun 22: 139–145.
34. Manoussakis MN, Spachidou MP, Maratheftis CI (2010) Salivary epithelial cells from Sjogren's syndrome patients are highly sensitive to anoikis induced by TLR-3 ligation. J Autoimmun 35: 212–218.
35. Salomonsson S, Jonsson MV, Skarstein K, Brokstad KA, Hjelmstrom P, et al. (2003) Cellular basis of ectopic germinal center formation and autoantibody production in the target organ of patients with Sjogren's syndrome. Arthritis Rheum 48: 3187–3201.
36. Okuma A, Hoshino K, Ohba T, Fukushi S, Aiba S, et al. (2013) Enhanced apoptosis by disruption of the STAT3-IkappaB-zeta signaling pathway in epithelial cells induces Sjogren's syndrome-like autoimmune disease. Immunity 38: 450–460.
37. Casciola-Rosen LA, Anhalt G, Rosen A (1994) Autoantigens targeted in systemic lupus erythematosus are clustered in two populations of surface structures on apoptotic keratinocytes. J Exp Med 179: 1317–1330.
38. O'Brien BA, Geng X, Orteu CH, Huang Y, Ghoreishi M, et al. (2006) A deficiency in the in vivo clearance of apoptotic cells is a feature of the NOD mouse. J Autoimmun 26: 104–115.
39. Clancy RM, Neufing PJ, Zheng P, O'Mahony M, Nimmerjahn F, et al. (2006) Impaired clearance of apoptotic cardiocytes is linked to anti-SSA/Ro and -SSB/La antibodies in the pathogenesis of congenital heart block. J Clin Invest 116: 2413–2422.
40. Allina J, Stanca CM, Garber J, Hu B, Sautes-Fridman C, et al. (2008) Anti-CD16 autoantibodies and delayed phagocytosis of apoptotic cells in primary biliary cirrhosis. J Autoimmun 30: 238–245.
41. Selmi C, Meroni PL, Gershwin ME (2012) Primary biliary cirrhosis and Sjogren's syndrome: Autoimmune epithelitis. J Autoimmun 39: 34–42.
42. Fragoulis GE, Vakrakou AG, Papadopoulou A, Germenis A, Kanavakis E, et al. (2014) Impaired degradation and aberrant phagocytosis of necrotic cell debris in the peripheral blood of patients with primary Sjogren's syndrome. J Autoimmun http://dx.doi.org/10.1016/j.jaut.2014.08.004 [Epub ahead of print].
43. Ogden CA, Elkon KB (2006) Role of complement and other innate immune mechanisms in the removal of apoptotic cells. Curr Dir Autoimmun 9: 120–142.
44. Gaipl US, Kuhn A, Sheriff A, Munoz LE, Franz S, et al. (2006) Clearance of apoptotic cells in human SLE. Curr Dir Autoimmun 9: 173–187.
45. Ramos-Casals M, Brito-Zeron P, Soria N, Nardi N, Vargas A, et al. (2009) Mannose-binding lectin-low genotypes are associated with milder systemic and immunological disease expression in primary Sjogren's syndrome. Rheumatology (Oxford) 48: 65–69.
46. Gullstrand B, Martensson U, Sturfelt G, Bengtsson AA, Truedsson L (2009) Complement classical pathway components are all important in clearance of apoptotic and secondary necrotic cells. Clin Exp Immunol 156: 303–311.
47. Chen XW, Shen Y, Sun CY, Wu FX, Chen Y, et al. (2011) Anti-class a scavenger receptor autoantibodies from systemic lupus erythematosus patients impair phagocytic clearance of apoptotic cells by macrophages in vitro. Arthritis Res Ther 13: R9.
48. Shoenfeld Y, Szyper-Kravitz M, Witte T, Doria A, Tsutsumi A, et al. (2007) Autoantibodies against protective molecules–C1q, C-reactive protein, serum amyloid P, mannose-binding lectin, and apolipoprotein A1: prevalence in systemic lupus erythematosus. Ann N Y Acad Sci 1108: 227–239.
49. Kenyon KD, Cole C, Crawford F, Kappler JW, Thurman JM, et al. (2011) IgG autoantibodies against deposited C3 inhibit macrophage-mediated apoptotic cell engulfment in systemic autoimmunity. J Immunol 187: 2101–2111.
50. Litvack ML, Post M, Palaniyar N (2011) IgM promotes the clearance of small particles and apoptotic microparticles by macrophages. PLoS One 6: e17223.

Self DNA from Lymphocytes that have Undergone Activation-Induced Cell Death Enhances Murine B Cell Proliferation and Antibody Production

Qing Lu[1], Ji-Yang Wang[1,2], Luman Wang[1], Xuechao Jiang[1], Yiwei Chu[1,2]*

1 Key Laboratory of Medical Molecular Virology of MOE/MOH, Department of Immunology, School of Basic Medical Sciences, Fudan University, Shanghai, China,
2 Biotherapy Research Center of Fudan University, Shanghai, China

Abstract

Systemic lupus erythematosus (SLE) is characterized by prominent autoinflammatory tissue damage associated with impaired removal of dying cells and DNA. Self DNA-containing immune complexes are able to activate both innate and adaptive immune responses and play an important role in the maintenance and exacerbation of autoimmunity in SLE. In this study, we used DNA from lymphocytes that have undergone activation-induced cell death (ALD-DNA) and analyzed its role on the activation and differentiation of B cells from normal BALB/c mice as well as lupus-prone $MRL^{+/+}$ and MRL/lpr mice. We found that ALD-DNA directly increased the expression of costimulatory molecules and the survival of naïve B cells *in vitro*. Although ALD-DNA alone had little effect on the proliferation of naïve B cells, it enhanced LPS-activated B cell proliferation *in vitro* and *in vivo*. In addition, ALD-DNA increased plasma cell numbers and IgG production in LPS-stimulated cultures of naïve B cells, in part via enhancing IL-6 production. Importantly, B cells from lupus mice were hyperresponsive to ALD-DNA and/or LPS relative to normal control B cells in terminal plasma cell differentiation, as evidenced by increases in $CD138^{+}$ cell numbers, IgM production, and mRNA levels of B lymphocyte-induced maturation protein-1 (Blimp-1) and the X-box binding protein 1 (XBP1). Furthermore, ALD-DNA enhanced CD40-activated naïve B cell proliferation. Collectively, these data indicate that self DNA can serve as a DAMP (damage-associated molecular pattern) that cooperates with signals from both innate and adaptive immunity to promote polyclonal B cell activation, a common characteristic of autoimmune diseases.

Editor: Pierre Bobé, INSERM-Université Paris-Sud, France

Funding: The work was supported by grants from the Chinese Natural Sciences Foundation (Grant 30872337 [QL], 81273215 [YC] and 81330080 [QL]) (http://www.nsfc.gov.cn/). The funders had no role in study design, data collection and analysis, decision to publish, or preparation of the manuscript.

Competing Interests: The authors have declared that no competing interests exist.

* Email: yiwei_chu@126.com

Introduction

Systemic lupus Erythematosus (SLE) is a chronic-relapsing autoimmune disease of incompletely understood etiology and is characterized by polyclonal B cell activation and autoantibodies to components of the cell nucleus, such as DNA and the nucleosome, a complex composed of 180 bp of DNA and five histone molecules. These autoantibodies may induce inflammation and tissue damage, most prominently glomerulonephritis through immune complex deposition.

Autoimmunity results from the failure of tolerance to autoantigens. Although the origin of anti-dsDNA antibodies is at present controversial, exposure of the immune system to endogenous DNA can lead to the development of autoimmunity, as demonstrated by the finding that insufficient digestion of extracellular DNA in DNase I deficient mice causes SLE-like disease [1] and that mutations of *DNASE I* have been identified in humans with SLE [2]. In SLE patients and murine lupus, excessive apoptosis with a defect in clearance of apoptotic cells is implicated as one source of extracellular DNA [3–6]. Furthermore, DNA-containing immune complexes (ICs) in serum of SLE patients were shown to activate plasmacytoid dendritic cells to overproduce type I IFN and the serum type I IFN levels correlated with both SLE disease activity and severity [7,8].

A direct correlation was established between endogenous DNA and autoantibody production in studies with transgenic AM14 B cells specific for autologous IgG2a (rheumatoid factor, RF). ICs containing IgG2a mAbs specific for DNA or chromatins can directly activate autoreactive AM14 RF^{+} B cells to proliferate in a T-cell independent (TI) manner by dual engagement of the B cell receptor (BCR) and intracellular Toll-like receptor (TLR) 9. DNA component in antigen is a critical factor for these immunostimulatory ICs to activate autoreactive AM14 RF^{+} B cells [9]. TLR9 was first shown to uniquely recognize unmethylated CpG motif rich in microbial DNA and transmit mitogenic signals to B cells, although it was subsequently shown that TLR9 might also mediate mammalian DNA recognition. It has been proposed that the endosomal localization of nucleic acid-sensing TLRs may be an evolutionary strategy to protect them from access to self nucleic acids [10,11]. Thus, DNA containing ICs are actively involved in anti-nucleic acid and RF autoantibody production, and in the maintenance and exacerbation of autoimmunity [12].

B cells play an important role in protective immunity by producing large amounts of antibodies against invading pathogens. B cells are also responsible for the development and pathogenesis of both systemic and organ-specific autoimmune diseases, as highlighted by the clinical efficacy of B-cell depletion therapies [13,14]. B cells sense antigens through antigen-specific BCRs and innate pattern recognition receptors (PRRs) such as TLRs. In general, the antibody response against thymus dependent protein antigens (TD-Ags) requires the antigen-specific $CD4^+$ T helper cells, which provide help for antigen specific B-cell activation via CD40-CD40L interactions and by cytokines in the germinal centers (GCs). Here, activated B cells proliferate and undergo class switch recombination (CSR), affinity maturation, and differentiate into memory B cells or high affinity antibody-secreting plasma cells. The TI antibody response can be elicited by microbial products in the absence of helper T cells. Both LPS (TLR4 ligand) and unmethylated CpG DNA (TLR9 ligand) can trigger polyclonal activation of naïve mouse B cells and induce proliferation and differentiation into short-lived plasma cells [15]. However, human naïve B cells express low to undetectable levels of TLRs, and therefore require prior stimulation via BCR to respond to TLR ligands (microbial products) irrespective of the nature of T helper cells present [16]. In contrast to naïve B cells, human memory B cells have higher constitutively expressed TLRs and can respond directly to TLR stimulation to induce B cell proliferation and differentiation into plasma cells [16,17]. Requirement of cognate T cell help is usually a constraint for autoreactive B cell activation. The finding that microbial products such as LPS or CpG DNA could circumvent this control may explain at least in part the well-known association between infections and the flare or onset of autoantibody-mediated diseases [18].

A series of studies have revealed that injecting SLE-non-susceptible BALB/c mice with DNA from lymphocytes that have undergone activation-induced cell death (ALD-DNA) mixed with bacterial adjuvants could evoke SLE-like autoimmune diseases [19,20]. Indeed, DNA trapped in the plasma ICs from SLE patients showed size laddering and low molecular weight that were characteristic of the apoptotic process [21,22]. To better understand the immune properties of self DNA and its role in initiation and progression of B-cell autoimmunity, we used DNA from lymphocytes that had undergone activation-induced cell death (ALD-DNA) to directly stimulate B cells from normal BALB/c and two murine lupus-like models, $MRL^{+/+}$ and MRL/lpr. $MRL^{+/+}$ mice uniformly acquire lupus like disease, but disease is relatively mild and progression is slow. The genes predisposing to autoimmunity have not yet been clearly identified. The *lpr* mutation of *Fas* on the MRL genetic background accelerates and exacerbates disease in MRL/lpr mice [23]. Our results indicated that ALD-DNA cooperated with LPS in promoting B cell activation under normal and autoimmune conditions. Importantly, B cells from lupus mice showed heightened responsiveness to ALD-DNA and/or LPS in the terminal plasma cell differentiation and antibody production. Furthermore, ALD-DNA enhanced the proliferation of anti-CD40-activated naïve B cells. Taken together, our results indicate that self DNA can serve as a DAMP (damage-associated molecular pattern) that cooperates with signals from both innate and adaptive immunity to promote polyclonal B cell activation, a common characteristic of autoimmune diseases.

Materials and Methods

Ethics Statement

This work was conducted according to the guidelines for care of animals used for scientific purposes (Ministry of Health, P.R. China, 1998) and with the ethical approval of the Shanghai Medical Laboratory Animal Care and Use Committee (Permit number: 2009–0082) as well as the Ethical Committee of Fudan University (Permit number: 20120002). All experiments carried out in this study were strictly performed in a manner to minimize suffering of laboratory mice.

Mice

Female BALB/c, lupus-prone MRL/lpr, and nude mice were purchased from the Shanghai laboratory Animal Center (SLAC), Chinese Academy of Science (Shanghai, P. R. China). Female lupus-prone $MRL^{+/+}$ mice were kindly provided by Dr. Nan Shen, Joint Molecular Rheumatology Laboratory, Shanghai Ren Ji Hospital and Institute of Health Sciences, Shanghai JiaoTong University, Shanghai, China. All mice were housed in the animal facility of Fudan University under specific pathogen free conditions. BALB/c and nude mice used in this study were aged between 6 weeks to 8 weeks, whereas $MRL^{+/+}$ and MRL/lpr mice were sacrificed at 12-week-old and 16- to 20-week-old, respectively.

Lymphocyte purification and culture conditions

Single-cell suspensions were prepared by crushing spleens between frosted glass slides. Splenic resting B cells from BALB/c and $MRL^{+/+}$ mice were isolated by negative selection using anti-CD43-coated magnetic beads (Miltenyi Biotech, Bergisch Gladbach, Germany). The cell isolation was performed according to the manufacturer's protocol. Splenic B cells from MRL/lpr mice were obtained by positive selection using anti-CD19 MicroBeads (Miltenyi Biotech) according to the manufacturer's protocol. High purity of cells(≥98%) was confirmed by performing flow cytometric analysis. Purified B cells were cultured in RPMI 1640 medium supplemented with 10% FCS, 50 μM 2-mercaptoethanol, and penicillin/streptomycin (100 U/ml). Unless indicated otherwise, the concentrations of LPS (Sigma-Aldrich, St. Louis, MO), ALD-DNA, and anti-CD40 antibody (eBioscience, San Diego, CA) used for stimulation were 100 ng/ml, 50 μg/ml, and 1 μg/ml, respectively.

ALD-DNA preparation

Splenocytes from female BALB/c mice were cultured for 6 days in the presence of 5 μg/ml concanavalin A (Con A) (Sigma-Aldrich) to trigger activation-induced cell death (AICD). DNA was purified from Con A-activated splenocytes by extraction with phenol-chloroform-isoamyl alcohol (25/24/1) and ethanol precipitation followed by repeated extraction with Triton X-114 to remove endotoxin. The level of endotoxin was monitored using the Limulus amebocyte lysate assay (detection limit 0.1 EU/ml, BioWhittaker, Walkersville, MD, USA). The endotoxin levels before and after Triton X-114 extraction were 10.4 EU/mg DNA and <1 EU/mg DNA, respectively. The DNA concentration was determined by measuring absorbance at 260 nm. The A260/A280 ratio for all the DNA preparations was ≥1.9. The apoptotic DNA laddering was confirmed by performing agarose gel electrophoresis (Figure S1A). Endotoxin-free *Escherichia coli* genomic DNA was purchased from InvivoGen (San Diego, CA). Single-stranded (ss) DNA was prepared by boiling dsDNA for 10 min followed by immediate cooling on ice for 5 min.

B cell proliferation assay

Cell proliferation was analyzed by CFSE dilution assay or BrdU incorporation. For CFSE dilution assay, B cells were incubated with 1 μM CFSE (eBioscience) for 10 min at room temperature, and then washed with medium containing 10% FCS. CFSE-labeled B cells were cultured with ALD-DNA, LPS, *E. coli* DNA, ALD-DNA plus LPS, or *E. coli* DNA plus LPS for 3 days. The cells were analyzed using a CyAn ADP analyzer (Beckman-Coulter) and the Modfit software (Verity Software House, Topsham, ME).

For BrdU incorporation, ALD-DNA, anti-CD40 antibody, LPS, or a combination of these stimuli were added to the cultures for 3 days. In some cases, cells were pretreated with 20 μg/ml polymyxin B (PMB, Sigma-Aldrich) for 20 min at 37°C. Cells were harvested after 24-hour incubation with 10 μM BrdU (Roche Diagnostics, Mannheim, Germany). BrdU incorporation was analyzed using Cell proliferation ELISA Kit (Roche Diagnostics) according to the manufacturer's instruction.

In vivo assay of B cell proliferation

Nude mice were administered an intravenous injection containing either 50 μg ALD-DNA, or 1 μg LPS, or a combination of both dissolved in 200 μl PBS on day 1. An additional intraperitoneal injection of BrdU (2 mg; BD Biosciences, San Diego, CA) was administered 24 h before sacrificing the mice. Mice that were intravenously injected with sterile PBS were used to determine background values. After 3 days, spleens were collected and BrdU incorporation assay was performed using a FITC BrdU Flow kit (BD Pharmingen, San Diego, CA) according to the manufacturer's protocol.

Antibodies and flow cytometric analysis

Cells stimulated with ALD-DNA, LPS, or a combination of these stimuli for 3 days were stained with B220-APC (RA3-6B2, eBioscience), CD86-PE (GL1, eBioscience), MHC class II-FITC (2G9, BD Biosciences), or CD138-PE (281-2, BD Biosciences). CFSE-labeled B cells stimulated with ALD-DNA, *E. coli* DNA, LPS, anti-CD40, or different combinations of these stimuli for 3 days were stained with B220-APC (RA3-6B2, eBioscience) or CD138-APC (281-2, BD Biosciences). Appropriate isotype-matched antibodies were included as controls. Data were acquired on a CyAn ADP Analyzer and analyzed using Summit 5.2 software (both from Beckman-coulter). Dead cells and debris were excluded by forward scatter and side scatter (FSC/SSC) gating and propidium iodide staining (Sigma-Aldrich). For BrdU incorporation assay using a FITC BrdU Flow kit, cells were fixed, permeabilized, and treated with DNase prior to BrdU staining using a FITC-coupled anti-BrdU monoclonal antibody, as recommended by the manufacturer. The incorporated BrdU was measured in conjunction with DNA content by 7-AAD staining.

Detection of IL-6, IL-10, and antibodies by ELISA

To analyze antibody production, purified splenic B cells were cultured in ALD-DNA, LPS, or ALD-DNA plus LPS. The culture supernatant was collected from day 6 cultures, and the antibody levels were measured using Mouse IgM ELISA Ready-SET-Go (detection range, 0.39–25.00 ng/ml) for IgM and Mouse IgG ELISA Ready-SET-Go (detection range, 1.56–100.00 ng/ml) for IgG. For cytokine production, purified splenic B cells were cultured with ALD-DNA, LPS, *E. coli* DNA, a combination of ALD-DNA and LPS, or a combination of *E. coli* DNA and LPS for 72 h. Then supernatant was assayed using Mouse IL-6 ELISA Ready-SET-Go (detection range, 4–500 pg/ml) for IL-6 and Mouse IL-10 ELISA Ready-SET-Go (detection range, 32–4000 pg/ml) for IL-10, respectively. All kits were purchased from eBioscience and experimental procedures were performed following the manufacturer's instructions.

Analysis of Blimp-1, XBP1 and IL-6 mRNA expression by real-time PCR

Purified splenic B cells were cultured in the presence of LPS, ALD-DNA, or a combination of both for 6 h to induce IL-6, and 4 d to induce Blimp-1 and XBP1 expression. Total RNA was extracted using RNeasy Mini kit (Qiagen, Valencia, CA) and cDNA was generated using PrimeScript RT reagent Kit (TaKaRa, Dalian, China) as per manufacturer's instructions. Gene expression was analyzed by real-time PCR using the SYBR Premix Ex Taq (TaKaRa), according to manufacturer's instructions. The primer pairs used for real-time PCR were as follows: 5′-TGC TTA AAA CTC CAT GAC CTC-3′ and 5′-GCT ACA CAC CCT CAC CTC TG-3′ for Blimp-1; 5′-CAG GTG GAC ATG GGA TTC-3′ and 5′-TGC ACA TAA GGG AAA ACA AG-3′ for XBP1; 5′-TCC AAT GCT CTC CTA ACA GA-3′ and 5′-ACT AGG TTT GCC GAG TAG ATC-3′ for IL-6; 5′-ATG CTC CCC GGG CTG TAT-3′ and 5′-CAT AGG AGT CCT TCT GAC CCA TTC-3′for β-actin. All reactions were performed in triplicate in an ABI PRISM 7700 system and purity of the amplified PCR products was determined by a heat-dissociation protocol to enable detection of non-specific amplification. Target gene expression in each sample was calculated by the comparative Ct method using β-actin for normalization, and expressed relative to the untreated sample.

Statistical analysis

P values were determined by using the paired t test for *in vitro* experiments and a Mann-Whitney U-test (2-tailed Student's t-test using non parametric criteria for independent samples) for *in vivo* experiments. All analyses were performed using GraphPad Prism software. A value of $P<0.05$ was considered indicative of a significant difference.

Results

ALD-DNA enhances LPS induced survival and proliferation of naïve B cells

Initial experiments in which splenic resting B cells were stimulated with a range of ALD-DNA concentrations (25–100 μg/ml) revealed a weak but dose-dependent proliferative effect of ALD-DNA. We then examined whether ALD-DNA was able to collaborate with TLR4-derived signals and enhance LPS-induced B cell proliferation. The CFSE assay data indicated that ALD-DNA (25 μg/ml–100 μg/ml) cooperated with low doses of LPS to induce B cell proliferation (Figure S1B). The observed effects were additive or approximately additive and became less evident as the doses of LPS were increased, suggesting that the ALD-DNA-mediated enhancement was prominent on suboptimally activated B cells (Figure S1C). We further confirmed the cooperation of ALD-DNA and LPS for B cell survival and proliferation by performing additional *in vitro* and *in vivo* experiments. The flow cytometry analyses indicated that ALD-DNA alone enhanced the cell division (Figure 1A, $P=0.0002$) and survival (Figure 1B, $P=0.01$) of naïve B cells. In addition, ALD-DNA further enhanced LPS-induced proliferation (Figure 1A, $P=0.0003$) and survival (Figure 1B, $P=0.0002$). Analysis of the CFSE histograms revealed that the percentage of B cells that underwent four rounds of division was considerably higher in the presence of both ALD-DNA and LPS (39.1%) than in the presence of ALD-DNA (13.6%) or LPS (28.1%) alone (Figure 1A). The percentage of gated live cells in cell culture samples stimulated by both ALD-DNA and LPS (25.1%) was considerably higher than those for cells stimulated with ALD-DNA (11.1%) or LPS (17.9%), or for control cells (7.4%) (Figure 1B). To investigate whether ALD-DNA was able to enhance LPS induced B cell proliferation in a TI-manner *in vivo*, we injected ALD-DNA, LPS or both into nude mice and analyzed cell division by BrdU incorporation. Consistent with the results of *in vitro* experiments, we found a significant increase in the BrdU$^+$ proliferating B cells after injecting both ALD-DNA and LPS (7.4%) as compared with ALD-DNA (3.1%) or LPS (4.5%) alone (Figure 1C, n = 6, $P<0.05$). These data indicate that ALD-DNA and LPS are able to promote B cell proliferation both under *in vitro* and *in vivo* conditions.

ALD-DNA directly induces CD86 and MHC class II expression on B cells

B cell activation is often accompanied by up-regulation of MHC class II and CD86 expression, which facilitate antigen presentation to and activation of helper T cells. We therefore analyzed the effect of ALD-DNA on the expression of these molecules. As shown in the left panels of Figure 2A, LPS up-regulated CD86 expression in a dose-dependent manner. ALD-DNA stimulation increased the percentage of CD86$^+$ B cells to 36.8% as compared with the control cells that were stimulated with medium alone (11.7%; top two panels of Figure 2A). Furthermore, addition of ALD-DNA resulted in an increase in CD86 expression induced by LPS at suboptimal concentrations (Figure 2A, right panels). ALD-DNA also up-regulated MHC class II expression, although the effect was not as strong as that induced by bacterial DNA (Figure 2B). These results indicate that ALD-DNA can directly stimulate B cells to up-regulate CD86 and MHC class II expression, however, the immunostimulatory effect is less potent than that induced by bacterial DNA.

ALD-DNA and LPS synergize for inducing IgG production in naive B cells

After demonstrating that ALD-DNA enhanced LPS-induced survival, proliferation and the up-regulation of CD86 expression, we next analyzed the effect of ALD-DNA on the antibody

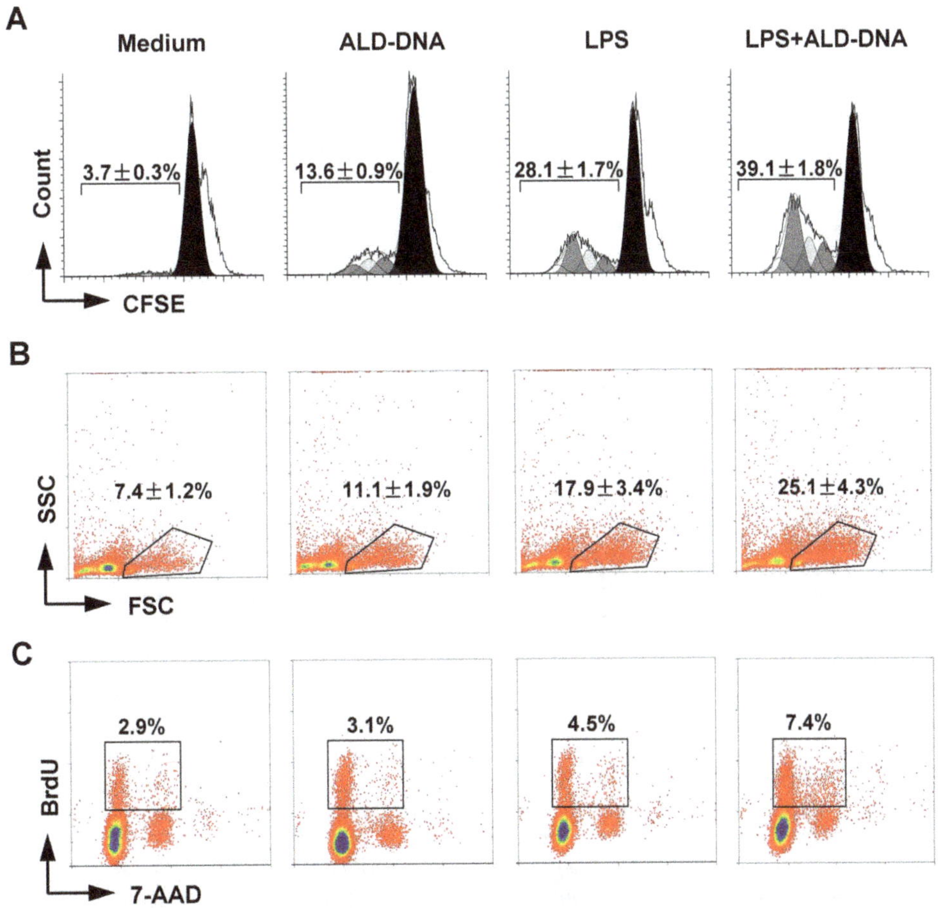

Figure 1. Enhancement of LPS-stimulated B cell survival and division by ALD-DNA. (**A**) CFSE-labeled B cells were stimulated with ALD-DNA (50 μg/ml) in the presence or absence of LPS (100 ng/ml) for 72 h. Division progression of B cells was determined by dilution of CFSE. Representative histogram plots show the percentage of proliferating (CFSE-low) B cells after each treatment (mean values ±SEM, n = 6). Shaded areas show the cell division peaks predicted by the ModFit software. (**B**) Flow cytometry dot plots showing the gate used to select living cells and eliminate cell debris, and showing the viability of B cells (mean values ±SEM, n = 11) under different culture conditions as described above for 72 h. (**C**) Nude mice were administered one intravenous injection of indicated stimuli at day 1 and an additional intraperitoneal injection of BrdU 24 h before sacrifice. After 72 h, spleens were collected, and B220$^+$ B cells with incorporated BrdU combined with total DNA content (with 7-AAD) were analyzed by FACS. The region gates applied to the 7-AAD versus BrdU dot plot indicate the cell subsets that were resided in the S phase of the cell cycle. Results represent 6 mice/experimental group from two separate experiments.

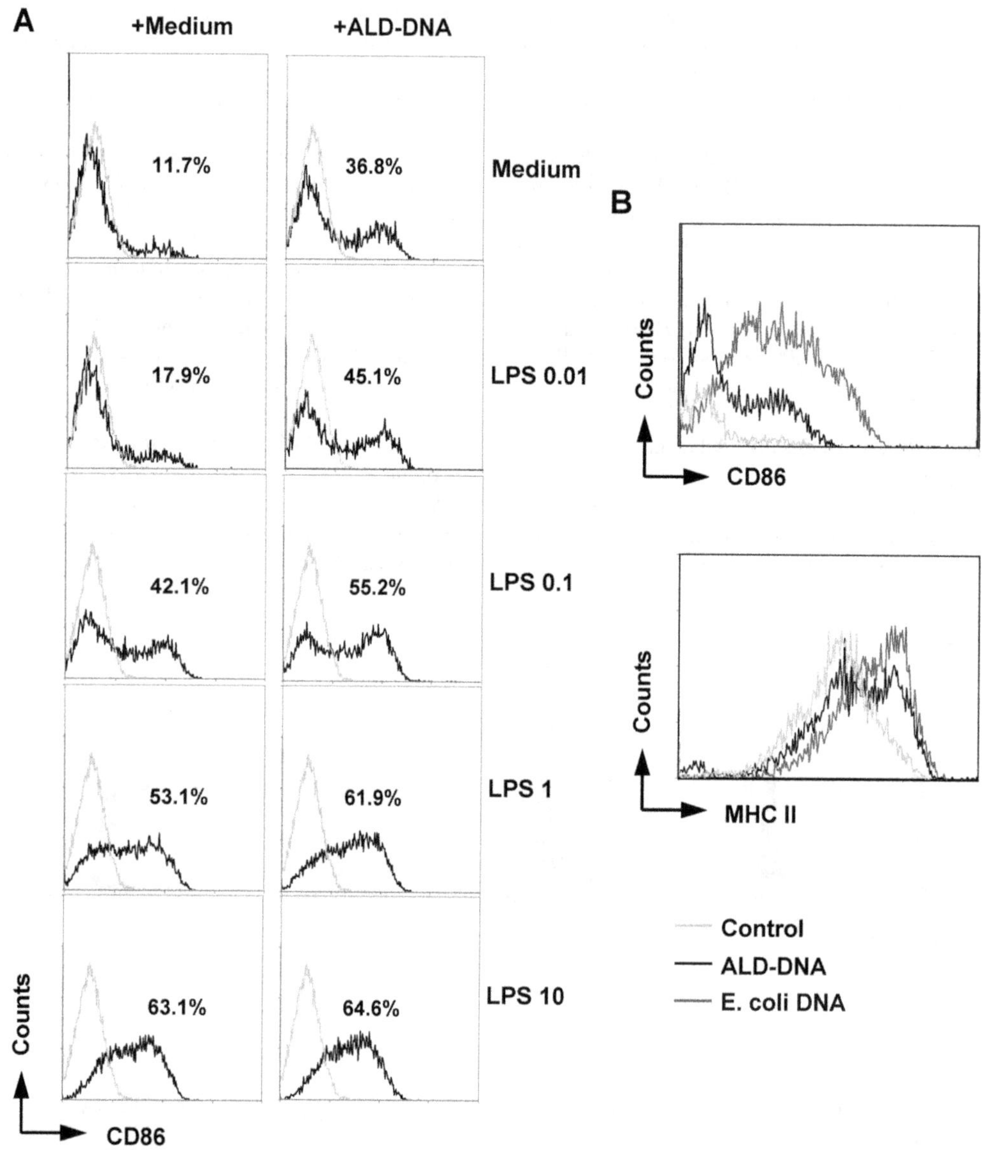

Figure 2. Up-regulation of CD86 and MHC class II expression in naïve B cells by ALD-DNA stimulation. (**A**) Naïve B cells were incubated with ALD-DNA (50 μg/ml) in the presence or absence of LPS ranging from 0.01 μg/mL to 10 μg/ml for 72 h. The numbers of CD86-expressing B cells after each treatment were determined by flow cytometry. (**B**) Naive B cells were stimulated with ALD-DNA or *E. coli* single-stranded (ss) DNA (both at 50 μg/ml) for 72 h. CD86 and MHC class II expression was determined by performing flow cytometry. Histogram plots show the mean fluorescence intensity (MFI) of these surface molecules. The data are representative of three independent experiments.

production by LPS-activated B cells. LPS stimulation preferentially increased the production of IgM (Figure 3, lift panel). Addition of ALD-DNA did not further increase LPS-induced IgM production. However, LPS-induced IgG production was significantly higher (Figure 3, right panel, $P = 0.007$) with ALD-DNA stimulation (IgG yield: 160.5±32.6 ng/ml; n = 5) as compared with that of cell cultures stimulated with LPS alone (IgG yield: 55.4±18.6 ng/ml; n = 5).

Effect of ALD-DNA on LPS-driven plasma cell differentiation in naïve B cells

We next analyzed the effect of ALD-DNA on the generation of $CD138^+$ plasma cells. Stimulation with a suboptimal dose of LPS resulted in the induction of a small proportion of $B220^-CD138^+$ cells (1.08%; Figure 4A). Addition of ALD-DNA to LPS-stimulated culture led to about 1.9-fold increase in this population (2.04%; Figure 4A). Molecular events that control plasma cell differentiation include expression of the transcription factors Blimp-1 and XBP1 [24]. ALD-DNA did not up-regulate Blimp-1 and XBP1 mRNA expression in naïve B cells (Figure 4B). In addition, ALD-DNA did not enhance LPS-induced Blimp-1 and XBP1 mRNA expression (Figure 4B). Therefore, although ALD-DNA increased the proportion of LPS-induced plasma cells, it did not seem to affect the expression of transcription factors that played essential roles in plasma cell differentiation.

We assessed whether ALD-DNA and LPS together enhance the survival of plasma cells. IL-6 has been shown to be a potent *in vitro* and *in vivo* growth factor for murine plasmacytosis [25,26]. In addition, IL-6 as a nonswitching factor enhanced IgG production in IgG-committed B cells of a particular subclass

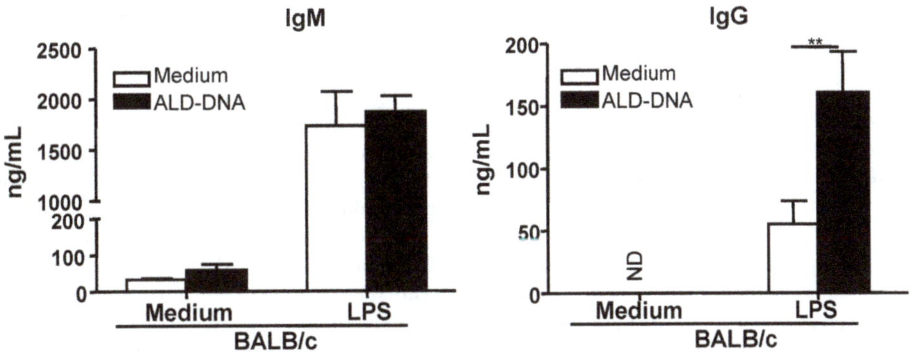

Figure 3. Synergistic enhancement of LPS-driven IgG production in naive B cells by ALD-DNA stimulation. Naive B cells were cultured for 6 days in media containing ALD-DNA (50 μg/ml) with or without LPS (100 ng/ml). Cell culture supernatants were collected, and the levels of IgM and IgG were measured by ELISA. Bars represent the means ±SEM of three independent experiments (n = 5). ND (not detected). $^{**}P<0.01$.

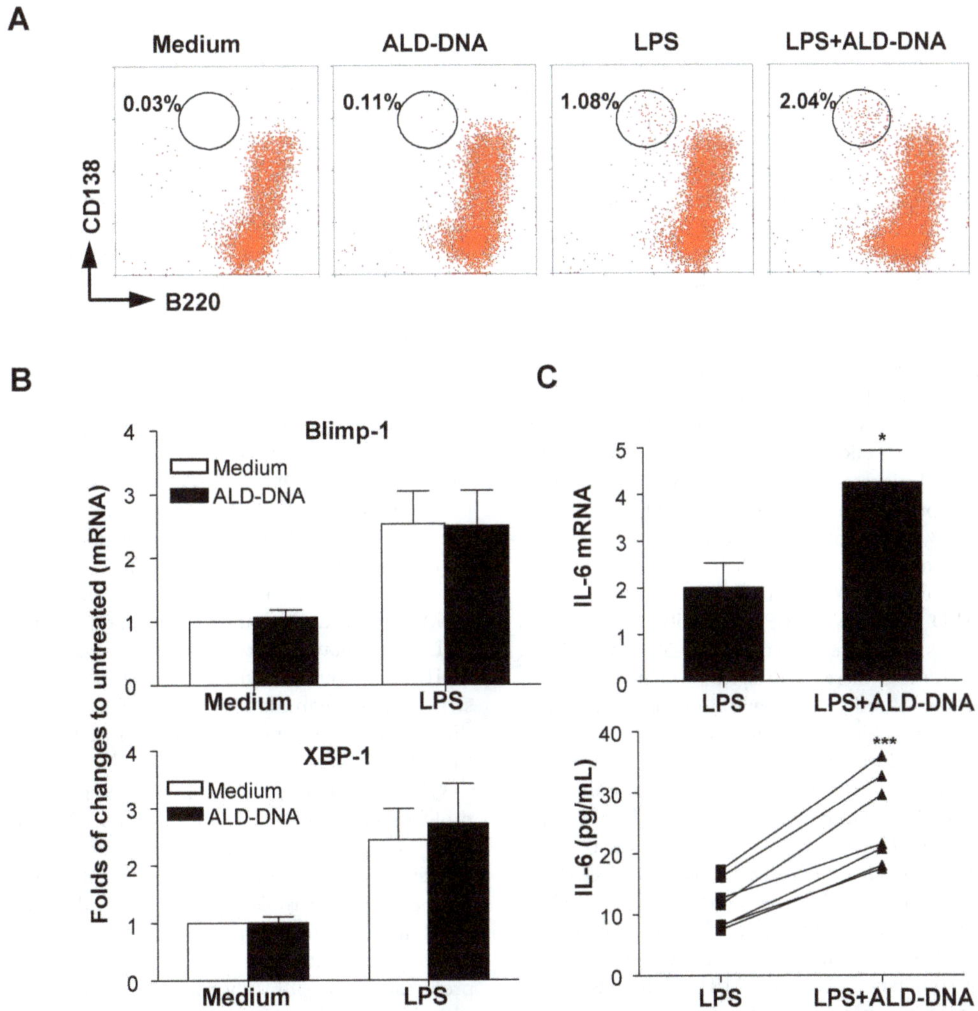

Figure 4. Effect of ALD-DNA on CD138, Blimp-1, XBP1, and IL-6 expression in naïve B cells. Naïve B cells were cultured in media containing ALD-DNA (50 μg/ml), LPS (100 ng/ml), or both for different periods as described below. (**A**) After 72 h stimulation, Cells were analyzed for B220 and CD138 surface expression by flow cytometry. The number indicates the percentage of $B220^{-}CD138^{+}$ cells in the gate. Similar results were obtained in three independent experiments. (**B**) Expression of Blimp-1 and XBP1 mRNA from B cells cultured for 96 hours was examined by real-time PCR. Fold induction relative to their untreated controls is shown (means ±SEM, n = 5). (**C**) Expression of IL-6 mRNA in B cells after 6 h stimulation was examined by real-time PCR. Fold induction relative to their untreated controls is shown (means ±SEM, n = 5); The amounts of IL-6 protein in the culture supernatants of B cells after 72 h stimulation were measured by ELISA (n = 6, a line linked two dots represents a pair observation). Up-regulation of IL-6 protein was undetectable in all samples after ALD-DNA treatment. $^{*}P<0.05$ as compared to the LPS, $^{***}P<0.001$ as compared to the LPS.

[27]. We therefore measured IL-6 mRNA and protein expression after 6 h and 3 days of cultures, respectively. ALD-DNA enhanced the LPS-induced IL-6 mRNA transcription (Figure 4C, upper panel, $P = 0.02$) and protein secretion (Figure 4C, lower panel, $P = 0.0001$) by naïve B cells. These data indicate that ALD-DNA is able to increase the proportion of plasma cells and IgG production in LPS stimulated cultures in part by enhancing the secretion of IL-6.

ALD-DNA and LPS cooperate to stimulate B cells from lupus mice

To assess the cooperative effect of LPS and ALD-DNA under autoimmune conditions, splenic B cells isolated from lupus-prone $MRL^{+/+}$ and MRL/lpr mice that had developed a lupus-like disease were stimulated with ALD-DNA and/or LPS *in vitro*. As shown in Figure 5A (lower panels, MRL/lpr),ALD-DNA alone induced a 2.9-fold increase in the number of $B220^{+}CD138^{+}$ plasmablasts over those enumerated in the control. LPS induced a higher number of $B220^{+}CD138^{+}$ plasmablasts (4.5%), which were further enhanced by the addition of ALD-DNA (6.9%). LPS also induced viable cell numbers (36.1%) that were at least twice as high as those induced by ALD-DNA stimulation (16.2%), as determined by flow cytometry gated on FSC/SSC plots (data not shown). B cells from $MRL^{+/+}$ mice responded to ALD-DNA and/or LPS stimulation by generation of the $B220^{-}CD138^{+}$ plasma cells (Figure 5A, upper panels), in contrast to the generation of the $B220^{+}CD138^{+}$ plasmablasts by MRL/lpr B cells (Figure 5A, lower panels). Therefore, B cells from MRL/lpr and $MRL^{+/+}$ mice both responded to ALD-DNA and LPS to undergo B cell terminal differentiation although these cells were driven to different stages of plasma cell generation.

The differentiation of activated B cells into plasma cells is regulated by transcriptional cell programs. Consistent with the findings of increased percentages of $CD138^{+}$ cells after ALD stimulation, the real-time PCR analysis revealed that ALD-DNA stimulation significantly increased XBP1 and to a lesser extent, Blimp-1 mRNA expression in LPS stimulated lupus B cells (Figure 5B, $P<0.05\%$) but not normal BALB/c B cells (Figure 4B). ALD-DNA alone also caused slight increases in XBP1 and Blimp-1 mRNA expression in lupus B cells.

The effect of ALD-DNA and/or LPS on antibody production by lupus B cells was also investigated (Figure 5C). ALD-DNA induced a similar 1.5-fold increase in IgM production in both $MRL^{+/+}$ and MRL/lpr B cells as compared to their unstimulated controls. B cells from two lupus mice showed robust response to LPS stimulation and produced high amount of IgM as compared to normal BALB/c mice (Figure 5C and Figure 3). The presence of ALD-DNA markedly enhanced LPS-induced IgM production by lupus B cells (Figure 5C, upper panel) but not normal BALB/c B cells (Figure 3, lift panel). It is intriguing to note that MRL/lpr B cells produced lower amount of IgM than did $MRL^{+/+}$ B cells in response to ALD-DNA and/or LPS (Figure 5C, upper panel). In contrast, MRL/lpr B cells produced greater amount of IgG, even in the absence of stimulation, than did $MRL^{+/+}$ B cells. ALD-DNA did not further enhance LPS-induced IgG production by either $MRL^{+/+}$ or MRL/lpr B cells (Figure 5C, lower panel). Collectively, ALD-DNA and LPS together promoted the differentiation of plasma cells and the production of IgM but not IgG by lupus B cells.

Cooperation between ALD-DNA and CD40 signal

We have thus far provided evidence that ALD-DNA can cooperate with LPS to activate B cells obtained from normal and autoimmune mice. To investigate whether ALD-DNA can also cooperate with signals from helper T cells, we analyzed the effect of ALD-DNA on B cell proliferation induced by CD40 ligation. As shown in Figure 6A, ALD-DNA caused a significant increase in BrdU incorporation by naive B cells stimulated with an anti-CD40 antibody. The increased BrdU incorporation might result from accelerated cell cycle progression, elevated cell survival, or both. To distinguish these possibilities, we monitored cell division by performing CFSE dilution assay. About 1.45-fold more cells underwent four rounds of cell divisions in the presence of anti-CD40 antibody plus ALD-DNA as compared with cells stimulated with anti-CD40 antibody alone (Figure 6B). The enhancement of ALD-DNA on CD40-stimulated naïve B cell proliferation was not blocked by LPS inhibitor PMB (Figure 6A), indicating that the observed effect of ALD-DNA was not mediated by endotoxin contamination. Taken together, these results show that self DNA may serve as an endogenous adjuvant in CD40-mediated B cell response.

Discussion

Excessive apoptosis with deficiency in clearance of apoptotic cells was related to the extracellular source of DNA in patients with SLE as well as murine lupus. Additionally, primary lymphocyte necrosis occurred in patients with SLE [28,29], and SLE is characterized by prominent inflammatory tissue damage. DAMPs including genomic and mitochondrial DNA, RNA, histones, and high mobility group box 1 (HMGB1), all which are described as non-infectious endogenous TLR ligands, may be released into circulation or within tissues causing and accelerating inflammation [30–34]. Ishii et al. reported that genomic DNA released from dying cells stimulated DC maturation and boosted both antigen specific antibody and $CD8^{+}$ T-cell immune response [35]. However, while bacterial genomic DNA triggered direct B-cell activation, vertebrate genomic DNA did not, and the difference in CpG status was considered to be the cause of the mitogenicity of bacterial DNA [36].

In the current study, we found that ALD-DNA alone or in the presence of suboptimal doses of LPS enhanced the survival and proliferation of B cells and increased expression of MHC class II and CD86 molecules in naïve B cells. Moreover, ALD-DNA increased a number of plasma cells and IgG production in LPS stimulated cultures in part by enhancing the secretion of IL-6. To our knowledge, this is the first study to demonstrate that mammalian DNA from apoptotic cells can directly stimulate normal naïve B cells and modulate their function.

While we found that ALD-DNA promoted LPS-triggered proliferation of naïve B cells, Dil and Marshall reported that CpG ODN and LPS did not synergistically induce naïve B cell proliferation, but significantly stimulated IL-10 production [37]. Furthermore, microbial product-induced IL-10 production appears to mitigate exaggerated B cell responses to pathogenic microbes by potently inhibiting CpG- or LPS-induced B cell proliferation [16,38]. Therefore, CpG ODN and LPS are not synergy in B cell proliferation due to the synergistic induction of large amounts of IL-10 [37]. Consistent with these findings, we observed that bacterial genomic DNA also greatly enhanced LPS-triggered IL-10 production (Figure S2C), but to a lesser extent than CpG ODN [37]. Bacterial DNA and LPS had neither additive nor synergetic effect on naïve B cell proliferation, although both stimulants were potent mitogens for B cells (Figure S2A). In addition, the immunosuppressive effect of IL-10 on CpG ODN-stimulated Ig-secreting cell generation was also previously reported [16]. Similarly, we found that stimulation with bacterial

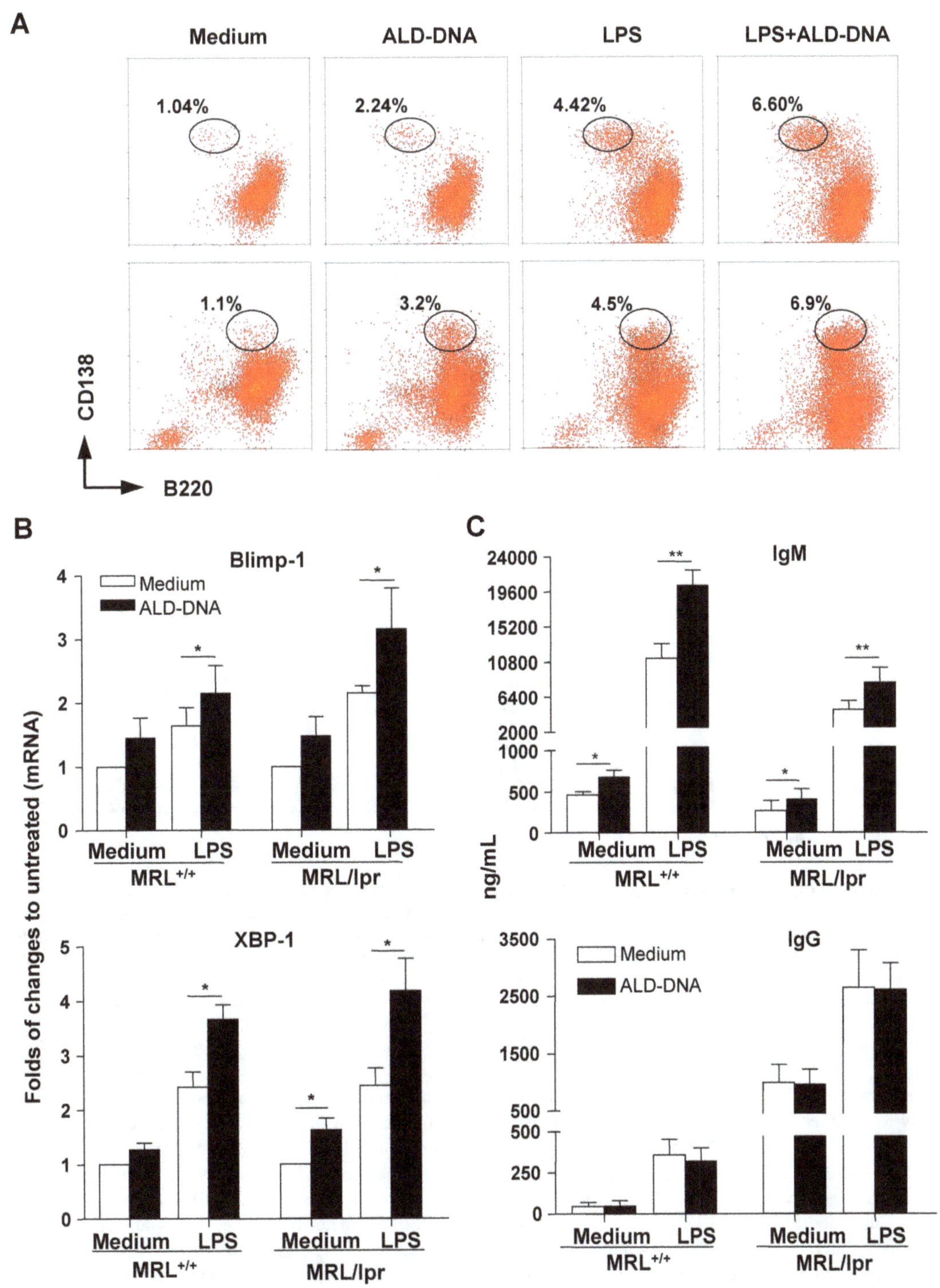

Figure 5. Promotion of plasma cell differentiation and Ig production in lupus B cells by ALD-DNA. Splenic B cells from 16- to 20-week-old MRL/lpr mice and 12-week-old $MRL^{+/+}$ mice were cultured in media alone, or in the presence of ALD-DNA (50 μg/ml), LPS (100 ng/ml), or both for different periods as indicated below. (**A**) After 72 h stimulation, viable cells were analyzed for B220 and CD138 surface expression by flow cytometry. Representative dot plots showed the frequencies of plasmablasts ($B220^{+}CD138^{hi}$, lower panels, MRL/lpr, n = 6) or plasma cells ($B220^{-}CD138^{+}$, upper panels, $MRL^{+/+}$, n = 6) generated after each treatment. (**B**) Expression of Blimp-1 and XBP1 mRNA from lupus B cells cultured for 96 h was examined by real-time PCR. Results are expressed as the fold induction of gene transcription relative to their untreated controls (means ±SEM, n = 6). (**C**) Ig production in cell culture supernatants harvested on day 6 was determined by ELISA. Bars represent the means ±SEM of three independent experiments (n = 6). *$P<0.05$, **$P<0.01$.

DNA along with LPS did not enhance differentiation into plasma cells (Figure S2B). In contrast, stimulation with ALD-DNA alone had no effect on IL-10 expression and slightly increased LPS-triggered IL-10 production (Figure S3). Taken together, the data indicate that ALD-DNA is functionally distinct from CpG ODN and bacterial genomic DNA, and is able to enhance

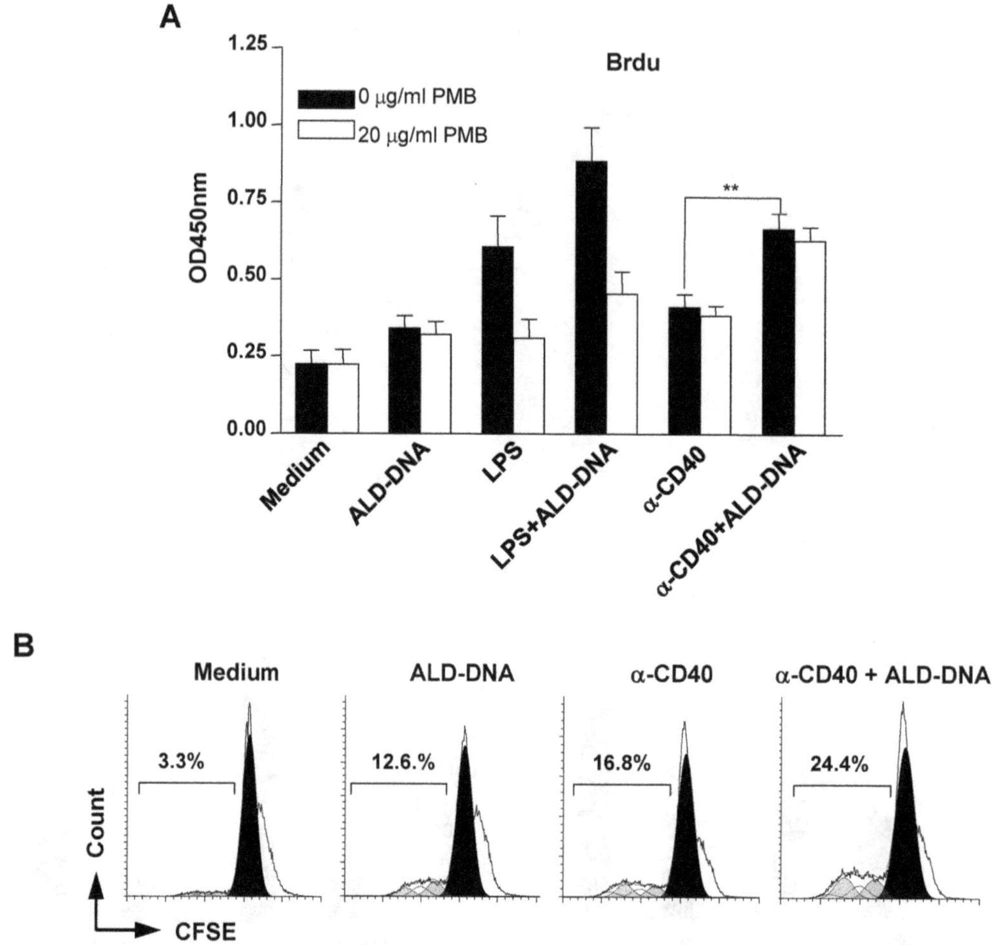

Figure 6. Enhancement of CD40-stimulated naïve B cell proliferation by ALD-DNA. (**A**) Naïve B cells were pre-incubated for 20 min with polymyxin B (PMB; 20 μg/ml) before the addition of ALD-DNA (50 μg/ml), LPS (100 ng/ml), anti-CD40 (1 μg/ml), LPS (100 ng/ml) plus ALD-DNA (50 μg/ml), or anti-CD40 (1 μg/ml) plus ALD-DNA (50 μg/ml). After 72 h stimulation, cell proliferation was detected by performing BrdU incorporation assay using ELISA. Data are presented as the means ±SEM of three independent experiments. (**B**) CFSE-labeled naïve B cells were cultured in media containing ALD-DNA, anti-CD40, or both (at the concentrations as described above) for 72 h. Cell division was monitored by measuring the dilution of CFSE. Shaded areas show the cell division peaks predicted by the ModFit software. Results from one representative experiment of three are shown. $^{**}P<0.01$.

LPS-mediated proliferation and plasma cell generation in part due to its weak ability to enhance LPS-triggered IL-10 production.

Remarkably, we found that ALD-DNA treated lupus B cells were able to induce surface CD138 and secrete IgM (Figure 5). ALD-DNA slightly increased XBP1 and Blimp-1 mRNA expression. These data suggested that ALD-DNA at least partially activated plasma cell differentiation and promoted a subset of lupus B cells to become IgM-secreting plasmablasts/plasma cells. In contrast, ALD-DNA alone had little effect on the increases in $CD138^+$ cell numbers, antibody production and mRNA levels of XBP1 and Blimp-1 in normal naïve B cells (Figure 3 and 4). Therefore, lupus B cells appear to be more sensitive to ALD-DNA stimulation than normal B cells. Furthermore, ALD-DNA enhanced LPS-triggered plasmablast/plasma cell differentiation program of lupus B cells, as evidenced by increases in $CD138^+$ cell numbers, XBP1 and Blimp-1 mRNA expression as well as IgM production (Figure 5).

The ELISA data indicated that ALD-DNA enhanced LPS-induced IgG, but not IgM, production in normal naïve B cells (Figure 3). In striking contrast, ALD-DNA promoted LPS-induced IgM, but not IgG, production in lupus B cells (Figure 5). Therefore, ALD-DNA had distinct effect on antibody production in normal and lupus B cells, at least under these *in vitro* culture conditions. IL-6 is a survival factor for plasma cells [25,26] and acts as a nonswitching factor to enhance IgG production by committed B cells [27]. ALD-DNA promoted LPS-induced IL-6 expression in normal naïve B cells and this finding may in part account for the increased IgG production. Conversely, ALD-DNA did not enhance LPS-induced IL-6 expression (ALD-DNA plus LPS and LPS alone induced IL-6 at concentrations of 59 pg/ml and 63.2 pg/ml, respectively; data not shown) in lupus B cells.

The mechanisms that enable ALD-DNA to selectively stimulate IgM production by lupus B cells, but not normal B cells, remain unclear. Moreover, lupus B cells showed higher responsiveness than normal B cells to ALD-DNA and/or LPS stimulation to undergo terminal differentiation and yielded higher antibody production. These differential effects might be partially attributable to the distinct B cell subset composition. Enlargement of marginal zone (MZ) B cell population was reported in different mouse models of lupus such as $MRL^{+/+}$, MRL/lpr, NZB/W F1, Palmerston North (PN) and BAFF transgenic mice [39–41]. Our result also confirmed this abnormality (Figure S4). MZ B cells are programmed for efficient differentiation into mature plasma cells with the ability to secrete massive quantities of IgM in response to TLR agonists such as LPS [42]. In addition, MZ B cells have an enhanced secretory apparatus [43] and lower activation thresholds [44]. These unique capacity might allow MZ B cells to respond to TLR ligands that occur at low concentrations and have low-affinity, including less favorable CpG sequences found in hypomethylated mammalian DNA [40]. Additionally, we used CD19 microbeads to purify splenic B cells from MRL/lpr mice that had actively developed a lupus-like disease, in order to avoid loss of any B cell subpopulations. Thus B cells isolated from 16-week-old MRL/lpr mice might have a cell population shift toward antigen-activated B cells, antibody producing plasmablasts [45], and memory B cells, in contrast to predominantly resting B cells isolated from normal BALB/c and prediseased $MRL^{+/+}$ mice. Therefore the differential responsiveness to ALD-DNA and/or LPS stimulation cannot be simply ascribed to distinct cell activation states *in vivo*.

Normal MZ B-cell repertoires contain a high frequency of autoreactive B cells including anti-DNA [46]. An expansion of the MZ B-cell subset is common in several genetically distinct murine lupus models, implying a role of MZ B cells involved in disease pathogenesis. Furthermore, MRL/lpr mice have a high frequency of apoptotic lymphocytes in secondary lymphoid organs with a macrophage defect in apoptotic cell phagocytosis [4]. Impaired removal of dying cells resulted in deposition and accumulation of apoptotic DNA in the formation of IgM ICs in the splenic marginal zone [5]. It has been noted that DNA released from necrotic/apoptotic cells complexes with HGMB1 can facilitate the entry of nucleic acids into cells to activate endosomal TLR9 [47]. It is possible that apoptotic DNA when bound to natural IgM in the formation of ICs may increase its availability not only to MZ but also follicular (FO) B cells through engagement of FcμR on the surface of B cells [48], and this may occur at the prediseased stage in lupus prone mice.

Thus, cooperation of self DNA and low levels of LPS represent an attractively cooperative model of DAMPs and PAMPs, and may serve two important roles: firstly, to aid quick and efficient clearance of infections before they become pathogenic, and secondly, in some circumstances, initiate polyclonal B cell response often characteristic of autoimmune diseases either at the origin [49] or in an amplification loop [50–52].

We have analyzed the cooperation effects of stimulation with ALD-DNA and LPS, the ligand for TLR4. In contrast to murine B cells, human B cells express TLR1/2, TLR7, TLR9 but not TLR4 [16,53]. However, terminally differentiated plasma cells isolated from human peripheral blood have been shown to express all TLRs including TLR4 with the exception of TLR10, and their antibody production and secretion can be enhanced after engagement of TLRs [53]. Synergistic activation of B cells by different PRRs like TLR9 and TLR2 [54] or TLR9 and NOD-like receptors (NLRs) [55] has been reported. It would be interesting to explore whether ALD-DNA can cooperate with innate PPR ligands (in addition to TLR4 ligand LPS) that modulate B cell activation, and to compare the responsiveness of B cell subsets as well as plasma cells to these stimuli. Such studies will help us understand the potential roles of self DNA in human B-cell autoimmunity development and aid in designing novel therapeutic strategies for SLE.

Notably, ALD-DNA also enhanced CD40 activated naïve B cell proliferation (Figure 6). GCs are candidate locations where B cells may receive signals from CD40 and apoptotic DNA as well as bacterial products. In GCs of some patients with SLE, tingible body macrophages were defective in uptake of apoptotic cells, and apoptotic nuclear debris was attached on the surfaces of follicular dendritic cells [56,57]. Activated B cells express CD40 ligand CD154 in both patients with SLE and lupus prone mice [58,59]. Our results implicated that DNA might enhance CD40 signaling in B cells activated by homotypic CD40-CD154 interactions. It is possible that DNA in conjunction with signaling from either CD40 or PRRs may promote positive selection of autoreactive B cells that are generated by random somatic hypermutation of Ig genes during TD GC reaction or TI extrafollicular response [60–62].

In conclusion, the current study has demonstrated that self DNA can serve as a DAMP that cooperates with signals from both innate and adaptive immunity to promote polyclonal B cell activation, a common characteristic of autoimmune diseases. Importantly, B cells from lupus mice showed heightened responses to ALD-DNA and/or LPS in the terminal plasma cell differentiation and antibody production, indicating that self DNA could be a contributing factor to hyperactive B-cell compartments in SLE. Further elucidation of the molecular and cellular mechanisms by which ALD-DNA contributes to B cell activation would provide new insights for the development of novel therapeutic strategies for SLE.

Supporting Information

Figure S1 Dose-specific effects of ALD-DNA and/or LPS on naïve B cell proliferation. (**A**) DNA purified from ConA-activated lymphocytes that had undergone AICD (size standards, lane 1; ALD-DNA, lane 2 and 3). (**B**) CFSE-labeled naïve B cells were stimulated with ALD-DNA (0 μg/mL, 25 μg/mL, 50 μg/mL, or 100 μg/mL) in the presence or absence of 100 ng/ml LPS for 72 h. (**C**) CFSE-labeled naïve B cells were stimulated with LPS (0 μg/mL, 0.01 μg/mL, 0.1 μg/mL, or 1 μg/mL) in the presence or absence of 50 μg/ml ALD-DNA for 72 h. The frequency of proliferating ($B220^+$ CFSE-low) B cells (**B and C**) was determined by performing flow cytometry analysis. Data, pooled from three independent experiments, are shown as bar graphs (means ±SEM).

Figure S2 Effects of bacterial DNA on LPS-induced proliferation, plasma cell generation, and IL-10 production. (**A**) CFSE-labeled naïve B cells were stimulated with *E. coli* ssDNA (0 μg/mL, 10 μg/mL, 50 μg/mL, or 100 μg/ml) in the presence or absence of 100 ng/ml LPS for 72 hours. The frequency of proliferating ($B220^+$CFSE-low) B cells was determined by performing flow cytometry analysis. Data, pooled from three independent experiments, are shown as bar graphs (means ±SEM, n = 5). $^{**}P<0.01$ as compared to LPS or *E. coli* DNA, and $^{***}P<0.001$ as compared to LPS or *E. coli* DNA. (**B**) CFSE-labeled naïve B cells were stimulated with *E. coli* ssDNA (10 μg/mL or 50 μg/ml) in the presence or absence of 100 ng/ml LPS for 72 h. Cells were analyzed by flow cytometry for CD138 surface expression. Representative dot plots of three independent experiments show the percentages of $CD138^+$ plasma cells generated under different culture conditions. (**C**) Naïve B cells were cultured in media containing *E. coli* ssDNA (50 μg/ml) with or without LPS (100 ng/ml) for 72 h, and cell culture supernatants were collected for analysis of IL-10 by ELISA. Data, pooled from three independent experiments, are shown as bar graphs (mean ±SEM, n = 4).$^{*}P<0.05$ as compared to LPS.

Figure S3 Enhancement of LPS-induced IL-10 production in naïve B cells by ALD-DNA. Naïve B cells were cultured in media containing ALD-DNA (50 μg/ml) in the presence or absence of LPS (100 ng/ml) for 72 h, and cell culture supernatants were collected for analysis of IL-10 by ELISA. Data, pooled from three independent experiments, are shown as bar graphs (mean ±SEM, n = 4). ND (not detected). *$P<0.05$ as compared to LPS.

Figure S4 Frequency of MZ B cells in normal and MRL$^{+/+}$ lupus mice. Splenic B cells were isolated from normal BALB/c and MRL$^{+/+}$ mice by negative selection using anti-CD43-coated magnetic beads. The frequency of MZ B cells (CD21^{hi} CD23^{lo}) was determined by flow cytometry.

Acknowledgments

We thank Dr. Rui He for study design. We also thank Dr. Feifei Luo and Jing Qian for excellent technique support.

Author Contributions

Conceived and designed the experiments: QL JW LW XJ YC. Performed the experiments: QL LW XJ. Analyzed the data: QL JW LW XJ YC. Contributed reagents/materials/analysis tools: QL YC. Wrote the paper: QL JW YC.

References

1. Napirei M, Karsunky H, Zevnik B, Stephan H, Mannherz HG, et al. (2000) Features of systemic lupus erythematosus in Dnase1-deficient mice. Nat Genet 25: 177–181.
2. Yasutomo K, Horiuchi T, Kagami S, Tsukamoto H, Hashimura C, et al. (2001) Mutation of DNASE1 in people with systemic lupus erythematosus. Nat Genet 28: 313–314.
3. Emlen W, Niebur J, Kadera R (1994) Accelerated *in vitro* apoptosis of lymphocytes from patients with systemic lupus erythematosus. J Immunol 152: 3685–3692.
4. Qian Y, Conway KL, Lu X, Seitz HM, Matsushima GK, et al. (2006) Autoreactive MZ and B-1 B-cell activation by Faslpr is coincident with an increased frequency of apoptotic lymphocytes and a defect in macrophage clearance. Blood 108: 974–982.
5. Finke D, Randers K, Hoerster R, Hennig H, Zawatzky R, et al. (2007) Elevated levels of endogenous apoptotic DNA and IFN-alpha in complement C4-deficient mice: implications for induction of systemic lupus erythematosus. Eur J Immunol 37: 1702–1709.
6. Su KY, Pisetsky DS (2009) The role of extracellular DNA in autoimmunity in SLE. Scand J Immunol 70: 175–183.
7. Means TK, Latz E, Hayashi F, Murali MR, Golenbock DT, et al. (2005) Human lupus autoantibody-DNA complexes activate DCs through cooperation of CD32 and TLR9. J Clin Invest 115: 407–417.
8. Dall'era MC, Cardarelli PM, Preston BT, Witte A, Davis JC Jr (2005) Type I interferon correlates with serological and clinical manifestations of SLE. Ann Rheum Dis 64: 1692–1697.
9. Leadbetter EA, Rifkin IR, Hohlbaum AM, Beaudette BC, Shlomchik MJ, et al. (2002) Chromatin-IgG complexes activate B cells by dual engagement of IgM and Toll-like receptors. Nature 416: 603–607.
10. Barton GM, Kagan JC, Medzhitov R (2006) Intracellular localization of Toll-like receptor 9 prevents recognition of self DNA but facilitates access to viral DNA. Nat Immunol 7: 49–56.
11. Yasuda K, Yu P, Kirschning CJ, Schlatter B, Schmitz F, et al. (2005) Endosomal translocation of vertebrate DNA activates dendritic cells via TLR9-dependent and -independent pathways. J Immunol 174: 6129–6136.
12. Kono DH, Haraldsson MK, Lawson BR, Pollard KM, Koh YT, et al. (2009) Endosomal TLR signaling is required for anti-nucleic acid and rheumatoid factor autoantibodies in lupus. Proc Natl Acad Sci USA 106: 12061–12066.
13. Anolik JH, Barnard J, Cappione A, Pugh-Bernard AE, Felgar RE, et al. (2004) Rituximab improves peripheral B cell abnormalities in human systemic lupus erythematosus. Arthritis Rheum 50: 3580–3590.
14. Jacob N, Stohl W (2010) Autoantibody-dependent and autoantibody-independent roles for B cells in systemic lupus erythematosus: past, present, and future. Autoimmunity 43: 84–97.
15. Vinuesa CG, Chang PP (2013) Innate B cell helpers reveal novel types of antibody responses. Nat Immunol 14: 119–126.
16. Bernasconi NL, Onai N, Lanzavecchia A (2003) A role for Toll-like receptors in acquired immunity: upregulation of TLR9 by BCR triggering in naive B cells and constitutive expression in memory B cells. Blood 101: 4500–4504.
17. Bernasconi NL, Traggiai E, Lanzavecchia A (2002) Maintenance of serological memory by polyclonal activation of human memory B cells. Science 298: 2199–2202.
18. Phan TG, Amesbury M, Gardam S, Crosbie J, Hasbold J, et al. (2003) B cell receptor-independent stimuli trigger immunoglobulin (Ig) class switch recombination and production of IgG autoantibodies by anergic self-reactive B cells. J Exp Med 197: 845–860.
19. Zhang W, Xu W, Xiong S (2011) Macrophage differentiation and polarization via phosphatidylinositol 3-kinase/Akt-ERK signaling pathway conferred by serum amyloid P component. J Immunol 187: 1764–1777.
20. Cai Y, Zhang W, Xiong S (2013) Mannose-binding lectin blunts macrophage polarization and ameliorates lupus nephritis. PLoS One 8: e62465.
21. Sano H, Takai O, Harata N, Yoshinaga K, Kodama-Kamada I, et al. (1989) Binding properties of human anti-DNA antibodies to cloned human DNA fragments. Scand J Immunol 30: 51–63.
22. Sano H, Morimoto C (1982) DNA isolated from DNA/anti-DNA antibody immune complexes in systemic lupus Erythematosus is rich in guanine-cytosine content. J Immunol 128: 1341–1345.
23. Santiago-Raber ML, Laporte C, Reininger L, Izui S (2004) Genetic basis of murine lupus. Autoimmun Rev 3: 33–39.
24. Oracki SA, Walker JA, Hibbs ML, Corcoran LM, Tarlinton DM (2010) Plasma cell development and survival. Immunol Rev 237: 140–159.
25. Nordan RP, Potter M (1986) A macrophage-derived factor required by plasmacytomas for survival and proliferation *in vitro*. Science 233: 566–569.
26. Suematsu S, Matsuda T, Aozasa K, Akira S, Nakano N, et al. (1989) IgG1 plasmacytosis in interleukin 6 transgenic mice. Proc Natl Acad Sci USA 86: 7547–7551.
27. Kawano Y, Noma T, Kou K, Yoshizawa I, Yata J (1995) Regulation of human IgG subclass production by cytokines: human IgG subclass production enhanced differentially by interleukin-6. Immunology 84: 278–284.
28. Eisner MD, Amory J, Mullaney B, Tierney L Jr, Browner WS (1996) Necrotizing lymphadenitis associated with systemic lupus erythematosus. Semin Arthritis Rheum 26: 477–482.
29. Gergely P Jr, Grossman C, Niland B, Puskas F, Neupane H, et al. (2002) Mitochondrial hyperpolarization and ATP depletion in patients with systemic lupus erythematosus. Arthritis Rheum 46: 175–190.
30. Jiang N, Pisetsky DS (2005) The effect of inflammation on the generation of plasma DNA from dead and dying cells in the peritoneum. J Leukoc Biol 77: 296–302.
31. Pisetsky DS (2013) Immune activation by histones: Plusses and minuses in inflammation. Eur J Immunol 43: 3163–3166.
32. Karikó K, Ni H, Capodici J, Lamphier M, Weissman D (2004) mRNA is an endogenous ligand for Toll-like receptor 3. J Biol Chem 279: 12542–12550.
33. Scaffidi P, Misteli T, Bianchi ME (2002) Release of chromatin protein HMGB1 by necrotic cells triggers inflammation. Nature 418: 191–195.
34. Zhang Q, Raoof M, Chen Y, Sumi Y, Sursal T, et al. (2010) Circulating mitochondrial DAMPs cause inflammatory responses to injury. Nature 464: 104–107.
35. Ishii KJ, Suzuki K, Coban C, Takeshita F, Itoh Y, et al. (2001) Genomic DNA released by dying cells induces the maturation of APCs. J Immunol 167: 2602–2607.
36. Krieg AM, Yi AK, Matson S, Waldschmidt TJ, Bishop GA, et al. (1995) CpG motifs in bacterial DNA trigger direct B-cell activation. Nature 374: 546–549.
37. Dil N, Marshall AJ (2009) Role of phosphoinositide 3-kinase p110 delta in TLR4- and TLR9-mediated B cell cytokine production and differentiation. Mol Immunol 46: 1970–1978.
38. Marcelletti JF (1996) IL-10 inhibits lipopolysaccharide-induced murine B cell proliferation and cross-linking of surface antigen receptors or ligation of CD40 restores the response. J Immunol 157: 3323–3333.
39. Liu J, Karypis G, Hippen KL, Vegoe AL, Ruiz P, et al. (2006) Genomic view of systemic autoimmunity in MRLlpr mice. Genes Immun 7: 156–168.
40. Brummel R, Lenert P (2005) Activation of marginal zone B cells from lupus mice with type A(D) CpG-oligodeoxynucleotides. J Immunol 174: 2429–2434.
41. Mackay F, Woodcock SA, Lawton P, Ambrose C, Baetscher M, et al. (1999) Mice transgenic for BAFF develop lymphocytic disorders along with autoimmune manifestations. J Exp Med 190: 1697–1710.
42. Genestier L, Taillardet M, Mondiere P, Gheit H, Bella C, et al. (2007) TLR agonists selectively promote terminal plasma cell differentiation of B cell subsets specialized in thymus-independent responses. J Immunol 178: 7779–7786.
43. Gunn KE, Brewer JW (2006) Evidence that marginal zone B cells possess an enhanced secretory apparatus and exhibit superior secretory activity. J Immunol 177: 3791–3798.
44. Martin F, Kearney JF (2002) Marginal-zone B cells. Nat Rev Immunol 2: 323–335.
45. William J, Euler C, Shlomchik MJ (2005) Short-lived plasmablasts dominate the early spontaneous rheumatoid factor response: differentiation pathways, hypermutating cell types, and affinity maturation outside the germinal center. J Immunol 174: 6879–6887.

46. Martin F, Kearney JF (2000) B-cell subsets and the mature preimmune repertoire: marginal zone and B1 B cells as part of a "natural immune memory". Immunol Rev175: 70–79.
47. Tian J, Avalos AM, Mao SY, Chen B, Senthil K, et al. (2007) Toll-like receptor 9-dependent activation by DNA-containing immune complexes is mediated by HMGB1 and RAGE. Nat Immunol 8: 487–496.
48. Ouchida R, Mori H, Hase K, Takatsu H, Kurosaki T, et al. (2012) Critical role of the IgM Fc receptor in IgM homeostasis, B-cell survival, and humoral immune responses. Proc Natl Acad Sci USA 109: E2699–2706.
49. Klinman DM (1990) Polyclonal B cell activation in lupus-prone mice precedes and predicts the development of autoimmune disease. J Clin Invest 86: 1249–1254.
50. Arce E, Jackson DG, Gill MA, Bennett LB, Banchereau J, et al. (2001) Increased frequency of pre-germinal center B cells and plasma cell precursors in the blood of children with systemic lupus erythematosus. J Immunol 167: 2361–2369.
51. Hoyer BF, Moser K, Hauser AE, Peddinghaus A, Voigt C, et al. (2004) Short-lived plasmablasts and long-lived plasma cells contribute to chronic humoral autoimmunity in NZB/W mice. J Exp Med 199: 1577–1584.
52. Cassese G, Lindenau S, de Boer B, Arce S, Hauser A, et al. (2001) Inflamed kidneys of NZB/W mice are a major site for the homeostasis of plasma cells. Eur J Immunol 31: 2726–2732.
53. Dorner M, Brandt S, Tinguely M, Zucol F, Bourquin JP, et al. (2009) Plasma cell toll-like receptor (TLR) expression differs from that of B cells, and plasma cell TLR triggering enhances immunoglobulin production. Immunology 128: 573–579.
54. Tuvim MJ, Gilbert BE, Dickey BF, Evans SE (2012) Synergistic TLR2/6 and TLR9 activation protects mice against lethal influenza pneumonia. PLoS One 7: e30596.
55. Petterson T, Jendholm J, Månsson A, Bjartell A, Riesbeck K, et al. (2011) Effects of NOD-like receptors in human B lymphocytes and crosstalk between NOD1/NOD2 and Toll-like receptors. J Leukoc Biol 89: 177–187.
56. Baumann I, Kolowos W, Voll RE, Manger B, Gaipl U, et al. (2002) Impaired uptake of apoptotic cells into tingible body macrophages in germinal centers of patients with systemic lupus erythematosus. Arthritis Rheum 46: 191–201.
57. Gaipl US, Munoz LE, Grossmayer G, Lauber K, Franz S, et al. (2007) Clearance deficiency and systemic lupus erythematosus (SLE). J Autoimmun 28: 114–121.
58. Grammer AC, Slota R, Fischer R, Gur H, Girschick H, et al. (2003) Abnormal germinal center reactions in systemic lupus erythematosus demonstrated by blockade of CD154-CD40 interactions. J Clin Invest 112: 1506–1520.
59. Higuchi T, Aiba Y, Nomura T, Matsuda J, Mochida K, et al. (2002) Cutting Edge: Ectopic expression of CD40 ligand on B cells induces lupus-like autoimmune disease. J Immunol 168: 9–12.
60. Schroeder K, Herrmann M, Winkler TH (2013) The role of somatic hypermutation in the generation of pathogenic antibodies in SLE. Autoimmunity 46: 121–127.
61. Puga I, Cols M, Barra CM, He B, Cassis L, et al. (2012) B cell-helper neutrophils stimulate the diversification and production of immunoglobulin in the marginal zone of the spleen. Nat Immunol 13: 170–180.
62. Dörner T, Giesecke C, Lipsky PE (2011) Mechanisms of B cell autoimmunity in SLE. Arthritis Res Ther 13: 243–255.

The Coexistence of Antiphospholipid Syndrome and Systemic Lupus Erythematosus in Colombians

Juan-Sebastian Franco[1,2*], Nicolás Molano-González[1], Monica Rodríguez-Jiménez[1], Yeny Acosta-Ampudia[1], Rubén D. Mantilla[1,2], Jenny Amaya-Amaya[1,2], Adriana Rojas-Villarraga[1,2], Juan-Manuel Anaya[1,2*]

1 Center for Autoimmune Diseases Research (CREA), School of Medicine and Health Sciences, Universidad del Rosario, Bogotá, Colombia, 2 Mederi, Hospital Universitario Mayor, Bogotá, Colombia

Abstract

Objectives: To examine the prevalence and associated factors related to the coexistence of antiphospholipid syndrome (APS) and systemic lupus erythematosus (SLE) in a cohort of Colombian patients with SLE, and to discuss the coexistence of APS with other autoimmune diseases (ADs).

Method: A total of 376 patients with SLE were assessed for the presence of the following: 1) confirmed APS; 2) positivity for antiphospholipid (aPL) antibodies without a prior thromboembolic nor obstetric event; and 3) SLE patients without APS nor positivity for aPL antibodies. Comparisons between groups 1 and 3 were evaluated by bivariate and multivariate analysis.

Results: Although the prevalence of aPL antibodies was 54%, APS was present in just 9.3% of SLE patients. In our series, besides cardiovascular disease (AOR 3.38, 95% CI 1.11–10.96, $p = 0.035$), pulmonary involvement (AOR 5.06, 95% CI 1.56–16.74, $p = 0.007$) and positivity for rheumatoid factor (AOR 4.68, 95%IC 1.63–14.98, $p = 0.006$) were factors significantly associated with APS-SLE. APS also may coexist with rheumatoid arthritis, Sjögren's syndrome, autoimmune thyroid diseases, systemic sclerosis, systemic vasculitis, dermatopolymyositis, primary biliary cirrhosis and autoimmune hepatitis.

Conclusions: APS is a systemic AD that may coexist with other ADs, the most common being SLE. Awareness of this polyautoimmunity should be addressed promptly to establish strategies for controlling modifiable risk factors in those patients.

Editor: Jose Crispin, Beth Israel Deaconess Medical Center, United States of America

Funding: This work was supported by the School of Medicine and Health Sciences, Universidad del Rosario, Bogota, Colombia. The funders had no role in study design, data collection and analysis, decision to publish, or preparation of the manuscript.

Competing Interests: The authors have indicated that they have no conflicts of interest regarding the content of this article.

* Email: francoa.juan@gmail.com (JSF); juan.anaya@urosario.edu.co (JMA)

Introduction

Autoimmune diseases (ADs) are chronic conditions initiated by the loss of immunological tolerance to self-antigens, and they represent a heterogeneous group of disorders that affect specific target organs or multiple systems. Because of the chronic condition of these diseases, they constitute a significant burden on the health care system, with direct and indirect economic costs and quality of life impairment [1–4].

The fact that ADs share several subphenotypes, physiopathological mechanisms, environmental factors, and genetic factors has been called the "autoimmune tautology" and indicates that ADs share common physiopathological mechanisms and a common origin [1–9].

The clinical evidence of the autoimmune tautology highlights the coexistence of distinct ADs within an individual, which corresponds to polyautoimmunity, defined as the presence of more than one AD in a single patient [1,10]. When three or more ADs coexist, this condition is called multiple autoimmune syndrome (MAS) [11]. Factors significantly associated with polyautoimmunity include female gender and familial autoimmunity (i.e., the presence of diverse ADs in multiple members of a nuclear family) [10,12]. Polyautoimmunity represents the effect of a single genotype on diverse phenotypes [1].

Several subphenotypes are shared by ADs, including cutaneous involvement (i.e., photosensibility, alopecia, Raynaud's phenomenon), arthralgia and arthritis, fatigue, and even cardiovascular disease (CVD) [1,2]. Polyautoimmunity has been reported in most ADs, including systemic lupus erythematosus (SLE) [10,13], in which one of the most frequent coexistent disease is antiphospholipid syndrome (APS) [13]. Therefore, the purposes of this study were to examine the prevalence and associated factors of the coexistence of SLE and APS in a cohort of Colombian patients with SLE, as well as to discuss on the coexistence of APS with other ADs.

Patients and Methods

Study population

A cross-sectional analytical study was conducted in 376 Colombian patients with SLE. The subjects have been systematically followed at the Center for Autoimmune Diseases Research (CREA) in Bogota, Colombia. All of the subjects fulfilled the 1997 update of the American College of Rheumatology (ACR) classification criteria for SLE [14].

The patient socio-demographic and cumulative clinical and laboratory data, as well as a household description, were obtained by interview, standardized report form, physical examination and chart review as previously reported [15]. The data were collected in an electronic and secure database. The socio-demographic variables included age at SLE onset, disease duration, educational and socioeconomic status, current occupation, smoking habits, coffee consumption, expositional factors and physical activity. The age at onset (AOD) of the disease was defined as the first subjective experience of the symptom(s) and/or sign(s) described in any of the items of the classification criteria [16]. The duration of disease was considered as the difference between the AOD and the date of the first participation in the study. The educational level was recorded as the number of years of education and was divided into two groups (equal to or more than 9 years and less than 9 years of education) based on the "General Law of Education" in Colombia [17,18]. The socioeconomic status was categorized on the basis of national legislation and was divided into low (1 and 2), intermediate (3) and high (4–6) status [19]. The smoking habits were assessed as never smoking; 1–6, 6–15, and >15 packages/year; or cessation of cigarette consumption. Coffee intake was asked as yes or not and measured in cups per day (i.e., 1–2, 2–4, >4).

Ethics statement

This study was performed in compliance with Act 008430/1993 of the Ministry of Health of the Republic of Colombia, which classified it as minimal-risk research. All of the patients voluntarily accepted to participate in the study by reading and signing the informed consent. The institutional review board of the Universidad del Rosario approved the study design.

Clinical variables

Clinical and laboratory variables were registered as present or absent at any time during the course of the disease as previously reported [15,20]. In particular, lupus nephritis was defined as active urinary sediment, or proteinuria >500 mg/24 h or positive renal biopsy (ISN/RNP). Pulmonary compromise was considered in the presence of pulmonary hypertension, or pulmonary embolism or diffuse alveolar hemorrhage. Pleuritis was defined as the presence of pleural rub and/or effusion and/or typical pleuritic pain, and confirmed by chest X-ray or computed tomography. Neurologic involvement included the presence of seizures without any other definable cause, or psychosis lacking any other definable cause, or other conditions such as peripheral neuropathy, stroke, transverse myelitis, chorea, or other central nervous system lesions directly attributable to SLE in the absence of other causes. Autoimmune hemolytic anemia (hematocrit <35%, reticulocyte count >4%, and positive Coombs test), leukopenia (white cells <4000/mm3) and thrombocytopenia (platelets <100000/mm3) were also assessed. Other manifestations such as polyautoimmunity [1,10], MAS [11], familial autoimmunity, and familial autoimmune disease [12] were also included.

CVD represents a broad spectrum of manifestations (i.e., subphenotypes) such as hypertension (HTN), myocardial infarction (MI), peripheral vascular disease (PVD), and cerebrovascular accidents (i.e., stroke). Since atherosclerosis (AT), the usual cause of CVD, starts when the endothelium becomes damaged, and is considered to be an autoimmune-inflammatory disease, CVD was assessed by characterizing the following five subphenotypes: HTN, defined as having blood pressure ≥140/90 mm Hg recorded as an average of two measurements, with at least a 15-minute interval between the measurements or the use of any antihypertensive medication [21]; a history of stroke; a coronary event [i.e., unstable angina, MI]; a thrombotic event (other than MI and carotid involvement, requiring anticoagulant treatment); and carotid disease (by the Doppler criteria or intima-media thickness ≥0.9). The traditional risk factors assessed and included were smoking [22], type 2 diabetes mellitus [23] and dyslipidemia [24].

Concerning pharmacological treatment, the current or past use of steroid therapy (i.e., prednisolone, methylprednisolone, deflazacort), antimalarials (i.e., cloroquine, hydroxychloroquine), immunosupressors (i.e., azathioprine, mycophenolate mofetil and cyclophosphamide) and biological therapy (i.e., rituximab) were also recorded.

APS polyautoimmunity assessment

All of the patients were systematically assessed and classified for the presence of the following: 1) confirmed APS according to the 2006 update of the classification criteria [i.e., a thromboembolic event and positivity for anti-cardiolipin (aCL) IgG/IgM in medium or high titer, anti-beta 2-glycoprotein 1 (B2GPI) IgG/IgM antibodies or lupus anticoagulant (LAC), on two or more occasions] [25]; 2) positivity for antiphospholipid (aPL) antibodies (i.e., aCL IgG/IgM, B2GPI IgG/IgM or LAC) without a prior thromboembolic nor obstetric event; and 3) SLE patients without APS nor positivity for aPL antibodies.

Laboratory measurements

The relevant laboratory variables associated with SLE were registered. Patients underwent measurement of the following antibodies by ELISA using commercial kits (QUANTA Lite, INOVA Diagnostics, San Diego, CA, USA): anti-double strand DNA antibodies (anti-dsDNA), precipitating antibodies to extractable nuclear antigens (ENAs: Sm, U1-RNP, Ro/SS-A, La/SS-B), aCL IgG and IgM, B2GPI IgG and IgM antibodies and rheumatoid factor (RF) IgM. The positive cut-off values were >300 UI for anti-dsDNA; >40 UI aCL (IgG and IgM), and B2GPI (IgG and IgM); >20 UI ENAs; and >6 UI for RF. Additionally, the antinuclear antibodies (ANAs) were measured by indirect immunofluorescence on HEp-2 cell (NOVA Lite^{TM} Hep-2 ANA kit, INOVA Diagnostics, San Diego, CA, USA), according to the manufacturer's instructions. Other autoantibodies, including lupus anticoagulant, anti-Scl 70, -centromere, -mitochondrial, and -smooth muscle antibodies, were recorded. White blood cell and platelet count, hemoglobin levels, mean corpuscular volume, complement (i.e., C3 and C4 levels), venereal disease research laboratory results, and creatinine levels were extracted from each patient's clinical record.

Statistical analysis

First, univariate descriptive statistics were performed. The categorical variables were described by the frequencies. The quantitative continuous variables were described as the mean and standard deviation, as well as the median and interquartile range. The comparisons between group 1 (i.e., confirmed APS) and 3 (i.e., SLE patients with neither APS nor positive aPL autoantibodies) in

Table 1. Demographic and clinical characteristics of 376 patients with SLE.

Characteristic	*Median, range*
Age(y)	36, 25–46
Age at SLE onset (y)	27, 19–38
Duration of disease (y)	5, 2–11
Sociodemographic characteristics	***%(n/N)***
Female	91.8 (345/376)
LEL	13.8 (51/369)
Low SES	24.2 (86/355)
Ever smoking	36.3 (134/369)
Coffee intake	61.8 (225/364)
Clinical variables	***%(n/N)***
Female	91.8 (345/376)
Arthritis	74.7 (281/376)
Malar rash	44.4 (167/376)
Photosensitivity	57.2 (215/376)
Oral ucers	30.6 (115/376)
Alopecia	49.7 (187/376)
Serositis	30 (113/376)
Renal involvement	44.9 (168/376)
Neurological involvement	40.9 (154/376)
Pulmonary involvement	10.4 (39/376)
Haematological involvement	79.1 (295/376)
CVD	38.5(145/376)
Pregnancy loss	20.5 (70/342)
Poliautoimmunity	31.1 (112/376)
AITD	11.97 (45/376)
SS	9.04 (34/376)
RA	6.12 (23/376)
MAS	7.98 (30/376)
Familial autoimmunity	19.68 (74/376)
APS assessment	***%(n/N)***
Group 1 (APS)	9.3 (35/376)
Group 2 (aPL antibodies)	30.8 (116/376)
Group 3 (SLE without APS nor aPL)	59.8 (225/376)
Medication	***%(n/N)***
Steroid therapy	87.3 (281/322)
Antimalarials	86 (277/322)
Immunosupressors[a]	51.1 (164/321)
Laboratory findings	***%(n/N)***
ANA (+)	100 (376/376)
Anti dsDNA (+)	66.1 (236/357)
Anti Sm (+)	39.9 (144/361)
Anti Ro (+)	49.45 (180/364)
Anti La (+)	25.6 (93/363)
Anti RNP (+)	44.5 (161/362)
LAC (+)	51.45 (71/158)
aCL IgG (+)	33.3 (120/360)
aCL IgM (+)	39.8 (140/352)
B2GPI IgG (+)	11.3 (33/293)
B2GPI IgM (+)	13.5 (39/288)
RF IgM (+)	42.1 (120/285)

Table 1. Cont.

Characteristic	*Median, range*
Hypocomplementemia[b]	66.4 (209/315)

APS: antiphospholipid syndrome; aCL: anticardiolipin antibodies; AITD: autoimmune thyroid disease; ANA: antinuclear antibodies; B2GPI: anti-β2 glycoprotein I antibodies; CVD: cardiovascular disease; LAC: lupus anticoagulant; LEL: low educational level; MAS: multiple autoimmune syndrome; RA: rheumatoid arthritis; RF: rheumatoid factor; SS: Sjogren's sindrome; SES: socioeconomic status; y: years.
[a]Immunosupressors based on treatment with mycophenolate mophetil and/or cyclophosphamide and/or azathioprine.
[b]Hypocomplementemia defined as the presence of low C3 or C4.

relation to the other categorical variables, were assessed by chi square tests or Fisher's exact tests when facing small sample sizes. The comparisons between the two groups in relation to the continuous variables were performed with the Kruskal-Wallis test. A logistic regression model with APS and SLE polyautoimmunity as the dependent variable was fit (group 1 vs. group 3). As the independent factors, the model included the variables that were statistically significant in the bivariate analyses and those variables that were biologically plausible. The model was adjusted by gender and duration of the disease. The adequacies of the logistic models were assessed using the Hosmer–Lemeshow goodness-of-fit test. The Nagelkerke R2 (i.e., the pseudo-R2) was used to estimate the percentage of variance explained by the models. The adjusted odds ratios (AOR) were calculated with 95% confidence intervals (CI). The Wald statistical test was used to evaluate the significance of the individual logistic regression coefficients for each independent variable. The statistical analyses were performed in R 3.0.2 [26].

Results

Of the 376 patients with SLE, 91.8% were women. Thirty-five patients fulfilled the classification criteria for APS, with a prevalence of 9.3%, representing the second most common polyautoimmunity, preceded by autoimmune thyroid disease, which disclosed a prevalence of 12%. The range of time elapsed from the SLE onset to the diagnosis of APS was 1 to 7 years. All of the patients had SLE prior to the diagnosis of APS. Out of the 35 patients with APS-SLE, 51.4% had a prior thromboembolic event, 40% pregnancy loss and 8.5% had both. Among the non-criteria manifestations, 9 (26%) patients had pulmonary involvement, of whom 6 had pulmonary hypertension and 3 pulmonary embolism, 6 (17%) patients had thrombocytopenia, and 5 (14%) livedo reticularis. Regarding CVD, this was present in 22 (63%) patients, of whom 18 had thrombosis and 10 hypertension (29%). There were 2 additional patients with prior thromboembolic and/or obstetric manifestations and positivity for aPL below medium or high titers that were excluded from further analysis, but in whom a "seronegative" APS could not be rule out. The most frequently found aPL antibody was LAC, with a prevalence rate of 51.5%, followed by aCL IgM with 40% and IgG with 33%. B2GPI IgG and IgM were positive in 11% and 13% of the patients, respectively. Of the SLE patients, 60% had neither APS nor positivity for aPL antibodies. The characteristics of the cohort are illustrated in Table 1. Socioeconomic status, smoking and coffee intake had no significant influence of the coexistence of SLE-APS. Although SLE disease activity index (SLEDAI) was calculated upon study entry, this variable was not included in the analysis.

Factors associated with APS polyautoimmunity

There was no difference in the patient age, AOD or duration of SLE. CVD, Sjögren's syndrome (SS), pulmonary involvement and positivity for RF were risk factors significantly associated with APS. The presence of alopecia was negatively associated with APS (Table 2).

The adjusted effects of the risk factors for APS polyautoimmunity

As expected, CVD was associated with APS-SLE. The main subphenotypes associated with CVD in APS-SLE were thrombosis and hypertension. Additional variables influencing this condition were pulmonary involvement and positivity for RF, regardless of gender and duration of the disease. Alopecia was confirmed to be negatively associated with APS (Table 3). A second logistic regression model was fit to evaluate the effect of aPL alone (i.e.,

Table 2. Factors associated with APS in SLE (bivariate analysis).

Variable	*SLE + APS %(n/N)*	*SLE %(n/N)*	*OR (95% CI)*	*p*
Gender	91.4 (32/35)	92.9 (211/227)	0.81 (0.22–2.9)	0.746
CVD	62.2 (23/37)	36.1 (82/227)	2.74 (1.42–6.1)	0.002
Abortion	46.8 (15/32)	13.9 (29/308)	4.97 (2.45–11.83)	<0.001
SS	25.7 (9/35)	7.5 (17/227)	3.88 (1.77–10.47)	<0.001
Alopecia	28.6 (10/35)	55.5 (126/227)	0.30 (0.15–0.70)	0.003
Pulmonary involvement	25.7 (9/35)	9.7 (22/227)	2.97 (1.38–7.73)	0.006
RF IgM (+)	57.1 (16/28)	34.5 (59/171)	2.29 (1.12–5.55)	0.02

APS: antiphospholipid syndrome; OR: odds ratio; 95% CI: 95% confidence interval; CVD: cardiovascular disease; RF: rheumatoid factor; SLE: systemic lupus erythematosus; SS: Sjögren's syndrome.

Table 3. Adjusted factors associated with APS in SLE polyautoimmunity (multivariate analysis).

Characteristics	*β*	*AOR*	*95% CI*	*p**
CVD	1.218	3.38	1.11–10.96	0.035
Alopecia	−1.556	0.21	0.06–0.64	0.009
Pulmonary involvement	1.62	5.06	1.56–16.74	0.007
RF IgM (+)	1.543	4.68	1.63–14.98	0.006

AOR: adjusted odds ratio; 95% CI: 95% confidence interval; CVD: cardiovascular disease; RF: rheumatoid factor.
*Variables statistically significant are shown.

group 2) on the expression of SLE without APS nor positivity for aPL antibodies (i.e., group 3). An association between aPL and RF was observed, but not with clinical features.

Discussion

In our series, the coexistence of APS with SLE was 9.3% and was associated with a distinctive subphenotype characterized by a higher risk of CVD, pulmonary involvement and positivity for RF.

The interplay between SLE and APS has been analyzed over the years, since APS was initially not considered to be a systemic AD and was thought to occur only in patients with SLE [27–29]. Furthermore, APS has been found to be associated with systemic manifestations (e.g., non-thrombotic renal disease, migraine, livedo reticularis, pulmonary hypertension, MI) and laboratory features (e.g., positive ANAs, hypocomplementemia) also present in patients with SLE, complicating the clear differentiation between these entities [27–29]. However, rather than being the spectrum of the same disease, the coexistence of APS and SLE is a reflection of complex disease traits and highlights the common mechanisms shared by ADs [1,4].

The association between CVD and SLE mortality was first established by Urowitz et al. [30], with the description of the bimodal pattern of mortality in SLE patients, with an early death due to active disease and infections, and a late death secondary to CVD. Despite a reduction in SLE mortality over the years, CVD remains prevalent among these patients, affecting up to 28% of patients after four decades of disease duration [31,32]. Traditional risk factors have been described for CVD in SLE (e.g., HTN, dyslipidemia) [33]. However, Esdaile et al. [34] demonstrated that these factors do not fully account for the accelerated AT in these patients, suggesting that there are factors related with the disease involved in the development of CVD. Among the novel risk factors described, polyautoimmunity with APS has been associated with CVD. In fact, APS has been reported as a non-traditional risk factor for CVD in SLE [15]. Other studies have reported similar results, as well as an increased accrual of damage measured by the SLE Damage Index [35–38]. Different mechanisms involving the role of aPL in the process of AT have been described, and these include overexpression of tissue factor, annexin I and II, cytokines and other mediators of endothelial dysfunction [39–41]; oxidative perturbations and mitochondrial dysfunction [42]; and cross-reactivity with oxidized low-density lipoproteins, accelerating their influx into macrophage and AT development [43]. Recently, Perez-Sanchez et al. [44] found a close relationship between patients with APS and those with polyautoimmunity of SLE and APS in the groups of genes belonging to the cluster of AT, highlighting the role of novel risk factors in the development of CVD among these patients.

The pulmonary involvement described in SLE and APS may be similar, and include pulmonary hypertension, pulmonary embolism and diffuse alveolar hemorrhage [45–47]. In our results, the association with pulmonary involvement was driven by the presence of pulmonary hypertension. aPL has been associated with the development of pulmonary hypertension in patients with SLE [48–51]. The positivity for RF seem to have a dual role in autoimmunity with a protective effect by interfering with the binding complement system to immune complexes, or a harmful effect by enhancing immune mediated tissue damage [52]. In SLE, positivity for RF has been found to have a protective role in the development of lupus nephritis [53–55]. In our results, we found that the positivity for FR IgM was associated with the coexistence of APS and SLE, as well as with the positivity for aPL antibodies. Similarly, Spadaro et al. [52] previously reported the relationship between different isotypes of RF in patients with APS and SLE polyautoimmunity. Positivity for RF IgG was negatively associated with serosal and hematological involvement, and negatively correlated with aCL IgG titer, suggesting that RF IgG is related with the absence of APS; on the other hand, RF IgM was associated with aCL IgM positivity, implying a possible relation with APS [52]. The interplay of RF isotypes in ADs and polyautoimmunity requires further investigation.

As already mentioned, APS was primarily recognized in patients with SLE and was, therefore, considered to be an overlap syndrome (i.e., "secondary" APS). The major difference between polyautoimmunity and overlap syndrome is that the former is the presence of two or more well-defined autoimmune conditions (i.e., overt clinical manifestations mediated by T or B cell responses) fulfilling the validated classification criteria whereas the latter is the partial presence of signs and symptoms of diverse ADs [1]. An overlap syndrome may evolve towards a well-defined phenotype or remain as an undifferentiated AD for years (i.e., the presence of some subphenotypes) [1]. The international consensus statement on an update of the classification criteria for definite APS advised against using the term "secondary" APS because no difference was found in the clinical consequences of aPL antibodies among the patients in this category (Evidence Level I) [25]. The consensus is that, rather than distinguishing patients by "primary" and "secondary" APS, documenting the coexistence of SLE (or other ADs) is more advantageous for classification [25]. In agreement with this argument, we have proposed the term "polyautoimmunity" instead of secondary AD to refer to the coexistence of two or more ADs [10].

Besides SLE, APS has been described in most ADs, including rheumatoid arthritis, SS, autoimmune thyroid diseases, systemic sclerosis (SSc), systemic vasculitis, dermatopolymyositis, primary biliary cirrhosis (PBC) and autoimmune hepatitis (AIH) [35–37,56–89]. Moreover, the coexistence of APS with other ADs may be associated with a modified clinical course, especially in SSc (i.e., associated with pulmonary arterial hypertension and MI), PBC (i.e., higher Mayo risk score) and AIH (i.e., associated with

Table 4. Polyautoimmunity in APS.

AD	APS	aCL % (n/N)		LAC	B2GPI	Commentary	Ref.
	% (n/N)	IgG	IgM	% (n/N)	% (n/N)		
SLE	6.5 (44/679)	-	-	-	-	The patients with SLE/APS polyautoimmunity were more likely to die from cardiovascular disease (i.e., myocardial infarction, acute coronary syndrome). These patients had a higher SDI score and poorer survival, which did not reach statistical significance.	[35]
	19.2 (5/26)	25 (5/20)		27.8 (5/18)	-	The SLE patients with intracranial hemorrhage had polyautoimmunity, including APS, more frequently than did the controls. Thrombocytopenia was found to be an independent risk factor for intracranial hemorrhage.	[56]
	19 (19/100)	53 (53/100)		2 (2/100)	84 (84/100)	IgG aCL and B2GPI correlated with a previous history of arthritis.	[57]
	8.4 (8/95)	13.4 (13/95)	2.1 (2/85)	-	-	The occurrence of aCL positivity was significantly associated with venous/arterial thrombosis and abortion. Thrombocytopenia was more frequent among the aCL positive patients; however, it did not reach statistical significance.	[58]
	12.4 (16/129)	15.5 (20/129)	13.9 (18/129)	-	10.1 (13/129)	In a mestizo cohort of SLE patients, aCL positivity was significantly associated with venous/arterial thrombosis and fetal loss.	[59]
	9.2 (12/130)	18.5 (24/130)		-	-	The occurrence of aCL positivity was present before the diagnosis of SLE and prior to the development of the clinical features of APS. The aCL positivity was associated with a higher number of the ACR criteria and early AOD of SLE as well as cutaneous, serosal, neuropsychiatric and renal involvement.	[60]
	12 (20/166)*	-	-	-	-	Polyautoimmunity with APS increased the risk of pregnancy loss, especially after week 20 of gestation.	[61]
	28.4 (50/176)	-	-	-	-	APS and damage (measured by SDI) were significantly associated with higher mortality in SLE patients.	[36]
	14.1 (28/198)	36.9 (73/198)	17.7 (35/198)	21.7 (43/198)	-	The independent predictor factors for diminished survival with SLE duration of 15 years were AOD, renal involvement and APS polyautoimmunity.	[37]
RA	3.6 (3/84)	8.3 (7/84)	2.4 (2/84)	-	7.1 (6/84)	The prevalence of aPL antibodies in RA was reported. No correlation was found with the clinical features.	[62]
	-	12.4 (12/97)	11.3 (11/97)	1 (1/97)	12.4 (12/97)	There was a negative association between aPL antibodies and anti-CCP antibodies.	[63]
	-	20.2 (35/173)	15.6 (27/173)	-	-	The presence of aCL antibodies was associated with rheumatoid nodules. The patients with aCL antibodies had more cutaneous manifestations (e.g., livedo reticularis, purpura, cutaneous ulcers); however, this association was not significant.	[64]
	-	8.9 (15/168)	4.2 (7/168)	5.9 (10/168)	-	The RA patients with positivity for aPL antibodies and high levels of homocysteine might be at a higher risk for thrombotic events.	[65]

Table 4. Cont.

AD	APS	aCL % (n/N)		LAC	B2GPI	Commentary	Ref.
	% (n/N)	IgG	IgM	% (n/N)	% (n/N)		
	-	6.8 (7/102)	0.9 (1/102)	-	-	A significant correlation was found between the aCL and anti-CCP antibody levels.	[66]
	-	11.9 (22/184)	4.3 (8/184)	3.8 (7/184)	-	The RA patients with positivity for aCL and a history of arterial/venous thrombosis were found to have lower levels of free protein S.	[67]
SS	4.1 (3/74)	32.4 (24/74)	6.8 (5/74)	10.8 (8/74)	4.1 (3/74)	The aPL-antibody positive patients were associated with polyautoimmunity. They had peripheral neuropathy and the presence of hypergammaglobulinemia.	[68]
	3 (3/100)	1 (1/100)	3 (3/100)	9 (9/100)	5 (5/100)	LAC was associated with a significantly higher risk for deep venous thrombosis, stroke and/or myocardial infarction. No significant association was found with the clinical features.	[69]
	3.1 (4/130)	10.8 (14/130)	6.2 (8/130)	9.2 (12/130)	-	The presence of aPL antibodies was associated with a higher prevalence of ANAs positivity.	[70]
	1.0 (4/402)	4.7 (19/402)	1.5 (6/402)	4.7 (19/402)	-	APS is an infrequent, but not exceptional, polyautoimmunity in SS.	[71]
	-	12.7 (8/63)	6.3 (4/63)	-	-	The presence of aCL antibodies was associated with RNP positivity. No relationship was found with the clinical features or extra glandular manifestations.	[72]
AITD	-	35.5 (11/31)	35.5 (11/31)	-	-	There was an increased incidence of aCL in patients with AITD. None of the patients had clinical features of APS.	[73]
	-	43.8 (57/130)	10 (13/130)	-	-	The prevalence of aPL is increased in AITD. There was no correlation between aPL titer and the titer of thyroid autoantibodies.	[74]
	-	10.1 (7/69)	5.8 (4/69)	-	-	The patients with aCL did not exhibit a higher titer of thyroid autoantibodies.	[75]
	-	10.5 (2/19)	10.5 (2/19)	-	-	The patients with Hashimoto's thyroiditis had an increased incidence of aCL. There was no correlation with thyroid autoantibodies titer.	[76]
SSc	2.7 (3/108)	11.1 (12/108)	2.7 (3/108)	-	6.5 (7/108)	The SSc patients with aCL positivity were associated with pulmonary hypertension. The patients with PAH had higher titers of aCL; however, this association was not significant.	[77]
	-	19.1 (13/68)	20.6 (14/68)	-	-	Anticentromere antibodies, anti-ScL-70 and smoking were significantly associated with severe ischemia and amputation in SSc, whereas no relationship was found with aCL.	[78]
	-	12.2 (10/82)	3.7 (3/82)	-	-	No association was found between aCL and the clinical features of SSc.	[79]

Table 4. Cont.

AD	APS	aCL % (n/N)		LAC	B2GPI	Commentary	Ref.
	% (n/N)	IgG	IgM	% (n/N)	% (n/N)		
	-	20.8 (10/48)	35 (17/48)	23.8 (5/21)	-	The presence of IgM aCL was significantly associated with higher cutaneous involvement (e.g., the number of lesions, plaques and body areas affected) and ANA and RF positivity in the patients with localized SSc compared to the controls.	[80]
	-	17.5 (20/40)	5 (2/40)	5 (2/40)	50 (20/40)	The aPL-antibody patients had a tendency to Raynaud's phenomenon, cutaneous ulcerations and pulmonary hypertension; however, this correlation was not significant.	[81]
	-	8.6 (9/105)	11.4 (12/105)	-	-	The SSc patients with aCL were significantly associated with ischemia or myocardial necrosis (i.e., on the electrocardiogram and/or scintigraphic findings). There was a higher prevalence of digital pitting scars, acroosteolysis and pulmonary involvement; however, it did not reach statistical significance.	[82]
	1.4 (1/72)	9.7 (7/72)		-	-	No correlation was found between aPL antibodies and the clinical features of SSc.	[83]
Systemic vasculitis	6.3 (12/144)	8 (12/144)		5.6 (8/144)	-	The presence of aPL antibodies might influence the clinical course for systemic vascularity.	[84]
DM/PM	3.1 (3/97)	-	-	-	-	The prevalence of polyautoimmunity with APS was reported in a cohort of DM/PM.	[85]
	-	2.7 (1/36)	5.6 (2/36)	-	-	The prevalence of aCL in ADs was reported	[86]
PBC	1.4 (1/31)	-	-	-	-	The prevalence of MAS in the patients with AIH/PBC polyautoimmunity was evaluated. AITD was found to be the most prevalent AD. There was no correlation with the therapy response.	[87]
	-	27.3 (27/99)	27.3 (27/99)	-	2 (2/99)	IgG aCL were significantly associated with the presence of cirrhosis, a higher Mayo risk score and thrombocytopenia.	[88]
AIH	-	38.9 (23/59)	23.7 (14/59)	-	3.4 (2/59)	IgG aCL were significantly associated with the presence of cirrhosis and disease activity (in the clinical features and the laboratory).	[89]

AD: autoimmune disease; aCL: anticardiolipin antibodies; AIH: autoimmune hepatitis; AITD: autoimmune thyroid disease; anti-CCP: anti-cyclic citrullinated peptides antibodies; AOD: age at onset of disease; APS: antiphospholipid syndrome; B2GPI: anti-beta 2 glycoprotein I antibodies; DM/PM: dermatopolymyositis; LAC: lupus anticoagulant; MAS: multiple autoimmune syndrome; PBC: primary biliary cirrhosis; SDI: systemic lupus erythematosus damage index; SLE: systemic lupus erythematosus; SS: Sjögren's syndrome; SSc: scleroderma; RA: rheumatoid arthritis; RF: rheumatoid factor.

*Correspond to 166 pregnancies in 125 women followed in the Hopkins Lupus Cohort.

cirrhosis and disease activity) (Table 4). Therefore, APS should be addressed in patients with the aforementioned ADs.

Although our study sample size was not negligible, as a cross-sectional study, it would have been more valuable to have had an appropriate follow up to address the association of APS and SLE polyautoimmunity by the inclusion of other measurements such as antibodies isotypes (e.g., B2GPI IgA [90], RF IgG), serologic biomarkers and genetic markers.

Conclusions

APS is considered a systemic AD, and may coexist with other ADs, SLE being the most frequent. The coexistence of APS and SLE is associated with a more severe subphenotype characterized by a higher CVD rate and pulmonary involvement. CVD is a major cause of morbidity and mortality in SLE patients. Novel risk factors related to autoimmunity are recognized because the traditional risk factors do not completely explain the high CVD rates. APS polyautoimmunity should be addressed in every SLE patient to identify the higher risk population and encourage prevention strategies and early therapeutic intervention. APS should be included as a non-traditional risk factor for CVD in SLE and other ADs in further studies.

Acknowledgments

We thank all patients for their participation in the study, and colleagues at the Center for Autoimmune Diseases Research (CREA) for their fruitful discussions and contributions.

Author Contributions

Conceived and designed the experiments: JMA. Performed the experiments: JSF NMG YAA MRJ JMA. Analyzed the data: JSF NMG MRJ JAA JMA. Contributed reagents/materials/analysis tools: JMA JSF NMG YAA MRJ RDM ARV. Wrote the paper: JSF NMG MRJ YAA RDM JAA ARV JMA.

References

1. Anaya JM (2014) The diagnosis and clinical significance of polyautoimmunity. Autoimmun Rev 4–5: 4–7.
2. Anaya JM, Rojas-Villarraga A, Shoenfeld Y (2013) From the mosaic of autoimmunity to the autoimmune tautology. In: Anaya JM, Rojas-Villarraga A, Shoenfeld Y, Levy R, Cervera R, editors. Autoimunity From bench to bedside. Bogotá: Editorial Universidad del Rosario. pp. 237–245.
3. Anaya JM, Rojas-Villarraga A, García-Carrasco M (2012) The autoimmune tautology: from polyautoimmunity and familial autoimmunity to the autoimmune genes. Autoimmune Dis 2012.
4. Anaya JM (2010) The autoimmune tautology. Arthritis Res Ther 12: 147.
5. Shoenfeld Y, Isenberg DA (1989) The mosaic of autoimmunity. Immunol Today 10: 123–6.
6. Anaya JM, Corena R, Castiblanco J, Rojas-Villarraga A, Shoenfeld Y (2007) The kaleidoscope of autoimmunity: multiple autoimmune syndromes and familial autoimmunity. Expert Rev Clin Immunol 3: 623–35.
7. Anaya JM (2012) Common mechanisms of autoimmune diseases (the autoimmune tautology). Autoimmun Rev 11: 781–4.
8. Cifuentes RA, Restrepo-Montoya D, Anaya JM (2012) The autoimmune tautology: an in silico approach. Autoimmune Dis 2012: 792106.
9. Rojas-Villarraga A, Castellanos-delahoz J, Perez-Fernandez O, Amaya-Amaya J, Franco JS, et al. (2013) The autoimmune ecology. In: Anaya JM, Shoenfeld Y, Rojas-Villarraga A, Levy R, Cervera R, editors. Autoimmunity From bench to bedside. Bogotá: Editorial Universidad del Rosario. pp. 322–41.
10. Rojas-Villarraga A, Amaya-Amaya J, Rodriguez-Rodriguez A, Mantilla RD, Anaya J-M (2012) Introducing polyautoimmunity: secondary autoimmune diseases no longer exist. Autoimmune Dis 2012: 254319.
11. Anaya J-M, Castiblanco J, Rojas-Villarraga A, Pineda-Tamayo R, Levy RA, et al. (2012) The multiple autoimmune syndromes. A clue for the autoimmune tautology. Clin Rev Allergy Immunol 43: 256–64.
12. Cárdenas-Roldán J, Rojas-Villarraga A, Anaya JM (2013) How do autoimmune diseases cluster in families? A systematic review and meta-analysis. BMC Med 11: 73.
13. Rojas-Villarraga A, Toro C-E, Espinosa G, Rodríguez-Velosa Y, Duarte-Rey C, et al. (2010) Factors influencing polyautoimmunity in systemic lupus erythematosus. Autoimmun Rev 9: 229–32.
14. Klippel J, Lahita R, Esdaile JM, Hahn BH, Urowitz MB, et al. (1999) Guidelines for referral and management of systemic lupus erythematosus in adults. American College of Rheumatology Ad Hoc Committee on Systemic Lupus Erythematosus Guidelines. Arthritis Rheum 42: 1785–96.
15. Amaya-Amaya J, Sarmiento-Monroy JC, Caro-Moreno J, Molano-González N, Mantilla RD, et al. (2013) Cardiovascular disease in latin american patients with systemic lupus erythematosus: a cross-sectional study and a systematic review. Autoimmune Dis 2013: 794383.
16. Hochberg MC (1997) Updating the American College of Rheumatology revised criteria for the classification of systemic lupus erythematosus. Arthritis Rheum 40: 1725.
17. Ministry of Education (1992) Law of Higher Education – Law 30 of 1992. Government of Colombia. Available: http://www.mineducacion.gov.co/1621/articles-86437_Archivo_pdf.pdf. Accessed 2014 Jul 10.
18. Ministry of Education (1994) Law 115 of 1994. Government of Colombia. Available: http://www.mineducacion.gov.co/1621/articles-85906_archivo_pdf.pdf. Accessed 2014 Jul 10.
19. Calixto OJ, Anaya JM (2014) Socioeconomic status. The relationship with health and autoimmune diseases. Autoimmun Rev 13: 641–54.
20. Anaya JM, Cañas C, Mantilla RD, Pineda-Tamayo R, Tobón GJ, et al. (2011) Lupus nephritis in Colombians: contrasts and comparisons with other populations. Clin Rev Allergy Immunol 40: 199–207.
21. Jones DW, Hall JE (2004) Seventh report of the Joint National Committee on Prevention, Detection, Evaluation, and Treatment of High Blood Pressure and evidence from new hypertension trials. Hypertension 43: 1–3.
22. Toloza SMA, Uribe AG, McGwin G, Alarcón GS, Fessler BJ, et al. (2004) Systemic lupus erythematosus in a multiethnic US cohort (LUMINA). XXIII. Baseline predictors of vascular events. Arthritis Rheum 50: 3947–57.
23. American Diabetes Association (2014) Diagnosis and classification of diabetes mellitus. Diabetes Care 37 (Suppl 1): S81–90.
24. Stone NJ, Bilek S, Rosenbaum S (2005) Recent National Cholesterol Education Program Adult Treatment Panel III update: adjustments and options. Am J Cardiol 96: 53E–59E.
25. Miyakis S, Lockshin MD, Atsumi T, Branch DW, Brey RL, et al. (2006) International consensus statement on an update of the classification criteria for definite antiphospholipid syndrome (APS). J Thromb Haemost 4: 295–306.
26. Team RC (2013) R: A language and environment for statistical computing.
27. Agmon-Levin N, Shoenfeld Y (2014) The spectrum between antiphospholipid syndrome and systemic lupus erythematosus. Clin Rheumatol 33: 293–5.
28. Taraborelli M, Andreoli L, Tincani A (2012) Much more than thrombosis and pregnancy loss: the antiphospholipid syndrome as a "systemic disease". Best Pract Res Clin Rheumatol 26: 79–90.
29. Agmon-Levin N, Mosca M, Petri M, Shoenfeld Y (2012) Systemic lupus erythematosus one disease or many? Autoimmun Rev 11: 593–5.
30. Urowitz MB, Bookman AA, Koehler BE, Gordon DA, Smythe HA, et al. (1976) The bimodal mortality pattern of systemic lupus erythematosus. Am J Med 60: 221–5.
31. Nikpour M, Gladman DD, Urowitz MB (2013) Premature coronary heart disease in systemic lupus erythematosus: what risk factors do we understand? Lupus 22: 1243–50.
32. Urowitz MB, Gladman DD, Tom BDM, Ibañez D, Farewell VT (2008) Changing Patterns in Mortality and Disease Outcomes for Patients with Systemic Lupus Erythematosus. J Rheumatol 35: 2152.
33. Nikpour M, Urowitz MB, Gladman DD (2009) Epidemiology of atherosclerosis in systemic lupus erythematosus. Curr Rheumatol Rep 11: 248–54.
34. Esdaile JM, Abrahamowicz M, Grodzicky T, Li Y, Panaritis C, et al. (2001) Traditional Framingham risk factors fail to fully account for accelerated atherosclerosis in systemic lupus erythematosus. Arthritis Rheum 44: 2331–7.
35. Mok CC, Chan PT, Ho LY, Yu KL, To CH (2013) Prevalence of the antiphospholipid syndrome and its effect on survival in 679 Chinese patients with systemic lupus erythematosus: a cohort study. Medicine (Baltimore) 92: 217–22.
36. Signorelli FV, Salles GF, Papi JA (2011) Antiphospholipid syndrome as predictor of mortality in Brazilian patients with systemic lupus erythematosus. Lupus 20: article 419.
37. Ruiz-Irastorza G, Egurbide M-V, Ugalde J, Aguirre C (2004) High impact of antiphospholipid syndrome on irreversible organ damage and survival of patients with systemic lupus erythematosus. Arch Intern Med 164: 77–82.
38. Soares M, Reis L, Papi JAS, Cardoso CRL (2003) Rate, pattern and factors related to damage in Brazilian systemic lupus erythematosus patients. Lupus 12: 788–94.
39. Cuadrado MJ, López-Pedrera C, Khamashta MA, Camps MT, Tinahones F, et al. (1997) Thrombosis in primary antiphospholipid syndrome: a pivotal role for monocyte tissue factor expression. Arthritis Rheum 40: 834–41.
40. Cugno M, Borghi MO, Lonati LM, Ghiadoni L, Gerosa M, et al. (2010) Patients with antiphospholipid syndrome display endothelial perturbation. J Autoimmun 34: 105–10.
41. López-Pedrera C, Cuadrado MJ, Herández V, Buendia P, Aguirre MA, et al. (2008) Proteomic analysis in monocytes of antiphospholipid syndrome patients:

deregulation of proteins related to the development of thrombosis. Arthritis Rheum 58: 2835–44.
42. Perez-Sanchez C, Ruiz-Limon P, Aguirre MA, Bertolaccini ML, Khamashta MA, et al. (2012) Mitochondrial dysfunction in antiphospholipid syndrome: implications in the pathogenesis of the disease and effects of coenzyme Q(10) treatment. Blood 119: 5859–70.
43. Hasunuma Y, Matsuura E, Makita Z, Katahira T, Nishi S, et al. (1997) Involvement of beta 2-glycoprotein I and anticardiolipin antibodies in oxidatively modified low-density lipoprotein uptake by macrophages. Clin Exp Immunol 107: 569–73.
44. Perez-Sanchez C, Barbarroja N, Messineo S, Ruiz-Limon P, Rodriguez-Ariza A, et al. (2014) Gene profiling reveals specific molecular pathways in the pathogenesis of atherosclerosis and cardiovascular disease in antiphospholipid syndrome, systemic lupus erythematosus and antiphospholipid syndrome with lupus. Ann Rheum Dis DOI: 10.1136/annrheumdis-2013-204600.
45. Paran D, Fireman E, Elkayam O (2004) Pulmonary disease in systemic lupus erythematosus and the antiphospholpid syndrome. Autoimmun Rev 3: 70–5.
46. Pego-Reigosa JM, Medeiros DA, Isenberg DA (2009) Respiratory manifestations of systemic lupus erythematosus: old and new concepts. Best Pract Res Clin Rheumatol 23: 469–80.
47. Stojanovich L (2006) Pulmonary manifestations in antiphospholipid syndrome. Autoimmun Rev 5: 344–8.
48. Cefle A, Inanc M, Sayarlioglu M, Kamali S, Gul A, et al. (2011) Pulmonary hypertension in systemic lupus erythematosus: relationship with antiphospholipid antibodies and severe disease outcome. Rheumatol Int 31: 183–9.
49. Asherson RA, Higenbottam TW, Dinh Xuan AT, Khamashta MA, Hughes GR (1990) Pulmonary hypertension in a lupus clinic: experience with twenty-four patients. J Rheumatol 17: 1292–8.
50. Alarcón-Segovia D, Pérez-Vázquez ME, Villa AR, Drenkard C, Cabiedes J (1992) Preliminary classification criteria for the antiphospholipid syndrome within systemic lupus erythematosus. Semin Arthritis Rheum 21: 275–86.
51. Alarcón-Segovia D, Delezé M, Oria CV, Sánchez-Guerrero J, Gómez-Pacheco L, et al. (1989) Antiphospholipid antibodies and the antiphospholipid syndrome in systemic lupus erythematosus. A prospective analysis of 500 consecutive patients. Medicine (Baltimore) 68: 353–65.
52. Spadaro A, Riccieri V, Terracina S, Rinaldi T, Taccari E, et al. (2000) Class specific rheumatoid factors and antiphospholipid syndrome in systemic lupus erythematosus. Lupus 9: 56–60.
53. Skare TL, Silva MBG, Holler AP, Chavez PA (2009) Protective role of rheumatoid factor in lupus nephritis. Clin Exp Rheumatol 27: 895.
54. Feldman D, Ginzler E, Kaplan D (1989) Rheumatoid factor in patients with systemic lupus erythematosus. J Rheumatol 16: 618–22.
55. Hill GS, Hinglais N, Tron F, Bach JF (1978) Systemic lupus erythematosus. Morphologic correlations with immunologic and clinical data at the time of biopsy. Am J Med 64: 61–79.
56. Gao N, Wang ZL, Li MT, Han SM, Dang YQ, et al. (2013) Clinical characteristics and risk factors of intracranial hemorrhage in systemic lupus erythematosus. Lupus 22: 453–60.
57. Gould T, Tikly M, Asherson R, Loizou S, Singh S (2006) Prevalence and clinical correlates of anti-phospholipid antibodies in South Africans with systemic lupus erythematosus. Scand J Rheumatol 35: 29–34.
58. Vianna JL, Haga HJ, Tripathi P, Cervera R, Khamashta MA, et al. (1992) Reassessing the status of antiphospholipid syndrome in systemic lupus erythematosus. Ann Rheum Dis 51: 160–1.
59. Aguirre V, Cuchacovich R, Barria L, Aris H, Trejo C, et al. (2001) Prevalence and isotype distribution of antiphospholipid antibodies in Chilean patients with systemic lupus erythematosus (SLE). Lupus 10: 75–80.
60. McClain MT, Arbuckle MR, Heinlen LD, Dennis GJ, Roebuck J, et al. (2004) The prevalence, onset, and clinical significance of antiphospholipid antibodies prior to diagnosis of systemic lupus erythematosus. Arthritis Rheum 50: 1226–32.
61. Clowse ME, Magder LS, Witter F, Petri M (2006) Early risk factors for pregnancy loss in lupus. Obstet Gynecol 107: 293–9.
62. Palomo I, Pinochet C, Alarcón M, Sandoval R, Gonzalez J, et al. (2006) Prevalence of antiphospholipid antibodies in Chilean patients with rheumatoid arthritis. J Clin Lab Anal 20: 190–4.
63. Jeleniewicz R, Majdan M, Targońska-Stępniak B, Dryglewska M (2012) Prevalence of antiphospholipid antibodies in rheumatoid arthritis patients and relationship with disease activity. Pol Arch Med Wewn 122: 480–6.
64. Wolf P, Gretler J, Aglas F, Auer-Grumbach P, Rainer F (1994) Anticardiolipin antibodies in rheumatoid arthritis: their relation to rheumatoid nodules and cutaneous vascular manifestations. Br J Dermatol 131: 48–51.
65. Seriolo B, Fasciolo D, Sulli A, Cutolo M (2001) Homocysteine and antiphospholipid antibodies in rheumatoid arthritis patients: relationships with thrombotic events. Clin Exp Rheumatol 19: 561–4.
66. Vittecoq O, Jouen-Beades F, Krzanowska K, Bichon-Tauvel I, Menard JF, et al. (2000) Prospective evaluation of the frequency and clinical significance of antineutrophil cytoplasmic and anticardiolipin antibodies in community cases of patients with rheumatoid arthritis. Rheumatology (Oxford) 39: 481–9.
67. Seriolo B, Accardo S, Garnero A, Fasciolo D, Cutolo M (1999) Anticardiolipin antibodies, free protein S levels and thrombosis: a survey in a selected population of rheumatoid arthritis patients. Rheumatology (Oxford) 38: 675–8.
68. Fauchais A, Lambert M, Launay D, Queyrel V, Nguyen N, et al. (2004) Antiphospholipid antibodies in primary Sjögren's syndrome: prevalence and clinical significance in a series of 74 patients. Lupus 13: 245–8.
69. Pasoto SG, Chakkour HP, Natalino RR, Viana VST, Bueno C, et al. (2012) Lupus anticoagulant: a marker for stroke and venous thrombosis in primary Sjögren's syndrome. Clin Rheumatol 31: 1331–8.
70. Cervera R, García-Carrasco M, Font J, Ramos M, Reverter JC, et al. (1997) Antiphospholipid antibodies in primary Sjögren's syndrome: prevalence and clinical significance in a series of 80 patients. Clin Exp Rheumatol 15: 361–5.
71. Ramos-Casals M, Nardi N, Brito-Zerón P, Aguiló S, Gil V, et al. (2006) Atypical autoantibodies in patients with primary Sjögren syndrome: clinical characteristics and follow-up of 82 cases. Semin Arthritis Rheum 35: 312–21.
72. Jedryka-Goral A, Jagiello P, D'Cruz DP, Maldykowa H, Khamashta MA, et al. (1992) Isotype profile and clinical relevance of anticardiolipin antibodies in Sjogren's syndrome. Ann Rheum Dis 51: 889–91.
73. Paggi A, Caccavo D, Ferri GM, Di Prima MA, Amoroso A, et al. (1994) Anticardiolipin antibodies in autoimmune thyroid diseases. Clin Endocrinol (Oxf) 40: 329–33.
74. Nabriski D, Ellis M, Ness-Abramof R, Shapiro M, Shenkman L (2000) Autoimmune thyroid disease and antiphospholipid antibodies. Am J Hematol 64: 73–5.
75. Díez JJ, Doforno RA, Iglesias P, Sastre J, Gómez-Pan A, et al. (1993) Anticardiolipin antibodies in autoimmune thyroid disease. J Clin Lab Immunol 40: 125–34.
76. Osundeko O, Hasinski S, Rose LI (2001) Anticardiolipin antibodies in Hashimoto's disease. Endocr Pract 7: 181–3.
77. Assous N, Allanore Y, Batteux F, Meune C, Toulon P, et al. (2005) Prevalence of antiphospholipid antibodies in systemic sclerosis and association with primitive pulmonary arterial hypertension and endothelial injury. Clin Exp Rheumatol 23: 199–204.
78. Herrick AL, Heaney M, Hollis S, Jayson MI (1994) Anticardiolipin, anticentromere and anti-Scl-70 antibodies in patients with systemic sclerosis and severe digital ischaemia. Ann Rheum Dis 53: 540–2.
79. Enzenauer RJ, Collier DH, Lopez LR (2006) Anticardiolipin antibodies in scleroderma. J Clin Rheumatol 12: 324–6.
80. Sato S, Fujimoto M, Hasegawa M, Takehara K (2003) Antiphospholipid antibody in localised scleroderma. Ann Rheum Dis 62: 771–4.
81. Touré AO, Ly F, Sall A, Diatta A, Gadji M, et al. (2013) Antiphospholipid antibodies and systemic scleroderma. Turkish J Haematol 30: 32–6.
82. Picillo U, Migliaresi S, Marcialis MR, Ferruzzi AM, Tirri G (1997) Clinical setting of patients with systemic sclerosis by serum autoantibodies. Clin Rheumatol 16: 378–83.
83. Gupta R, Thabah MM, Gupta S, Shankar S, Kumar A (2009) Clinical significance of antiphospholipid antibodies in Indian scleroderma patients. Rheumatol Int 30: 277–9.
84. Rees JD, Lança S, Marques PV, Gómez-Puerta JA, Moco R, et al. (2006) Prevalence of the antiphospholipid syndrome in primary systemic vasculitis. Ann Rheum Dis 65: 109–11.
85. Sherer Y, Livneh A, Levy Y, Shoenfeld Y, Langevitz P (2000) Dermatomyositis and polymyositis associated with the antiphospholipid syndrome-a novel overlap syndrome. Lupus 9: 42–6.
86. Merkel PA, Chang Y, Pierangeli SS, Convery K, Harris EN, et al. (1996) The prevalence and clinical associations of anticardiolipin antibodies in a large inception cohort of patients with connective tissue diseases. Am J Med 101: 576–83.
87. Efe C, Wahlin S, Ozaslan E, Berlot AH, Purnak T, et al. (2012) Autoimmune hepatitis/primary biliary cirrhosis overlap syndrome and associated extrahepatic autoimmune diseases. Eur J Gastroenterol Hepatol 24: 531–4.
88. Zachou K, Liaskos C, Rigopoulou E, Gabeta S, Papamichalis P, et al. (2006) Presence of high avidity anticardiolipin antibodies in patients with autoimmune cholestatic liver diseases. Clin Immunol 119: 203–12.
89. Liaskos C, Rigopoulou E, Zachou K, Georgiadou S, Gatselis N, et al. (2005) Prevalence and clinical significance of anticardiolipin antibodies in patients with type 1 autoimmune hepatitis. J Autoimmun 24: 251–60.
90. Murthy V, Willis R, Romay-Penabad Z, Ruiz-Limón P, Martínez-Martínez LA, et al. (2013) Value of isolated IgA anti-β2 -glycoprotein I positivity in the diagnosis of the antiphospholipid syndrome. Arthritis Rheum 65: 3186–93.

21

A Non-Invasive Laboratory Panel as a Diagnostic and Prognostic Biomarker for Thrombotic Microangiopathy: Development and Application

Tao Zhang[1], Huimei Chen[1,2]*, Shaoshan Liang[1], Dacheng Chen[1], Chunxia Zheng[1], Caihong Zeng[1], Haitao Zhang[1], Zhihong Liu[1]*

1 National Clinical Research Center of Kidney Diseases, Jinling Hospital, Nanjing University School of Medicine, Nanjing 210002, P. R. China, **2** Jiangsu Key Laboratory of Molecular Medicine, Nanjing University School of Medicine, Nanjing, 210093, P. R. China

Abstract

Background: Thrombotic microangiopathy (TMA) in the kidney is a histopathologic lesion that occurs in a number of clinical settings and is often associated with poor renal prognosis. The standard test for the diagnosis of TMA is the renal biopsy; noninvasive parameters such as potential biomarkers have not been developed.

Methods: We analyzed routine parameters in a cohort of 220 patients with suspected TMA and developed a diagnostic laboratory panel by logistic regression. The levels of candidate markers were validated using an independent cohort (n = 46), a cohort of systemic lupus erythematosus (SLE) (n = 157) and an expanded cohort (n = 113), as well as 9 patients with repeat biopsies.

Results: Of the 220 patients in the derivation cohort, 51 patients with biopsy-proven TMA presented with a worse renal prognosis than those with no TMA (P = 0.002). Platelet and L-lactate dehydrogenase (LDH) levels showed an acceptable diagnostic value of TMA (AUC = 0.739 and 0.756, respectively). A panel of 4 variables - creatinine, platelets, ADAMTS13 (a disintegrin and metalloprotease with thrombospondin type 1 repeats 13) activity and LDH - can effectively discriminate patients with TMA (AUC = 0.800). In the validation cohort, the platelet and LDH levels and the 4-variable panel signature robustly distinguished patients with TMA. The discrimination effects of these three markers were confirmed in patients with SLE. Moreover, LDH levels and the 4-variable panel signature also showed discrimination values in an expanded set. Among patients undergoing repeat biopsy, increased LDH levels and panel signatures were associated with TMA status when paired evaluations were performed. Importantly, only the 4-variable panel was an independent prognostic marker for renal outcome (hazard ratio = 3.549; P<0.001).

Conclusions: The noninvasive laboratory diagnostic panel is better for the early detection and prognosis of TMA compared with a single parameter, and may provide a promising biomarker for clinical application.

Editor: Nancy Lan Guo, West Virginia University, United States of America

Funding: This work was supported in part by National Basic Research Program of China 973 Program No.2012CB517600 (No.2012CB517606) (to Z.L.)(http://www.973.gov.cn/AreaMana.aspx), National Natural Science Foundation (NSF) Grant 81370788 (to H.C.) (http://www.nsfc.gov.cn/), The National Key Technology R&D Program (2011BAI10B04) (to Z.L.) (http://kjzc.jhgl.org/) and Six Talent Peaks Project of Jiangsu Province (2012-WSN-071) (to H.C.) (http://archives.nuist.edu.cn/rcgf/). The funders had no role in study design, data collection and analysis, decision to publish, or preparation of the manuscript.

Competing Interests: The authors have declared that no competing interests exist.

* Email: chenhuimei@nju.edu.cn (HC); liuzhihong@nju.edu.cn (ZL)

Introduction

Thrombotic microangiopathy (TMA) is a pathological lesion that results in thrombosis in capillaries and arterioles, due to an endothelial injury [1–3]. TMA lesions in the kidney usually present in two different forms with considerable overlap: (1) glomerular involvement with capillary thrombi, capillary loops with double contours and mesangiolysis with microhemorrhage, that is most frequently seen in patients with hemolytic uremic syndrome; or (2) predominant arteriolar involvement with thrombi and fibrinoid necrosis, particularly in thrombotic thrombocytopenic purpura and malignant hypertension [4,5].

TMA lesions occur in a number of other kidney diseases as well, including IgA nephropathy, systemic lupus erythematosus (SLE), antiphospholipid antibody syndrome, systemic sclerosis, pre-eclampsia, infections, medications and post transplantation [2,6,7]. The presence of TMA in the kidney has been proven to be associated with poor renal prognosis [8,9]. Nephrologists often face a typical situation in which patients are suspected of having TMA lesions on the basis of renal disorders. In such cases, it is difficult to decide on an early therapy before the results of a renal biopsy are obtained [10]. While the interpretation of the renal biopsy has become more standardized and the invasive procedure safer over time, bleeding and subsequent functional impairment nevertheless still occur, especially in the patients with coagulopathy [11].

Heterogeneous disorders with TMA are usually characterized by microangiopathic hemolytic anemia (MAHA) [12], thrombocytopenia and/or ischemic organ failure. It is questionable as to whether these abnormalities can predict TMA, since they are also observed in patients without TMA, and studies have been inconsistent [13,14]. Hence, we enrolled cohorts of patients with renal damage and MAHA and/or thrombocytopenia to determine whether a single parameter or a diagnostic panel could predict the histological TMA. In addition, the association between the noninvasive prediction and a poor renal outcome was further investigated.

Methods

Ethics statement

The study was approved by the Ethics Committee of Jinling Hospital. Because this study was retrospective, the Ethics Committee agreed to waive the requirement for the informed consent, and the data were analyzed anonymously.

Patient selection and study design

We enrolled a cohort of suspected patients from the Research Institute of Nephrology, Jinling Hospital, Nanjing University School of Medicine, PR China during July 2011 to July 2012 (n = 266). The enrollment criteria were: renal damage (proteinuria, hematuria or renal dysfunction) and microangiopathic hemolytic anemia (hemoglobin level below 120 g/L for males, 110 g/L for females, at least 5 schistocytes per high power field in a peripheral blood smear, elevated LDH above 240 u/L [normal 60–240 u/L]) or thrombocytopenia (platelet counts below 100×10^9/L of blood at any time in the course of the disease) [15]. Patients were randomly divided into two cohorts: (1) derivation cohort (n = 220) and (2) validation cohort (n = 46).

In addition, 157 patients diagnosed with SLE were selected from the suspected patients, and 113 patients were enrolled in an expanded group for external validation. SLE was defined according to the 1997 American College of Rheumatology revised criteria for SLE [16]. The independent patients were enrolled in the expanded group according to the criteria: (1) renal damage (proteinuria, hematuria or renal dysfunction) and (2) fever (temperature of >38°C, no infection), elevated LDH (more than 240 u/L) or non-renal anemia. The information and profiles of patients during the follow-up sessions were also reviewed through October 2013.

Definitions

TMA in the kidney was defined by the histologic feature of occlusive fibrin-platelet thrombi in at least one glomerulus or one arteriole, with one or more of the following: (1) glomerular endothelial swelling and detachment, capillary wall thickening and double contour formation, mesangial lysis with microhemorrhage, and erythrocytolysis, and/or (2) obliterative arteriolopathy defined as luminal occlusion with mural myxoid or fibrinoid change, thickening of the vessel wall, with or without erythrocytolysis, luminal thrombosis and concentric spindle cell proliferation or hypercellularity [2,5].

All patients accepted adjunctive treatments, including protecting the organ function, symptomatic and immunosuppressive treatment. Glomerularfiltration rate was estimated (eGFR) using the simplified MDRD (Modification of Diet in Renal Disease) formula. End stage renal disease (ESRD) was defined as eGFR< 15 mL/min/1.73 m^2 or a need for permanent dialysis therapy. During follow-up, the combined event defined as ESRD or a doubling of the serum creatinine level and death. The renal survival rate was defined as the percentage of patients who had preservation of renal function independent of ESRD and death, while the survival rate was defined as the percentage of live patients.

Laboratory features

Physical exams and routine laboratory tests were performed on the suspected patients. Serum ADAMTS13 activity was measured by the Fluorescence Resonance Energy Transfer (FRET) assay (United States Patent No.7270976) [17]. Serum anti-ADAMTS13 IgG antibodies (Sekisui Diagnostics, USA), vWF (von Willebrand factor) (Sunbiote, Shanghai, China), thrombomodulin (Diaclone Research, Besancon, France), E-selectin (R&D Systems, Minneapolis, Minnesota, USA) and soluble vascular cellular adhesion molecule-1 (sVCAM-1, VCAM) (R&D Systems, Minneapolis, Minnesota, USA) were measured using enzyme linked immunosorbent assays. The concentrations of endothelial cells in the circulation were sorted using a magnetic microbead sorting system (MACS, Miltenyi Biotec, Germany), according to the manufacturer's instructions [18].

Statistical analysis

All data were given a numerical code and statistical analysis was performed using SPSS software, version 19.0 or RMS software, version 2.12.2. Comparisons of proportions or mean values between patients with or without TMA in the kidney were calculated by the Mann-Whitney test or chi-square ($\chi2$) test.

Logistic regression was used to identify 6 parameters - hemoglobin, platelets, serum creatinine, LDH, ADAMTS13 activity and THBD - that discriminated between patients with and without TMA in the kidney. Regression estimated from this panel defined a diagnostic signature or individual predictors, and the greatest area under the receiver-operating-characteristic (ROC) curve as the best-fitting model was used. The area under the curve (AUC) was calculated, and sensitivity and specificity were used to evaluate the ability of these to discriminate TMA in the kidney. The best sub-set panel was then fit to 1000 additional bootstrap samples. Cross-validated measures of discrimination (i.e., the AUC), model fit (i.e., calibration-curve intercept and slope) and a locally estimated scatterplot-smoothed (loess) calibration plot were obtained [19].

Cumulative incidence of poor renal outcome was calculated using Kaplan-Meier survival probabilities (1- survival probabilities) and comparisons were made using the log-rank test. Cox regression was performed to test the association of the pathologic findings and the 4-variable panel signature with the renal outcome. A two-tailed P value less than 0.05 is considered to be statistically significant.

Results

In the derivation cohort of 220 patients, 51 (23.2%) patients were histologically proven to have TMA by renal biopsy. Compared with patients without TMA, the patients with TMA presented a worse renal outcome (P = 0.002, log-rank test; Figure 1) at the 12-month follow-up, with a renal survival rate of 54.9% (P = 0.015; Table 1).

Correlation between laboratory parameters and TMA lesions

The levels of serum creatinine, LDH and thrombomodulin (THBD) were significantly higher in patients with TMA than those

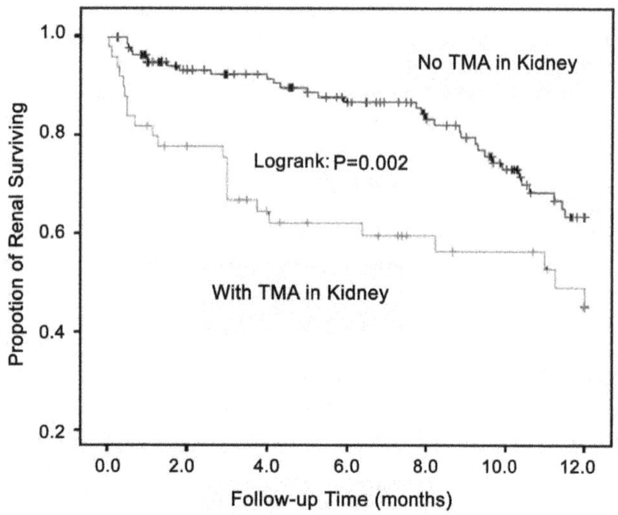

Figure 1. Comparison of renal outcome in suspected patients. After 12 months of follow-up, the patients with TMA had a worse outcome of renal survival than those without TMA (Log rank: P = 0.002).

without TMA, while levels of hemoglobin, platelets and ADAMTS13 activity were remarkably lower (all $P<0.05$; Table 1). With a cutoff of 0.05 (P value, in Table 1), 6 laboratory parameters were included in the next binary logistic regression analysis. The ROC curve showed that these 6 parameters individually can distinguish patients with TMA in the derivation set (all $P<0.05$; Figure 2A). Only the platelet and LDH levels showed acceptable discrimination values ($0.7\leq AUC<0.8$), while levels of hemoglobin, serum creatinine, ADAMSTS13 activity and THBD had low discrimination accuracy ($0.5\leq AUC<0.7$). With the use of the cutoff point of 97.5×10^9/L, platelets had 82.4% sensitivity and 60.9% specificity, and with the cutoff point of 289 u/L, LDH had 67.3% sensitivity and 74.1% specificity (Table S1 in File S1).

In an independent validation cohort, platelet and LDH levels also could discriminate patients with TMA from those without TMA (Figure 2B; Table S2 in File S1). Thus, the levels of platelets and LDH showed acceptable predictive probabilities of patients with TMA in the kidney.

Correlation between the 4-variable panel and TMA lesions

Furthermore, multiple logistic regression analysis in the derivation set indicated that levels of serum creatinine (SCr), platelets (PLT), LDH and ADAMTS13 activity were valid predictors of renal TMA lesions (all $P<0.05$; Table 2), with the final panel signature:

$$-0.371-0.002\times \text{ADAMTS13activity}$$
$$+0.140\times \text{SCr}+0.004\times \text{LDH}-0.010\times \text{PLT}$$

The units of measurement are as listed in Table 1. In the equation, −0.371 was the intercept, and −0.002, 0.140, 0.004 and −0.010 were the slopes (coefficients), respectively, for the ADAMTS13 activity, SCr (mg/dL), LDH and PLT values in the best-fitting logistic-regression model. The intercept and slopes have no intrinsic units of measurement.

The ROC curve showed that this 4-variable model yielded an AUC of 0.800 (95% confidence interval [CI], 0.723 to 0.877; $P<0.001$), suggesting a good discrimination between patients with TMA in the kidney and those without TMA (Figure 3A). With the use of the cutoff point of 0.248, this diagnostic panel has 81.6% sensitivity and 66.9% specificity. The diagnostic panel for the prediction of TMA was validated in the independent cohort, with an AUC of 0.815 ($P<0.001$; Figure 3B). The use of the cut-off of 0.248 predicted the presence of TMA with 80.0% sensitivity and 61.5% specificity.

Bootstrap validation of this 4-variable panel yielded a cross-validated estimate of the AUC of 0.777, which is an estimate of the expected value of the AUC in the combined derivation and validation cohorts. The calibration-curve intercept and slope were 0.07 and 0.64, respectively. It was revealed that the predicted probabilities of a biopsy showing TMA in the kidney tended to be relatively higher than the actual probabilities (Figure 3C). The loess-smoothed estimates of the unadjusted and cross-validated calibration curves were overlaid on a diagonal reference line representing good model calibration ($P=0.489$). The close correspondence of the two curves to the reference line shows good fit and reflects the above interpretation of the intercept and slope estimates of the calibration curve (Figure 3C).

Evaluation of LDH, platelet and the 4- variable panel in extra cohorts

Since renal TMA lesions occur in a number of kidney diseases, we focused on a specific condition and 157 renal patients diagnosed with SLE were selected in extra validation (Table S3 in File S1). All levels of platelets, LDH and the 4-variable panel could discriminate patients with TMA in SLE. The ability of discrimination in the 4-variable panel was higher than the levels of platelets and LDH, with an AUC of 0.872 (Figure 4A). With the use of the cutoff point of 0.248, the diagnostic panel has 74.1% sensitivity and 83.6% specificity.

To further enhance the application of these markers, we enrolled another independent group of 113 patients and determined the association between the levels of LDH, platelets and the 4-variable panel and TMA lesions (Table S4 in File S1). ROC curve analysis showed that the levels of LDH and the 4-variable panel yielded an AUC of 0.843 and 0.825, showing a good discrimination of TMA (both $P<0.001$; Figure 4B). However, platelet levels could not predict patients with TMA lesions in this cohort ($P=0.068$).

Evaluation of LDH and the 4-variable panel in patients with repeat biopsy

We then analyzed, in a subset of 9 patients who underwent repeat renal biopsy, levels of LDH and the 4-variable panel in paired blood samples taken at the time of the first and second biopsy (Table S5 in File S1). It is interesting to note that the 4-variable panel signature plummeted from 0.248 or higher in the same subset of patients when they presented with TMA at the first biopsy, but with no TMA at second biopsy (Figure 5A). On the contrary, for the only patient who had no TMA at first biopsy but exhibited TMA at the second biopsy, the 4-variable panel dramatically increased to greater than 0.248. For the other 5 patients, the 4-variable signature was significantly decreased after treatment ($P=0.030$), although they each presented without TMA at the two biopsies and the signature was 0.248 or less.

A similar pattern of LDH changes were observed in the patients with repeat biopsy, and increased LDH levels were associated with TMA status (Figure 5B). However, an LDH value of 289 u/L was

Table 1. Clinical laboratory data for suspected patients in derivation cohort (n = 220).

	TMA	No TMA	P Value
Number of patients	**51**	**169**	
Age (year)	26 (963)	28 (1370)	0.450
Male (n, %)	10 (19.6)	45 (26.6)	0.310
Clinical diagnosis			
HUS/TTP (n, %)	15 (29.4)	0 (0)	<0.001
Primary glomerulonephritis & acute interstitial nephritis (n, %)	0 (0)	22 (13.0)	0.003
Autoimmune diseases (n, %)	29 (56.9)	144 (85.2)	<0.001
SLE (n, %)	27/29 (93.1)	130/144 (90.3)	1.000
Pregnancy/postpartum (n, %)	5 (9.8)	1 (0.6)	0.003
Malignant hypertension (n, %)	1 (2.0)	0 (0)	0.232
Post-transplantation (n, %)	1 (2.0)	2 (1.2)	0.549
Laboratory profiles			
Urine protein (g/24 h)	1.5 (0.310.6)	2.5 (0.29.8)	0.073
Erythrocyturia ($\times10^4$/mL)	18 (110000)	24 (19000)	0.364
Hemoglobin (g/L)	74.2±16.1	87.1±21.6	<0.001
Platelets ($\times10^9$/L)	73 (10275)	108 (34441)	<0.001
Serum creatinine (umol/L)	347.2 (52.21697.5)	162.7 (33.61556.0)	<0.001
Globulin (g/L)	22.0±5.7	23.3±6.6	0.289
C3 (g/L)	0.62±0.29	0.57±0.30	0.219
C4 (g/L)	0.16±0.10	0.14±0.10	0.098
L-lactate dehydrogenase (u/L)	418 (1292920)	267 (64878)	<0.001
ADAMTS13 antibody (Au/mL)	16.6 (2.184.9)	16.6 (1.681.3)	0.862
ADAMTS13 activity (ng/mL)	616±331	772±255	0.001
NEC (/ml)	19.7±6.8	20.7±8.9	0.654
E-selectin (ng/mL)	65.2±37.3	73.1±72.8	0.636
VCAM (ng/mL)	2011±1070	2460±1340	0.073
Thrombomodulin (ng/mL)	6.3±4.3	4.4±2.8	<0.001
vWF (%)	184±127	215±120	0.080
After 12-months of follow up			
Renal survival rate (%)	54.9 (28/51)	74.6 (126/169)	0.015
Survival rate (%)	94.1 (48/51)	98.2 (166/169)	0.138

Values are expressed as medians (range), means ± standard deviation or percentages. *P* values were calculated by Mann-Whitney U test, Fisher's exact test or chi-square test as appropriate. HUS: hemolytic uremic syndrome; TTP: thrombotic thrombocytopenic purpura; SLE: systemic lupus erythematosus; C3: Complement component 3; C4: Complement component 4; ADAMTS13: A Disintegrin and Metalloprotease with ThromboSpondin type 1 repeats 13; NEC: normal endothelial cells; VCAM: vascular cell adhesion molecule; vWF: von Willebrand factor.

not a good cut-off level to discriminate TMA status in this group of patients.

Association of LDH levels and the 4-variable panel with renal survival

To further evaluate whether LDH levels and the 4-variable panel can serve as a predictor of renal survival in patients with suspected TMA, we performed a Kaplan-Meier survival analysis. As suspected, patients with a higher 4-variable panel signature had a statistically significant worse renal outcome (P<0.001, log-rank test; Figure 6A). However, the pattern of increased LDH concentrations was not associated with a poorer renal outcome (P = 0.183, log-rank test; Figure 6B).

Furthermore, the renal survival was only 53.9% in patients with a panel signature of more than 0.248, but was 79.5% in patients with a panel signature of less than 0.248. The Cox proportional hazard survival regression model revealed that TMA lesions increased the risk for a poor renal outcome, with a hazard ratio of 2.235 (95% CI 1.306 to 3.826, P = 0.003), while a panel signature 0.248 or greater had a hazard ratio of 3.549 (95% CI 2.034 to 3.549, P<0.001). These two diagnostic factors showed a similar predictive effect on renal outcome (P = 0.964).

Discussion

Histological TMA in the kidney has been frequently described in association with a large number of underlying diseases [20–22]. Although the causes of TMA in the kidney are unclear, it has been reported that there is a significantly worse renal outcome among patients with TMA [16,22]. Kaplan et al. [23] reported that death rates were as high as 25% and progression to ESRD occurred in half of the patients with TMA within 10 years after diagnosis. In agreement with published studies [24], we confirmed that patients

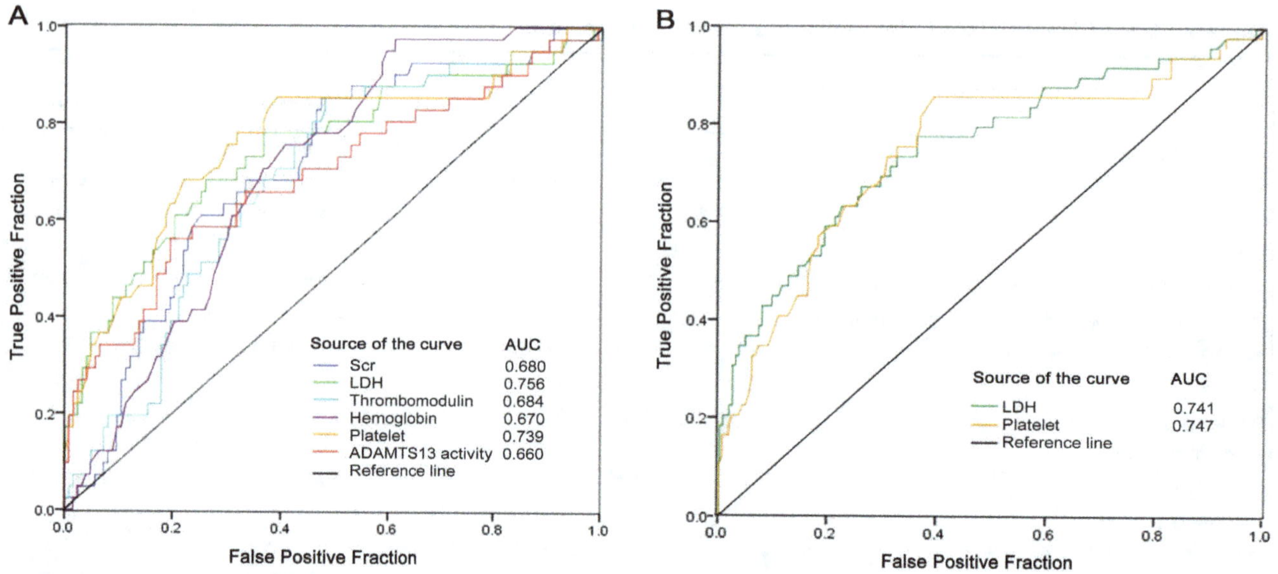

Figure 2. Receiver operating characteristic curves of laboratory parameters. (A) The fraction of true positive results (sensitivity) and the fraction of false positive results (1-specificity) for LDH, HGB, SCr, PLT, THBD and ADAMTS13 activity were developed in 220 patients (all P≤0.001), and the levels of platelet and LDH showed acceptable discrimination, with AUC 0.739 and 0.756, respectively. (B) The levels of platelet and LDH could discriminate patients with TMA from those with no TMA in the validation cohort (n = 46), with AUC 0.747 and 0.741, respectively.

with renal biopsy-proven TMA presented with a poor outcome in the kidney and the patients with TMA had a 2.24-fold higher risk of renal failure than those without TMA.

The renal biopsy represents the gold standard in the management of patients with TMA, but a noninvasive diagnostic method for detection of TMA would be a valuable clinical application. Few studies have focused on the prediction of the histopathologic lesions, although abnormalities in the urinalysis and an increase in serum creatinine have been observed in patients with TMA lesions [25]. In addition, reports have demonstrated that laboratory variables were involved in clinical conditions associated with TMA [26–28], including hemolytic uremic syndrome and thrombotic thrombocytopenic purpura. Increased levels of LDH are associated with the severity of hemolysis and tissue ischemia, which might increase the risk of tissue lesions [29]. A deficiency of ADAMTS13 was related to thrombus formation and was subsequently noted in patients with thrombocytopenic purpura, who often suffered from TMA lesions in the kidney [30,31].

This study is the first to demonstrate the potential of routine laboratory parameters to be used in the detection of TMA without renal biopsy. Six parameters - serum creatinine, platelets, hemoglobin, THBD, ADAMTS13 activity and LDH - had moderate diagnostic value for TMA. The strengths of this study are that we developed a diagnostic panel based on 4 laboratory variables (levels of serum creatinine, LDH, platelets and ADAMTS13 activity). This panel can noninvasively and accurately predict histological TMA. This is supported by the high AUC values of 0.800 derived from patients with and without TMA (sensitivity 81.6%; specificity 66.9%). Similar effects were noted when the predictive panel was validated using an independent population. The cross-validation further revealed that the 4-variable model tended to have high sensitivity, but a relatively low specificity. To the best of our knowledge, this is the first noninvasive biomarker that can detect TMA in the kidney. In addition, each individual parameter of the 5 or 6 variable model could not reach statistical significance (P<0.05, data not shown). The model of fewer variables could discriminate patients with TMA in derivation cohort, including the levels of LDH and platelets, but this effect was not proven by all different validation cohorts.

The 3 markers, LDH, platelets and the 4-variable panel, were further evaluated in a group of patients with SLE and expanded sets of patients. SLE is often reported with TMA lesions in the kidney [6,22], and there were 157 patients diagnosed with SLE

Table 2. Results of logistic regression analysis (n = 220).

Variable	B	S.E	Sig.	Exp (B)	95% CI
					Lower-Upper
Serum creatinine	0.140	0.060	0.020	1.150	1.022–1.295
LDH	0.004	0.001	0.002	1.004	1.001–1.006
Platelet	−0.010	0.004	0.021	0.990	0.981–0.998
ADAMTS 13 Activity	−0.002	0.001	0.014	0.998	0.996–1.000

Abbreviations: B: coefficient of regression; S.E.: Standard Error; Sig: P value; Exp (B): odds ratio; CI: confidence interval. LDH: L-lactate dehydrogenase; ADAMTS 13: a disintegrin and metalloprotease with thrombospondin type 1 repeats 13.

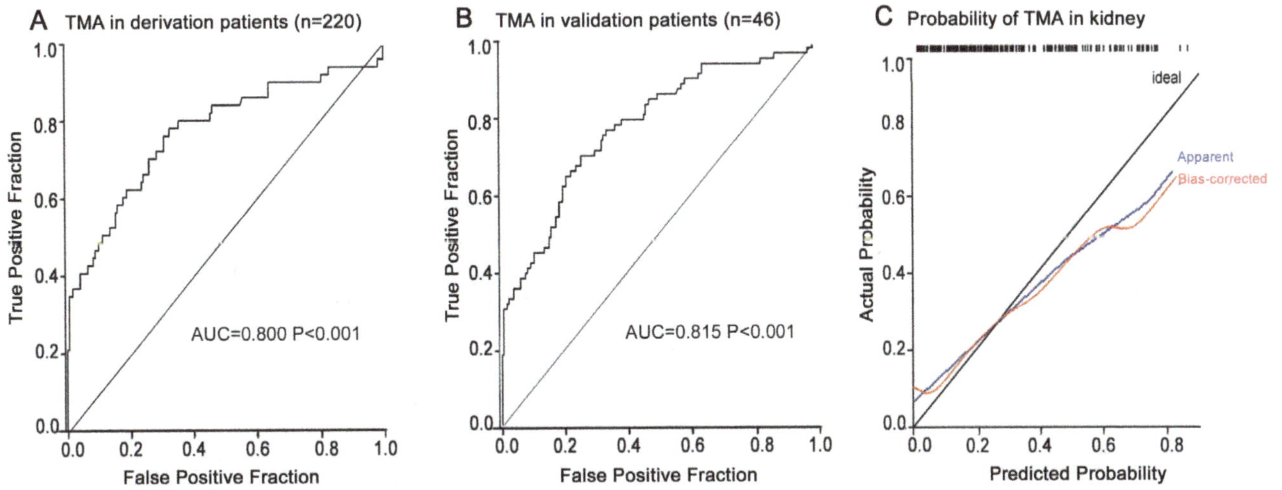

Figure 3. Receiver operating characteristic curves and calibration curve for a diagnostic panel. (A) The diagnostic panel was developed in the derivation group of 220 suspected patients, with AUC 0.800, P<0.001. (B) This marker was validated in 46 independent patients, with AUC 0.815, P<0.001. (C) Bootstrap validation shows the calibration curve of the diagnostic panel. Cross-validated estimates of the AUC, calibration-curve intercept and slope were 0.777, 0.07 and 0.64, respectively. The loess-smoothed estimates of the cross-validated and unadjusted calibration curves are overlaid on a diagonal reference line representing good model calibration.

among the suspected patients investigated. Focusing on one particular disease, all 3 markers showed discrimination values for patients with TMA. Because some patients with TMA exhibit little or no signs of clinical manifestations [31–33], we expanded the application of these markers. LDH levels and the 4-variable panel still demonstrated good discrimination, while platelets did not. Thus, LDH levels and the 4-variable panel might have wide usage in different cohorts of patients. In addition, data from patients with a repeat biopsy confirmed the association of increased LDH levels and the 4-variable signature with TMA status.

Another important finding of our study was that the 4-variable panel also serves as a prognostic biomarker for renal patients. The increased signature of the 4-variable panel was an independent prognostic parameter. The prognostic value of the 4-variable panel was similar with the histological diagnosis of TMA. As a noninvasive biomarker, the 4-variable panel showed an advantage in clinical application. However, LDH levels did not exhibit a prognostic value for renal outcome. Therefore, the 4-variable panel might not only diagnose TMA but also help predict renal

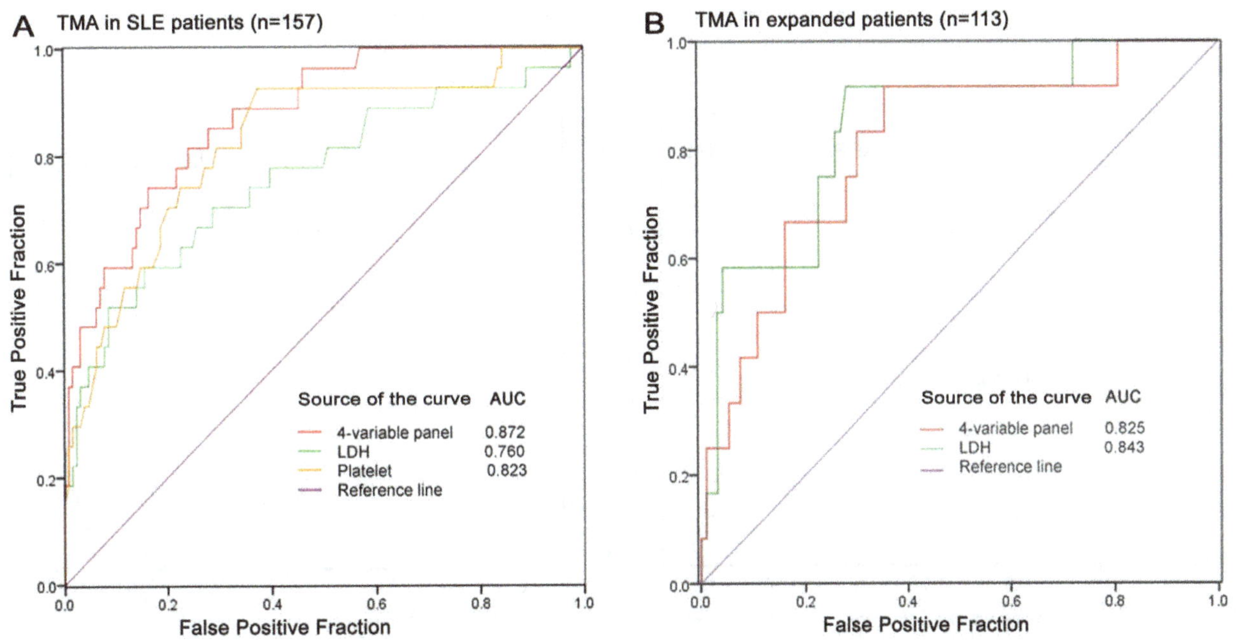

Figure 4. Evaluation of LDH, platelet and 4-variable panel in extra cohorts. (A) All levels of platelet, LDH and the 4-variable panel were evaluated in 157 suspected patients diagnosed with SLE and could discriminate patients with TMA, with an AUC of 0.823, 0.76 and 0.872, respectively. (B) To further validate in another independent group of 113 patients and ROC curve analysis showed that the levels of LDH and the 4-variable panel yielded an AUC of 0.843 and 0.825, showing an good discrimination of TMA (both P<0.001).

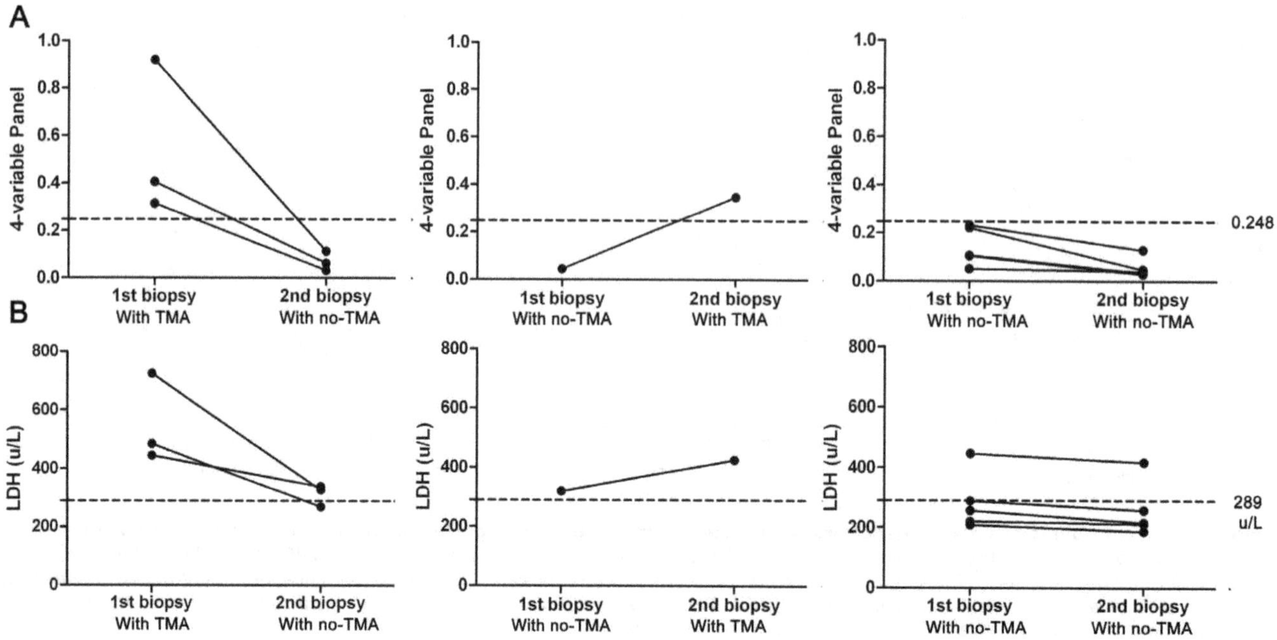

Figure 5. Evaluation of LDH and 4-variable panel in patients with repeat biopsy. (A)We analyzed paired first and second levels of LDH and 4-variable panel in a subset of 9 patients, who underwent repeat renal biopsy. The first figure shows 4-variable panel signature plummeted from 0.248 or greater in the same subset of patients, when three patients presented TMA at first biopsy but no TMA at second biopsy. In the second figure, only one patient had no TMA at first biopsy and TMA at second biopsy and 4-variable panel dramatically increased to 0.348. For other 5 patients, 4-variable signature was significantly decreased after treatment, although they consistently presented without TMA at two biopsies and the signature was 0.248 or less. (B) Similar pattern of LDH changes was observed in the patients with repeat biopsy, and increased LDH levels were associated with TMA status.

outcome with a higher accuracy than other single laboratory parameter.

Although our current assay may become a promising diagnostic tool for TMA, we acknowledge three potential limitations of this study. It is retrospective and will need to be validated with a prospective cohort of patients. Furthermore, the evaluation of prognosis was rendered difficult because of the variable nature of the treatments received. In addition, the number of patients with certain diseases was small and some validations were calculated using non-independent data, which prevented an in-depth

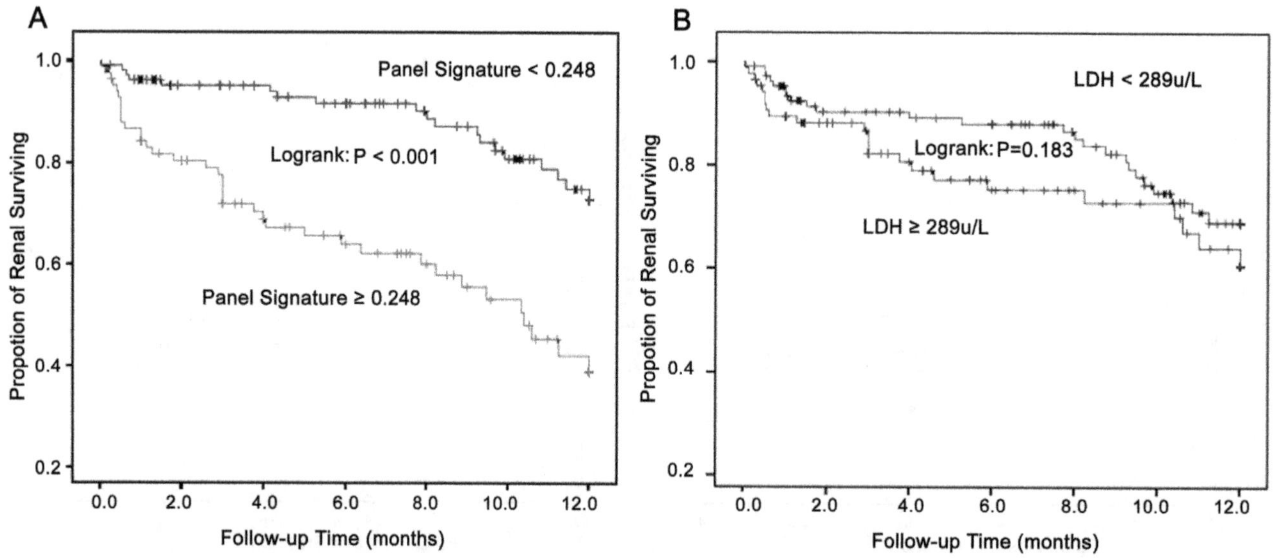

Figure 6. Association of LDH levels and 4-variable panel with renal survival. (A) Using the cutoff value of 0.248, suspected patients were divided into two groups by more or less than the value and the renal survival of two groups followed up 12 months was significantly different (P< 0.001). (B) The pattern of increased LDH concentrations (more than the cutoff point of 289 u/L) associated statistically poorer renal outcome was not observed (P = 0.183).

evaluation of the usefulness of the diagnostic panel for specifically predicting TMA in the kidney.

Conclusions

In conclusion, our results provide compelling evidence for the potential use of laboratory parameters as a noninvasive diagnostic and prognostic tool for TMA in the kidney. The 4-variable panel showed an advantage for the early detection of renal TMA lesions without renal biopsy and in directly predicting renal prognosis. In order for this concept to be incorporated into routine clinical practice in the near-future, validation is needed in large-scale prospective trials.

Supporting Information

File S1 Includes table S1–S5. **Table S1,** Diagnosis of TMA in kidney among patients (n = 220). **Table S2,** Laboratory variables in the validation group of internal patients (n = 46). **Table S3,** Clinical laboratory data for suspected patients with SLE (n = 157). **Table S4,** Clinical laboratory data for patients in expanded group (n = 113). **Table S5,** The laboratory feature of patients with/without TMA in the kidney at first renal biopsy and repeat biopsy.

Acknowledgments

We thank all the patients and their families who participated in this study.

Author Contributions

Conceived and designed the experiments: TZ HC ZL. Performed the experiments: TZ HC DC CZ SL CZ. Analyzed the data: TZ HC ZL. Contributed reagents/materials/analysis tools: DC SL HZ. Contributed to the writing of the manuscript: TZ HC ZL.

References

1. Moake JL (2002) Thrombotic microangiopathies. N Engl J Med 347: 589–600.
2. El Karoui K, Hill GS, Karras A, Jacquot C, Moulonguet L, et al. (2012) A clinicopathologic study of thrombotic microangiopathy in IgA nephropathy. J Am Soc Nephrol 23: 137–148.
3. Goldberg RJ, Nakagawa T, Johnson RJ, Thurman JM (2010) The role of endothelial cell injury in thrombotic microangiopathy. Am J Kidney Dis 56: 1168–1174.
4. van den Born BJ, van der Hoeven NV, Groot E, Lenting PJ, Meijers JC, et al. (2008) Association between thrombotic microangiopathy and reduced ADAMTS13 activity in malignant hypertension. Hypertension 51: 862–866.
5. Laurence J (2000) Pathological and therapeutic distinctions in HUS/TTP. Lancet 355: 497; author reply 497–498.
6. Hughson MD, Nadasdy T, McCarty GA, Sholer C, Min KW, et al. (1992) Renal thrombotic microangiopathy in patients with systemic lupus erythematosus and the antiphospholipid syndrome. Am J Kidney Dis 20: 150–158.
7. Eremina V, Jefferson JA, Kowalewska J, Hochster H, Haas M, et al. (2008) VEGF inhibition and renal thrombotic microangiopathy. N Engl J Med 358: 1129–1136.
8. Garg AX, Suri RS, Barrowman N, Rehman F, Matsell D, et al. (2003) Long-term renal prognosis of diarrhea-associated hemolytic uremic syndrome: a systematic review, meta-analysis, and meta-regression. JAMA 290: 1360–1370.
9. Reynolds JC, Agodoa LY, Yuan CM, Abbott KC (2003) Thrombotic microangiopathy after renal transplantation in the United States. Am J Kidney Dis 42: 1058–1068.
10. Clark WF (2012) Thrombotic microangiopathy: current knowledge and outcomes with plasma exchange. Semin Dial 25: 214–219.
11. Stiles KP, Yuan CM, Chung EM, Lyon RD, Lane JD, et al. (2000) Renal biopsy in high-risk patients with medical diseases of the kidney. Am J Kidney Dis 36: 419–433.
12. Symmers WS (1952) Thrombotic microangiopathic haemolytic anaemia (thrombotic microangiopathy). Br Med J 2: 897–903.
13. George JN, Vesely SK, James JA (2007) Overlapping features of thrombotic thrombocytopenic purpura and systemic lupus erythematosus. South Med J 100: 512–514.
14. D'Angelo WA, Fries JF, Masi AT, Shulman LE (1969) Pathologic observations in systemic sclerosis (scleroderma). A study of fifty-eight autopsy cases and fifty-eight matched controls. Am J Med 46: 428–440.
15. Cataland SR, Yang SB, Witkoff L, Kraut EH, Lin S, et al. (2009) Demographic and ADAMTS13 biomarker data as predictors of early recurrences of idiopathic thrombotic thrombocytopenic purpura. Eur J Haematol 83: 559–564.
16. Hochberg MC (1997) Updating the American College of Rheumatology revised criteria for the classification of systemic lupus erythematosus. Arthritis Rheum 40: 1725.
17. Peng J, Gong L, Si K, Bai X, Du G (2011) Fluorescence resonance energy transfer assay for high-throughput screening of ADAMTS1 inhibitors. Molecules 16: 10709–10721.
18. White LE, Cui Y, Shelak CM, Lie ML, Hassoun HT (2012) Lung endothelial cell apoptosis during ischemic acute kidney injury. Shock 38: 320–327.
19. Austin PC, Tu JV (2004) Bootstrap methods for developing predictive models. Am Stat 58: 131–137.
20. Baliga RS, Wingo CS (2003) Quinine induced HUS-TTP: an unusual presentation. Am J Med Sci 326: 378–380.
21. Noris M, Remuzzi G (2010) Thrombotic microangiopathy after kidney transplantation. Am J Transplant 10: 1517–1523.
22. Hu WX, Liu ZZ, Chen HP, Zhang HT, Li LS, et al. (2010) Clinical characteristics and prognosis of diffuse proliferative lupus nephritis with thrombotic microangiopathy. Lupus 19: 1591–1598.
23. Kaplan B, Meier-Kriesche HU (2002) Death after graft loss: an important late study endpoint in kidney transplantation. Am J Transplant 2: 970–974.
24. Michael M, Elliott EJ, Craig JC, Ridley G, Hodson EM (2009) Interventions for hemolytic uremic syndrome and thrombotic thrombocytopenic purpura: a systematic review of randomized controlled trials. Am J Kidney Dis 53: 259–272.
25. Droz D, Nochy D, Noel LH, Heudes D, Nabarra B, et al. (2000) Thrombotic microangiopathies: renal and extrarenal lesions. Adv Nephrol Necker Hosp 30: 235–259.
26. Vesely SK, George JN, Lammle B, Studt JD, Alberio L, et al. (2003) ADAMTS13 activity in thrombotic thrombocytopenic purpura-hemolytic uremic syndrome: relation to presenting features and clinical outcomes in a prospective cohort of 142 patients. Blood 102: 60–68.
27. Park YA, Waldrum MR, Marques MB (2010) Platelet count and prothrombin time help distinguish thrombotic thrombocytopenic purpura-hemolytic uremic syndrome from disseminated intravascular coagulation in adults. Am J Clin Pathol 133: 460–465.
28. Cataland SR, Yang S, Wu HM (2012) The use of ADAMTS13 activity, platelet count, and serum creatinine to differentiate acquired thrombotic thrombocytopenic purpura from other thrombotic microangiopathies. Br J Haematol 157: 501–503.
29. Cohen JA, Brecher ME, Bandarenko N (1998) Cellular source of serum lactate dehydrogenase elevation in patients with thrombotic thrombocytopenic purpura. J Clin Apher 13: 16–19.
30. Furlan M, Robles R, Solenthaler M, Wassmer M, Sandoz P, et al. (1997) Deficient activity of von Willebrand factor-cleaving protease in chronic relapsing thrombotic thrombocytopenic purpura. Blood 89: 3097–3103.
31. Galbusera M, Noris M, Rossi C, Orisio S, Caprioli J, et al. (1999) Increased fragmentation of von Willebrand factor, due to abnormal cleavage of the subunit, parallels disease activity in recurrent hemolytic uremic syndrome and thrombotic thrombocytopenic purpura and discloses predisposition in families. The Italian Registry of Familial and Recurrent HUS/TTP. Blood 94: 610–620.
32. George JN (2006) Clinical practice. Thrombotic thrombocytopenic purpura. N Engl J Med 354: 1927–1935.
33. Hastings MC, Wyatt RJ, Ault BH, Jones DP, Lau KK, et al. (2007) Diagnosis of de novo localized thrombotic microangiopathy by surveillance biopsy. Pediatr Nephrol 22: 742–746.

22

Association between Polymorphisms of the IKZF3 Gene and Systemic Lupus Erythematosus in a Chinese Han Population

Xinze Cai[1,2], Ying Qiao[1], Cheng Diao[1], Xiaoxue Xu[1], Yang Chen[1], Shuyan Du[1], Xudong Liu[1], Nan Liu[1], Shuang Yu[1], Dong Chen[1], Yi Jiang[1,2,3]*

1 Central Laboratory, First Affiliated Hospital of China Medical University, Shenyang, China, **2** Department of Immunology, College of Basic Medical Sciences, China Medical University, Shenyang, China, **3** Department of Dermatology, First Affiliated Hospital of China Medical University, Shenyang, China

Abstract

Objective: It has been reported that IKAROS family of zinc finger 3 (IKZF3)-deficient mice spontaneously develop human systemic lupus erythematosus (SLE)-like phenotypes and produce anti-dsDNA Ab leading to immune complex-mediated glomerulonephritis. Polymorphism of the IKZF3 gene corresponds with the susceptibility to several immune-related diseases. Our intention was to establish an association between polymorphisms in the IKZF3 gene and SLE in the Chinese Han population.

Methods: The study involved obtaining blood samples for DNA extraction and genotyping the 4 selected single-nucleotide polymorphisms (SNPs) in IKZF3, including rs12150079, rs9909593, rs907091, and rs2872507, by performing PCR restriction fragment length polymorphism analysis (PCR-RFLP). A group of 366 SLE patients were compared to 455 healthy controls.

Results: A significant decrease in frequencies of the rs907091 CC genotype and C allele appeared in the SLE patients unlike that observed in the controls ($p = 0.001$ and 0.015, respectively). The frequencies of the rs12150079 genotype and allele were different between the SLE patients and the control individuals, although the significance was only marginal ($p = 0.046$ and 0.049, respectively). In addition, a significantly low frequency of the GGCG haplotype was observed in the SLE patients, suggesting that it may provide protection against SLE ($p = 0.011$).

Conclusion: To the best of our knowledge, this is the first study to demonstrate an important association between polymorphisms in IKZF3 and SLE in the Chinese Han population. A strong association between rs907091 in the IKZF3 gene and SLE was identified.

Editor: Frederic Rieux-Laucat, Pavillon Kirmisson, France

Funding: The work was supported by a grant from the National Natural Science Foundation of China (No. 30571701; 30600541; 81401330). The funders had no role in study design, data collection and analysis, decision to publish, or preparation of the manuscript.

Competing Interests: The authors have declared that no competing interests exist.

* Email: xzcai@mail.cmu.edu.cn

Introduction

Systemic lupus erythematosus (SLE) is a chronic autoimmune disease with a wide spectrum of manifestations and severity. [1] Disease incidence is roughly 5.2 individuals per 100,000 persons per year and a higher incidence of SLE is seen among females, with a gender bias of roughly 9:1. [2] The disease is caused by dysregulation of T cell responses and B cell activation, and is characterized by the formation of immune complexes which usually cause injuries of multiple organs and tissues such as skin, joints and kidneys. [3] Although it has been reported that SLE is affected by several factors including genetic and environmental ones, the pathogenesis of SLE has not been clarified clearly to date.

IKAROS family of zinc finger3 (IKZF3, also known as AIOLOS) encodes a zinc finger protein that is expressed at its highest levels in mature peripheral B cells and has chromatin remodeling and histone deacetylase activities through interacting with Ikaros proteins. [4,5] In the periphery of mice homozygous for IKZF3-null mutation, B cells exhibit an activated cell surface phenotype and elevated serum IgG and IgE are detected in IKZF3-deficient mice. [6] It is demonstrated that IKZF3-deficient mice spontaneously develop human SLE-like phenotypes and produce anti-dsDNA Ab leading to immune complex-mediated glomerulonephritis. [7] With the development in genetic study, several single nucleotide polymorphisms (SNPs) in IKZF3 gene have been identified as being related to the susceptibility to immune-related diseases, including rheumatoid arthritis, ankylosing spondylitis, asthma and lupus. [3,8–11] Association between SLE and variants in the region of IKZF3 has been recently identified in genome-wide association scan (GWAS) of SLE by testing a multiethnic population [11].

Therefore, in this study, we aimed to determine the association between IKZF3 polymorphisms and susceptibility to SLE in a Chinese population. In accordance with our aim, we analyzed 4 SNPs, including rs12150079, rs9909593, rs907091, and rs2872507.

Methods

Patients and Healthy Controls

366 patients with SLE diagnosed according to the criteria of the 1982 American College of Rheumatology were enrolled. [12] At the same time, 455 healthy controls without autoimmune disease or cancer were recruited, who were sex- and age-matched with the patients. The study participants were from the Chinese Han population and the age range was from 16 to 65.

Ethics Statement

The Medical Ethics Committee of the First Affiliated Hospital of China Medical University approved the study. Written informed consent was obtained from all the participants, including the guardians on behalf of the children enrolled in our study.

SNP Selection

Haplotype-tagging SNPs (tagSNPs) were selected using HapMap dbSNP (www.hapmap.ncbi.nlm.nih.gov) and Haploview (www. Broadinstitute.org/haploview/haploview), complemented by National Center for Biotechnology Information's dbSNP (www.ncbi.nlm.nih.gov/projects/SNP), using LD-based tagSNP selection with a pairwise algorithm LDSelect available in Haploview (Tagger). [13,14] A chromosomal region including IKZF3 gene and 4,000 bp upstream and 1,500 bp downstream (to capture the 5′ and 3′UTR) was searched, and all SNPs identified in Chinese Han population with a minor allele frequency (MAF) of 10% or greater were included in the algorithm. Among these tagSNPs, we selected rs12150079, rs9909593 and rs907091 as candidate SNPs. We also selected rs2872507 as a candidate SNP as it had been demonstrated earlier to be associated with RA [9].

Genotyping

Genomic DNA was extracted via the conventional phenol-chloroform extraction method. Both the quality and quantity of the extracted DNA were then determined using spectrophotometry. The IKZF3 SNPs (rs12150079, rs9909593, rs907091, and rs2872507) were analyzed by restriction fragment length polymorphism (RFLP). [15] Primers used in PCR-RFLP were: for rs12150079, 5′-CATCTGCTTGGCAGTTCA-3′ (forward) and 5′-TGTTTCTGGTTTGGTGGA-3′ (reverse); for rs9909593, 5′-GCAGGAGGATTGATTG-3′ (forward) and 5′-ATTACCGCCACATTTA-3′ (reverse); for rs907091, 5′-TGTCATTTAGATTAGGGAGA-3′ (forward) and 5′-ACATAGCCAGAGGAGAAC-3′ (reverse); for rs2872507, 5′-TTTCCAAAATAAAGCAGTTC-3′ (forward) and 5′-ATGCCTAAAAGTAGCATCAA-3′ (reverse). The restriction enzymes for the SNPs above were Tth111 I, Blp I, Msp I and Nco I respectively (New England Biolabs). Direct sequencing was performed by using randomly selected subjects to validate the accuracy of the SNP genotyping assays (20% of the cases).

Statistical analysis

Data were managed and stored using the SPSS software (version 16.0). Call rates were compared between SLE patient and control groups by the chi-square test. Hardy-Weinberg equilibrium (HWE) of the IKZF3 SNPs in the control subjects was evaluated using chi-square test. The frequencies of the alleles and genotypes were also compared between patient and control groups by the chi-square test. The odds ratio (OR) and 95% confidence intervals (95% CI) were estimated. The haplotypes comprising rs12150079, rs9909593, rs907091, and rs2872507 for each individual were assigned using the online software platform SHEsis (www.analysis2.bio-x.cn/myanalysis.php). All tests were two-tailed, and p values<0.05 were considered as statistically significant.

Results

The 4 SNP (rs12150079, rs9909593, rs907091, and rs2872507) call rates in the patients and control individuals and their HWE p-values are shown in Table 1. The genotype frequencies of 4 SNPs were in agreement with the Hardy-Weinberg equilibrium in control group (p>0.05). There was no different concerning the call rates between the SLE group and the control (p>0.05).

The results of genotypic and allelic frequency analysis for the 4 SNPs in SLE patients and controls are shown in Table 2. With respect to the frequencies of rs907091, the SLE patients and the controls exhibited a significant difference. The frequency of the rs907091 CC genotype was much lower in SLE patients than in the controls, while the frequency of the rs907091 T allele was higher in patients (p = 0.001, odds ratio (OR) 0.38, 95% CI 0.21 to 0.68; p = 0.015, odds ratio (OR) 0.78, 95% CI 0.61 to 0.95, respectively). The results also show that the frequencies of the rs12150079 genotype and allele were different between the SLE patients and the control individuals, although the significance was only marginal (p = 0.046, odds ratio (OR) 1.78, 95% CI 1.01 to 3.14; p = 0.049, odds ratio (OR) 1.25, 95% CI 1.00 to 1.57, respectively). No difference in the genotype and allele frequencies in rs9909593 and rs2872507 was observed between the SLE and the control groups (p>0.05).

The online software platform SHEsis was used to analyze the haplotype data and probabilities in Table 3. Haplotypes were constructed in both SLE and control groups and the haplotypes with frequency of >1% were built from all the four SNPs. The results show that the GGCG haplotype frequency was significantly low in the SLE patients, unlike that observed in the controls (p = 0.011, odds ratio (OR) 0.42, 95% CI 0.21 to 0.84). In addition, a higher frequency of the GGTG haplotype was observed in the SLE patients than that in the controls (p = 0.027, odds ratio (OR) 2.10, 95% CI 1.07 to 4.12). No difference was detected between the SLE patients and the control individuals with respect the other 3 haplotypes (p>0.05).

Discussion

To our knowledge, this is the first report to determine the association between IKZF3 polymorphisms (rs12150079, rs9909593, rs907091 and rs2872507) and SLE susceptibility in a Chinese Han population. We confirmed that rs907091 and rs12150079 SNPs may have a relationship with SLE. The haplotype GGCG was found to protect against SLE, whereas the haplotype GGTG was associated with susceptibility to SLE.

SLE is prototypic, systemic, autoimmune disease, characterized by a diverse array of autoantibody production, complement activation and immune-complex deposition, and shows extremely heterogeneous clinical features varying in the severity. [3,16] It appears that genetic factor is closely involved in the pathogenesis of SLE. Although the etiology of SLE remains incompletely understood, there is accumulating evidence showing the important role of IKZF3 in SLE [7,11,17].

Human IKZF3, which is mapped in chromosome 17, consists of 509 amino acid protein and forms homo or heterodimers with the

Table 1. The 4 SNP call rates in patients and control individuals and HWE p-values.

SNP	Call rate (%)		HWE p-value	
	SLE	Control	SLE	Control
rs12150079	95.6%	98.9%	0.71	0.38
rs9909593	91.8%	92.7%	0.03	0.25
rs907091	92.1%	96.0%	0.01	0.68
rs2872507	94.8%	98.5%	0.18	0.27

Ikaros proteins in T and B lymphocytes. The physiological effect of IKZF3 deficiency is an increase in B cells precursors and spontaneous production of autoantibodies. [18] It was shown that B cell dysfunction, autoantibodies production, tissue injury, and SLE development existed in IKZF3-deficient mice. [7] Recently, multiple susceptibility loci of IKZF3 was successfully identified in case-control study of SLE [11].

In the present study, we investigated the effect of 4 SNPs of the IKZF3 gene on SLE in Chinese Han population. Among the tagSNPs identified in Chinese Han population with MAF of 10% or greater, we selected rs12150079, rs9909593 and rs907091 as candidate SNPs; another polymorphism, rs2872507, was found to be associated with rheumatoid arthritis; [9] therefore, these SNPs were analyzed in our study. Considering that results on the association of gene polymorphisms with disease can be influenced by many factors, we aimed to ensure the correctness of our results. First, we selected SLE patients strictly according to the criteria of the 1982 American College of Rheumatology and excluded the ones who did not fit the criteria. [12] Second, we chose unrelated healthy individuals from the same geographic region as the controls; all the study participants were similar with respect to their age, sex and ethnicity. Finally, to verify the results of genotyping by PCR-RFLP, we repeated the sequencing of 20% of the samples. Direct sequencing was performed by using randomly selected 90 subjects (20% of the cases) to validate the accuracy of the SNP genotyping assays. Only 2 subjects failed in direct sequencing and the percentage of effective validation was close to 98% (Figure 1 and Figure 2). These approaches ensured the accuracy of the results of this study.

As stated in our study, the frequency of presence of the CC genotype and C allele of rs907091 in SLE patients ($p = 0.001$, odds ratio (OR) 0.38, 95% CI 0.21 to 0.68; $p = 0.015$, odds ratio (OR) 0.78, 95% CI 0.61 to 0.95) presented a significant decrease, suggesting a protective factor to SLE. Although the significance was only marginal, the frequency of presence of the AA genotype and A allele of rs12150079 in SLE patients ($p = 0.046$, odds ratio

Table 2. Frequencies of alleles and genotypes of IKZF3 polymorphisms in SLE patients and control individuals.

SNP	Genotype	SLE (%)	Control (%)	χ^2	P	Odds Ratio (95% CI)
	Allele	(N = 366)	(N = 455)			
rs12150079	GG	180 (51.4)	255 (56.7)			reference
	AG	140 (40.0)	172 (38.2)	1.11	0.292	1.17 (0.87–1.57)
	AA	30 (8.6)	23 (5.1)	3.99	0.046	1.78 (1.01–3.14)
	G	500 (71.4)	682 (75.8)			reference
	A	200 (28.6)	218 (24.2)	3.86	0.049	1.25 (1.00–1.57)
rs9909593	AA	123 (36.7)	175 (41.5)			reference
	AG	175 (52.2)	185 (43.8)	3.53	0.06	1.34 (0.99–1.84)
	GG	37 (11.0)	62 (14.7)	0.42	0.518	0.86 (0.54–1.37)
	A	421 (62.8)	535 (63.4)			reference
	G	249 (37.2)	309 (36.6)	0.05	0.825	0.97 (0.79–1.20)
rs907091	TT	168 (49.9)	197 (45.1)			reference
	CT	153 (45.4)	190 (43.5)	0.14	0.704	0.94 (0.70–1.27)
	CC	16 (4.7)	50 (11.4)	10.84	0.001	0.38 (0.21–0.68)
	T	489 (72.6)	584 (66.8)			reference
	C	185 (27.4)	290 (33.2)	5.87	0.015	0.76 (0.61–0.95)
rs2872507	GG	170 (49.0)	227 (50.7)			reference
	AG	153 (44.1)	177 (39.5)	0.92	0.339	1.15 (0.86–1.55)
	AA	24 (6.9)	44 (9.8)	1.35	0.245	0.73 (0.42–1.24)
	G	493 (71.0)	631 (70.4)			reference
	A	201 (29.0)	265 (29.6)	0.07	0.789	0.97 (0.78–1.21)

Table 3. Frequencies of the haplotypes formed by rs12150079, rs9909593, rs907091 and rs2872507 SNPs in SLE patients and healthy control individuals.

Haplotype	SLE (%)	Control (%)	χ2	P	Odds Ratio (95% CI)
AGCA	101.13 (16.6)	168.69 (20.7)	1.43	0.231	0.85 (0.64–1.11)
GATG	363.19 (59.7)	507.62 (62.2)	1.15	0.283	1.14 (0.90–1.44)
GGCA	38.71 (6.4)	52.68 (6.5)	0.12	0.733	1.08 (0.70 1.66)
GGCG	10.81 (1.8)	36.42 (4.5)	6.42	0.011	0.42 (0.21–0.84)
GGTG	21.03 (3.5)	14.90 (1.8)	4.89	0.027	2.10 (1.07–4.12)

(OR) 1.78, 95% CI 1.01 to 3.14; p = 0.049, odds ratio (OR) 1.25, 95% CI 1.00 to 1.57) presented a moderate increase, indicating a potential susceptibility factor to this disease. Further studies on the influence of rs12150079 variants on SLE will require genetic analysis of a very large cohort. As different populations had different genetic backgrounds, which could cause ethnic heterogeneity, the genetic analysis of multiethnic study on the 4 SNPs will still be required. FASTSNP () is a web server that allows users to efficiently identify and prioritize high-risk SNPs according to their putative functional effects. We used FastSNP to predict the function for the different variants. We found that rs12150079 SNP might be a promoter in the regulatory region and rs9909593 might be an intronic enhancer.

Haplotype analysis revealed that the haplotype GGCG conferred a reduced risk of SLE, whereas GGTG was associated with susceptibility to SLE. By analyzing the results presented in Table 2 and Table 3, it is possible that the haplotype GGCG, which provides protection to SLE, results from the rs907091 C allele. As with other studies regarding the association of gene polymorphisms in SLE, our study still has limitations. This study only investigated SLE patients from a Chinese Han population. In addition, SLE is a heterogenetic disease and the environment is very important for the disease; gene-gene and gene-environment interactions are needed to clarify the impact of the gene on SLE. [19] Therefore, further research should be carried out in a larger number of samples and include analysis of the combined effect of multiple loci other than one single SNP or a single gene. Function analysis of the gene and the SNPs is also required to clarify the pathogenesis of SLE.

The previous published GWA scan of multiethnic population consisting of European and African American showed that rs9913957, rs8076347 and rs8079075 in IKZF3 gene contributed to the SLE susceptibility, and rs2872507 was most likely associated with RA in European, Japanese and Korean populations. In our study, a chromosomal region including IKZF3 gene and 4,000 bp upstream and 1,500 bp downstream was searched using HapMap and Haploview, and all SNPs identified in Chinese Han population with MAF of 10% or greater were included in the algorithm. Among these tagSNPs, we selected rs12150079, rs9909593 and rs907091 as candidate SNPs, which have not been analyzed in SLE before. We also selected rs2872507 as a candidate SNP as its MAF in Chinese Han population is over 10% and it had been demonstrated earlier to be associated with RA in European, Japanese and Korean populations (the other three, rs9913957, rs8076347 and rs8079075, were with low MAF = 0% in Chinese Han population).

Three newly identified variants in the 11q23.3 region were shown independent association with SLE by performing GWAS on Chinese Han populations from Hong Kong and Anhui. [20] It was shown that they had little LD with variants found in previous studies, suggesting complex biological mechanisms for the involvement of this region in SLE pathogenesis. So it would be important that focusing on the variants in our study with proven association with SLE from the previous work via meta-analysis and further replication in independent cohorts. Additionally, several SNPs (such as rs9913957, rs8076347 and rs8079075) in IKZF3 were previously reported as risk loci for SLE in other ancestries, but these SNPs are all with low MAF (0%) in Chinese Han population. More work will be required to extensively evaluate the role of the rare variants. Although we identified a strong association between rs907091 in the IKZF3 gene and SLE, we still could not determine the potential causal variants in LD with it. Better understanding whether the SNP is functionally relevant or is merely correlated with other unexamined causal polymorphisms will require mechanistic and fine-mapping experiments. Fine mapping and resequencing of this region in Chinese Han population are needed if researchers are to more precisely refine this association and determine the loci associated with risk.

We regret to analyze the few tagSNPs because of the limited working condition and analysis capacity and show the unsatisfac-

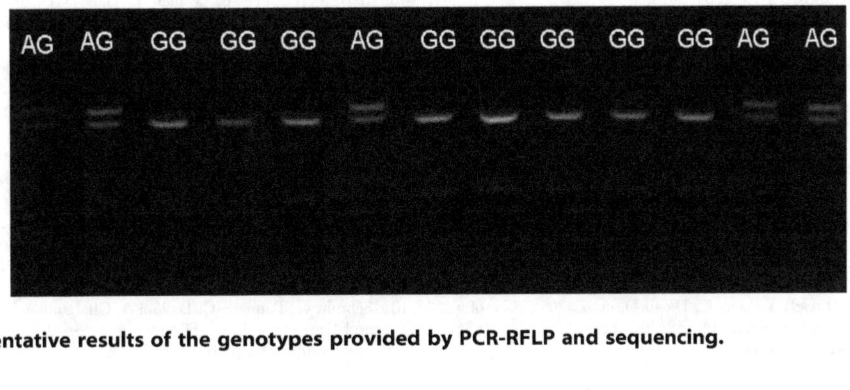

Figure 1. The representative results of the genotypes provided by PCR-RFLP and sequencing.

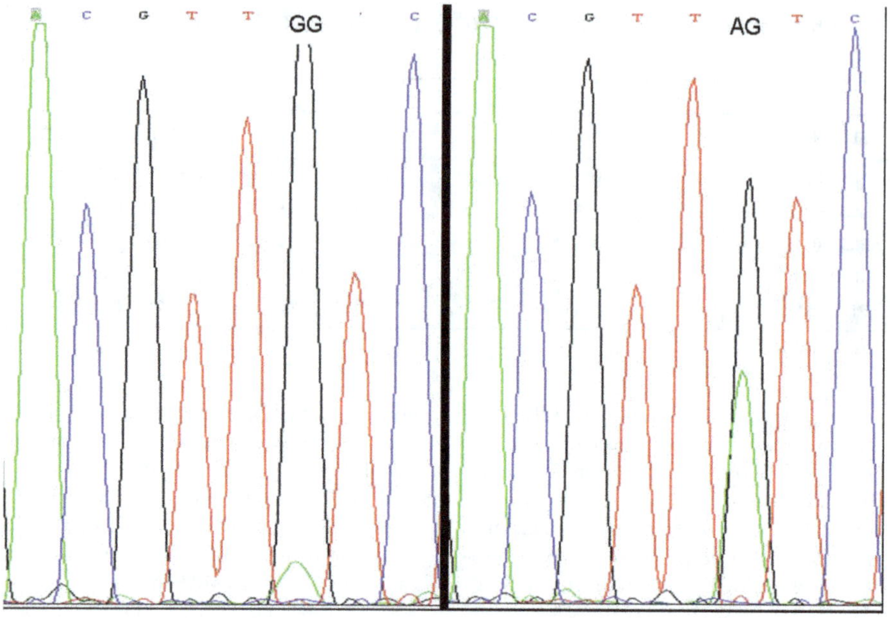

Figure 2. The representative results of the genotypes provided by PCR-RFLP and sequencing.

tory results and conclusions, which may be caused by the insufficient samples. Expanding the sample size of SLE and analyzing more SNPs of IKZF3 will be an emphasis in our future work. Another limitation is that we only analyzed the SNP with MAF>10% in Chinese Han population. It is possible that some variants with minor allele frequencies <10% also play a role in SLE risk but were not detected.

In conclusion, a strong association between rs907091 in IKZF3 gene and SLE was identified in our study. The CC genotype and C allele of rs907091 were confirmed as protective factors to SLE. Moreover, we also believe that further studies are required to determine whether rs12150079 and haplotype GGCG could influence SLE. These data should be useful to the improvements of the diagnosis, prognosis and therapy for SLE.

Acknowledgments

We especially thank all SLE patients who participated for making this study possible.

Author Contributions

Conceived and designed the experiments: XZC YQ. Performed the experiments: XZC YQ XDL NL DC. Analyzed the data: XZC CD. Contributed reagents/materials/analysis tools: XXX YC SYD SY. Contributed to the writing of the manuscript: XZC YJ. Collected blood samples of the patients and controls: SYD SY.

References

1. Lim LS, Lee SJ, Feldman BM, Gladman DD, Pullenayegum E, et al. (2014) A systematic review of the quality of prognosis studies in systemic lupus erythematosus. Arthritis Care Res (Hoboken). [Epub ahead of print].
2. De S, Barnes BJ (2014) B cell transcription factors: Potential new therapeutic targets for SLE. Clin Immunol 152: 140–151.
3. Zhang J, Zhu Q, Meng F, Lei H, Zhao Y (2014) Association study of TLR-9 polymorphisms and systemic lupus erythematosus in northern Chinese Han population. Gene 533: 385–388.
4. Morgan B, Sun L, Avitahl N, Andrikopoulos K, Ikeda T, et al. (1997) Aiolos, a lymphoid restricted transcription factor that interacts with Ikaros to regulate lymphocyte differentiation. EMBO J 16: 2004–2013.
5. Koipally J, Renold A, Kim J, Georgopoulos K (1999) Repression by Ikaros and Aiolos is mediated through histone deacetylase complexes. EMBO J 18: 3090–3100.
6. Wang JH, Avitahl N, Cariappa A, Friedrich C, Ikeda T, et al. (1998) Aiolos regulates B cell activation and maturation to effector state. Immunity 9: 543–553.
7. Sun J, Matthias G, Mihatsch MJ, Georgopoulos K, Matthias P (2003) Lack of the transcriptional coactivator OBF-1 prevents the development of systemic lupus erythematosus-like phenotypes in Aiolos mutant mice. J Immunol 170: 1699–1706.
8. Qiu R, Zhang H, Zhao H, Li J, Guo C, et al. (2013) Genetic variants on 17q21 are associated with ankylosing spondylitis susceptibility and severity in a Chinese Han population. Scand J Rheumatol 42: 469–472.
9. Kurreeman FA, Stahl EA, Okada Y, Liao K, Diogo D, et al. (2012) Use of a multiethnic approach to identify rheumatoid- arthritis-susceptibility loci, 1p36 and 17q12. Am J Hum Genet 90: 524–532.
10. Marinho S, Custovic A, Marsden P, Smith JA, Simpson A (2012) 17q12-21 variants are associated with asthma and interact with active smoking in an adult population from the United Kingdom. Ann Allergy Asthma Immunol 108: 402–411.
11. Lessard CJ, Adrianto I, Ice JA, Wiley GB, Kelly JA, et al. (2012) Identification of IRF8, TMEM39A, and IKZF3-ZPBP2 as susceptibility loci for systemic lupus erythematosus in a large-scale multiracial replication study. Am J Hum Genet 90: 648–660.
12. Yu C, Gershwin ME, Chang C (2014) Diagnostic criteria for systemic lupus erythematosus: a critical review. J Autoimmun 48–49: 10–3.
13. Barrett JC, Fry B, Maller J, Daly MJ (2005) Haploview: analysis and visualization of LD and haplotype maps. Bioinformatics 21: 263–265.
14. Carlson CS, Eberle MA, Rieder MJ, Yi Q, Kruglyak L, et al. (2004) Selecting a maximally informative set of single-nucleotide polymorphisms for association analyses using linkage disequilibrium. Am J Hum Genet 74: 106–120.
15. Wilson AG, di Giovine FS, Blakemore AI, Duff GW (1992) Single base polymorphism in the human tumour necrosis factor alpha (TNF alpha) gene detectable by NcoI restriction of PCR product. Hum Mol Genet 1: 353.
16. Akahoshi M, Nakashima H, Sadanaga A, Miyake K, Obara K, et al. (2008) Promoter polymorphisms in the IRF3 gene confer protection against systemic lupus erythematosus. Lupus 17: 568–574.
17. Narvi E, Nera KP, Terho P, Mustonen L, Granberg J, et al. (2007) Aiolos controls gene conversion and cell death in DT40 B cells. Scand J Immunol 65: 503–513.
18. Schmitt C, Tonnelle C, Dalloul A, Chabannon C, Debre P, et al. (2002) Aiolos and Ikaros: regulators of lymphocyte development, homeostasis and lymphoproliferation. Apoptosis 7: 277–284.

23

Leptin Enhances Availability of Apoptotic Cell-Derived Self-Antigen in Systemic Lupus Erythematosus

Gil Amarilyo[1]ᵠ, Noriko Iikuni[1]ᵠ, Aijing Liu[1]ᵠ, Giuseppe Matarese[2,3], Antonio La Cava[1*]

1 University of California Los Angeles, California, Los Angeles, United States of America, 2 Università di Salerno, Baronissi, Italy, 3 IRCCS MultiMedica, Milan, Italy

Abstract

In systemic lupus erythematosus (SLE), the availability of self-antigen promotes and fuels self-reactive immune responses. Apoptotic cells represent a major source of self-antigens, and an impairment of the removal of apoptotic material containing self-antigen can contribute to the development of autoimmunity. To address whether the adipocytokine leptin - which favors autoimmune responses through little understood mechanisms - could modulate the handling of apoptotic cells in SLE, we evaluated the ability of leptin to modulate the capacity of macrophages to phagocytose apoptotic bodies in (NZB×NZW)F_1 lupus mice. It was found that leptin promoted phagocytosis of apoptotic cells by macrophages by modulating cAMP levels in macrophages. This finding associated with an increased availability of antigen that favored the development of T cell responses to apoptotic-derived antigen. As leptin promotes macrophage phagocytosis of apoptotic bodies in SLE and subsequent availability of apoptotic-derived antigen to T cells, an inhibition of this process via leptin blockade might have a therapeutic potential in SLE.

Editor: Pierre Bobé, INSERM-Université Paris-Sud, France

Funding: The authors have no support or funding to report.

Competing Interests: The authors have declared that no competing interests exist.

* Email: alacava@mednet.ucla.edu

ᵠ These authors contributed equally to this work.

Introduction

Apoptotic cell death and subsequent clearance of apoptotic bodies have an important role in the maintenance of immune tolerance. A dysregulation of apoptosis and/or an altered clearance of apoptotic material can lead to the development of autoimmunity. [1] For example, a defective clearance of apoptotic cell-derived material has been described in systemic lupus erythematosus (SLE) patients and in lupus-prone mice [2–3].

SLE is a systemic autoimmune disease in which autoreactive immune responses attack multiple tissues, causing inflammation and tissue damage that can lead to a significant loss of organ function. The reasons why the course of SLE can alternate periods of illness with remissions are not well understood, although there is consensus that those aspects may be driven by factors that modulate the inflammatory state of the patient. [4] As a consequence of this gap of information, the treatment of SLE mainly relies on the use of immunosuppressive drugs that inhibit immune responses in a rather non-specific manner, to reduce inflammation [5].

Leptin is an adipocytokine that regulates metabolism [6] and modulates immune responses. [7] Leptin has structural similarities with the cytokines of the long-chain helical family, and displays proinflammatory properties that are most evident in inflammation and in autoimmunity. [7–8] The levels of this adipocytokine are increased in infection and in inflammation, or after exposure to inflammatory stimuli such as LPS, TNF-α, and IL-1. [7] Circulating leptin is also elevated in most SLE patients, and appears to contribute to proinflammatory events associated with the disease [9–10].

Since the generation and availability of self-antigen are important elements in the development and maintenance of tissue inflammation in SLE, we investigated how leptin influenced those aspects in the pathogenesis of SLE. In particular, we focused on the fact that the clearance of apoptotic cells by macrophages is critical for the control of tissue homeostasis, and that an impairment in the uptake of apoptotic cells can lead to the generation of autoantibodies to nuclear antigens and the activation of (auto)immune cells. [11–12] We found that leptin promoted availability of apoptotic cell-derived antigen in lupus mice which, in turn, favored expansion of antigen-reactive T cells.

Materials and Methods

Mice

(NZB×NZW) F_1 (NZB/W), C57Bl6 (B6), DO.11.10 transgenic mice (that carry a TCR specific for $OVA_{323-339}$ peptide), and leptin-receptor-deficient (*db/db*) ($B6^{db/db}$) mice were purchased from The Jackson Laboratory (Bar Harbor, ME) and housed at the University of California Los Angeles (UCLA). The study was carried out in strict accordance with the recommendations in the Guide for the Care and Use of Laboratory Animals of the National Institutes of Health with a protocol approved by the UCLA Animal Research Committee. Female mice, aged 8–10 weeks, were used in the experiments.

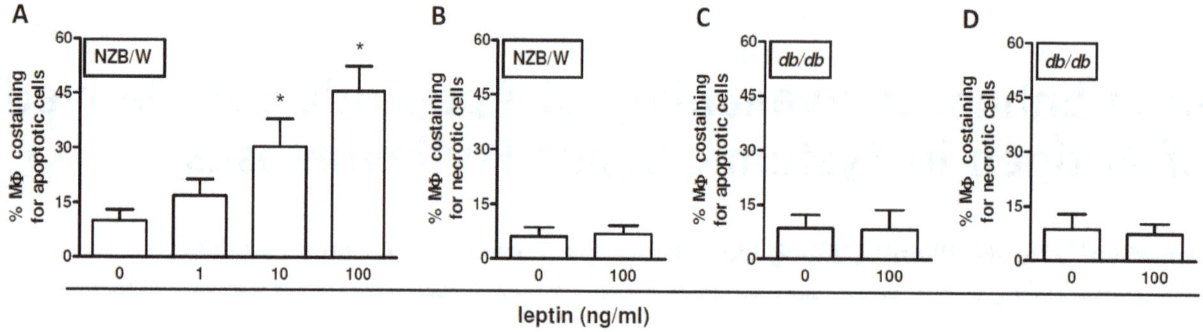

Figure 1. Leptin modulates the uptake of apoptotic cells *in vitro* from lupus macrophage. Peritoneal macrophages (MΦ) from NZB/W lupus mice (A–B) or leptin-receptor-deficient (non-autoimmune) *db/db* mice (C–D) were co-cultured *ex vivo* with 1×10^7 CFSE-labeled apoptotic cells (A, C) or necrotic cells (B, D) in the presence of scalar doses of leptin (*x* axis). After 2 h, cells were stained with PE-labeled anti-mouse CD11b Ab and the labeled phagocytosed material within macrophages (PE-positive) was visualized as co-staining in flow cytometry. Additional details are reported in the Methods. *p<0.01 vs no (0) leptin.

Reagents

Recombinant mouse leptin was purchased from R&D Systems (Minneapolis, MN). Anti-leptin Ab was from Cell Sciences (Canton, MA). Before use, reagents were treated with Pierce High Capacity Endotoxin Removal Resin (Thermo Scientific, Rockford, IL).

Flow cytometry

Phenotypic analyses were performed with combinations of fluorochrome-conjugated Ab (all from eBioscience, San Diego, CA) using standard techniques and acquired with a FACSCalibur flow cytometer (BD Biosciences, San Jose, CA). Data analysis was done using FloJo software (Tree Star Inc., Ashland, OR).

Cell preparation

Jurkat T cells purchased from the American Type Culture Collection (ATCC, Manassas, VA) were labeled with CFSE (carboxyfluorescein succinimidyl ester; Sigma-Aldrich, St. Louis, MO) and made apoptotic (as confirmed in flow cytometry by annexin V and 7-aminoactinomycin (7-AAD) staining using BD Biosciences kit) following exposure for 10 min at 254 nm UV and subsequent incubation for 2 h in medium. Necrotic cell death was induced by incubation at 55°C for 15 min. [13] Each of these treatments consistently resulted in >85% cell death, as determined by changes in forward and side scatter characteristics in flow cytometry (not shown).

Phagocytosis *in vivo*

To recruit macrophages into the peritoneum, mice were injected i.p. with 3 ml of 3% thioglycolate. Although thioglycolate treatment associated with a ~10-fold increase in the number of circulating macrophages, it did not influence their surface expression of leptin receptor (assessed by flow cytometry as MFI, not shown). Contralateral i.p. injection of recombinant mouse leptin (6 consecutive doses of 2 μg/g at 12-h intervals) or vehicle was given starting at the time of thioglycolate treatment. At day 3 post-injection, mice were infused i.p. with 1×10^7 CFSE-labeled apoptotic Jurkat cells. After 30 min, peritoneal cells were recovered. To remove erythrocytes and non-phagocytosed bodies, cells were incubated on polystyrene dishes for 1 h, and then washed. For determination of macrophage uptake of apoptotic

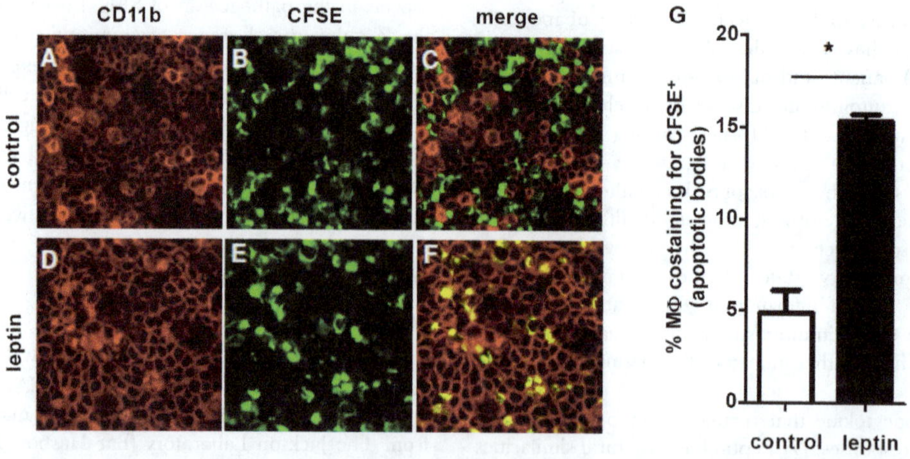

Figure 2. Leptin promotes phagocytosis by lupus macrophages *in vivo*. NZB/W mice were injected i.p. with thioglycolate prior to injection of either vehicle (A–C) or 2 μg/g leptin (D–F) at 12-h intervals. After 72 h, 1×10^6 CFSE-positive apoptotic cells were injected i.p. After 30 min, uptake of apoptotic cells by $CD11b^+$ macrophages (PE) in peritoneal fluid of recipient animals was visualized *ex vivo* by confocal microscopy as colocalization of PE-positive macrophages (red) and CFSE-positive (green) apoptotic bodies within the same cell (yellow). Representative of three experiments (n = 6 per group). Original magnification: 10x. (G) Cumulative flow cytometry of peritoneal macrophages costaining for apoptotic cells. *p<0.01 vs control.

cells (CFSE+) by flow cytometry, collected cells were stained with PE-conjugated anti-mouse CD11b Ab. For confocal microscopy, cells were resuspended in 1% cold BSA/PBS, centrifuged in a Shandon Cytospin 3 centrifuge (Thermo Fisher Scientific, Waltham, MA), and dried sediments were fixed with −20°C acetone, blocked with 3% BSA/PBS, and stained with anti-mouse CD11b Ab before visualization with a LSM 310 laser scanning confocal microscope (Carl Zeiss Inc., Toronto, Canada).

Phagocytosis *in vitro*

Three days after thioglycolate injection, peritoneal macrophages were collected from abdominal cavities and co-cultured in serum-free HL-1 medium (Lonza, Anaheim, CA) with CFSE-labeled apoptotic Jurkat T cells (1×10^7 cells) in the presence of scalar doses of leptin. After 2 h, cells were stained with anti-mouse CD11b Ab (BioLegend, San Diego, CA). Macrophage uptake of apoptotic cells was assessed by flow cytometry as co-staining for CFSE and anti-CD11b Ab.

Measurement of cAMP

cAMP levels were detected using the Cyclic AMP EIA Kit (Cayman Chemical Co., Ann Arbor, MI), according to the manufacturer's instructions.

Antigen presentation assay

After 1 h adherence of peritoneal macrophages at 37°C in HL-1 medium, non-adherent cells were removed by washing, and macrophages cultured for 2 h at 37°C with 20 µg/ml ovalbumin (OVA), labeled with TAMRA (5-carboxytetramethylrhodamine; Genaxxon Bioscience, Ulm, Germany). Adherent cells were then washed, sorted for TAMRA dye positivity, and induced to apoptose by treatment with 1 µg/ml lipopolysaccharide (LPS) (Sigma-Aldrich) for 4 h followed by addition of 5 mM ATP (Sigma-Aldrich) for another 45 min. Harvested material was washed before use as source of OVA-containing apoptotic bodies.

To study OVA-TCR transgenic T cell responses to OVA-containing apoptotic bodies, OVA-TCR transgenic DO11.10 mice were immunized s.c. with 2 µg OVA (Sigma-Aldrich) emulsified 1:1 in complete Freund adjuvant (CFA) (Sigma-Aldrich). After 72 h, mice were sacrificed, splenocytes stained with CFSE, and cocultured with TAMRA-labeled apoptotic bodies containing OVA (see above) in the presence of scalar doses of leptin or vehicle for 48 h before staining with clonotype-specific KJ1.26 Ab (eBioscience) and flow cytometry for enumeration of OVA-specific T cells.

Statistical analyses

Two-sided *t* test was used for two-group comparisons. Statistical analyses were done using Prism 5 software (GraphPad, San Diego). A p-value <0.05 was considered significant.

Results and Discussion

Leptin promotes lupus macrophage phagocytosis *in vitro*

In SLE, the impaired clearance of apoptotic cells causes an accumulation of cellular material that contains self-antigen. [1–2,14] To test a possible role of leptin in this process, we co-cultured - in the presence of scalar doses of leptin - purified macrophages derived from NZB/W lupus mice (obtained according to the protocol shown in figure S1) together with CFSE-labeled apoptotic cells. After 2 h in co-culture, a dose-dependent increase in the uptake of apoptotic cells by lupus macrophages was observed in the presence of increasing concentrations of leptin (figure 1A). Leptin did not modulate the phagocytic capacity of macrophages for non-apoptotic cells (figure 1B). Specificity of the results was indicated by lack of effects of leptin on macrophages in leptin-deficient (*db/db*) macrophages (figure 1C–D).

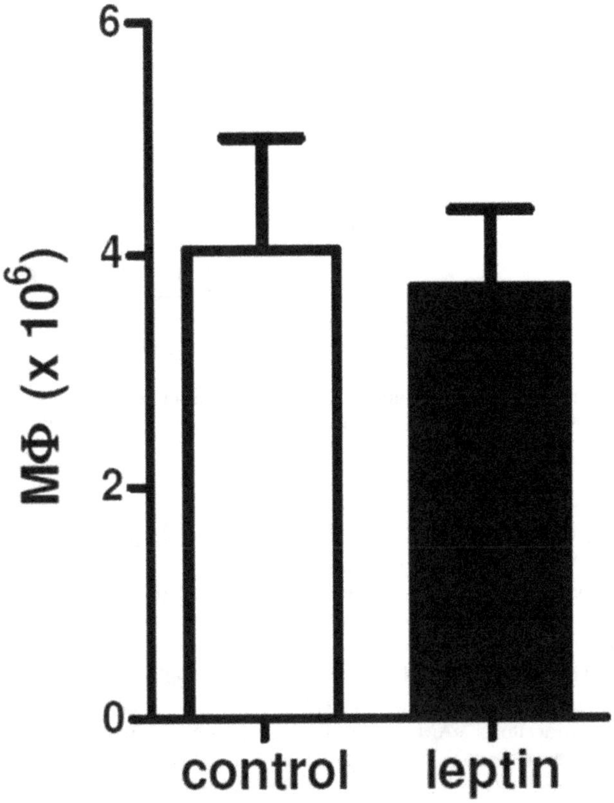

Figure 3. Leptin does not influence peritoneal macrophage recruitment. Total number of peritoneal macrophages recovered three days after i.p. thioglycolate in NZB/W mice in that had been injected i.p. with vehicle (control) or leptin. Further details can be found in the Methods. p not significant.

Leptin promotes lupus macrophage phagocytosis *in vivo*

Since the above findings suggested an ability of leptin to promote phagocytosis in macrophages, we determined whether similar effects could also be observed *in vivo*. To this aim, labeled apoptotic cells were injected i.p. into two groups of NZB/W mice that had been pre-treated with thioglycolate 3 days earlier. One group of mice received leptin in addition to apoptotic cells, the other (control) group of mice received vehicle together with apoptotic cells. It was found that leptin-treated mice had a significant increase in macrophage phagocytosis of apoptotic cells when compared to control mice that had been treated with vehicle (figure 2A–F). In particular, leptin-treated mice displayed a ~3-fold increase in the frequency of phagocytosed apoptotic cells as compared to controls (figure 2G). Those effects of leptin on macrophages were lupus-specific as not observed in control C57Bl.6 mice under the same experimental conditions (not shown) and were not due to a modulation of macrophages recruitment *in vivo*, because the total numbers of peritoneal macrophages were comparable between animals treated with leptin or with vehicle (figure 3).

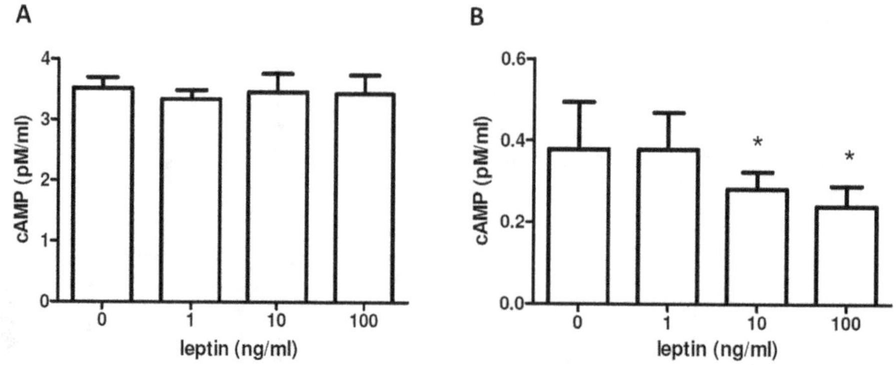

Figure 4. Effects of leptin on cAMP levels in macrophages. cAMP was measured as intracellular (A) and in supernatant (B) of NZB/W macrophages cultured 1 h with scalar doses of leptin (see Methods for further details). Representative of three experiments in triplicate. *$p<0.05$ vs control (0)

Leptin modulates cAMP levels in macrophages

cAMP is produced during phagocytosis [15], where it acts as second messenger in a signaling cascade that leads to downstream activation of the suppression of phagocytosis and facilitation of the production of proinflammatory mediators [16].

The analysis of the levels of cAMP in macrophages cultured in the presence of scalar doses of leptin showed no significant changes in intracellular cAMP expression (figure 4A). However, cAMP levels were reduced in supernatants of cultured macrophages in the presence of increasing concentrations of leptin (figure 4B), suggesting a transient effect of leptin on macrophage production of cAMP that is not maintained over time.

The uptake of apoptotic cells induced by leptin in macrophages promotes proliferation of T cells reactive to apoptotic-cell antigen

Macrophages that phagocytose apoptotic cells contain the self-antigen that is present in apoptotic bodies. [17] Self-antigens are known to represent driving factors in the generation and maintenance of autoimmune responses. [18] Considering that our results had indicated an ability of leptin to facilitate the uptake of apoptotic cells by macrophages (figures 1 and 2), we assessed the impact of availability of intracellular (apoptotic-derived) antigen to macrophages on the proliferation of T cells reactive to that antigen. Macrophages from DO11.10 mice (carrying the DO11.10 transgenic TCR reactive to OVA) were fed OVA, stained with TAMRA, and made apoptotic (see Methods for more details). Apoptotic bodies containing OVA ($TAMRA^+$) were then incubated with CFSE-labeled splenocytes from OVA-immunized DO11.10 mice for 2 h in the presence of scalar doses of leptin. Flow cytometry for $CD11b^+TAMRA^+CFSE^+$ cells showed that leptin had promoted phagocytosis of OVA-containing apoptotic bodies in the splenic macrophages (figure 5A). Additionally, the increased frequency of DO11.10 clonotype-specific $KJ1.26^+$ T cells reactive to OVA 48 h after treatment with leptin in the cocultures of splenocytes with OVA-loaded macrophages indicated a promoting activity of leptin on the proliferation of the splenic OVA-reactive T cells (figure 5B). This finding is consistent with our recent observations that showed that leptin could promote survival and proliferation of autoreactive $CD4^+$ T cells [19–20].

Since leptin levels are abnormally elevated in NZB/W lupus mice and in SLE patients, [9–10] these results suggest the possibility that leptin could sustain autoimmune responses by facilitating availability of apoptotic material that contains antigen

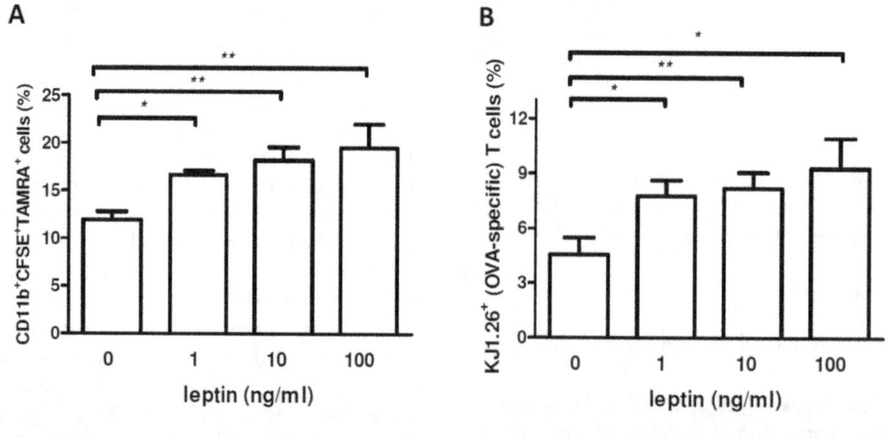

Figure 5. Increased macrophage uptake of apoptotic cells induced by leptin promotes proliferation of self antigen-reactive T cells. TAMRA-labeled apoptotic bodies containing OVA (see Methods) were co-cultured with CFSE-labeled macrophages for 2 h, followed by staining with APC-labeled anti-CD11b Ab and flow cytometry. (A) Frequency of $TAMRA^+CFSE^+$ $CD11b^+$ cells (macrophages positive for OVA-containing apoptotic bodies) in OVA-TCR transgenic mice (DO11.10) after culture in the presence of scalar doses of leptin. (B) Flow cytometry staining with clonotype-specific KJ1.26 Ab (OVA-specific TCR) 48 h after co-incubation of OVA-immunized DO11.10 (OVA-TCR transgenic) mouse splenocytes with macrophages containing OVA-loaded apoptotic bodies ($TAMRA^+$). *$p<0.05$, **$p<0.01$ vs control ($n=5$).

that can be recognized by antigen-specific T cells. In this sense, our findings extend mechanistically the prior work that showed an enhanced phagocytosis in murine macrophages induced by leptin [21], where (type 1) macrophages (M1) expressing the leptin receptor responded to leptin, producing pro-inflammatory IL-6 and TNF-α [22].

In summary, this manuscript shows that leptin can promote, via cAMP, the phagocytosis of apoptotic bodies and subsequent proliferation of T cells reactive to apoptosis-derived antigen. These results imply that limiting the above processes, e.g. via leptin blockade, could have effects in the modulation of autoimmune responses in SLE.

Supporting Information

Figure S1 Experimental protocol. Mice were injected i.p. with 3 ml 3% thioglycolate for i.p. recruitment of macrophages. Treated mice were then divided into two groups: one receiving six injections of 2 μg/g of leptin per body weight at 12-h intervals, the other group receiving vehicle at the same time points. After 72 h, peritoneal macrophages were recovered for experimental use.

Author Contributions

Conceived and designed the experiments: ALC. Performed the experiments: GA NI AL. Analyzed the data: GA NI AL ALC. Contributed reagents/materials/analysis tools: GM. Contributed to the writing of the manuscript: ALC.

References

1. Lenardo M, Chan KM, Hornung F, McFarland H, Siegel R, et al. (1999) Mature T lymphocyte apoptosis-immune regulation in a dynamic and unpredictable antigenic environment. Annu Rev Immunol 17: 221–253.
2. Muñoz LE, van Bavel C, Franz S, Berden J, Herrmann M, et al. (2008) Apoptosis in the pathogenesis of systemic lupus erythematosus. Lupus 17: 371–375.
3. Potter PK, Cortes-Hernandez J, Quartier P, Botto M, Walport MJ (2003) Lupus-prone mice have an abnormal response to thioglycolate and an impaired clearance of apoptotic cells. J Immunol 170: 3223–3232.
4. Petri M (2001) Long-term outcomes in lupus. Am J Manag Care 7: S480–485.
5. Wong M, La Cava A (2011) Lupus, the current therapeutic approaches. Drugs Today (Barc) 47: 289–302.
6. Ahima RS, Prabakaran D, Mantzoros C, Qu D, Lowell B, et al. (1996) Role of leptin in the neuroendocrine response to fasting. Nature 382: 250–252.
7. La Cava A, Matarese G (2004) The weight of leptin in immunity. Nat Rev Immunol 4: 371–379.
8. Iikuni N, Lam QL, Lu L, Matarese G, La Cava A (2008) Leptin and inflammation. Curr Immunol Rev 4: 70–79.
9. Garcia-Gonzalez A, Gonzalez-Lopez L, Valera-Gonzalez IC, Cardona-Muñoz EG, Salazar-Paramo M, et al. (2002) Serum leptin levels in women with systemic lupus erythematosus. Rheumatol Int 22: 138–141.
10. McMahon M, Skaggs BJ, Sahakian L, Grossman J, FitzGerald J, et al. (2011) High plasma leptin levels confer increased risk of atherosclerosis in women with systemic lupus erythematosus, and are associated with inflammatory oxidised lipids. Ann Rheum Dis 70: 1619–1624.
11. Katsiari CG, Liossis SN, Sfikakis PP (2010) The pathophysiologic role of monocytes and macrophages in systemic lupus erythematosus: a reappraisal. Semin Arthritis Rheum 39: 491–503.
12. Ramirez-Ortiz ZG, Pendergraft WF 3rd, Prasad A, Byrne MH, Iram T, et al. (2013) The scavenger receptor SCARF1 mediates the clearance of apoptotic cells and prevents autoimmunity. Nat Immunol 14: 917–926.
13. Cocco RE, Ucker DS (2001) Distinct modes of macrophage recognition for apoptotic and necrotic cells are not specified exclusively by phosphatidylserine exposure. Mol Biol Cell 12: 919–930.
14. Janko C, Schorn C, Grossmayer GE, Frey B, Herrmann M, et al. (2008) Inflammatory clearance of apoptotic remnants in systemic lupus erythematosus (SLE). Autoimmun Rev 8: 9–12.
15. Ogmundsdóttir HM, Weir DM (1980) Mechanisms of macrophage activation. Clin Exp Immunol 40: 223–234.
16. Ballinger MN, Welliver T, Straight S, Peters-Golden M, Swanson JA (2010) Transient increase in cyclic AMP localized to macrophage phagosomes. PLoS One 5: e13962.
17. Suber T, Rosen A (2009) Apoptotic cell blebs: repositories of autoantigens and contributors to immune context. Arthritis Rheum 60: 2216–2219.
18. Bach JF, Koutouzov S, van Endert PM (1998) Are there unique autoantigens triggering autoimmune diseases? Immunol Rev 164: 139–155.
19. Galgani M, Procaccini C, De Rosa V, Carbone F, Chieffi P, et al. (2010) Leptin modulates the survival of autoreactive $CD4^+$ T cells through the nutrient/energy-sensing mammalian target of rapamycin signaling pathway. J Immunol 185: 7474–7479.
20. Amarilyo G, Iikuni N, Shi FD, Liu A, Matarese G, et al. (2013) Leptin promotes lupus T-cell autoimmunity. Clin Immunol 149: 530–533.
21. Jiang JX, Mikami K, Shah VH, Torok NJ (2008) Leptin induces phagocytosis of apoptotic bodies by hepatic stellate cells via a Rho guanosine triphosphatase-dependent mechanism. Hepatology 48: 1497–1505.
22. Kredel LI, Batra A, Stroh T, Kühl AA, Zeitz M, et al. (2013) Adipokines from local fat cells shape the macrophage compartment of the creeping fat in Crohn's disease. Gut 62: 852–862.

A Multilocus Genetic Study in a Cohort of Italian SLE Patients Confirms the Association with STAT4 Gene and Describes a New Association with HCP5 Gene

Cinzia Ciccacci[1], Carlo Perricone[2], Fulvia Ceccarelli[2], Sara Rufini[1], Davide Di Fusco[1], Cristiano Alessandri[2], Francesca Romana Spinelli[2], Enrica Cipriano[2], Giuseppe Novelli[1], Guido Valesini[2], Paola Borgiani[1*], Fabrizio Conti[2]

1 Department of Biomedicine and Prevention, Section of Genetics, School of Medicine, University of Rome "Tor Vergata", Rome, Italy, **2** Lupus Clinic, Reumatologia, Dipartimento di Medicina Interna e Specialità Mediche, Sapienza Università di Roma, Rome, Italy

Abstract

Background: Systemic lupus erythematosus (SLE) is an autoimmune disease with complex pathogenesis in which genes and environmental factors are involved. We aimed at analyzing previously identified loci associated with SLE or with other autoimmune and/or inflammatory disorders (STAT4, IL10, IL23R, IRAK1, PSORS1C1, HCP5, MIR146a, PTPN2, ERAP1, ATG16L1, IRGM) in a sample of Italian SLE patients in order to verify or confirm their possible involvement and relative contribution in the disease.

Materials and methods: Two hundred thirty-nine consecutive SLE patients and 278 matched healthy controls were enrolled. Study protocol included complete physical examination, and clinical and laboratory data collection. Nineteen polymorphisms were genotyped by allelic discrimination assays. A case-control association study and a genotype-phenotype correlation were performed.

Results: STAT4 was the most associated gene [$P = 3 \times 10^{-7}$, OR = 2.13 (95% CI: 1.59–2.85)]. IL10 confirmed its association with SLE [rs3024505: P = 0.02, OR = 1.52 (95% CI: 1.07–2.16)]. We describe a novel significant association between HCP5 locus and SLE susceptibility [rs3099844: P = 0.01, OR = 2.06 (95% CI: 1.18–3.6)]. The genotype/phenotype correlation analysis showed several associations including a higher risk to develop pericarditis with STAT4, and an association between HCP5 rs3099844 and anti-Ro/SSA antibodies.

Conclusions: STAT4 and IL10 confirm their association with SLE. We found that some SNPs in PSORS1C1, ATG16L1, IL23R, PTPN2 and MIR146a genes can determine particular disease phenotypes. HCP5 rs3099844 is associated with SLE and with anti-Ro/SSA. This polymorphism has been previously found associated with cardiac manifestations of SLE, a condition related with anti-Ro/SSA antibodies. Thus, our results may provide new insights into SLE pathogenesis.

Editor: Jose Crispin, Beth Israel Deaconess Medical Center, United States of America

Funding: The authors have no support or funding to report.

* Email: borgiani@med.uniroma2.it

These authors contributed equally to this work.

Introduction

Systemic lupus erythematosus (SLE) is a chronic autoimmune disease characterized by the production of autoantibodies against intracellular, nucleic acid and cell surface antigens. The disease is relapsing and affects multiple organ systems including the skin, kidneys, lungs, heart and the central nervous system. The pathogenesis of SLE is complex, with several susceptibility genes and environmental factors involved in its development and clinical manifestations. Familial aggregation and a higher rate of concordance for SLE in monozygotic than in dizygotic twins [1,2] provide support for a strong role of genetic factors in the pathogenesis of this disorder.

During last decade, many genes were described for their potential role in predisposing to SLE [3]. The list of involved genes has increased with the advent of Genome Wide Association (GWA) studies. These studies confirmed genetic associations of over 40 genes [3]. The number of genes emphasizes the complexity of the inheritability of SLE. Most of the identified genes encode proteins that participate in key pathogenic pathways, including Toll-like receptor and type I interferon signaling pathways, immune regulation pathways and those that control the clearance of immune complexes [4].

Interestingly, SLE and other autoimmune diseases share many of the risk loci identified, suggesting the involvement of common pathways in autoimmune diseases [5]. Moreover, the existence of common genetic susceptibility was already suggested by the clustering of multiple autoimmune diseases within families, including families with SLE [2,6]. This genetic overlap is exemplified by the well-known associations of certain HLA loci with multiple autoimmune disease as well as non-HLA risk loci in different pathways such as IL2RA, STAT4, PTPN22 and IFIH1 [7,8]. In this context, in a previous paper, we have described for the first time, an association between SLE and the TRAF3IP2 gene [9], a gene involved in psoriasis and psoriatic arthritis [10], but also described in cutaneous complications in inflammatory bowel diseases [11].

Here, our aim was to analyze a number of previously identified loci associated with SLE or with other autoimmune and/or inflammatory diseases (STAT4, IL10, IL23R, IRAK1, PSORS1C1, HCP5, MIR146a, PTPN2, ERAP1, ATG16L1, IRGM) in a sample of Italian SLE patients in order to confirm or verify their possible involvement and their relative contribution in SLE susceptibility. The genes were chosen due their role in different pathways involved in SLE pathogenesis. We therefore performed a case/control study and a genotype-phenotype correlation analysis.

Materials and Methods

Sample collection

Two hundred and thirty-nine SLE consecutive Caucasian patients ≥18 years of age affected with SLE were retrospectively enrolled at the Lupus Clinic of the Rheumatology Unit, Sapienza University of Rome (Sapienza Lupus Cohort). SLE diagnosis was performed according to the revised 1997 American College of Rheumatology (ACR) criteria. This cohort was already described in Perricone et al. 2013 [9]. Briefly, 21 (8.8%) were males and 218 (91.2%) females, mean age ± SD was 42.7±11.4 years, mean age at diagnosis ±SD was 30.9±11.6 years. Musculo-skeletal was the most frequent involvement (71.0% of patients), 96.6% had positive ANA, and 73.3% had positive anti-dsDNA. Study protocol included complete physical examination and blood drawing. The clinical and laboratory data were collected in a standardized, computerized, electronically-filled form including demographics, past medical history with date of diagnosis, co-morbidities, and previous and concomitant treatments.

The evaluation of clinical and laboratory parameters was performed at the Lupus Clinic of Sapienza University of Rome. Clinical and laboratory features were assessed with a dichotomous score (present = 1; absent = 0).

Written informed consent was obtained from each patient and the ethic committee of Sapienza University of Rome approved the study design.

Two hundred seventy-eight age- and ethnicity-matched healthy subjects, enrolled at University of Rome Tor Vergata, served as controls.

Clinical laboratory analysis

Among the laboratory tests, the following parameters were evaluated: complete blood count [CBC], including erythrocytes, leucocytes and platelets count, erythrocyte sedimentation rate [ESR], C-reactive protein [CRP] levels, serum levels of creatinine and complement C3 and C4, anti-nuclear (ANA), anti-double-stranded DNA (anti-dsDNA), ENA, anti-Sm, anti-RNP, anti-Ro/SSA, anti-La/SSB, anti-CL IgG and IgM, anti-β_2GPI IgG and

Table 1. Results of allelic association analysis.

Gene	SNP	SLE MAF*%	Controls MAF%	P	OR
STAT4	rs7574865	0.35	0.2	3×10^{-7}	2.13 (1.59–2.85)
IL10	rs1800872	0.26	0.31	0.09	0.79 (0.6–1.04)
	rs3024505	0.17	0.12	0.02	1.52 (1.07–2.16)
HCP5	rs9469003	0.18	0.19	0.67	0.93 (0.65–1.32)
	rs3099844	0.1	0.05	0.01	2.06 (1.18–3.6)
IL23R	rs11209026	0.053	0.078	0.1	0.66 (0.4–1.09)
	rs11803505	0.34	0.34	1	1 (0.77–1.31)
	rs7517847	0.4	0.39	0.65	1.06 (0.82–1.87)
PSORS1C1	rs2233945	0.2	0.17	0.26	1.19 (0.87–1.63)
IRGM	rs13361189	0.09	0.11	0.38	0.79 (0.46–1.34)
	rs4958847	0.13	0.16	0.43	0.84 (0.54–1.3)
ATG16L1	rs2241880	0.46[§]	0.43[§]	0.39	0.87 (0.64–1.19)
PTPN2	rs2542151	0.14	0.11	0.38	1.29 (0.73–2.3)
	rs7234029	0.13	0.15	0.48	0.81 (0.45–1.46)
ERAP1	rs30187	0.36	0.38	0.65	0.93 (0.67–1.28)
	rs27524	0.38	0.38	0.89	1.02 (0.79–1.32)
MIR146A	rs2910164	0.3	0.27	0.49	1.1 (0.84–1.45)
	rs2431697	0.41	0.42	0.63	0.93 (0.68–1.26)
IRAK1	rs3027898	0.29	0.26	0.3	1.17 (0.87–1.6)

* MAF: Minor allele frequency,
[§]Allele A.

Table 2. Genotypes distribution for rs7574865 STAT4 SNP revealed an allele dose additive effect.

	SLE Patients	Controls			Mantel–Haenszel test of linearity
	n = 234	n = 243	P	OR (95% CI)	
GG	104	150			5.3×10^{-7}
GT	95	87	0.02	1.57 (1.07–2.31)	
TT	35	6	2.4×10^{-7}	8.4 (3.42–20.72)	

GT+TT *vs* GG: P = 0.00016, OR = 2 (1.4–2.9).

IgM, and LA. To be positive, each of these tests had to be positive in at least 2 occasions 12 weeks apart all along patient clinical history.

ANA were determined by means of indirect immunofluorescence (IIF) on Hep-2 (titer ≥1:160 or ++ on a scale from + to ++++); anti-dsDNA with ELISA assays (considering levels higher than the cut-off of the reference laboratory) or IIF on Crithidia Luciliae, ENA (including anti-Ro/SSA, anti-La/SSB, anti-Sm, anti-RNP) by ELISA assay considering titers above the cut-off of the reference laboratory, anti-CL of IgG or IgM isotype, by ELISA, in serum or plasma at medium or high titers [e.g.,>40 standardized international units (GPL/MPL units) or above the 99th percentile], anti-β_2GPI of IgG or IgM isotype, by ELISA, in serum or plasma (above the 99th percentile), and finally LAC was assessed according to the guidelines of the International Society on Thrombosis and Hemostasis (Scientific Subcommittee on lupus anticoagulant/phospholipid-dependent antibodies) [12].

All subjects underwent blood drawing (5 ml supplemented with 0.5% EDTA) in order to perform genetic analysis.

DNA extraction and genotyping

Genomic DNA was isolated from peripheral blood mononuclear cells using a Qiagen blood DNA mini kit. A panel of SNPs was selected on the basis of literature data in 11 genes involved in immune response, autophagy and inflammation, already described as associated with any kind of autoimmune disease. The selected SNPs were the following: rs7574865 (STAT4), rs1800872 and rs3024505 (IL10), rs9469003 and rs3099844 (HCP5), rs11209026, rs11803505 and rs7517847 (IL23R), rs2233945 (PSORS1C1), rs13361189 and rs4958847 (IRGM), rs2241880 (ATG16L1), rs2542151 and rs7234029 (PTPN2), rs30187 and rs27524 (ERAP1), rs2910164 and rs2431697 (MIR146A) and rs3027898 (IRAK1). Genotyping was performed by allelic discrimination assay by TaqMan assays (Applied Biosystems, Foster City, CA, USA) and ABI PRISM 7000. Each assay was run with positive (samples previously confirmed by direct sequencing as heterozygous and/or variant homozygous) and negative controls.

Statistical analysis

The Hardy–Weinberg equilibrium was verified for all SNPs by the Pearson χ^2 test.

Differences in alleles/genotypes/haplotypes frequencies between cases and control were evaluated by Pearson χ^2 test. Haplotypes were inferred using Arlequin, version 3.11 [13]. Odds ratios (ORs) with 95% CI were calculated. A genotype-phenotype correlation analysis has been performed considering the heterozygotes and variant homozygotes together (1degree of freedom [df]). A binary logistic regression analysis (stepwise) was carried out considering the presence/absence of SLE as dependent variable and all genetics associated factors as independent variables. All statistical analyses were performed by the SPSS 13.0 program (SSPS Inc., IL, USA).

Results

Case/control association analysis

We studied 19 polymorphisms in 11 genes. Deviations from Hardy–Weinberg equilibrium were not observed. In Table 1, we reported the comparisons of the allele frequencies between cases and controls for all studied polymorphisms. Among the studied genes, STAT4 resulted, as expected, the most associated with a $P = 3\times10^{-7}$ and OR = 2.13 (95% CI 1.59–2.85). Moreover, the Mantel–Haenszel test for linear association highlights that there was an additive effect of STAT4 risk allele ($P = 5.3\times10^{-7}$): subjects with one risk allele presented an OR = 1.57, while subjects with two risk alleles reached an OR = 8.4 (95% CI 3.42–20.72, Table 2). Furthermore, IL10 confirmed the association with SLE in our cohort with the rs3024505 SNP (P = 0.02 and OR = 1.52 [95% CI 1.07–2.16]).

Moreover, for the first time, we described an association between HCP5 locus and SLE susceptibility: the variant allele of rs3099844 resulted a risk allele with P = 0.01 and OR = 2.06 (95% CI 1.18–3.6). No significant associations were observed for all the other studied SNPs.

A binary logistic regression analysis was carried out considering the three associated SNPs as independent variables and the presence/absence of SLE as dependent variable (Table 3). This

Table 3. Final model of binary logistic regression analysis (stepwise method) considering only associated genetic factors.

	B	P	OR (95%CI)	R^2 (Cox & Snell)
STAT4_rs7574865	0.931	<0.0001	2.54 (1.58–4.06)	0.059
HCP5_rs3099844	0.835	0.022	2.31 (1.13–4.71)	

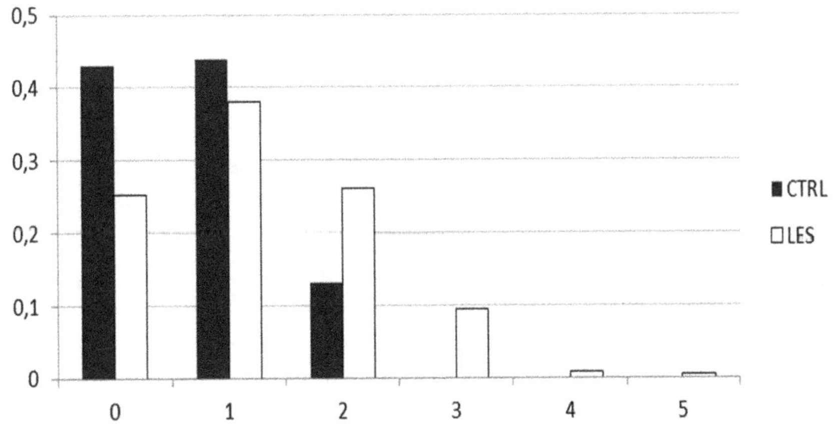

Figure 1. Counting of risk alleles in cases and controls. The risk alleles considered are the variant alleles of rs7574865, rs3099844 and rs3024505 SNPs.

analysis confirmed the involvement of STAT4 and HCP5. This model explains the 5.9% of genetic susceptibility (Cox and Snell R^2).

Haplotypes analysis

We inferred the haplotypes distribution for IL10, IL23R, HCP5, IRGM, PTPN and ERAP1 genes. However, we did not find any significant association comparing the distribution in cases and controls (data not shown). Only for IL10 we observed a significant difference comparing the TC (composed by the variant allele of rs3024505 and wildtype allele of rs1800872) *vs* CA (composed by the wild-type allele of rs3024505 and the variant allele of rs1800872) haplotype ($P = 0.012$ and $OR = 1.7$ [95% CI 1.12–2.56]), but this evidence does not improve consistently the statistical significance obtained considering only the rs3024505 SNP.

Number of risk alleles

We counted the number of risk alleles, considering as risk alleles the variant alleles of rs7574865 (STAT4), rs3024505 (IL10), and rs3099844 (HCP5) SNPs, and we evaluated the different risk allele number distribution between cases and controls (Figure 1, Table 4). As expected the class with no risk allele was significantly more present in controls than in patients ($P = 0.0008$, $OR = 0.45$). On the contrary, the class with two risk alleles was significantly more present in cases than in controls ($P = 0.0003$, $OR = 3.78$). Finally, genetic profiles with three or more risk alleles were present only in SLE patients ($P<0.0001$).

Genotype-phenotype correlation analysis

A genotype/phenotype correlation analysis between the genotypes and clinical characteristics of SLE patients was performed. Results of this analysis were reported in Table 5. STAT4, that showed the strongest association with the disease, was also associated with a higher risk to develop pericarditis, while HCP5 SNPs resulted associated with anti-Ro/SSA, anti-dsDNA and aCL.

Interestingly, some SNPs that did not associate with the disease, showed association with particular disease phenotypes. For example, PTPN2 SNP resulted associated with a higher risk to develop pericarditis and serositis, while ATG16L1 SNP resulted protective towards pericarditis. IL23R SNPs resulted associated with a higher risk to develop aphthous/ulcer and with a minor risk to develop malar rash. MIR146A SNP resulted associated with a higher risk to develop arthritis and with C3 consumption. PSORS1C1 resulted associated with the presence of LAC and decreased C4.

Moreover, PSORS1C1 resulted also associated with age at diagnosis (table 6): indeed the average age at onset is significantly lower in patients with rs2233945 SNP variant (28.6 vs 32.2 years, $P = 0.042$).

Table 4. Counting of risk alleles in cases and controls.

Number of risk alleles	Controls	SLE patients	Comparisons	P	OR
0	49	59	0 *vs* others	0.0008	0.45 (0.28–0.72)
1	50	89	1 *vs* 0	0.13	1.47 (0.88–2.47)
2	15	61	2 vs 0	0.0003	3.78 (1.71–6.67)
3		22	(3+4+5) *vs* 0	<0.0001	ND
4		2			
5		1			
Total	114	234			

$P_{tot} = 8*10^{-6}$.
(3df).
The risk alleles considered are the variant alleles of rs7574865, rs3099844 and rs3024505 SNPs.

Table 5. Association between disease phenotypes and studied polymorphisms.

Phenotype	Gene	Locus	P	OR (95% CI)
Pericarditis	ATG16L1	rs2241880	0.024	0.43 (0.2–0.9)
	STAT4	rs7574865	0.015	2.32 (1.17–4.6)
	PTPN2	rs2542151	0.032	2.35 (1.07–5.18)
Serositis	PTPN2	rs2542151	0.022	2.49 (1.13–5.5)
Aphthous/ulcers	IL23R	rs7517847	0.046	2.13 (1.0–4.52)
	IL23R	rs11209026	0.045	2.6 (0.99–6.86)
Arthritis	MIR146A	rs2910164	0.024	1.93 (1.09–3.4)
Malar Rash	IL23R	rs11209026	0.048	0.44 (0.19–1.01)
aCL	IL10	rs3024505	0.027	0.49 (0.26–0.93)
	HCP5	rs3099844	0.005	0.34 (0.15–0.74)
	Mir146a	rs2431697	0.035	2.03 (1.05–3.95)
ENA	STAT4	rs7574865	0.018	1.93 (1.12–3.36)
C3 (below normal values)	MIR146A	rs2910164	0.029	1.91 (1.06–3.4)
Anti-Ro/SSA	PSORS1C1	rs2233945	0.024	0.48 (0.25–0.91)
	HCP5	rs9469003	0.007	0.37 (0.18–0.78)
	HCP5	rs3099844	0.016	2.28 (1.15–4.52)
LAC	PSORS1C1	rs2233945	0.008	2.44 (1.25–4.76)
C4 (below normal values)	PSORS1C1	rs2233945	0.009	2.24 (1.22–4.12)
Anti-dsDNA	HCP5	rs3099844	0.047	0.5 (0.25–1)

Discussion

In the last years, the advent of genome wide association studies and the technological possibility to detect polymorphisms in large samples have revolutionized the field of human genetics by identification and confirmation of common gene variants that confer susceptibility to a plethora of diseases. A number of studies support the concept that common risk genes underlie multiple autoimmune disorders and suggest the involvement of common pathways of pathogenesis among different diseases [14]. In this study, we have examined specific genes, involved in autoimmunity, in inflammation and in autophagy to evaluate their involvement in SLE susceptibility. We aimed at confirming the association between STAT4, IL10 and IRAK1 [15–19] in a monocentric Italian cohort with SLE. Other genes, such as IL23R, PSORS1C1, HCP5, were found to be associated with psoriasis and rheumatoid arthritis [20–23]. Regarding genes involved in autophagy, we have chosen IRGM and ATG16L1 as candidate genes, since they were associated with Crohn's disease [24]. PTPN2 was associated with Crohn's disease [25] and type I diabetes [26]; ERAP1 was associated with psoriasis [27] and multiple sclerosis [28].

In our study, only three genes resulted associated with the disease development: STAT4, IL10 and HCP5. Indeed, we confirmed the STAT4 rs7574865 variant allele as a risk factor for SLE susceptibility, with an OR even higher than previously described (OR = 2.13 [95% CI 1.59–2.85]). Moreover, we observed an allele-dose risk effect, whereby individuals with two STAT4 alleles have 8.4-fold risk to develop the disease compared with wild-type subjects, while heterozygous subjects show 1.57-fold risk. Considering the fact that, usually, each risk factor gives a moderate contribution to SLE susceptibility, in our cohort, this SNP has a considerable weight. STAT4 is a member of the STAT family of transcription factors, and is involved in mediating responses to IL12 in lymphocytes, and regulating the differentiation of T helper cells. The STAT4 rs7574865 polymorphism, located within the third intron of the gene, shows the strongest association with several autoimmune conditions [29,30], such as SLE, RA, type 1 and 2 diabetes, systemic sclerosis, inflammatory bowel diseases, primary Sjogren's syndrome (SS), juvenile idiopathic arthritis, primary antiphospholipid syndrome, autoimmune thyroid diseases, multiple sclerosis, psoriasis, granulomatosis with polyangiitis, giant cell arteritis [31].

The STAT4 gene can be activated and phosphorylated upon ligation of the type I IFN receptor by IFN-α, and subsequently induce downstream transcription of IFN-α-induced genes [32]. It has been recently showed that a great number of genes target for STAT4 are enriched to functional pathways in the type I interferon system, and have key roles in the inflammatory

Table 6. PSORS1C1 SNP correlates with age at onset.

	Mean Age at diagnosis	N	Standard Deviation	P
CC	32.19	124	11.46	0.042
CA+AA	28.65	69	11.57	

response. Thus, by participating in transcription complex with other co-factors, STAT4 harbors the potential of regulating a large number of target genes, which may contribute to their strong association with SLE [33].

The other interesting result is the association between a gene variant in HCP5 gene and SLE susceptibility that was never described before. Indeed, this is the first study, by our knowledge, that evaluated the involvement of this gene in SLE susceptibility. Moreover, HCP5 SNPs resulted associated with anti-Ro/SSA and anti-dsDNA antibodies. The rs3099844 polymorphism has been previously described as involved in Steven Johnson Syndrome and Toxic Epidermal Necrolysis susceptibility [34–36], but also in another autoimmune condition, primary sclerosing cholangitis [37]. In this condition, anti-ENA including anti-SSA can be found in up to 11.5% of patients and anti-dsDNA at a lesser extent (1–3% of patients). However, the most interesting study is a genome-wide association study showing an association between the rs3099844 and the cardiac manifestations of systemic lupus erythematosus [38]. As it is well known, this clinical condition is associated with the presence of anti-Ro/SSA antibodies [39–43]. Altogether, these data suggest a strong evidence of an association of such polymorphism with the anti-Ro/SSA antibodies, and further studies are awaited to clarify the specific underlying mechanisms. Another SNP in the HCP5 gene (rs2395029) was previously associated with psoriasis and psoriatic arthritis [23]. HCP5 gene (major histocompatibility complex P5), located in HLA region, is expressed primarily in cells of the immune system such as spleen, blood and thymus consistent with a potential role in autoimmunity [23]. This allele was associated with lower viral load set point following HIV-1 infection. This is of interest, since anti-Ro/SSA antibodies have been described in HIV infected subjects [44,45]. Hence, it is possible that HCP5 carriers mount a strong immune reaction to viral infection that, in genetically susceptible individuals, could lead to excessive inflammation. On the other hand, sera from SLE and SS patients were also found to present reactivity with HIV-1 p24 antigen [46], suggesting a specific pattern of nonrandom cross-reactivity between virus p24 and autoimmune sera. Moreover, both a direct interaction between the SSB and HIV-1 trans-activation response element as well as the involvement of the SSB autoantigen in HIV-1 gene expression have been reported previously [47,48]. Thus, there exist a relationship between the anti-Ro/SSA, anti-La/SSB antibodies and HIV [49] of which HCP5 may represent the bridge.

Finally, besides the confirmation of STAT4 and the newly described association with HCP5, we confirmed the risk effect of IL10 rs3024505 variant allele on SLE development. Polymorphisms in this gene were described as associated with several autoimmune disease, including SLE, rheumatoid arthritis, psoriasis and Crohn's disease, highlighting that IL10 is one of the common risk genes. IL10, primarily produced by monocytes and lymphocytes, is a multifunctional cytokine in immune-regulation and inflammation. A number of studies have been conducted to investigate the association of the IL10 gene polymorphisms with SLE susceptibility, although with conflicting results [18]. Considering the three associated SNPs, we also observed a cumulative genetic effect that distinguish cases from controls (Figure 1). A similar analysis in a previous study, described a different genetic risk scores in males and females [50].

Regarding the other genes, although we did not find any association with the development of the disease, some of the examined polymorphisms resulted associated with particular phenotypes, suggesting that these genes probably do not affect the disease susceptibility but modulate the phenotype. Of course, this lack of association does not mean that these genes are not involved with the disease; indeed, we cannot exclude that other SNPs in these same genes, not investigated in our study, could be associated. Interestingly, PSORS1C1 gene, which maps in the HLA region, resulted associated with LAC, decreased C4, and with an early-onset of the disease. PSORS1C1 gene is one of psoriasis susceptibility loci [51], but it is also associated with systemic sclerosis [52] and has been suggested to play an important role in the development of RA [53]. We also described an association between MiR-146a and the development of arthritis complications. It is known that MiR-146a is a negative regulator of the IFN pathway, and under-expression of MiR-146a conduces to alterations in the type I IFN pathway in lupus patients by targeting the key signaling proteins [54]. Autophagy has been described as a critical homeostatic mechanism in T lymphocytes, influencing proliferation and differentiation [55], and there are studies in the literature which highlighted the association between SLE and autophagy genes [56,57]. However, in our study, we did not find any association of the disease with ATG16L1 and IRGM genetic variants. Of course, this lack of association could be due to the SNPs selection and other SNPs in the same gene could associate with the disease. Nonetheless, it is interesting to note that rs2241880 in ATG16L1 resulted associated with a minor risk to develop pericarditis as a complication. Admittedly, a limitation of our study is the relatively small number of samples; however, it should be underlined that this a monocentric cohort of patients of the same ethnicity, strictly followed and clinically well characterized.

In conclusion, our study confirms the role of STAT4 and IL10 in SLE susceptibility and describes for the first time the association between a HCP5 genetic variant and SLE susceptibility. These results confirm the importance of the adaptive and innate arms of the immune system in establishing SLE risk. However, each of the identified alleles accounts for only a fraction of the overall genetic risk, and functional studies are necessary to clearly explain their involvement with SLE pathogenesis.

Author Contributions

Conceived and designed the experiments: CC CP GN GV PB F. Conti. Performed the experiments: CC CP F. Ceccarelli SR DDF CA FRS EC. Analyzed the data: CC CP PB F. Ceccarelli. Contributed reagents/materials/analysis tools: CC SR DDF PB. Wrote the paper: CC CP PB F. Ceccarelli.

References

1. Deapen D, Escalante A, Weinrib L, Horwitz D, Bachman B, et al. (1992) A revised estimate of twin concordance in systemic lupus-erythematosus. Arthritis Rheum 35: 311–318.
2. Alarcón-Segovia D, Alarcón-Riquelme ME, Cardiel MH, Caeiro F, Massardo L, et al.; Grupo Latinoamericano de Estudio del Lupus Eritematoso (GLADEL) (2005) Familial aggregation of systemic lupus erythematosus, rheumatoid arthritis, and other autoimmune diseases in 1177 lupus patients from the GLADEL cohort. Arthritis Rheum 52: 1138–1147.
3. Cui Y, Sheng Y, Zhang X (2013) Genetic susceptibility to SLE: recent progress from GWAS. J Autoimmun 41:25–33.
4. Deng Y1, Tsao BP (2010) Genetic susceptibility to systemic lupus erythematosus in the genomic era. Nat Rev Rheumatol 6:683–92.
5. Delgado-Vega A, Sánchez E, Löfgren S, Castillejo-López C, Alarcón-Riquelme ME (2010) Recent findings on genetics of systemic autoimmune diseases. Curr Opin Immunol 22:698–705. doi:10.1016/j.coi.2010.09.002.
6. Ramos PS, Criswell LA, Moser KL, Comeau ME, Williams AH, et al. (2011) International Consortium on the Genetics of Systemic Erythematosus A comprehensive analysis of shared loci between systemic lupus erythematosus (SLE) and sixteen autoimmune diseases reveals limited genetic overlap. PLoS Genet 7:e1002406.

7. Gregersen PK, Olsson LM (2009) Recent advances in the genetics of autoimmune disease. Annu Rev Immunol 27:363–391.
8. Perricone R, Perricone C, Shoenfeld Y (2011) Autoimmunity: when the immune system becomes the self-ish giant. Autoimmun Rev 10:575–6.
9. Perricone C, Ciccacci C, Ceccarelli F, Di Fusco D, Spinelli FR, et al. (2013) TRAF3IP2 gene and systemic lupus erythematosus: association with disease susceptibility and pericarditis development. Immunogenetics 65:703–9.
10. Hüffmeier U, Uebe S, Ekici AB, Bowes J, Giardina E, et al. (2010) Common variants at TRAF3IP2 are associated with susceptibility to psoriatic arthritis and psoriasis. Nat Genet 42:996–9.
11. Ciccacci C, Biancone L, Di Fusco D, Ranieri M, Condino G, et al. (2013) TRAF3IP2 gene is associated with cutaneous extraintestinal manifestations in inflammatory bowel disease. J Crohns Colitis 7:44–52.
12. Miyakis S, Lockshin MD, Atsumi T, Branch DW, Brey RL, et al. (2006) International consensus statement on an update of the classification criteria for definite antiphospholipid syndrome (APS). J Thromb Haemost 4:295–306.
13. Excoffier L, Lischer HE (2010) Arlequin suite ver. 3.5: a new series of programs to perform population genetics analyses under Linux and Windows. Mol Ecol Resour 10:564–7.
14. Gregersen PK, Behrens TW (2006) Genetics of autoimmune disease — disorders of immune homeostasis. Nat Rev Genet 7:917–28.
15. Zheng J, Yin J, Huang R, Petersen F, Yu X (2013) Meta-analysis reveals an association of STAT4 polymorphisms with systemic autoimmune disorders and anti-dsDNA antibody. Hum Immunol 74:986–92.
16. Wang C, Sandling JK, Hagberg N, Berggren O, Sigurdsson S, et al. (2013) Genome-wide profiling of target genes for the systemic lupus erythematosus-associated transcription factors IRF5 and STAT4. Ann Rheum Dis 72:96–103.
17. Schotte H, Willeke P, Becker H, Poggemeyer J, Gaubitz M, et al. (2014) Association of extended interleukin-10 promoter haplotypes with disease susceptibility and manifestations in German patients with systemic lupus erythematosus. Lupus 23:378–85.
18. Liu P, Song J, Su H, Li L, Lu N, et al. (2013) IL-10 gene polymorphisms and susceptibility to systemic lupus erythematosus: a meta-analysis. PLoS One 8:e69547.
19. Kaufman KM, Zhao J, Kelly JA, Hughes T, Adler A, et al. (2013) Argentine Collaborative Group; BIOLUPUS network, Fine mapping of Xq28: both MECP2 and IRAK1 contribute to risk for systemic lupus erythematosus in multiple ancestral groups. Ann Rheum Dis 72:437–44.
20. Song GG, Bae SC, Choi SJ, Ji JD, Lee YH (2012) Associations between interleukin-23 receptor polymorphisms and susceptibility to rheumatoid arthritis: a meta-analysis. Mol Biol Rep 39:10655–63.
21. Zhai Y, Xu K, Huang F, Peng H, Feng CC, et al. (2012) Association of interleukin 23 receptor gene polymorphisms (rs10489629, rs7517847) with rheumatoid arthritis in European population: a meta-analysis. Mol Biol Rep 39:8987–94.
22. Sun H, Xia Y, Wang L, Wang Y, Chang X (2013) PSORS1C1 may be involved in rheumatoid arthritis. Immunol Lett 153:9–14. doi:10.1016/j.imlet.2013.06.001.
23. Liu Y, Helms C, Liao W, Zaba LC, Duan S, et al. (2008) A genome-wide association study of psoriasis and psoriatic arthritis identifies new disease loci. PLoS Genet 4:e1000041.
24. Latiano A, Palmieri O, Valvano MR, D'Incà R, Cucchiara S, et al. (2008) Replication of interleukin 23 receptor and autophagy-related 16-like 1 association in adult- and pediatric-onset inflammatory bowel disease in Italy. World J Gastroenterol 14:4643–51.
25. Glas J, Wagner J, Seiderer J, Olszak T, Wetzke M, et al. (2012) PTPN2 gene variants are associated with susceptibility to both Crohn's disease and ulcerative colitis supporting a common genetic disease background. PLoS One 7:e33682.
26. Espino-Paisan L, de la Calle H, Fernández-Arquero M, Figueredo MA, de la Concha EG, et al. (2011) A polymorphism in PTPN2 gene is associated with an earlier onset of type 1 diabetes. Immunogenetics 63:255–8.
27. Genetic Analysis of Psoriasis Consortium & the Wellcome Trust Case Control Consortium 2, Strange A, Capon F, Spencer CC, Knight J, et al. (2010) A genome-wide association study identifies new psoriasis susceptibility loci and an interaction between HLA-C and ERAP1. Nat Genet 42:985–90.
28. Guerini FR, Cagliani R, Forni D, Agliardi C, Caputo D, et al. (2012) A functional variant in ERAP1 predisposes to multiple sclerosis. PLoS One 7:e29931.
29. Korman BD, Kastner DL, Gregersen PK, Remmers EF (2008) STAT4: genetics, mechanisms, and implications for autoimmunity. Curr Allergy Asthma Rep 8:398–403.
30. Perricone C, Ceccarelli F, Valesini G (2011) An overview on the genetic of rheumatoid arthritis: a never-ending story. Autoimmun Rev 10:599–608.
31. Liang YL, Wu H, Shen X, Li PQ, Yang XQ, et al. (2012) Association of STAT4 rs7574865 polymorphism with autoimmune diseases: a meta-analysis. Mol Biol Rep 39:8873–82.
32. Kariuki SN, Niewold TB (2010) Genetic regulation of serum cytokines in systemic lupus erythematosus. Transl Res 155:109–17.
33. Wang C, Sandling JK, Hagberg N, Berggren O, Sigurdsson S, et al. (2013) Genome-wide profiling of target genes for the systemic lupus erythematosus-associated transcription factors IRF5 and STAT4. Ann Rheum Dis 72:96–103. doi:10.1136/annrheumdis-2012-201364.
34. Borgiani P, Di Fusco D, Erba F, Marazzi MC, Mancinelli S, et al. (2014) HCP5 genetic variant (rs3099844) contributes to Nevirapine-induced Stevens Johnsons Syndrome/Toxic Epidermal Necrolysis susceptibility in a population from Mozambique. Eur J Clin Pharmacol. 70:275–8. doi:10.1007/s00228-013-1622-5.
35. Tohkin M, Kaniwa N, Saito Y, Sugiyama E, Kurose K, et al. (2013) Japan Pharmacogenomics Data Science Consortium. A whole-genome association study of major determinants for allopurinol-related Stevens-Johnson syndrome and toxic epidermal necrolysis in Japanese patients. Pharmacogenomics J 13:60–9.
36. Génin E, Schumacher M, Roujeau JC, Naldi L, Liss Y, et al. (2011) Genome-wide association study of Stevens-Johnson Syndrome and Toxic Epidermal Necrolysis in Europe. Orphanet J Rare Dis 6:52.
37. Karlsen TH, Franke A, Melum E, Kaser A, Hov JR, et al. (2010) Genome-wide association analysis in primary sclerosing cholangitis. Gastroenterology 138:1102–11.
38. Clancy RM, Marion MC, Kaufman KM, Ramos PS, Adler A (2010) International Consortium on Systemic Lupus Erythematosus Genetics, Identification of candidate loci at 6p21 and 21q22 in a genome-wide association study of cardiac manifestations of neonatal lupus. Arthritis Rheum 62:3415–24.
39. Julkunen H, Kurki P, Kaaja R, Heikkila R, Immonen I, et al. (1993) Isolated congenital heart block. Long-term outcome of mothers and characterization of the immune response to SS-A/Ro and to SS-B/La. Arthritis Rheum 36:1588–1598.
40. Salomonsson S, Dorner T, Theander E, Bremme K, Larsson P, et al. (2002) A serologic marker for fetal risk of congenital heart block. Arthritis Rheum 46:1233–1241.
41. Fritsch C, Hoebeke J, Dali H, Ricchiuti V, Isenberg DA, et al. (2006) 52-kDa Ro/SSA epitopes preferentially recognized by antibodies from mothers of children with neonatal lupus and congenital heart block. Arthritis Res Ther 8:R4.
42. Eronen M, Miettinen A, Walle TK, Chan EK, Julkunen H (2004) Relationship of maternal autoimmune response to clinical manifestations in children with congenital complete heart block. Acta Paediatr 93:803–809.
43. Salomonsson S, Dzikaite V, Zeffer E, Eliasson H, Ambrosi A, et al. (2011) A population-based investigation of the autoantibody profile in mothers of children with atrioventricular block. Scand J Immunol 74:511–517.
44. Muller S, Richalet P, Laurent-Crawford A, Barakat S, Rivière Y, et al. (1992) Autoantibodies typical of non-organ-specific autoimmune diseases in HIV-seropositive patients. AIDS 6:933–942.
45. Argov S, Schattner A, Burstein R, Handzel ZT, Shoenfeld Y, et al. (1991) autoantibodies in male homosexuals and HIV infection. Immunol Lett 30:31–35.
46. Deas JE, Liu LG, Thompson JJ, Sander DM, Soble SS, et al. (1998) Reactivity of sera from systemic lupus erythematosus and Sjogren syndrome patients with peptides derived from human immunodeficiency virus p24 capsid antigen. Clin Diagn Lab Immunol 5:181–185.
47. Svitkin YV, Pause A, Sonenberg N (1994) La autoantigen alleviates translational repression by the 5′ leader sequence of the human immunodeficiency virus type 1 mRNA. J Virol 68:7001–7007.
48. Chang YN, Kenan DJ, Keene JD, Gatignol A, Jeang KT (1995) Direct interactions between autoantigen La and human immunodeficiency virus leader RNA. J Virol 69:618–619.
49. Billaut-Mulot O, Cocude C, Kolesnitchenko V, Truong MJ, Chan EK, et al. (2001) SS-56, a novel cellular target of autoantibody responses in Sjögren syndrome and systemic lupus erythematosus. J Clin Invest 108:861–869.
50. Hughes T, Adler A, Merrill JT, Kelly JA, Kaufman KM, et al. (2012) Analysis of autosomal genes reveals gene-sex interactions and higher total genetic risk in men with systemic lupus erythematosus. Ann Rheum Dis 71:694–9.
51. Chang YT, Liu HN, Shiao YM, Lin MW, Lee DD, et al. (2005) A study of PSORS1C1 gene polymorphisms in Chinese patients with psoriasis. Br J Dermatol 153:90–6.
52. Allanore Y, Saad M, Dieudé P, Avouac J, Distler JH, et al. (2011) Genome-wide scan identifies TNIP1, PSORS1C1, and RHOB as novel risk loci for systemic sclerosis. PLoS Genet 7:e1002091.
53. Sun H, Xia Y, Wang L, Wang Y, Chang X (2013) PSORS1C1 may be involved in rheumatoid arthritis. Immunol Lett 153:9–14. doi:10.1016/j.imlet.2013.06.001.
54. Tang Y, Luo X, Cui H, Ni X, Yuan M, et al. (2009) MicroRNA-146A contributes to abnormal activation of the type I interferon pathway in human lupus by targeting the key signaling proteins. Arthritis Rheum 60:1065–75. doi:10.1002/art.24436.
55. Pierdominici M, Vomero M, Barbati C, Colasanti T, Maselli A, et al. (2012) Role of autophagy in immunity and autoimmunity, with a special focus on systemic lupus erythematosus. FASEB J 26:1400–12. doi:10.1096/fj.11-194175.
56. Zhou XJ, Lu XL, Lu JC, Yang HZ, Qin LX, et al. (2011) Genetic association of PRDM1-ATG5 intergenic region and autophagy with systemic lupus erythematosus in a Chinese population. Ann Rheum Dis 70:1330–7.
57. Järvinen TM, Hellquist A, Zucchelli M, Koskenmies S, Panelius J, et al. (2012) Replication of GWAS-identified systemic lupus erythematosus susceptibility genes affirms B-cell receptor pathway signalling and strengthens the role of IRF5 in disease susceptibility in a Northern European population. Rheumatology (Oxford) 51:87–92.

Permissions

All chapters in this book were first published in PLOS ONE, by The Public Library of Science; hereby published with permission under the Creative Commons Attribution License or equivalent. Every chapter published in this book has been scrutinized by our experts. Their significance has been extensively debated. The topics covered herein carry significant findings which will fuel the growth of the discipline. They may even be implemented as practical applications or may be referred to as a beginning point for another development.

The contributors of this book come from diverse backgrounds, making this book a truly international effort. This book will bring forth new frontiers with its revolutionizing research information and detailed analysis of the nascent developments around the world.

We would like to thank all the contributing authors for lending their expertise to make the book truly unique. They have played a crucial role in the development of this book. Without their invaluable contributions this book wouldn't have been possible. They have made vital efforts to compile up to date information on the varied aspects of this subject to make this book a valuable addition to the collection of many professionals and students.

This book was conceptualized with the vision of imparting up-to-date information and advanced data in this field. To ensure the same, a matchless editorial board was set up. Every individual on the board went through rigorous rounds of assessment to prove their worth. After which they invested a large part of their time researching and compiling the most relevant data for our readers.

The editorial board has been involved in producing this book since its inception. They have spent rigorous hours researching and exploring the diverse topics which have resulted in the successful publishing of this book. They have passed on their knowledge of decades through this book. To expedite this challenging task, the publisher supported the team at every step. A small team of assistant editors was also appointed to further simplify the editing procedure and attain best results for the readers.

Apart from the editorial board, the designing team has also invested a significant amount of their time in understanding the subject and creating the most relevant covers. They scrutinized every image to scout for the most suitable representation of the subject and create an appropriate cover for the book.

The publishing team has been an ardent support to the editorial, designing and production team. Their endless efforts to recruit the best for this project, has resulted in the accomplishment of this book. They are a veteran in the field of academics and their pool of knowledge is as vast as their experience in printing. Their expertise and guidance has proved useful at every step. Their uncompromising quality standards have made this book an exceptional effort. Their encouragement from time to time has been an inspiration for everyone.

The publisher and the editorial board hope that this book will prove to be a valuable piece of knowledge for researchers, students, practitioners and scholars across the globe.

List of Contributors

Ning-Sheng Lai, Kuang-Yung Huang, Chien-Hsueh Tung and Ming-Chi Lu
Division of Allergy, Immunology and Rheumatology, Dalin Tzu Chi Hospital, Buddhist Tzu Chi Medical Foundation, Chiayi, Taiwan

Ning-Sheng Lai, Kuang-Yung Huang and Ming-Chi Lu
School of Medicine, Tzu Chi University, Hualien, Taiwan

Tzung-Yi Tsai and Malcolm Koo
Department of Medical Research, Dalin Tzu Chi Hospital, Buddhist Tzu Chi Medical Foundation, Chiayi, Taiwan

Tzung-Yi Tsai
Department of Nursing, Tzu Chi College of Technology, Hualien, Taiwan
Department of Environmental and Occupational Health, College of Medicine, National Cheng Kung University, Tainan, Taiwan

Malcolm Koo
Dalla Lana School of Public Health, University of Toronto, Toronto, Ontario, Canada

Lihua Shi, Kelly Maurer, Patrícia Costa Reis, Li Song and Kathleen E. Sullivan
The Division of Allergy Immunology, The Children's Hospital of Philadelphia, Philadelphia, Pennsylvania, United States of America

Zhe Zhang and Angela M. Yu
The Center for Biomedical Informatics, The Children's Hospital of Philadelphia, Philadelphia, Pennsylvania, United States of America

Wei Wang and Zhi Wei
Department of Computer Science, New Jersey Institute of Technology, Newark, New Jersey, United States of America

Ehtisham Akhter and Michelle Petri
Division of Rheumatology, Johns Hopkins University School of Medicine, Baltimore, Maryland, United States of America

Eleni I. Kampylafka, Haralampos Alexopoulos, Michalis L. Kosmidi, Panayiotis G. Vlachoyiannopoulos, Marinos C. Dalakas, Haralampos M. Moutsopoulos and Athanasios G. Tzioufas
Department of Pathophysiology, School of Medicine, National and Kapodistrian University of Athens, Athens, Greece

Demosthenes B. Panagiotakos
Department of Nutrition and Dietetics, Harokopio University, Athens, Greece

Yasuhito Hamaguchi, Manabu Fujimoto, Takashi Matsushita, Kenzo Kaji, Kazuhiro Komura, Minoru Hasegawa and Kazuhiko Takehara
Department of Dermatology, Kanazawa University Graduate School of Medical Science, Kanazawa, Japan

Masanari Kodera
Department of Dermatology, Social Insurance Chukyo Hospital, Nagoya, Japan

Eiji Muroi
Department of Dermatology, Nagasaki University Graduate School of Biomedical Sciences, Nagasaki, Japan

Keita Fujikawa
Unit of Translational Medicine, Department of Immunology and Rheumatology, Nagasaki University Graduate School of Biomedical Sciences, Nagasaki, Japan

Mariko Seishima
Department of Dermatology, Ogaki Municipal Hospital, Ogaki, Japan

Hidehiro Yamada
Division of Rheumatology, Department of Internal Medicine, and Allergy, St. Marianna University, Kawasaki, Japan

Ryo Yamada
Center for Genomic Medicine, Graduate School of Medicine, Kyoto University, Kyoto, Japan

Shinichi Sato
Department of Dermatology, Faculty of Medicine, University of Tokyo, Tokyo, Japan

Masataka Kuwana
Division of Rheumatology, Department of Internal Medicine, Keio University School of Medicine, Tokyo, Japan

Xue Yang, Yu Xue, Dandan Xuan, Shucong Zheng and Hejian Zou
Division of Rheumatology, Huashan Hospital, Fudan University, Shanghai, China

Xue Yang, Yu Xue, Dandan Xuan, Shucong Zheng and Hejian Zou
Institute of Rheumatology, Immunology and Allergy, Fudan University, Shanghai, China

Xue Yang, Yu Xue, Dandan Xuan, Shucong Zheng and Hejian Zou
Institute of Molecular and Translational Medicine, Huashan Hospital, Fudan University

Ji Yang
Department of Dermatology, Zhongshan Hospital, Fudan University, Shanghai, China

Yiwei Chu
Department of Immunology, Shanghai Medical College, Fudan University, Shanghai, China

Fei-Yan Deng, Shu-Feng Lei, Yong-Hong Zhang and Zeng-Li Zhang
Center for Genetic Epidemiology and Genomics, Soochow University, Suzhou, Jiangsu, P. R. China

Shu-Feng Lei and Yong-Hong Zhang
Department of Epidemiology, School of Public Health, Soochow University, Suzhou, Jiangsu, P. R. China

Yu-Fan Guos
Department of Rheumatology, the First Affiliated Hospital of Soochow University, Suzhou, Jiangsu, P. R. China

Karim Sacre, Marie-Paule Chauveheid and Thomas Papo
Département de Médecine Interne, Hôpital Bichat, Université Paris Diderot, PRES Sorbonne Paris Cité, Assistance Publique Hôpitaux de Paris, Paris, France

Karim Sacre and Thomas Papo
INSERM U1149, Paris, France

Karim Sacre and Thomas Papo
Département Hospitalo-Universitaire FIRE (Fibrosis, Inflammation and Remodelling in Renal and Respiratory Diseases), Paris, France

Brigitte Escoubet
Département de Physiologie, Hôpital Bichat, Université Paris Diderot, PRES Sorbonne Paris Cité, Assistance Publique Hôpitaux de Paris, INSERM U1138, Paris, France

Blandine Pasquet and Florence Tubach
Département d'Epidémiologie et Recherche Clinique, Hôpital Bichat, Université Paris Diderot, PRES Sorbonne Paris Cité, Assistance Publique Hôpitaux de Paris, INSERM CIE 801, Paris, France

Maria- Christina Zennaro
Département de Cardiologie, Hôpital Européen Georges Pompidou, Université Paris Descartes, PRES Sorbonne Paris Cité, Assistance Publique-Hôpitaux de Paris, INSERM, UMRS 970, Paris, France

Christophe Richez
Service de Rhumatologie, Hôpital Pellegrin, CHU de Bordeaux, Bordeaux, France

Christophe Richez and Pierre Duffau
UMR-CNRS 5164, Université Victor Segalen Bordeaux 2, Bordeaux, France

Christophe Richez, Rocco J. Richards, Zachary Weitzner, Ian R. Rifkin and Tamar Aprahamian
Department of Medicine-Renal Section, Boston University School of Medicine, Boston, Massachusetts, United States of America

Pierre Duffau
Service de Médecine Interne, Hôpital Saint André, CHU de Bordeaux, Bordeaux, France

Christopher D. Andry
Department of Medicine-Pathology, Boston University School of Medicine, Boston, Massachusetts, United States of America

Ralph Brinks and Sandra Landwehr
German Diabetes Center, Institute of Biometry and Epidemiology, Duesseldorf, Germany

Ralph Brinks, Rebecca Fischer-Betz and Matthias Schneider
University Hospital, Polyclinics for Rheumatology, Duesseldorf, Germany

Sandra Landwehr and Guido Giani
Heinrich-Heine-University, Institute for Statistics in Medicine, Duesseldorf, Germany

Ming-Wei Lin and Stephen Adelstein
Department of Clinical Immunology, Royal Prince Alfred Hospital, Sydney, New South Wales, Australia

Ming-Wei Lin and Stephen Adelstein
Discipline of Medicine, Sydney Medical School, The University of Sydney, Sydney, New South Wales, Australia

Joshua W. K. Ho
Division of Genetics, Department of Medicine, Brigham and Women's Hospital, Harvard Medical School, Boston, Massachusetts, United States of America

Leonard C. Harrison
The Walter and Eliza Hall Institute of Medical Research, Department of Clinical Immunology and Burnet Clinical Research Unit The Royal Melbourne Hospital, Parkville, Victoria, Australia

Cristobal G. dos Remedios
Discipline of Anatomy, Bosch Institute, The University of Sydney, Sydney, New South Wales, Australia

Xuebing Feng, Dandan Wang, Jingjing Chen, Lin Lu, Bingzhu Hua, Xia Li and Lingyun Sun
Department of Rheumatology, The Affiliated Drum Tower Hospital of Nanjing University Medical School, Nanjing, Jiangsu, China

Betty P. Tsao
Division of Rheumatology, David Geffen School of Medicine at UCLA, Los Angeles, California, United States of America

Aline Lá zara Resende, Luciene Machado dos Reis, Cristiane Bitencourt Dias, Melani Ribeiro Custódio, Vanda Jorgetti and Viktoria Woronik
Nephrology Division, Sao Paulo University Medical School, Sao Paulo, Brazil

Chun-Chou Tsai, Chun-Ching Chiu, Huai-Sheng Hsu and Tsai- Ching Hsu
Institute of Microbiology and Immunology, Chung Shan Medical University, Taichung, Taiwan

Chun-Ching Chiu
Department of Neurology and Department of Medical Intensive Care Unit, Chunghua Christian Hospital, Chunghua, Taiwan

Jeng-Dong Hsu
Department of Pathology, School of Medicine, Chung Shan Medical University, Taichung, Taiwan
Department of Pathology, Chung Shan Medical University Hospital, Taichung, Taiwan

Bor-Show Tzang
Department of Biochemistry, School of Medicine, Chung Shan Medical University, Taichung, Taiwan
Institute of Biochemistry and Biotechnology, Chung Shan Medical University, Taichung, Taiwan

Bor-Show Tzang and Tsai- Ching Hsu
Clinical Laboratory, Chung Shan Medical University Hospital, Taichung, Taiwan

Xinzhou Zhang, Hualin Ma and Jianrong Huang
Department of Nephrology, Shenzhen People's Hospital, Second Clinical Medical College, Jinan University, Shenzhen, China

Yong Dai
Clinical Medical Research Center, Shenzhen People's Hospital, Second Clinical Medical College, Jinan University, Shenzhen, China

Barbara Dema, Chao Jiang, Tiffany K. Ricks, Jörg Scheffel and Juan Rivera
Laboratory of Molecular Immunogenetics, National Institute of Arthritis and Musculoskeletal and Skin Diseases, National Institutes of Health, Bethesda, Maryland, United States of America

Christophe Pellefigues, Karim Sacre, Thomas Papo and Nicolas Charles
Institut National de la Santé et de la Recherche Mé dicale U699, Université Paris Diderot, Paris, France

Sarfaraz Hasni
Office of the Clinical Director, National Institute of Arthritis and Musculoskeletal and Skin Diseases, National Institutes of Health, Bethesda, Maryland, United States of America

Karim Sacre, Delphine Gobert and Thomas Papo
Department of Internal Medicine, Hôpital Bichat, Assistance Publique-Hôpitaux de Paris, Université Paris Diderot, Faculté de Médecine site Bichat, Paris, France

Mathieu Jablonski and Eric Daugas
Department of Nephrology, Hôpital Bichat, Assistance Publique-Hôpitaux de Paris, Université Paris Diderot, Faculté de Médecine site Bichat, Paris, France

Nathalie Gault
Clinical Research Unit, Hôpital Bichat, Assistance Publique- Hôpitaux de Paris, Université Paris Diderot, Faculté de Mé decine site Bichat, Paris, France

Gabor Illei
Sjogren's Syndrome Clinic, National Institute of Dental and Craniofacial Research, National Institutes of Health, Bethesda, Maryland, United States of America

Michael M. Bonelli
Lymphocyte Biology Section, National Institute of Arthritis and Musculoskeletal and Skin Diseases, National Institutes of Health, Bethesda, Maryland, United States of America

Rivka C. Stone, Di Feng and Betsy J. Barnes
Department of Biochemistry and Molecular Biology, New Jersey Medical School, UMDNJ, Newark, New Jersey, United States of America

Rivka C. Stone, Di Feng and Betsy J. Barnes
New Jersey Medical School - University Hospital Cancer Center, UMDNJ, Newark, New Jersey, United States of America

Peicheng Du
High Performance and Research Computing, Department of Information Systems and Technology, UMDNJ, Newark, New Jersey, United States of America

Kopal Dhawan and Robert Donnelly
Molecular Resource Facility, New Jersey Medical School, UMDNJ, Newark, New Jersey, United States of America

Lars Rönnblom and Maija-Leena Eloranta
Department of Medical Sciences, Section of Rheumatology, Uppsala University, Uppsala, Sweden

María-Belén Bautista-Caro, Irene Arroyo-Villa, Concepción Castillo-Gallego, Eugenio de Miguel, Diana Peiteado, Chamaida Plasencia-Rodríguez, Alejandro Villalba, Emilio Martín-Mola and María-Eugenia Miranda-Carús
Department of Rheumatology, Hospital Universitario La Paz-IdiPAZ, Madrid, Spain

Sánchez-Mateos and Amaya Puig-Kröger
Laboratorio de Inmuno-Oncología, Hospital General Universitario Gregorio Marañón, Madrid, Spain

Menelaos N. Manoussakis, George E. Fragoulis, Aigli G. Vakrakou and Haralampos M. Moutsopoulos
Department of Pathophysiology, School of Medicine, University of Athens, Athens, Greece

Menelaos N. Manoussakis
Hellenic Pasteur Institute, Athens, Greece

Qing Lu, Ji-Yang Wang, Luman Wang, Xuechao Jiang and Yiwei Chu
Key Laboratory of Medical Molecular Virology of MOE/MOH, Department of Immunology, School of Basic Medical Sciences, Fudan University, Shanghai, China

Ji-Yang Wang and Yiwei Chu
Biotherapy Research Center of Fudan University, Shanghai, China

Juan-Sebastian Franco, Nicolá s Molano-González, Monica Rodríguez-Jiménez, Yeny Acosta-Ampudia, Rubén D. Mantilla, Jenny Amaya-Amaya, Adriana Rojas-Villarraga and Juan-Manuel Anaya
Center for Autoimmune Diseases Research (CREA), School of Medicine and Health Sciences, Universidad del Rosario, Bogotá, Colombia

Juan-Sebastian Franco, Rubén D. Mantilla, Jenny Amaya-Amaya, Adriana Rojas-Villarraga and Juan-Manuel Anaya
Mederi, Hospital Universitario Mayor, Bogotá, Colombia

Tao Zhang, Huimei Chen, Shaoshan Liang, Dacheng Chen, Chunxia Zheng, Caihong Zeng, Haitao Zhang and Zhihong Liu
National Clinical Research Center of Kidney Diseases, Jinling Hospital, Nanjing University School of Medicine, Nanjing 210002, P. R. China

Huimei Chen
Jiangsu Key Laboratory of Molecular Medicine, Nanjing University School of Medicine, Nanjing, 210093, P. R. China

Xinze Cai, Ying Qiao, Cheng Diao, Xiaoxue Xu, Yang Chen, Shuyan Du, Xudong Liu, Nan Liu, Shuang Yu, Dong Chen and Yi Jiang
Central Laboratory, First Affiliated Hospital of China Medical University, Shenyang, China

Xinze Cai and Yi Jiang
Department of Immunology, College of Basic Medical Sciences, China Medical University, Shenyang, China

Yi Jiang
Department of Dermatology, First Affiliated Hospital of China Medical University, Shenyang, China

Gil Amarilyo, Noriko Iikuni, Aijing Liu and Antonio La Cava
University of California Los Angeles, California, Los Angeles, United States of America

Giuseppe Matarese
Universitàdi Salerno, Baronissi, Italy
IRCCS MultiMedica, Milan, Italy

Cinzia Ciccacci, Sara Rufini, Davide Di Fusco, Giuseppe Novelli and Paola Borgiani
Department of Biomedicine and Prevention, Section of Genetics, School of Medicine, University of Rome "Tor Vergata", Rome, Italy

Carlo Perricone, Fulvia Ceccarelli, Cristiano Alessandri, Francesca Romana Spinelli, Enrica Cipriano, Guido Valesini and Fabrizio Conti
Lupus Clinic, Reumatologia, Dipartimento di Medicina Interna e Specialità Mediche, Sapienza Università di Roma, Rome, Italy

Index

www.ingramcontent.com/pod-product-compliance
Lightning Source LLC
LaVergne TN
LVHW060552210926
848485LV00005B/1303